AARP Books is an educational and public service project of the American Association of Retired Persons, which, with a membership of more than 26 million, is the largest association of persons fifty and over in the world today. Founded in 1958, AARP provides older Americans with a wide range of membership programs and services, including legislative representation at both federal and state levels. For further information about additional association activities, write to AARP, 1909 K Street, N.W., Washington, DC 20049.

PUBLISHER'S NOTE:

AARP PHARMACY SERVICE PRESCRIPTION DRUG HANDBOOK

An AARP Book
published by
American Association of Retired Persons, Washington, D.C.
Scott, Foresman and Company, Lifelong Learning Division, Glenview, Illinois

Library of Congress Cataloging-in-Publication Data

AARP pharmacy service prescription drug handbook.

  Includes index.
  1. Drugs—Dictionaries. 2. Chemotherapy—
Dictionaries. I. American Association of Retired
Persons. [DNLM: 1. Drugs—handbooks.
2. Prescriptions, Drugs—handbooks. QV 39 A113]
RS51.A28 1987   615.1   87-16661

ISBN 0-673-24842-9 (Scott, Foresman)

CONTENTS

PREFACE

In 1982, the AARP Pharmacy Service began providing the first voluntary patient prescription drug information leaflets in the United States to AARP members. The new Medication Information Leaflets for Seniors (MILS) were and are given routinely to the Pharmacy's mail-service customers with their prescription drug orders. The leaflets were written for easy understanding, and the information was carefully checked with the U.S. Food and Drug Administration and physicians and pharmacists in geriatric medicine. The MILS have become models for health care agencies seeking to provide information for older persons to use in working with their doctors and other health care providers to manage their own health programs better.

It is a logical step for the AARP Pharmacy Service to now produce this major reference work on prescription drugs for older persons, who consume more than 30 percent of the prescription drugs sold in the United States. As the largest private, non-profit mail-service pharmacy in the world, addressing specifically the needs of persons fifty years of age and older, the Service felt an obligation to make the information in this book available to a greater population of those who use prescription drugs and those who wish to monitor such drug use in older people they care for.

The Editorial Advisory Board members listed on the following pages provided invaluable guidance in the development and review of the manuscript for this book. Many of them are specialists in geriatric medicine, a field of medicine dealing specifically with diseases in older persons.

John R. McHugh, R.Ph., President

EDITORIAL ADVISORY BOARD

FRANK PARKER, M.D.
Professor and Chairman
Department of Dermatology
Oregon Health Sciences University
School of Medicine
Portland, Oregon

NEIL RESNICK, M.D.
Instructor in Medicine
Harvard Medical School
Beth Israel Hospital
Director, Harvard Continence Clinic
Director, Geriatric Consultation Service
Brigham and Women's Hospital
Boston, Massachusetts

LARRY F. RICH, M.S., M.D.
Associate Professor of Ophthalmology
Chief of Cornea and External Disease Service
Oregon Health Sciences University
Portland, Oregon

JOHN R. WALSH, M.D.
Chief of Gerontology Section
Veterans Administration Medical Center
Professor of Medicine
Oregon Health Sciences University
Portland, Oregon

JEANNE Y. WEI, M.D., Ph.D.
Director, Gerontology Research Laboratory
Gerontology and Cardiovascular Divisions
Beth Israel Hospital
Assistant Professor of Medicine
Harvard Medical School
Boston, Massachusetts

MICHAEL WEINTRAUB, M.D.
Associate Professor of Preventive Medicine,
  Pharmacology, and Medicine
University of Rochester
School of Medicine and Dentistry
Rochester, New York

SCOTT T. WEISS, M.S., M.D.
Associate Professor of Medicine
Harvard Medical School
Pulmonary Division
Beth Israel Hospital
Boston, Massachusetts

CHARLES S. WINANS, M.D.
Professor of Medicine
Section of Gastroenterology
University of Chicago Pritzker School of
  Medicine
Chicago, Illinois

LAWRENCE A. YANUZZI, M.D.
Surgeon Director in Ophthalmology
Manhattan Eye, Ear, and Throat Hospital
Associate Clinical Professor of Ophthalmology
Cornell University Medical College
New York, New York

NANCY J. OLINS, M.A.
Editorial Coordinator
AARP Pharmacy Service

OVERVIEW

As you leave your doctor's office, prescription in hand, you may not be able to decipher the handwriting indicating the name of the drug prescribed and the directions for its use. Even the label clearly typed by the pharmacist will provide you with scant information about the drug you will be swallowing or spraying, inserting or inhaling. A talk with your doctor or pharmacist may answer some of your questions, but you may later recall ones you forgot to ask, perhaps about side effects of the medicine or whether you can drink or drive while on the drug.

This book will provide you with the information you need to know about the medicines your doctor has prescribed. You will learn why a drug is being prescribed for a particular condition, what effects—both good and bad—you can expect from a drug, and how your eating habits and other aspects of your lifestyle can influence drug therapy. You will find out how a drug you are taking compares with other drugs used to treat the same condition and what other treatment options are available. In short, the information presented here will help you play a more active and positive role in maintaining your health.

As you can see from the Contents, the introductory material for this book contains five overview sections to increase your general knowledge about both prescription and over-the-counter (OTC) medicines. It is a good idea to familiarize yourself with this information before going on to read about specific products. These sections will arm you with information on proper ways to administer drugs, provide tips for remembering complicated drug schedules, and suggest appropriate questions to pose to your doctor and pharmacist. Also discussed are the use of nonprescription drugs, medicine considerations when traveling, and strategies for saving money on drugs without compromising on quality.

HOW TO USE THIS BOOK

The specific drug information is contained in thirteen major chapters, each covering a group of related medical conditions (such as digestive disorders or respiratory problems). Information about each of the related medical conditions covered in the chapter appears in brief medical guides. Each medical guide offers a quick overview of the particular medical condition and discusses its causes, diagnosis, and treatment, including drug and nondrug alternatives. Following each medical guide are drug charts. These drug charts summarize, in table form, important information about the medicines that may be prescribed for the condition discussed in the medical guide.

Not every available drug for every disorder is included. Instead, this book focuses on the several hundred drugs that are most commonly prescribed for and used by people over fifty. Drugs were selected based on information gathered from the AARP Pharmacy Service, the National Diagnostic and Therapeutic Index, other government and nongovernment statistical sources, and the judgments of the members of the Editorial Advisory Board.

None of the drugs included in this book must be administered by a doctor, though most must be prescribed by a doctor. Many of the OTC drug products you may have in your home will not appear here because you don't need a doctor's prescription to purchase them. Note, however, that limited exceptions have been made to this "prescription only" rule. Drug charts for aspirin and nonaspirin pain-killers are included because of their prominent therapeutic role in treating such conditions as arthritis and ministrokes, which are important problems in people over fifty. A drug chart is also included for calcium supplements, which are often recommended for older women. The last exception concerns vitamins and minerals. The designation of these products as "over-the-counter" or "prescription only" often depends on dosage strength; frequently used products in this category are listed, even if available without a prescription, to ensure that important vitamin combinations are included in this book.

The medical-condition index in the back of this book lists alphabetically all the medical conditions discussed in the text and can be used as a starting-off point in finding the medical guide that provides the information you want. Following the medical guides are the drug charts relevant to the condition being discussed. You might wish to look over and compare information on the various drugs available for treating your condition; you will find those charts all grouped together in one section of a chapter. The more you know about what you are taking—and what you are not—the more control you will have over your own health.

But you may be more interested in zeroing in on a specific drug than a specific illness. For example, you have been given a prescription for a medicine and want to know all about it before you take it. Or you may want to know, more specifically, if there are any special considerations for older people using this drug. To locate the appropriate drug chart, check the drug index, which appears right after the medical-condition index. The drug index lists medicines alphabetically by their generic (chemical) names (for example, tetracycline) and brand (trade) names (brand names of tetracycline, for example, include Achromycin, Sumycin, and Tetrex). The page numbers in boldface indicate where the drug chart appears; additional references to the drug are also listed.

To provide you with even more complete information about the drugs your doctor prescribes, a color identification section appears after page 916. The actual-size pictures in this section are organized according to the color of the drug and listed by both brand and generic names. To locate the picture of a particular drug, see the drug identification index on pages 908-916, which will direct you to the correct page as well as list the color and shape of the brand-name capsule or tablet (liquids, skin patches, and suppositories are not pictured).

A Guide to the Drug Charts

The opening section of each drug chart contains the most basic information about the medicine—generic name, brand name(s), dosage forms and strengths, and, where appropriate, how much of each ingredient it contains. (See page 5 for a further explanation of this). In some cases, not all available brands are included but the most common ones are. The number of drugs available changes regularly, with new drugs appearing on the market and others being removed. Note that the listing of dosage forms and strengths does *not* include information on how much of the drug you should take. That must be determined for you individually by your doctor and written on the prescription label.

The next section of the charts, the "Drug Profile," describes briefly what the medicine is used for and how it acts in the body.

The next section, "Before Using this Drug," alerts you to what information to give your doctor. The doctor should review your medical history and any allergic reactions or other problems you've had with similar drugs or those in a related class. Also, you should provide your doctor with a report on both prescription and OTC medicines you are currently taking. Drugs can interact in your body with other drugs, altering the effectiveness, toxicity, or side effects of either drug.

The section, "Special Restrictions While Taking this Drug," will help you get the most benefit from your medicine. It tells you, specifically, what drugs interact with your medicine and how to adjust your diet to help your medicine work more effectively. Information on medical examinations or tests you may need to take while on the drug are also outlined. In addition, any special restrictions on alcohol use, smoking, driving, sun exposure, exposure to excessive heat or cold, and exercise and exertion are discussed here. Other precautions are indicated when applicable to the particular drug.

The section on "Possible Side Effects" tells what type of side effects can be caused by the medicine and at what point to check with your doctor if you are experiencing any. Although the list of side effects is often long and can seem intimidating, keep in mind that many of the reactions are quite rare and may never happen to you.

In their concluding sections, the drug charts provide you with "Storage Instructions" for the medicine (improperly stored medicine can lose potency) and information on "Stopping or Interrupting Therapy." You may be tempted to discontinue taking the medicine when your symptoms begin to go away, but complete recovery may require longer treatment. Some drugs cannot be stopped abruptly; dosages must be diminished gradually.

Finally, the drug charts present "Special Considerations for Those over Sixty-Five." As a person ages, physical changes occur that may affect how long the drug remains in the body. This section lists side effects that are especially likely to occur in this age group and particular precautions to follow.

Although certain drugs are used to treat more than one type of medical condition, drug charts are not repeated in this book. Instead, cross references are provided in the appropriate chapters to direct you from a particular medical condition to a relevant drug that may be listed in a different part of the book.

Drug Categories and Dosage Forms

Drugs are classified and grouped together in the drug charts in categories the Editorial Advisory Board judged to be most helpful to consumers. The "Category" listing refers to the medicines in terms that are commonly used by doctors and readily understood by patients. Where the Advisory Board concluded that drugs of a particular class were similar, the drugs appear in the same drug chart. If the judgment of the board was that certain differences outweighed similarities between products, these drugs appear in different charts.

The dosage forms (for example, capsules, suppositories, tablets) of each product are listed in alphabetical order. If the particular form of the drug has just one active ingredient, the dosage strength is given next to that form; for example: Tablet: 300 mg. However, a dosage form of a particular drug may have two or more active ingredients; this is especially common for liquids. In those cases, the drug chart lists the amounts of each of the ingredients contained in the product.

The information on dosage strengths and forms may be useful to you in a number of situations. For example, if your doctor has instructed you to take two 250-mg tablets of your medicine three times a day and the drug chart indicates that the drug also comes in a 500-mg tablet, you might ask your doctor whether one higher-strength tablet would work as well as two lower-strength tablets. Or if you have trouble swallowing tablets and the drug chart indicates that your medicine also comes in liquid form, you might want to discuss a possible switch with your doctor.

The information in these charts is presented in a concise, easy-to-understand format for quick reference. But it should not be your sole source of facts; it is designed as a supplement to information provided by your doctor, pharmacist, or other health professional. If it raises any questions or does not completely satisfy your concerns, ask a qualified health professional for clarification.

ABBREVIATIONS USED IN THIS BOOK

g = gram (there are approximately 30 grams to an ounce)

mg = milligram (one thousandth of a gram)

μg = microgram (one millionth of a gram)

ml = milliliter (one thousandth of a liter, or approximately one thousandth of a quart)

WHAT YOU SHOULD KNOW ABOUT THE DRUGS YOU TAKE

You may think you are doing all you can for your health if you go for a medical examination when you have a problem, have any prescription you are given filled by a pharmacy, and then follow the instructions on the label (as best you can) for taking the medicine. However, research has shown that people often make errors when taking prescription drugs. These errors may have serious outcomes. Not only can they undermine the effectiveness of the drug, but they may also actually cause medical harm.

Mistakes can be avoided if you ask the right questions of your doctor, pharmacist, or other health professional, but many people are reluctant to do so. They do not know what to ask, or they are afraid of taking up too much of the professional's time, or they may be concerned that they will sound mistrustful. None of these is a good reason for being uninformed—or misinformed—about the medicines you take. The potential effects on your health are too great for you to be less than fully informed.

Questions to Ask

Below is a list of questions you should ask your doctor about any medicine prescribed. Be sure to have paper and a pencil handy to jot down the answers.
• What is the drug's name? Many drugs have a brand name and a generic name. Ask about both, and write them down for your own records.

• What exactly does the drug do? At what point should you start to see an effect, and what should you do if none is apparent?
• How much medicine should you take, and how often? Ask your doctor to write on the prescription that these instructions should be included on the drug label.
• How long should you take the drug?
• What should you do if you miss taking the drug at the specified time?
• Can this drug be prescribed in a generic form, which often costs less than the brand-name version? (See pages 10–12 for more information on generic vs. brand-name medicines.)
• If you will be taking the drug for some time, could it be prescribed in a large quantity that will remain fresh at the rate you use it? This can help save you money.
• What foods, drinks, or activities and what other medicines should you avoid while on this drug?
• Should this medicine be taken with food or on an empty stomach?
• What are the common side effects and what should you do if they occur? Which ones are severe enough to warrant consulting your doctor?
• Is any written information available about this drug? Pamphlets or magazine articles can help reinforce your doctor's instructions and your own notes.
• Is there a less expensive alternative available that will have the same therapeutic effect?
• Are there effective alternatives to treatment with drugs? Some conditions can be helped by changes in diet,

for example, or exercise, and you might want to explore those options first.

Your pharmacist is another valuable source of information in becoming a better informed consumer. You can raise the same types of issues mentioned above, as well as other specific concerns about your prescription:

• How much does the medicine cost?
• Is it available in a generic form?
• How should it be stored?
• Is it safe to crush a tablet or to open a capsule?
• Can this prescription be refilled?
• Can the medicine be put in a container that is easy to open?
• Is the medicine available in a more convenient or easy-to-use form?
• What does the extra labeling on the container mean?

Both your doctor and your pharmacist should be responsive to your questions and concerns about medicines, whether prescription or OTC. If you are dissatisfied with the time and attention you are receiving, consider finding a health professional who will answer your questions more fully.

Practical Pointers on Taking Drugs

Swallowing a pill may not be all there is to taking your medicine as the doctor ordered. Your medicine may come in different, less familiar forms, and you may be confused by different dosage schedules if more than one product is involved. If it is six o'clock in the evening, should you take three red tablets or two green capsules? Or is it time to get out the eye dropper or, perhaps, to change your skin patch?

As medical science becomes more sophisticated, taking medicine can be more complicated.

Storage Instructions Even the proper storage of drugs is not as simple as just lining them up in your bathroom medicine cabinet. Drugs should *not* be stored in the bathroom, where heat and moisture may affect them, but rather in a dry, cool place such as a bedroom or kitchen cabinet (*not* a cabinet above the stove). If directions call for the medicine to be refrigerated, do not place it in your freezer.

Remembering When There are some tricks for remembering which drugs to take when. One technique involves making a list each day of the different times of day—morning, afternoon, evening, and night—and writing down next to each time the name and amount of the drug(s) you are supposed to take. Then check off the time once you have taken the appropriate medicine(s). Another memory helper is to label the compartments of a small box with the different times of day. (Make sure the box seals tightly to protect your medicines from air and moisture.) Then, fill each section with the pills you are supposed to take at that time. (You can buy a special pillbox to serve the same function.) Alternatively, you might try using vials with different-colored caps that stand for different times of day (such as blue for morning, white for afternoon, red for evening, and black for bedtime). Your pharmacist may be able to provide you with special calendars and drug-reminder charts that will jog your memory if you are faced with confusing schedules involving several drugs.

Learning How Once you have figured out *when* to take your medicine, you are still left with the problem of *how*. Pill swallowing is something most people have mastered, more or less, but what if our medicine comes in a different form, for example, a *buccal* tablet? The term *buccal* relates to the cheek and mouth, and a buccal tablet is one that should be placed in the pouch between the cheek and the gum. After taking this kind of tablet, close your mouth and let the tablet dissolve completely—do not swallow or chew it. While the tablet is dissolving, don't eat, drink, or smoke. For a *sublingual* tablet—one that is placed under the tongue while it dissolves— the recommendations and warnings are the same. Note that a *controlled-release* tablet should never be crushed or chewed.

You have probably had experience using eye, ear, and nose drops, as well as nasal sprays, but here is a brief review of safe, effective methods for administering these products.

Eye Drops

• Wash your hands with soap and water.
• Lie down (or tilt back your head) and look up at the ceiling.
• Gently pull down your lower eyelid so that a pouch is formed.
• With the dropper in your other hand, approach the eye from the side.

Place the dropper close to the eye but not touching it.
• Place the prescribed number of drops into the eye pouch.
• Close your eye for a minute or two.
• Don't rub your eye. Instead, press gently with your fingers next to the bridge of your nose (on the same side as the eye into which you have inserted the drops) for about a minute. This helps prevent the eye drops from being drained from the eye.

If someone else administers the eye drops for you, have that person follow the steps outlined above, beginning with well-scrubbed hands.

Ear Drops

• Hold the bottle in your hands for a few minutes. This warms the drops to room temperature.
• Wash your hands with soap and water.
• Tilt your head or lie on your side, with the ear to be treated facing up. Gently pull the earlobe up and back.
• Place the prescribed number of drops into the ear. Do *not* insert the dropper into the ear.
• Stay in the same position for a few minutes after administering the drops.

This procedure can be done for you by somebody else, if necessary.

Nose Drops

• Blow your nose gently.
• Sit in a chair and tilt your head backward; alternatively, lie down with a pillow under your shoulders so that your head tips backward.
• Insert the nose dropper into the nostril about one third of an inch and

drop the prescribed number of drops into the nose.
• Stay in the same position for several minutes.

Nasal Sprays

• Blow your nose gently.
• While sitting down, tilt your head slightly forward.
• Shake the container well.
• Insert the spray tip firmly into the nostril and point it at the back and outer side of the nose. (Close the other nostril by pressing your finger against its side.)
• Keep your mouth closed, begin to breathe in, and release one spray of the medicine.
• Remove the spray tip from the nostril and bend your head backward for a few seconds.
• Hold your breath for a few seconds, then breathe out through your mouth.
• If necessary, repeat the procedure for the other nostril.

Transdermal Patches

A relatively new method of drug delivery is transdermal, which means "through the skin." This involves placing a medicated patch on the skin, often near the drug's target site (above the heart for nitroglycerin, for example, or on the abdomen for estrogen). Application instructions for the patch may differ somewhat for different products. In general, however, it should be applied to dry skin in a nonhairy area. Press the patch firmly in place for about ten to fifteen seconds, and then seal it by running your finger along its outside edge. At the

prescribed time, the patch should be removed and thrown away and the next one applied.

Other Dosage Forms

caplet A tablet that is shaped like a capsule.

controlled-release Medicine is effective only during that period of time when the active ingredients are released and absorbed by the body at high enough rates. Dosage forms that prolong the medicine's period of effectiveness are said to have a *controlled-release* property. Other names for that property are timed-release, sustained-release, extended-release, and long-acting.

cream A semisolid preparation in which particles of medicine are combined—dissolved or undissolved—in a mixture of oil and water. Creams are applied externally; in addition to their specific medical effects, they may also soften and lubricate the areas being treated. These preparations can neither be seen nor felt after they've been applied, and they can be easily washed off with water.

elixir A liquid preparation taken orally in which particles of medicine are thoroughly dissolved in an alcohol-based solution. Elixirs may also include a sweetener or other flavoring to improve the medicine's taste. The amount of drug per dose of the medicine is measured in milligrams.

enteric-coated tablet A tablet coated with a thin outer layer that is not broken down by stomach acid but is easily dissolved by the juices of the intestines. The purpose of this outer coating is either to protect the stomach from being irritated by the medicine or to prevent the medicine from being destroyed by stomach acid.

ointment A semisolid preparation in which particles of medicine are combined—dissolved or undissolved—in a mixture of oil or animal or vegetable fats and water. Ointments have a higher oil and lower water content than do creams. They are applied externally; in addition to their specific medical effects, they may also soften and lubricate the areas being treated. These preparations can be quite greasy and are not easily washed off with water.

solution A liquid preparation taken orally in which particles of medicine are thoroughly dissolved in water or a water substitute. The amount of drug per dose of medicine is measured in milligrams.

suspension A liquid preparation taken orally in which solid particles of medicine are mixed with water or a water substitute, but are not dissolved. It is important that the particles in a suspension be evenly distributed throughout the preparation; this can be accomplished by thoroughly shaking the medication just before taking it. The amount of drug per dose of the medicine is measured in milligrams.

syrup A liquid preparation taken orally in which particles of medicine are thoroughly dissolved in water or a water substitute. A sweetener or other flavoring is added to improve the medicine's taste. The amount of drug per dose of the medicine is measured in milligrams.

SAVING MONEY ON PRESCRIPTION DRUGS

"You get what you pay for" is an axiom that has stopped many a consumer from getting bilked in the marketplace. But when it comes to medicine, price is not a reliable guide to quality. In fact, the price of the same drug can vary tenfold or more, depending on where you purchase it and under what name it is being sold.

The first key to saving money on drugs is to have some understanding of how new drugs are marketed and the difference between generic and brand names. When a new drug is being tested, it is given its *generic* name by an organization known as the United States Adopted Name Council. (This name is, in most cases, a simplified version of the product's chemical formula.) Once the drug has been approved as safe and effective by the U.S. Food and Drug Administration (FDA), it is usually marketed by just one pharmaceutical company (the innovator), which obtains a patent for the product and gives it a *brand* name. When the patent expires, other companies are free to sell the drug under its generic name or under other brand names. (The antibiotic tetracycline, for example, can be sold either under the name tetracycline or under such brand names as Achromycin, Sumycin, and Tetrex.) An act passed by

Congress in 1984 enables pharmaceutical companies to get generic drugs on the market more speedily and at lower cost than was previously possible. Savings can then be passed on to the consumer.

Most generic drugs are less expensive than brand-name versions and just as safe and effective. Therefore, when your doctor gets ready to write you a prescription for a particular medicine, inquire whether the generic form of the drug is available. Not all brand-name drugs have generic equivalents available to consumers. If your doctor prescribes by the generic name whenever possible, you will be able to save money on almost every prescription you have filled. In some states, pharmacists may substitute a generic drug for the brand-name form unless the doctor says not to.

But don't count the money you save just yet! You still have some work to do, by phone or by foot. Different pharmacies may charge very different prices for the same medicine, so be prepared to shop around. Some stores will cite their prices over the telephone, sparing you legwork. A number of states require pharmacists to post the prices of frequently prescribed drugs—another aid to the consumer. You may decide to comparison shop for each prescription. That strategy will save you the most money.

No matter what you end up paying to fill your prescription, check your medical insurance policy. Some plans pay all or part of drug costs. The time it takes for you to do the paperwork may translate into big savings on your drug bills.

You may be tempted to cut costs by not having your prescription refilled even though your doctor has instructed you to do so. That is actually a counterproductive measure that can threaten both your pocketbook and your health. Even if you feel fine, your illness may recur if you do not take your medicine for the full length of time prescribed by your doctor.

A more reasonable way to save money on drugs is to consider curtailing your OTC drugs while you are taking a prescription drug. Let your doctor decide whether the nonprescription product is necessary—or wise—for you to take at that time.

BRAND (TRADE) AND GENERIC (CHEMICAL) NAMES OF THE MOST COMMON PRESCRIPTION DRUGS

The following table will familiarize you with the generic names of the forty brand-name drugs that, according to AARP Pharmacy Service statistics, are most commonly prescribed for persons fifty and over.

Brand (Trade) Name	Generic (Chemical) Name
Aldactazide	Spironolactone and hydrochlorothiazide
Aldomet	Methyldopa
Aldoril	Methyldopa and hydrochlorothiazide

Brand (Trade) Name	Generic (Chemical) Name
Apresoline	Hydralazine
Armour Thyroid	Thyroid hormone (dessicated)
Clinoril	Sulindac
Deltasone	Prednisone
Diabinese	Chlorpropamide
Dilantin	Phenytoin
Dyazide	Triamterene and hydrochlorothiazide
Esidrix	Hydrochlorothiazide
Feldene	Piroxicam
Inderal	Propranolol
Indocin	Indomethacin
Isordil	Isosorbide dinitrate
K-Tabs	Potassium chloride
Lanoxin	Digoxin
Lasix	Furosemide
Levothroid	L-thyroxine (Levothyroxine)
Lopressor	Metoprolol
Micro-K	Potassium chloride
Minipress	Prazosin
Motrin	Ibuprofen
Naprosyn	Naproxen
Nitrobid	Nitroglycerin
Norpace	Disopyramide
Pavabid	Papaverine
Persantine	Dipyridamole
Procardia	Nifedipine
Quinidex	Quinidine sulfate
Ser-Ap-Es	Hydralazine, reserpine, and hydrochlorothiazide
Slow-K	Potassium chloride
Sorbitrate	Isosorbide dinitrate
Synthroid	L-thyroxine (Levothyroxine)
Tagamet	Cimetidine
Timoptic	Timolol
Tenormin	Atenolol
Valium	Diazepam
Ventolin	Albuterol
Zyloprim	Allopurinol

A GUIDE TO OVER-THE-COUNTER MEDICINES

You can go into any pharmacy, buy a bottle off the shelf, and take it home with you. You do not need a doctor's prescription for it, so it must be safe. Right? Not necessarily. Although nearly everybody uses over-the-counter (OTC) medicines, often with good results, these drugs *can* cause adverse reactions. They may aggravate an already existing condition or, even worse, mask the symptoms of an underlying disease and delay proper treatment.

There are many good reasons to select OTC medicines. If your medical condition is simple enough for self-diagnosis (for example, a headache), treating it with an OTC product saves time and money. In addition, OTC medicine contains a lower amount of drug than prescription counterparts (for example, ibuprofen, corticosteroids, and antihistamines) and is therefore generally safer.

Before You Buy

To obtain the most benefit with the least risk, approach these products with caution. The elderly and anyone with a serious, long-term disorder (such as impaired liver or kidney function) should consult a doctor or pharmacist before taking a nonprescription drug. Your doctor should know about all the medicines you take, even those that may seem as harmless to you as vitamins.

Before you even buy the medicine, read the label carefully. This will tell you what symptoms the drug treats, who should *not* use the drug, the dosage, the ingredients, and possible side effects. If you decide to purchase the drug, follow the directions on the label. If you do not understand them, ask a health professional for clarification.

For the most part, OTC medicines do not cure disease but are designed to relieve its symptoms. If symptoms persist after a reasonable period of time, consult a doctor. The symptoms may not be trivial but, rather, signs of a serious condition that requires medical care.

Keep in mind, always, that nonprescription drugs are real medicines. The possibilities of overdose, serious side effects, and the interaction of one medicine with another exist. Check with your doctor or pharmacist before using an OTC product if you are on other medicine or if another nonprescription product fails to relieve your symptoms.

Drugs to Have Handy

To cut down on your round trips to the pharmacy for OTC items and to be prepared for emergency situations, there are certain products you should have on hand from a few basic categories. You should check with your doctor first to make sure these are all appropriate for you and to learn whether you should add other medicines based on your particular medical needs.

For headaches and other types of pain, you should have an *analgesic* (a pain reliever) handy, such as aspirin. If someone in your family has a "sensitive" stomach or is allergic to aspirin, a nonaspirin product like acetaminophen may be substituted. Acetaminophen would be the best choice for individuals with impaired kidney function or for persons who suffer from stomach distress with the other medicines. Be aware, also, that you should not give aspirin to children without first consulting a health professional. When given to a child with influenza or chicken pox, aspirin may induce Reye's syndrome.

For occasional heartburn or symptoms of indigestion, an *antacid* should be part of your medical supplies. If you are on a salt-restricted diet, certain antacids may be off limits because of their high salt content; some of the newer antacids contain relatively little salt. Antacids containing aluminum hydroxide and/or calcium carbonate are not good choices for people who tend to be constipated because such drugs can aggravate this problem. An antacid containing magnesium hydroxide would be a better selection. But if you tend to suffer from diarrhea, the aluminum or calcium varieties may be more appropriate for you. Because antacids can alter bodily functions, your doctor, pharmacist, or other health professional should help to decide what type you should purchase.

Itchiness can be annoying—and an *antipruritic* can be a welcome relief if you experience prickly heat, poison ivy, or mosquito bites. Ordinary calamine lotion is generally all you will need for this. (For serious cases, low-dose corticosteroid creams and ointments are available over the counter.)

An *antiseptic* is an important item to have in your medicine supply to cleanse minor wounds. The only one that's generally necessary is rubbing alcohol, or isopropyl (70 percent) alcohol. It should be applied after the wound is washed with soap and water.

Nasal congestion is another condition you should be prepared to cope with. As a *decongestant,* keep a nasal spray or nose drops to alleviate the stuffiness that commonly accompanies a cold. However, if you have high blood pressure or an overactive thyroid gland, you may not be a candidate for these medicines. Consult your doctor or pharmacist before making your purchase.

The best way to avoid constipation is to eat a diet that is high in fiber and to drink plenty of fluids. Too many people turn to *laxatives* to deal with constipation and become laxative abusers. After many years, such abuse can actually lead to constipation by causing the bowel to lose its ability to contract and propel its contents normally. However, if you do wish to have a laxative on hand, the safest choice for frequent use is a bulk laxative, such as Metamucil or Effersyllium. (People with diabetes need to be aware that some forms of Metamucil have a high sugar content.) These products are made up of vegetable fiber and act in much the same way as fiber in the diet. If you suffer only an occasional bout of constipation, milk of magnesia is reasonable to keep on hand.

For problems with loose, frequent bowel movements, you should have an *antidiarrheal remedy* available to use when needed. Follow your doctor's advice in choosing an appropriate OTC medicine. If the condition persists, ask your doctor whether you should try a more potent medicine—and whether you should be examined.

If you suffer from hemorrhoids, you should know that nonprescription *hemorrhoidal medicines* can often be effective.

Antifungal agents are used for such conditions as jock itch and athlete's foot and should be kept on hand if you are susceptible to these. Some of these drugs were originally prescription medicines and are now available over the counter.

There are certain OTC products you should avoid. These include mercury antiseptics, such as Mercurochrome, and OTC burn ointments, which cause allergic skin reactions in some people. (Instead, use ice water or cold running water to treat minor burns.)

Appropriately stocked with the right medicines (along with such first-aid equipment as bandages and gauze pads), your medicine cabinet can give you the peace of mind that you're ready to act quickly and effectively in dealing with common medical problems and emergency situations.

TRAVELING HEALTHY

You may look forward to your trips, near or far, as a great way to lift your spirits and improve your general mental health—but don't forget to take your physical health into account as well. Discuss your itinerary with your doctor, and ask about any potential health hazards it might entail. In ad-

dition, ask for a brief summary of your significant medical history, as well as a photocopy of your most recent electrocardiogram (whether or not you have heart disease).

This is also a good time to review and update prescriptions. Ask your doctor for the generic—or chemical—names of your medicines; this will help you identify them for foreign doctors in case you need medical care abroad. Be sure to take a list of all the medicines you are currently using.

Immunizations

You should also review your past immunizations with your doctor and find out which ones you will need before your trip. You may be surprised to learn you will need any. After all, aren't "shots" for kids? Not exclusively, since many adults lose the immunity they acquired during childhood and adolescence.

If you're traveling, some health professionals advise that you be immunized against the flu, tetanus, and diphtheria. You should also be immunized against pneumococcal pneumonia if you have chronic heart and lung disease or diabetes or are undergoing cancer chemotherapy. Travelers to many parts of Asia, Africa, and South America are advised to have immunizations for yellow fever, cholera, and typhoid. In many cases, injections of gamma globulin are recommended to lower the risk of hepatitis A. Your doctor may suggest that you be vaccinated against poliomyelitis, an illness still prevalent in many areas of the world. In some older people, polio can assume a severe and often fatal form.

As yet, there is no vaccine against malaria. But the disease can usually be prevented by taking one of the chloroquine antimalarial drugs weekly starting at least two weeks before entering a malarial area and continuing for eight weeks after leaving the area. If you're traveling to eastern or central Africa, the Amazon basin, or rural areas of Southeast Asia, you may need to take a second drug, Fansidar, to combat more resistant malarial parasites.

For advice on how to avoid the scourge of adventurous tourists, traveler's diarrhea, see chapter 3 (pages 333-334).

Taking It with You

Once you're well immunized and ready to pack for your trip, make sure to leave room for a "little black bag" of medicines and supplies. You may never need these but you'll feel better having them along. This personal medical kit (which you should keep with you on the plane) should contain the following items:

• An adequate supply of all your prescription medicines (in clearly labeled, plastic bottles)
• An extra pair of eyeglasses if you use them
• A copy of your current eyeglass or contact lens prescription if you use either
• Antacids
• Analgesics (aspirin, acetaminophen, or ibuprofen)
• Motion-sickness medicine (if desired)
• Nasal decongestant
• Antihistamine
• Antidiarrhea medicine
• Calamine lotion
• Insect repellant
• Sunscreen and sunglasses
• Thermometer in a well-protected case
• Bandages and adhesive tape

If you've ever experienced serious allergies or side effects from any medicines, take along a list of those products; if those reactions are potentially life threatening, you may need to wear an identification bracelet or necklace. A traveler who has a severe illness—such as heart disease, asthma, or a bleeding disorder—should have on hand a doctor's note outlining the condition and the medicines being used to treat it.

Finding a Doctor Abroad

No matter how well equipped you are, your supplies cannot meet every possible medical emergency. You may find yourself, far from home, needing medical assistance. Again, advance planning is the key. Two organizations can provide you with listings of qualified English-speaking doctors in different parts of the world. The International Association for Medical Assistance to Travelers (IAMAT, 736 Center St., Lewiston, N.Y. 14902; 716-754-4883) has a list covering 120 countries. There is no charge, but the organization relies on donations. You should write for the information at least eight weeks before your departure date. Intermedic (777 Third Ave., New York, N.Y. 10017; 212-486-8900) publishes a list of competent foreign doctors whose services are available to travelers for established fees. The list is for members only; annual membership is six dollars for an individual, ten dollars for a family. In addition, if you are an American Express card holder, the company provides a service called Global Assist that allows you to phone in from wherever you may be traveling to get a medical referral.

If this strategy does not work and you need a doctor fast, call the American Consulate or American Embassy; they are prepared to respond to American tourists in emergency situations. Your next plan of action (if that one fails) would be to locate the nearest university hospital or, if your medical condition warrants it, to take a plane to a larger city. You may be a long day's journey, or more, from home, but you are unlikely to be more than a few hours away from a well-equipped medical center that can meet your health needs.

You may need to adjust dosage schedules of medicines if you will be crossing a number of time zones. For people with diabetes on insulin injections, check sugar levels and use meal time rather than clock time to determine when to take your doses. For other medicine, check with your doctor about breaking up your doses into smaller ones to take them at slightly more frequent intervals.

Those persons unaccustomed to the rigors of travel should be especially careful to follow general health precautions—eat well, do not try to do too much, and avoid extremes of either heat or cold.

Chapter 1
Disorders of the Heart and Blood Vessels

HYPERTENSION

Hypertension, or high blood pressure, is one of the most common—and insidious—medical conditions in the Western world. Hypertension becomes more frequent with age, affecting as many as 30 percent to 50 percent of people in their fifties, sixties, and seventies. But this increase in blood pressure with age is not inevitable. In many nonindustrialized societies, blood pressure does not rise with age.

Although hypertension has no symptoms, it takes a high toll in illness and death. An elevation in blood pressure is the single most important risk factor for developing serious cardiovascular disease, including stroke and heart attack, and is a leading cause of heart and kidney failure.

But the good news is that hypertension is controllable. Over the past fifteen years, deaths from stroke have decreased by 45 percent, and heart attack deaths have declined by 31 percent. This encouraging trend has been attributed mostly to better diagnosis and treatment of hypertension.

CAUSES

Hypertension refers to an increase in the force required to pump the blood through the arteries. This increase in blood pressure may stem from either a greater volume of blood or a narrowing of the arteries. Only about one in ten cases of hypertension has a clear-cut cause—usually a disorder of the kidneys or of the adrenal glands, which sit atop the kidneys.

These cases of so-called secondary hypertension are often amenable to surgical correction, after which the blood pressure returns to normal.

In the majority of people with hypertension, however, no cause can be found. These people have what is known as essential, or primary, hypertension. (The word *essential* is an interesting relic of the last century, when doctors mistakenly believed that an increase in blood pressure was essential to keep blood flowing to the vital organs.) Some scientists believe that essential hypertension is caused by a defect in the body's ability to eliminate salt normally. Other explanations focus on potent hormones that raise blood pressure and on the nervous system.

Some people have the erroneous notion that hypertension is linked with emotional tension. Blood pressure does fluctuate throughout the day and can certainly rise temporarily when a person is upset. However, stress and tension do not cause high blood pressure, and a calm, peaceful existence will not cure it.

DIAGNOSIS

Because hypertension does not announce its presence with symptoms, doctors have to search for it. Hypertension is detected by measuring blood pressure with the familiar device called a sphygmomanometer, which consists of an inflatable cuff and a pressure gauge. When the blood pressure cuff is fully inflated, blood flow in the arm stops. As pressure in the cuff is gradually decreased, a health professional uses a stethoscope to listen to the sound of the blood flowing through an artery below the cuff. Several sounds are heard in sequence. The first whooshing sound represents the force of blood flow when the heart contracts, and the pressure at which this sound is heard is called the systolic blood pressure. A later, muffled sound signals blood flow between heartbeats, which marks the diastolic pressure.

Blood pressure is expressed as two numbers. If your doctor tells you that your blood pressure is, for example, 140 over 85, he or she means that your systolic blood pressure is 140 and your diastolic pressure is 85 (written as 140/85). The numbers represent millimeters of mercury, abbreviated *mm Hg*. Normal blood pressure in an adult is a diastolic pressure no higher than 90 mm Hg. This means that the odds of developing hypertension-related health problems are greater in people whose blood pressure rises above this number. It also means that treatment that reduces diastolic pressure to 90 mm Hg or less will decrease the likelihood of complications from hypertension.

After age sixty, it is not uncommon for the systolic pressure to rise without an increase in the diastolic pressure. This state is called isolated systolic hypertension. However, since it is not certain whether treating isolated systolic hypertension will avert the development of health problems, many doctors may not treat mildly elevated systolic pressure unless dia-

stolic pressure is also high. Recent studies have suggested that small doses of a diuretic may be a feasible, effective, and well-tolerated treatment for older persons who have isolated systolic hypertension.

One elevated measurement is not enough to confirm a diagnosis of hypertension. Many doctors will not treat hypertension unless readings are elevated on three separate occasions. This is because blood pressure can change with the person's situation and the time of day. In persons over age fifty, blood pressure must be measured in both a standing and a sitting position.

TREATMENT

A wide variety of medicines are effective in lowering blood pressure and reducing the complications of hypertension. In several large clinical studies, reducing high blood pressure with drugs significantly lowered the chances of illness or death from stroke or heart attack. The benefit was greatest in people over the age of sixty.

These antihypertensive drugs act by many methods, so a person whose blood pressure does not respond fully to one drug may have better luck with another. Even the best drugs, however, do not cure hypertension. You most likely will have to take your medicine for life.

People who experience troublesome side effects with one drug will often have fewer or no problems when switched to another. So be sure to be honest with your doctor if the medicine he or she prescribes seems to cause problems such as fatigue, dizziness, confusion, bad dreams, or loss of sexual interest.

The drug charts on pages 23–135 explain how the various blood pressure–lowering medicines work and what to expect from them.

The most important step you can take to control your hypertension is to take your medicine as your doctor prescribes. But there are other ways you can help yourself.

Your doctor will probably prescribe a moderate low-salt diet in addition to your medicine. If you are overweight, your doctor may suggest that you lose those extra pounds. For some people with hypertension, salt restriction and weight loss may bring blood pressure under control. For most people, dietary changes can at least play an important supporting role in the treatment of hypertension and may even lower your medication dose.

You can also improve your overall cardiovascular health by stopping smoking. Many doctors recommend regular exercise, such as brisk walking, to supplement drug therapy. Psychological methods for lowering blood pressure, such as relaxation and biofeedback, may have a modest effect on blood pressure but have not been shown to be strong enough to be used without drug treatment.

OUTLOOK

The dramatic reductions in stroke and heart disease that have occurred in the U.S. population as a whole have largely been brought about by better detection of high blood pressure and better treatments. You, too, can lower your risk of cardiovascular disease by having your blood pressure checked regularly. If your doctor diagnoses hypertension, you can greatly reduce the potential consequences by following the prescribed treatment. If you stick to your drug and diet treatment and your blood pressure returns to normal, your chances are better for a normal and active life.

CONDITION: **HYPERTENSION**

CATEGORY: **DIURETICS (THIAZIDES AND RELATED DRUGS)**

GENERIC (CHEMICAL) NAME	BRAND (TRADE) NAME	DOSAGE FORMS AND STRENGTHS
Chlorthalidone	HYGROTON THALITONE	Tablets: 25, 50, 100 mg Tablets: 25 mg
Chlorothiazide	DIURIL	Suspension: 250 mg per tsp Tablets: 250, 500 mg
Hydrochlorothiazide	ESIDRIX HydroDIURIL	Tablets: 25, 50, 100 mg Tablets: 25, 50, 100 mg
Hydroflumethiazide	DIUCARDIN	Tablets: 50 mg
Methyclothiazide	ENDURON	Tablets: 2.5, 5 mg
Metolazone	DIULO ZAROXOLYN	Tablets: 2.5, 5, 10 mg Tablets: 2.5, 5, 10 mg
Polythiazide	RENESE	Tablets: 1, 2, 4 mg
Trichloromethiazide	METAHYDRIN NAQUA	Tablets: 2, 4 mg Tablets: 2, 4 mg

DRUG PROFILE

Thiazide and thiazide-type diuretics are often used to help control high blood pressure. They work by increasing the amount of salt and water eliminated by the body (through urination) and by relaxing the walls of the smaller arteries so that they expand. With a smaller volume of blood (because water is eliminated) in a larger amount of space (because the artery walls are expanded), blood pressure decreases. These drugs may also be prescribed for swelling in certain parts of the body (the ankles, for example) because they help the body eliminate excess water. Thiazide diuretics are also used in the treatment of calcium stones because they decrease the amount of calcium eliminated through urination.

BEFORE USING THE DRUG

Let your doctor know *IF*

You have ever had allergic reactions or other problems with ■ any of the thiazide or thiazide-type diuretics ■ sulfonamides (sulfa drugs).

You have ever had any of the following medical problems: ■ diabetes ■ gout ■ kidney disease ■ liver disease ■ systemic lupus erythematosus ■ disease of the pancreas ■ allergies ■ asthma.

You are taking any of the following medicines: ■ other diuretics or other medicines for high blood pressure ■ corticosteroids or corticotropin (ACTH) ■ medicine for high cholesterol ■ medicine for diabetes ■ digoxin, digitoxin, or digitalis (heart medicines) ■ medicine for gout ■ lithium ■ methenamine (medicine to prevent urinary tract infections) ■ anticoagulants (blood thinners) ■ tetracycline.

SPECIAL RESTRICTIONS WHILE TAKING THIS DRUG

FOOD AND DRUG INTERACTIONS

Other Drugs	Do not take any other drugs, including over-the-counter (OTC) drugs, before checking with your doctor. OTC drugs for appetite suppression, asthma, colds, cough, hay fever, or sinus problems tend to increase blood pressure.
	If you are also taking cholestyramine (medicine for high cholesterol), take your thiazide drug at least one hour before taking cholestyramine.
Foods and Beverages	Your doctor may prescribe a special low-salt diet, which you should follow carefully because it will help your medicine work more effectively. You may also be advised to go on a weight-reduction diet. Thiazides

and related drugs may cause your body to lose large amounts of the mineral potassium. Your doctor may give you special instructions about eating or drinking foods that have a high potassium content (such as bananas and citrus fruit juices), taking a potassium supplement, or using salt substitutes. It is important that you follow your doctor's instructions exactly.

No special restrictions on alcohol use or smoking.

DAILY LIVING

Exertion and Exercise	Use caution when exercising or exerting yourself while taking this medicine because excessive sweating may cause you to become dehydrated and to feel dizzy, light-headed, or faint.
Sun Exposure/ Excessive Heat	Your skin may become more sensitive to sunlight and more likely to develop a sunburn while you are taking this medicine. It is a good idea to avoid too much sun, especially if you burn easily. Apply a sunscreen to exposed skin surfaces before going outdoors. Use caution during hot weather or when taking saunas or hot baths, since excessive sweating while taking this medicine may cause you to become dehydrated and to feel drowsy or faint.
Examinations or Tests	Many people have high blood pressure with no symptoms at all. It is important for you to keep all appointments with your doctor, even if you feel well, so that your blood pressure can be checked regularly. Blood tests at several weeks, and then again at several months, after starting therapy with this drug will probably be required.
Other Precautions	If you have diabetes, be aware that this medicine may raise blood-sugar levels. If you notice any change

when testing sugar levels in your blood or urine, let your doctor know.

When first starting on this type of medicine, you may feel tired and will probably experience both greater volume and frequency of urination. Until your individual pattern of urination has been established with this medicine, it may be wise to time carefully any activity that will put you out of convenient reach of a bathroom, such as bus or car travel. In addition, taking a diuretic at bedtime will probably interfere with sleep; you should discuss your dosage schedule with your doctor.

Check with your doctor if you become ill with flulike symptoms, such as cough, fever, or body aches; lose your appetite; vomit; or have diarrhea. This may cause you to lose a great deal of fluid, making it important not to take the diuretic for one or more doses.

Following mild fluid losses, some older people are more vulnerable to symptoms of weakness or dizziness upon standing or getting up.

No special restrictions on driving or exposure to excessive cold.

POSSIBLE SIDE EFFECTS

Although this list of adverse effects may seem somewhat intimidating, keep in mind that some are quite rare. Of course, should these or any other problems arise while you are on medication, it is always a good idea to consult your doctor.

IF YOU DEVELOP

increased skin sensitivity to sunlight (if severe) ■ dry mouth ■ increased thirst ■ dizziness or weakness upon standing or getting up ■ nausea or vomiting ■ severe stomach pain or cramps ■ joint or side pain ■ irregular heartbeat ■ weak

WHAT TO DO

Urgent Get in touch with your doctor immediately.

pulse ■ difficulty in breathing ■ decreased urination ■ mood changes ■ confusion ■ muscle
cramps or pain ■ tiredness or weakness

rash or hives ■ sore throat or fever ■ bleeding or bruising ■ yellowing of eyes or skin	**May be serious** Check with your doctor as soon as possible.
diarrhea ■ loss of appetite ■ upset stomach ■ male impotence ■ clumsiness	If symptoms are disturbing or persist, let your doctor know.

STORAGE INSTRUCTIONS

Store in a cool, dark place (not in a bathroom medicine cabinet). If your medicine is in a liquid form, make sure that it does not freeze.

STOPPING OR INTERRUPTING THERAPY

Since this drug does not cure high blood pressure but only controls it, you may have to take this medicine for the rest of your life. Do not stop taking it, even if you feel better. If you miss a dose, take it as soon as possible. If it is almost time for your next dose, skip the missed dose and resume your regular schedule. Do not take two doses at the same time.

SPECIAL CONSIDERATIONS FOR THOSE OVER SIXTY-FIVE

Older people are more likely to develop such side effects as confusion, weakness, clumsiness, dizziness when getting up from a reclining or sitting position, potassium deficiency, and dehydration. Thus, it is especially important to keep all doctor's appointments as well as appointments for laboratory tests. People over sixty-five should check with a doctor if they become ill with flulike symptoms, such as cough, fever, or body aches; lose their appetite; vomit; or have diarrhea because they may then be more vulnerable to fluid losses.

CONDITION: **HYPERTENSION**

CATEGORY: **DIURETICS (POTASSIUM-SPARING)**

GENERIC (CHEMICAL) NAME	BRAND (TRADE) NAME	DOSAGE FORMS AND STRENGTHS
Triamterene	DYRENIUM	Capsules: 50, 100 mg

DRUG PROFILE

Triamterene is a potassium-sparing diuretic that is used to treat edema (swelling due to excess fluid in the body). It is usually used along with other drugs to treat high blood pressure. Triamterene increases the amount of salt and water eliminated by the body; with the resulting smaller volume of blood, blood pressure usually decreases. Potassium-sparing diuretics maintain the body's level of potassium while they work.

BEFORE USING THIS DRUG

Let your doctor know *IF*

You have ever had allergic reactions or other problems with ■ triamterene.

You have ever had any of the following medical problems: ■ diabetes ■ gout ■ heart disease ■ kidney disease, including kidney stones ■ liver disease ■ disease of the pancreas ■ alcoholism.

You are taking any of the following medicines: ■ other diuretics or medicines for high blood pressure, especially captopril or enalapril ■ medicine for diabetes ■ medicine for gout ■ laxatives ■ lithium ■ potassium-containing medicines or supplements ■ aspirin, indomethacin, or other arthritis medicines (nonsteroidal anti-inflammatory drugs).

SPECIAL RESTRICTIONS WHILE TAKING THIS DRUG

FOOD AND DRUG INTERACTIONS

Other Drugs	Do not take any other drugs, including over-the-counter (OTC) drugs, before checking with your doc-

tor. OTC drugs for appetite suppression, asthma, colds, cough, hay fever, or sinus problems tend to increase blood pressure. Also check with your doctor before using any nonsteroidal anti-inflammatory drug (such as aspirin, indomethacin, or other arthritis medicines), since these drugs combined with triamterene may affect kidney function.

| Foods and Beverages | Your doctor may prescribe a special low-salt diet, which you should follow carefully because it will help your medicine work more effectively. You may also be advised to go on a weight-reduction diet. Since this medicine does not cause a loss of potassium from your body, it is not necessary to have extra potassium in your diet or take a potassium supplement; too much potassium can be harmful. Let your doctor know if you use salt substitutes; many of these products are high in potassium. |

No special restrictions on alcohol use or smoking.

DAILY LIVING

| Exertion and Exercise | Use caution when exercising or exerting yourself while taking this medicine because excessive sweating may cause you to become dehydrated and to feel dizzy, light-headed, or faint. |

| Sun Exposure/ Excessive Heat | Your skin may become more sensitive to sunlight and more likely to develop a sunburn while you are taking this medicine. It is a good idea to avoid too much sun, especially if you burn easily. Apply a sunscreen to exposed skin surfaces before going outdoors. Use caution during hot weather or while taking saunas or hot baths, since excessive sweating while taking this medicine may cause you to become dehydrated and to feel drowsy or faint. |

| Examinations or Tests | Many people have high blood pressure with no symptoms at all. It is important for you to keep all appointments with your doctor, even if you feel well, so that your blood pressure can be checked regularly. Periodic blood tests may be required. |

| Other Precautions | If you have diabetes, be aware that this medicine may raise blood-sugar levels. If you notice any change when testing sugar levels in your blood or urine, let your doctor know. |

When first starting on this type of medicine, you may feel tired and will probably experience both greater volume and frequency of urination. Until your individual pattern of urination has been established with this medicine, it may be wise to time carefully any activity that will put you out of convenient reach of a bathroom, such as bus or car travel. In addition, taking a diuretic at bedtime will probably interfere with sleep; you should discuss your dosage schedule with your doctor.

Check with your doctor if you become ill with flulike symptoms, such as cough, fever, or body aches; lose your appetite; vomit; or have diarrhea. This may cause you to lose a great deal of fluid, making it important not to take the diuretic for one or more doses.

Following mild fluid losses, some older people are more vulnerable to symptoms of weakness or dizziness upon standing or getting up.

| Helpful Hints | If this medicine upsets your stomach, taking it with milk, meals, or snacks should help. |

No special restrictions on driving or exposure to excessive cold.

POSSIBLE SIDE EFFECTS

Although this list of adverse effects may seem somewhat intimidating, keep in mind that some are quite rare. Of course, should these or any other problems arise while you are on medication, it is always a good idea to consult your doctor.

IF YOU DEVELOP	WHAT TO DO
irregular heartbeat ■ numbness or tingling in hands, feet, or lips ■ tiredness or weakness ■ confusion ■ difficulty in breathing ■ severe or continuing diarrhea ■ severe side pain ■ dry mouth ■ increased thirst ■ dizziness or weakness upon standing or getting up	**Urgent** Get in touch with your doctor immediately.
nervousness ■ heaviness of legs ■ tongue inflammation ■ cracked corners of mouth ■ rash or itching ■ sore throat or fever ■ bleeding or bruising ■ headache	**May be serious** Check with your doctor as soon as possible.
upset stomach ■ drowsiness ■ lack of energy ■ increased skin sensitivity to sunlight	If symptoms are disturbing or persist, let your doctor know.

STORAGE INSTRUCTIONS

Store in a cool, dark place (not in a bathroom medicine cabinet).

STOPPING OR INTERRUPTING THERAPY

Since this drug does not cure high blood pressure but only controls it, you may have to take this medicine for the rest of your life. Do not stop taking it, even if you feel better. If you miss a dose, take it as soon as possible. If it is almost time for your next dose, skip the missed dose and resume your regular schedule. Do not take two doses at the same time.

SPECIAL CONSIDERATIONS FOR THOSE OVER SIXTY-FIVE

Older people are more likely to develop problems caused by too much potassium in the body, such as irregular heartbeat, confusion, difficulty in breathing, and tiredness or weakness. Doctors may require regular checkups. People over sixty-five should check with a doctor if they become ill with flulike symptoms, such as cough, fever, or body aches; lose their appetite; vomit; or have diarrhea because they may then be more vulnerable to fluid losses.

CONDITION: **HYPERTENSION**

CATEGORY: **DIURETICS (POTASSIUM-SPARING)**

GENERIC (CHEMICAL) NAME	BRAND (TRADE) NAME	DOSAGE FORMS AND STRENGTHS
Spironolactone	ALDACTONE	Tablets: 25, 50, 100 mg

DRUG PROFILE

Spironolactone is a potassium-sparing diuretic that is used to treat high blood pressure, edema (swelling due to excess fluid in the body), conditions in which there is not enough potassium in the body, and certain hormonal disturbances. This drug increases the amount of salt and water eliminated by the body (through urination); with a smaller volume of blood (because water is eliminated), blood pressure usually decreases. Potassium-sparing diuretics maintain the body's level of potassium while they work.

BEFORE USING THIS DRUG

Let your doctor know *IF*

You have ever had allergic reactions or other problems with ■spironolactone.

You have ever had any of the following medical problems: ■ diabetes ■ heart disease ■ kidney disease ■ liver disease.

You are taking any of the following medicines: ■ other diuretics or medicines for high blood pressure ■ lithium ■ potassium-containing medicines or supplements ■ digoxin, digitoxin, or digitalis (heart medicines) ■ medicine for diabetes ■ medicine containing alcohol.

SPECIAL RESTRICTIONS WHILE TAKING THIS DRUG

FOOD AND DRUG INTERACTIONS

Other Drugs	Do not take any other drugs, including over-the-counter (OTC) drugs before checking with your doctor. OTC drugs for appetite suppression, asthma, colds, cough, hay fever, or sinus problems tend to increase blood pressure.
Foods and Beverages	Your doctor may prescribe a special low-salt diet, which you should follow carefully because it will help your medicine work more effectively. You may also be advised to go on a weight-reduction diet. Since this medicine does not cause a loss of potassium from your body, it is not necessary to have extra potassium in your diet or take a potassium supplement; too much potassium can be harmful. Let your doctor know if you use salt substitutes; many of these products are high in potassium.

No special restrictions on alcohol use or smoking.

DAILY LIVING

Exertion and Exercise	Use caution when exercising or exerting yourself while taking this medicine because excessive sweating may cause you to become dehydrated and to feel dizzy, light-headed, or faint.
Sun Exposure/ Excessive Heat	Your skin may become more sensitive to sunlight and more likely to develop a sunburn while you are taking this medicine. It is a good idea to avoid too much sun, especially if you burn easily. Apply a sunscreen to exposed skin surfaces before going outdoors. Use caution during hot weather or while taking saunas or

hot baths, since excessive sweating while taking this medicine may cause you to become dehydrated and to feel drowsy or faint.

Examinations or Tests	Many people have high blood pressure with no symptoms at all. It is important for you to keep all appointments with your doctor, even if you feel well, so that your blood pressure can be checked regularly.
Other Precautions	Tell any doctor or dentist you consult that you are taking this medicine, especially if you will be undergoing any type of surgery.

When first starting on this type of medicine, you may feel tired and will probably experience both greater volume and frequency of urination. Until your individual pattern of urination has been established with this medicine, it may be wise to time carefully any activity that will put you out of convenient reach of a bathroom, such as bus or car travel. In addition, taking a diuretic at bedtime will probably interfere with sleep; you should discuss your dosage schedule with your doctor.

Check with your doctor if you become ill with flulike symptoms, such as cough, fever, or body aches; lose your appetite; vomit; or have diarrhea. This may cause you to lose a great deal of fluid, making it important not to take the diuretic for one or more doses.

Following mild fluid losses, some older people are more vulnerable to symptoms of weakness or dizziness upon standing or getting up.

Helpful Hints	If this medicine upsets your stomach, taking it with milk, meals, or snacks should help.

No special restrictions on driving or exposure to excessive cold.

POSSIBLE SIDE EFFECTS

Although this list of adverse effects may seem somewhat intimidating, keep in mind that some are quite rare. Of course, should these or any other problems arise while you are on medication, it is always a good idea to consult your doctor.

IF YOU DEVELOP	WHAT TO DO
irregular heartbeat ■ numbness or tingling in hands, feet, or lips ■ tiredness or weakness ■ confusion ■ difficulty in breathing ■ severe or continuing vomiting or diarrhea ■ dry mouth ■ increased thirst ■ dizziness or weakness upon standing or getting up	**Urgent** Get in touch with your doctor immediately.
nervousness ■ heaviness of legs ■ fever ■ rash or itching ■ swelling of hands or feet	**May be serious** Check with your doctor as soon as possible.
upset stomach ■ female breast tenderness ■ male breast enlargement ■ male impotence ■ deepening voice ■ hair growth ■ clumsiness ■ headache	If symptoms are disturbing or persist, let your doctor know.

STORAGE INSTRUCTIONS

Store in a cool, dark place (not in a bathroom medicine cabinet).

STOPPING OR INTERRUPTING THERAPY

Since this drug does not cure high blood pressure but only controls it, you may have to take this medicine for the rest of your life. Do not stop taking it, even if you feel better. If you miss a dose, take it as soon as possible. If it is almost time for your next dose, skip the missed dose and resume your regular schedule. Do not take two doses at the same time.

SPECIAL CONSIDERATIONS FOR THOSE OVER SIXTY-FIVE

Older people are more likely to develop problems caused by too much potassium in the body, such as irregular heartbeat, confusion, difficulty in breathing, and tiredness or weakness. Doctors may require regular checkups. People over sixty-five should check with a doctor if they become ill with flulike symptoms, such as cough, fever, or body aches; lose their appetite; vomit; or have diarrhea because they may then be more vulnerable to fluid losses.

CONDITION: **HYPERTENSION**

CATEGORY: **DIURETICS (POTASSIUM-SPARING)**

GENERIC (CHEMICAL) NAME	BRAND (TRADE) NAME	DOSAGE FORMS AND STRENGTHS
Amiloride	MIDAMOR	Tablets: 5 mg

DRUG PROFILE

Amiloride is a potassium-sparing diuretic that is used with other drugs to treat high blood pressure or congestive heart failure. This drug decreases blood pressure by increasing the amount of salt and water eliminated by the body (through urination). Potassium-sparing diuretics maintain the body's level of potassium while they work.

BEFORE USING THIS DRUG

Let your doctor know *IF*

You have ever had allergic reactions or other problems with ■ amiloride.

You have ever had any of the following medical problems: ■ diabetes ■ heart disease ■ kidney disease ■ liver disease.

You are taking any of the following medicines: ■ other diuretics or medicines for high blood pressure ■ lithium ■ potassium-containing medicines or supplements ■ salt substitutes.

SPECIAL RESTRICTIONS WHILE TAKING THIS DRUG

FOOD AND DRUG INTERACTIONS

Other Drugs	Do not take any other drugs, including over-the-counter (OTC) drugs, before checking with your doctor. OTC drugs for appetite suppression, asthma,

colds, cough, hay fever, or sinus problems tend to increase blood pressure.

Foods and Beverages	Your doctor may prescribe a special low-salt diet, which you should follow carefully because it will help your medicine work more effectively. You may also be advised to go on a weight-reduction diet. Since this medicine does not cause a loss of potassium from your body, it is not necessary to have extra potassium in your diet or take a potassium supplement; too much potassium can be harmful. Let your doctor know if you use salt substitutes; many of these products are high in potassium.

No special restrictions on alcohol use or smoking.

DAILY LIVING

Exertion and Exercise	Use caution when exercising or exerting yourself while taking this medicine because excessive sweating may cause you to become dehydrated and to feel dizzy, light-headed, or faint.
Excessive Heat	Use caution during hot weather or while taking saunas or hot baths, since excessive sweating while taking this medicine may cause you to become dehydrated and to feel drowsy or faint.
Examinations or Tests	Many people have high blood pressure with no symptoms at all. It is important for you to keep all appointments with your doctor, even if you feel well, so that your blood pressure can be checked regularly. Periodic blood tests are usually required.
Other Precautions	When first starting on this type of medicine, you may feel tired and will probably experience both greater

volume and frequency of urination. Until your individual pattern of urination has been established with this medicine, it may be wise to time carefully any activity that will put you out of convenient reach of a bathroom, such as bus or car travel. In addition, taking a diuretic at bedtime will probably interfere with sleep; you should discuss your dosage schedule with your doctor.

Check with your doctor if you become ill with flulike symptoms, such as cough, fever, or body aches; lose your appetite; vomit; or have diarrhea. This may cause you to lose a great deal of fluid, making it important not to take the diuretic for one or more doses.

Following mild fluid losses, some older people are more vulnerable to symptoms of weakness or dizziness upon standing or getting up.

No special restrictions on driving, sun exposure, or exposure to excessive cold.

POSSIBLE SIDE EFFECTS

Although this list of adverse effects may seem somewhat intimidating, keep in mind that some are quite rare. Of course, should these or any other problems arise while you are on medication, it is always a good idea to consult your doctor.

IF YOU DEVELOP	WHAT TO DO
chest pain ■ irregular heartbeat ■ numbness or tingling in hands, feet, or lips ■ tiredness or weakness ■ confusion ■ difficulty in breathing ■ severe or continuing nausea, vomiting, or diarrhea ■ dry mouth ■ increased thirst ■ dizziness or weakness upon standing or getting up	**Urgent** Get in touch with your doctor immediately.
heaviness of legs	**May be serious** Check with your doctor as soon as possible.

diarrhea ■ nausea or vomiting ■ loss of appetite ■ constipation ■ stomach pain or feeling of full-ness ■ heartburn or indigestion ■ shortness of breath ■ cough ■ male impotence ■ diminished sex drive ■ muscle cramps or pain ■ tremors ■ headache ■ sleeplessness ■ drowsiness ■ depression ■ rash or itching ■ hair loss ■ taste changes ■ urinary frequency or other urinary problems

If symptoms are disturbing or persist, let your doctor know.

STORAGE INSTRUCTIONS

Store in a cool, dark place (not in a bathroom medicine cabinet).

STOPPING OR INTERRUPTING THERAPY

Since this drug does not cure high blood pressure but only controls it, you may have to take this medicine for the rest of your life. Do not stop taking it even if you feel better. If you miss a dose, take it as soon as possible. If it is almost time for your next dose, skip the missed dose and resume your regular schedule. Do not take two doses at the same time.

SPECIAL CONSIDERATIONS FOR THOSE OVER SIXTY-FIVE

Older people are more likely to develop problems caused by too much potassium in the body, such as irregular heartbeat, confusion, difficulty in breathing, and tired-ness or weakness. Regular checkups may be required. All doctor's appointments should be kept. People over sixty-five should consult a doctor if they become ill with flulike symptoms such as cough, fever, or body aches; lose their appetite; vomit; or have diarrhea because they may then be more vulnerable to fluid losses.

CONDITION: **HYPERTENSION**

CATEGORY: **DIURETICS (MISCELLANEOUS)**

GENERIC (CHEMICAL) NAME	BRAND (TRADE) NAME	DOSAGE FORMS AND STRENGTHS
Indapamide	LOZOL	Tablets: 2.5 mg

DRUG PROFILE

Indapamide is a diuretic that may be used alone or in combination with other antihypertensive drugs to control high blood pressure. Like the thiazide diuretics, indapamide works by increasing the amount of salt and water you eliminate through urination. Because of this action, it is also used to treat fluid accumulation in people who have congestive heart failure.

BEFORE USING THIS DRUG

Let your doctor know *IF*

You have ever had allergic reactions or other problems with ■ indapamide ■ thiazide or thiazide-type diuretics ■ sulfonamides (sulfa drugs).

You have ever had any of the following medical problems: ■ diabetes ■ gout ■ kidney disease ■ liver disease ■ systemic lupus erythematosus ■ high cholesterol ■ thyroid disorders.

You are taking any of the following medicines: ■ other diuretics or high blood pressure medicines ■ corticosteroids or corticotropin (ACTH) ■ digoxin, digitoxin, or digitalis (heart medicines) ■ lithium.

SPECIAL RESTRICTIONS WHILE TAKING THIS DRUG

FOOD AND DRUG INTERACTIONS

Other Drugs	Do not take any other drugs, including over-the-counter (OTC) drugs, before checking with your doctor. OTC drugs for appetite suppression, asthma, colds, cough, hay fever, or sinus problems tend to increase blood pressure. Barbiturates (sleep medicine, medicine for seizures) and narcotic pain-killers may increase risk of dizziness when sitting up or standing up.
Foods and Beverages	Your doctor may prescribe a special low-salt diet, which you should follow carefully because it will help your medicine work more effectively. You may also be advised to go on a weight-reduction diet. This medicine may cause your body to lose large amounts of the mineral potassium. Your doctor may give you special instructions about eating foods or drinking bever-

ages that have a high potassium content (such as bananas and citrus fruit juices), taking a potassium supplement, or using salt substitutes.

| Alcohol | Alcohol may increase the risk of dizziness when sitting up or standing up. |

No special restrictions on smoking.

DAILY LIVING

| Exertion and Exercise | Use caution when exercising or exerting yourself while taking this medicine because excessive sweating may cause you to become dehydrated and to feel dizzy, light-headed, or faint. |

| Excessive Heat | Use caution during hot weather or while taking saunas or hot baths, since excessive sweating while taking this medicine may cause you to become dehydrated and to feel drowsy or faint. |

| Examinations or Tests | Many people have high blood pressure with no symptoms at all. It is important for you to keep all appointments with your doctor, even if you feel well, so that your blood pressure can be checked regularly. Periodic blood and urine tests may be required. |

| Other Precautions | When first starting on this type of medicine, you may feel tired and will probably experience both greater volume and frequency of urination. Until your individual pattern of urination has been established with this medicine, it may be wise to time carefully any activity that will put you out of convenient reach of a bathroom, such as bus or car travel. In addition, taking a diuretic at bedtime will probably interfere with sleep; you should discuss your dosage schedule with your doctor. |

Check with your doctor if you become ill with flulike symptoms, such as cough, fever, or body aches; lose your appetite; vomit; or have diarrhea. This may cause you to lose a great deal of fluid, making it important not to take the diuretic for one or more doses.

Following mild fluid losses, some older people are more vulnerable to symptoms of weakness or dizziness upon standing or getting up.

No special restrictions on driving, sun exposure, or exposure to excessive cold.

POSSIBLE SIDE EFFECTS

Although this list of adverse effects may seem somewhat intimidating, keep in mind that some are quite rare. Of course, should these or any other problems arise while you are on medication, it is always a good idea to consult your doctor.

IF YOU DEVELOP	WHAT TO DO
severe or continuing vomiting or diarrhea ■ irregular heartbeat ■ weak pulse ■ dry mouth ■ increased thirst ■ anxiety ■ agitation ■ depression ■ tiredness or weakness ■ muscle cramps or pain	**May be serious** Check with your doctor as soon as possible.
upset stomach ■ loss of appetite ■ dizziness or light-headedness, especially when getting up from a reclining or sitting position ■ headache ■ sleep disturbances ■ blurred vision ■ changes in urination ■ constipation ■ diarrhea, nausea, or vomiting	If symptoms are disturbing or persist, let your doctor know.

STORAGE INSTRUCTIONS

Store in a cool, dark place (not in a bathroom medicine cabinet).

STOPPING OR INTERRUPTING THERAPY

Since this drug does not cure high blood pressure but only controls it, you may have to take this medicine for the rest of your life. Do not stop taking it even if you feel better. If you miss a dose, take it as soon as possible. If it is almost time for your next dose, skip the missed dose and resume your regular schedule. Do not take two doses at the same time.

SPECIAL CONSIDERATIONS FOR THOSE OVER SIXTY-FIVE

Older people are more likely to develop dizziness or light-headedness or signs of potassium loss, such as irregular heartbeat and weak pulse. Regular checkups may be required. People over sixty-five should consult a doctor if they become ill with flulike symptoms, such as cough, fever, or body aches; lose their appetite; vomit; or have diarrhea because they may then be more vulnerable to fluid losses.

CONDITION: **HYPERTENSION**

CATEGORY: **DIURETICS (COMBINATIONS)**

GENERIC (CHEMICAL) NAME	BRAND (TRADE) NAME	DOSAGE FORMS AND STRENGTHS
Triamterene and hydrochlorothiazide	DYAZIDE	Capsules: 50 mg triamterene and 25 mg hydrochlorothiazide
	MAXZIDE	Tablets: 75 mg triamterene and 50 mg hydrochlorothiazide

DRUG PROFILE

This combination of two diuretics in one tablet or capsule may be prescribed to control high blood pressure, while at the same time maintaining the body's potassium levels. Each tablet or capsule contains a thiazide diuretic as well as a potassium-sparing diuretic. This drug works by increasing the amount of salt and water eliminated through the body (through urination) and by relaxing the walls of the smaller arteries so that they expand. With a smaller volume of blood (because water is eliminated) in a larger amount of space (because the artery walls are expanded), blood pressure decreases. This drug may also be prescribed with other therapy for edema (swelling due to excess fluid in the body), because it helps the body to eliminate extra water.

BEFORE USING THIS DRUG

Let your doctor know *IF*

You have ever had allergic reactions or other problems with ■ triamterene ■ thiazide diuretics ■ sulfonamides (sulfa drugs).

You have ever had any of the following medical problems: ■ diabetes ■ gout ■ heart disease ■ kidney disease or stones ■ liver disease ■ systemic lupus erythematosus ■ disease of the pancreas.

You are taking any of the following medicines: ■ other diuretics or medicines for high blood pressure ■ corticosteroids or corticotropin (ACTH) ■ medicine for high cholesterol ■ medicine for diabetes ■ digoxin, digitoxin, or digitalis (heart medicines) ■ medicine for gout ■ laxatives ■ lithium ■ methenamine (medicine to prevent urinary tract infections) ■ phenobarbital ■ narcotics or other prescription pain-killers ■ anticoagulants (blood thinners) ■ aspirin, indomethacin, or other arthritis medicines (nonsteroidal anti-inflammatory drugs) ■ potassium-containing medicines or supplements.

SPECIAL RESTRICTIONS WHILE TAKING THIS DRUG

FOOD AND DRUG INTERACTIONS

Other Drugs	Do not take any other drugs, including over-the-counter (OTC) drugs, before checking with your doctor. OTC drugs for appetite suppression, asthma, colds, cough, hay fever, or sinus problems tend to increase blood pressure.
	Check with your doctor before using any nonsteroidal anti-inflammatory drugs such as indomethacin.
	Barbiturates (sleep medicine, medicine for seizures) and narcotic pain-killers may increase the risk of dizziness when sitting up or standing up.
Foods and Beverages	Your doctor may prescribe a special low-salt diet, which you should follow carefully because it will help

your medicine work more effectively. You should continue to drink a normal amount of fluids. This medicine may either increase or decrease potassium levels in your body. Your doctor may give you special instructions about eating foods or drinking beverages that have a high potassium content (such as bananas and citrus fruit juices), taking a potassium supplement, or using salt substitutes.

Alcohol	Alcohol may increase the risk of dizziness when sitting up or standing up.

No special restrictions on smoking.

DAILY LIVING

Exertion and Exercise	Use caution when exercising or exerting yourself while taking this medicine because excessive sweating may cause you to become dehydrated and to feel dizzy, light-headed, or faint.
Sun Exposure/ Excessive Heat	Your skin may become more sensitive to sunlight and more likely to develop a sunburn while you are taking this medicine. It is a good idea to avoid too much sun, especially if you burn easily. Apply a sunscreen to exposed skin surfaces before going outdoors. Use caution during hot weather or while taking saunas or hot baths, since excessive sweating while taking this medicine may cause you to become dehydrated and to feel drowsy or faint.
Examinations or Tests	Many people have high blood pressure with no symptoms at all. It is important for you to keep all appointments with your doctor, even if you feel well, so that your blood pressure can be checked regularly. Periodic blood tests are usually required.

Other Precautions

If you have diabetes, be aware that this medicine may raise blood-sugar levels. If you notice any change when testing sugar levels in your blood or urine, let your doctor know.

Tell any doctor or dentist you consult that you are taking this medicine, especially if you will be undergoing any type or surgery.

When first starting on this type of medicine, you may feel tired and will probably experience both greater volume and frequency of urination. Until your individual pattern of urination has been established with this medicine, it may be wise to time carefully any activity that will put you out of convenient reach of a bathroom, such as bus or car travel. In addition, taking a diuretic at bedtime will probably interfere with sleep; you should discuss your dosage schedule with your doctor.

Check with your doctor it you become ill with flulike symptoms, such as cough, fever, or body aches; lose your appetite; vomit; or have diarrhea. This may cause you to lose a great deal of fluid, making it important not to take the diuretic for one or more doses.

Following mild fluid losses, some older people are more vulnerable to symptoms of weakness or dizziness upon standing or getting up.

Your urine may appear blue, which is expected and not harmful.

No special restrictions on driving or exposure to excessive cold.

POSSIBLE SIDE EFFECTS

Although this list of adverse effects may seem somewhat intimidating, keep in mind that some are quite rare. Of course, should these or any other problems arise while you are on medication, it is always a good idea to consult your doctor.

IF YOU DEVELOP	**WHAT TO DO**
irregular heartbeat ■ numbness or tingling in hands, feet, or lips ■ tiredness or weakness ■ confusion ■ mood or mental changes ■ shortness of breath ■ weak pulse ■ muscle cramps or pain ■ nausea or vomiting ■ dry mouth ■ increased thirst ■ severe or continuing diarrhea	**Urgent** Get in touch with your doctor immediately.
headache ■ tongue inflammation ■ cracked corners of mouth ■ rash ■ sore throat or fever ■ bleeding or bruising ■ yellowing of eyes or skin ■ swelling of hands or feet	**May be serious** Check with your doctor as soon as possible.
upset stomach ■ loss of appetite ■ stomach cramps ■ headache ■ dizziness or light-headedness, especially when getting up from a reclining or sitting position ■ increased skin sensitivity to sunlight ■ blurred vision	If symptoms are disturbing or persist, let your doctor know.

STORAGE INSTRUCTIONS

Store in a cool, dark place (not in a bathroom medicine cabinet).

STOPPING OR INTERRUPTING THERAPY

Since this drug does not cure high blood pressure but only controls it, you may have to take this medicine for the rest of your life. Do not stop taking it, even if you feel better. If you miss a dose, take it as soon as possible. If it is almost time for your next dose, skip the missed dose and resume your regular schedule. Do not take two doses at the same time.

SPECIAL CONSIDERATIONS FOR THOSE OVER SIXTY-FIVE

Older people are more likely to develop dizziness, light-headedness, or problems caused by changing potassium levels, such as irregular heartbeat or weak pulse. People over sixty-five should consult a doctor if they become ill with flulike symptoms, such as cough, fever, or body aches; lose their appetite; vomit; or have diarrhea because they may then be more vulnerable to fluid losses.

CONDITION: **HYPERTENSION**

CATEGORY: **DIURETICS (COMBINATIONS)**

GENERIC (CHEMICAL) NAME	BRAND (TRADE) NAME	DOSAGE FORMS AND STRENGTHS
Spironolactone and hydrochlorothiazide	ALDACTAZIDE	Tablets: 25 mg spironolactone and 25 mg hydrochlorothiazide; 50 mg spironolactone and 50 mg hydrochlorothiazide

DRUG PROFILE

This combination of two diuretics in one tablet may be prescribed to control high blood pressure. Each tablet contains a thiazide diuretic as well as a potassium-sparing diuretic. This drug works by increasing the amount of salt and water eliminated by the body (through urination) and by relaxing the walls of the smaller arteries so that they expand. With a smaller volume of blood (because water is eliminated) in a larger amount of space (because the artery walls are expanded), blood pressure decreases. This drug may also be prescribed for edema (swelling due to excess fluid in the body) because it helps the body to eliminate extra water.

BEFORE USING THIS DRUG

Let your doctor know *IF*

You have ever had allergic reactions or other problems with ■ spironolactone ■ thiazide diuretics ■ sulfonamides (sulfa drugs).

You have ever had any of the following medical problems: ■ diabetes ■ gout ■ heart disease ■ liver disease ■ systemic lupus erythematosus ■ kidney disease ■ disease of the pancreas.

You are taking any of the following medicines: ■ other diuretics or medicines for high blood pressure ■ corticosteroids or corticotropin (ACTH) ■ colestipol (medicine for high cholesterol) ■ medicine for diabetes ■ digoxin, digitoxin, or digitalis (heart medicines) ■ medicine for gout ■ lithium ■ methenamine (medicine to prevent urinary tract infections) ■ anticoagulants (blood thinners) ■ aspirin ■ narcotics or other prescription pain-killers ■ potassium-containing medicines or supplements ■ laxatives ■ phenobarbital ■ indomethacin (medicine for arthritis).

SPECIAL RESTRICTIONS WHILE TAKING THIS DRUG

FOOD AND DRUG INTERACTIONS

Other Drugs	Do not take any other drugs, including over-the-counter (OTC) drugs, before checking with your doctor. OTC drugs for appetite suppression, asthma, colds, cough, hay fever, or sinus problems tend to increase blood pressure.
Foods and Beverages	Your doctor may prescribe a special low-salt diet, which you should follow carefully because it will help your medicine work more effectively. You may also be advised to go on a weight-reduction diet. You should continue to drink normal amounts of fluids.
	This medicine may either increase or decrease potassium levels in your body. Your doctor may give you special instructions about eating foods or drinking beverages that have a high potassium content (such as bananas and citrus fruit juices), taking a potassium supplement, or using salt substitutes.

No special restrictions on alcohol use or smoking.

DAILY LIVING

Exertion and Exercise	Use caution when exercising or exerting yourself while taking this medicine because excessive sweating may cause you to become dehydrated and to feel dizzy, light-headed, or faint.

Sun Exposure/ Excessive Heat	Your skin may become more sensitive to sunlight and more likely to develop a sunburn while you are taking this medicine. It is a good idea to avoid too much sun, especially if you burn easily. Apply a sunscreen to exposed skin surfaces before going outdoors. Use caution during hot weather or while taking saunas or hot baths, since excessive sweating while taking this medicine may cause you to become dehydrated and to feel drowsy or faint.
Examinations or Tests	Many people have high blood pressure with no symptoms at all. It is important for you to keep all appointments with your doctor, even if you feel well, so that your blood pressure can be checked regularly. Periodic blood tests may be required.
Other Precautions	Tell any doctor or dentist you consult that you are taking this medicine, especially if you will be undergoing any kind of surgery.

Although this drug has been shown to cause tumors in rats, no relationship has been shown in humans.

When first starting on this type of medicine, you may feel tired and will probably experience both greater volume and frequency of urination. Until your individual pattern of urination has been established with this medicine, it may be wise to time carefully any activity that will put you out of convenient reach of a bathroom, such as bus or car travel. In addition, taking a diuretic at bedtime will probably interfere with sleep; you should discuss your dosage schedule with your doctor.

Check with your doctor if you become ill with flulike symptoms, such as cough, fever, or body aches; lose your appetite; vomit; or have diarrhea. This may cause you to lose a great deal of fluid, making it important not to take the diuretic for one or more doses.

Following mild fluid losses, some older people are more vulnerable to symptoms of weakness or dizziness upon standing or getting up.

Helpful Hints	If this medicine upsets your stomach, taking it with milk, meals, or snacks should help.

No special restrictions on driving or exposure to excessive cold.

POSSIBLE SIDE EFFECTS

Although this list of adverse effects may seem somewhat intimidating, keep in mind that some are quite rare. Of course, should these or any other problems arise while you are on medication, it is always a good idea to consult your doctor.

IF YOU DEVELOP	WHAT TO DO
irregular heartbeat ■ numbness or tingling in hands, feet, or lips ■ tiredness or weakness ■ confusion ■ mood or mental changes ■ weak pulse ■ muscle cramps or pain ■ continuing nausea or vomiting ■ dry mouth ■ increased thirst ■ severe or continuing diarrhea ■ severe stomach pain	**Urgent** Get in touch with your doctor immediately.
blurred vision ■ rash ■ sore throat or fever ■ bleeding or bruising ■ yellowing of eyes or skin	**May be serious** Check with your doctor as soon as possible.
upset stomach ■ loss of appetite ■ female breast tenderness ■ male breast enlargement ■ male impotence ■ deepening voice ■ hair growth ■ clumsiness ■ headache ■ dizziness or lightheadedness, especially when getting up from a reclining or sitting position ■ increased skin sensitivity to sunlight	If symptoms are disturbing or persist, let your doctor know.

STORAGE INSTRUCTIONS

Store in a cool, dark place (not in a bathroom medicine cabinet).

STOPPING OR INTERRUPTING THERAPY

Since this drug does not cure high blood pressure but only controls it, you may have to take this medicine for the rest of your life. Do not stop taking it, even if you feel better. If you miss a dose, take it as soon as possible. If it is almost time for your next dose, skip the missed dose and resume your regular schedule. Do not take two doses at the same time.

SPECIAL CONSIDERATIONS FOR THOSE OVER SIXTY-FIVE

Older people are more likely to develop dizziness, light-headedness, or problems caused by changing body potassium levels, such as irregular heartbeat or weak pulse. People over sixty-five should consult a doctor if they become ill with flulike symptoms, such as cough, fever, or body aches; lose their appetite; vomit; or have diarrhea because they may then be more vulnerable to fluid losses.

CONDITION: **HYPERTENSION**

CATEGORY: **DIURETICS (COMBINATIONS)**

GENERIC (CHEMICAL) NAME	BRAND (TRADE) NAME	DOSAGE FORMS AND STRENGTHS
Amiloride and hydrochlorothiazide	MODURETIC	Tablets: 5 mg amiloride and 50 mg hydrochloro-thiazide

DRUG PROFILE

This combination of two diuretics in one tablet may be prescribed to control high blood pressure, while at the same time maintaining the body's potassium levels. Each tablet contains a thiazide diuretic as well as a potassium-sparing diuretic. This drug works by increasing the amount of salt and water eliminated through the body (through urination) and by relaxing the walls of the smaller arteries so that they expand. With a smaller volume of blood (because water is eliminated) in a larger amount of space (because the artery walls are expanded), blood pressure decreases. This drug is also used to treat fluid accumulation in people who have congestive heart failure.

BEFORE USING THIS DRUG

Let your doctor know *IF*

You have ever had allergic reactions or other problems with ■ amiloride ■ thiazide diuretics ■ sulfonamides (sulfa drugs).

You have ever had any of the following medical problems: ■ diabetes ■ gout ■ heart disease ■ kidney disease ■ liver disease ■ systemic lupus erythematosus ■ disease of the pancreas.

You are taking any of the following medicines: ■ other diuretics or medicine for high blood pressure ■ corticosteroids or corticotropin (ACTH) ■ colestipol (medicine for high cholesterol) ■ digoxin, digitoxin, or digitalis (heart medicines) ■ medicine for gout ■ lithium ■ methenamine (medicine to prevent urinary tract infections) ■ anticoagulants (blood thinners) ■ medicine for diabetes ■ potassium-containing medicines or supplements ■ salt substitutes.

SPECIAL RESTRICTIONS WHILE TAKING THIS DRUG

FOOD AND DRUG INTERACTIONS

Other Drugs	Do not take any other drugs, including over-the-counter (OTC) drugs, before checking with your doctor. OTC drugs for appetite suppression, asthma, colds, cough, hay fever, or sinus problems tend to increase blood pressure.
Foods and Beverages	Your doctor may prescribe a special low-salt diet, which you should follow carefully because it will help your medicine work more effectively. You may also be advised to go on a weight-reduction diet. This medicine may either increase or decrease potassium levels in your body. Your doctor may give you special instructions about eating foods or drinking beverages that have a high potassium content (such as bananas and citrus fruit juices), taking a potassium supplement, or using salt substitutes.

No special restrictions on alcohol use or smoking.

DAILY LIVING

Exertion and Exercise	Use caution when exercising or exerting yourself while taking this medicine because excessive sweating may cause you to become dehydrated and to feel dizzy, light-headed, or faint.
Sun Exposure/ Excessive Heat	Your skin may become more sensitive to sunlight and more likely to develop a sunburn while you are taking this medicine. It is a good idea to avoid too much sun, especially if you burn easily. Apply a sunscreen to exposed skin surfaces before going outdoors. Use caution during hot weather or while taking saunas or hot baths, since excessive sweating while taking this medicine may cause you to become dehydrated and to feel drowsy or faint.
Examinations or Tests	Many people have high blood pressure with no symptoms at all. It is important for you to keep all appointments with your doctor, even if you feel well, so that your blood pressure can be checked regularly. Periodic blood and urine tests are usually required.
Other Precautions	If you have diabetes, be aware that this medicine may raise blood-sugar levels. If you notice any change when testing sugar levels in your blood or urine, let your doctor know.
	When first starting on this type of medicine, you may feel tired and will probably experience both greater volume and frequency of urination. Until your individual pattern of urination has been established with this medicine, it may be wise to time carefully any activity that will put you out of convenient reach of a bathroom, such as bus or car travel. In addition, taking a diuretic at bedtime will probably interfere with sleep; you should discuss your dosage schedule with your doctor.

Check with your doctor if you become ill with flulike symptoms, such as cough, fever, or body aches; lose your appetite; vomit; or have diarrhea. This may cause you to lose a great deal of fluid, making it important not to take the diuretic for one or more doses.

Following mild fluid losses, some older people are more vulnerable to symptoms of weakness or dizziness upon standing or getting up.

No special restrictions on driving or exposure to excessive cold.

POSSIBLE SIDE EFFECTS

Although this list of adverse effects may seem somewhat intimidating, keep in mind that some are quite rare. Of course, should these or any other problems arise while you are on medication, it is always a good idea to consult your doctor.

IF YOU DEVELOP	WHAT TO DO
chest pain ■ irregular heartbeat ■ tiredness or weakness ■ numbness or tingling in hands, feet, or lips ■ confusion ■ weak pulse ■ shortness of breath ■ difficulty in breathing ■ depression ■ nervousness ■ muscle cramps or pain ■ nausea or vomiting ■ dry mouth ■ increased thirst ■ severe or continuing diarrhea	**Urgent** Get in touch with your doctor immediately.
sore throat or fever ■ bleeding or bruising ■ yellowing of eyes or skin	**May be serious** Check with your doctor as soon as possible.
upset stomach ■ loss of appetite ■ constipation ■ headache ■ dizziness or light-headedness, especially when getting up from a reclining or sitting position ■ increased skin sensitivity to sunlight ■ diminished sex drive ■ male impotence ■ sleep disturbances	If symptoms are disturbing or persist, let your doctor know.

STORAGE INSTRUCTIONS

Store in a cool, dark place (not in a bathroom medicine cabinet).

STOPPING OR INTERRUPTING THERAPY

Since this drug does not cure high blood pressure but only controls it, you may have to take this medicine for the rest of your life. Do not stop taking it, even if you feel better. If you miss a dose, take it as soon as possible. If it is almost time for your next dose, skip the missed dose and resume your regular schedule. Do not take two doses at the same time.

SPECIAL CONSIDERATIONS FOR THOSE OVER SIXTY-FIVE

Older people are more likely to develop problems caused by too much potassium in the body, such as irregular heartbeat, confusion, difficulty in breathing, and tiredness or weakness. People over sixty-five should get in touch with a doctor if they develop these symptoms. All doctor's appointments should be kept.

CONDITION: **HYPERTENSION**

CATEGORY: **NONDIURETICS (BETA-BLOCKERS)**

GENERIC (CHEMICAL) NAME	BRAND (TRADE) NAME	DOSAGE FORMS AND STRENGTHS
Acebutolol	SECTRAL	Capsules: 200, 400 mg
Atenolol	TENORMIN	Tablets: 50, 100 mg
Labetalol hydrochloride	NORMODYNE TRANDATE	Tablets: 100, 200, 300 mg Tablets: 100, 200, 300 mg
Metoprolol tartrate	LOPRESSOR	Tablets: 50, 100 mg
Nadolol	CORGARD	Tablets: 40, 80, 120, 160 mg

Pindolol	VISKEN	Tablets: 5, 10 mg
Propranolol hydrochloride	INDERAL	Tablets: 10, 20, 40, 60, 80, 90 mg
	INDERAL LA	Capsules: 80, 120, 160 mg
Timolol maleate	BLOCADREN	Tablets: 5, 10, 20 mg

DRUG PROFILE

Beta-adrenergic blocking drugs (beta-blockers) are a group of relatively new drugs that are used to control high blood pressure. By blocking certain nerve impulses, these medicines relax blood vessels, increase the supply of blood and oxygen to the heart, reduce the workload of the heart, and help the heart beat more regularly. Because of these effects, some beta-blockers are also useful for other conditions, such as angina, arrhythmias, migraine headaches, and hypertrophic subaortic stenosis (a disease of the heart muscle). They have also been found to improve a person's chance of survival for several years following a heart attack. Beta-blockers are sometimes used along with other high blood pressure medicines, especially the thiazide-type diuretics.

When used in the treatment of angina, beta-blockers prevent future attacks (they are not helpful during an acute attack of chest pain). Beta-blockers differ in the duration of action and when their peak effect occurs, and it is worthwhile to discuss with your doctor precisely how to time your doses in relation to the pattern of your attacks. If you suffer a side effect, such as depression or nightmares, with one beta-blocker, your doctor may be able to prescribe a different beta-blocker that will be equally effective. Beta-blockers may be used along with other anti-angina medicines.

BEFORE USING THIS DRUG

Let your doctor know *IF*

You have ever had allergic reactions or other problems with ■ any beta-blockers.

You have ever had any of the following medical problems: ■ history of allergy (including hay fever, hives, asthma, eczema) ■ slow heartbeat ■ bronchitis or emphysema ■ diabetes ■ any heart or blood vessel disease ■ kidney disease ■ liver disease ■ thyroid disease ■ Raynaud's syndrome (poor circulation in the fingers and toes) ■ intermittent claudication (limping) ■ glaucoma ■ myasthenia gravis ■ hypoglycemia (low blood sugar) ■ pheochromocytoma (adrenal gland tumor).

You are taking any of the following medicines: ■ any other medicine for high blood pressure ■ aminophylline, epinephrine, ephedrine, norepinephrine, isoproterenol, dyphylline, oxtriphylline, theophylline, phenylephrine (medicines for asthma or vasopressor drugs) ■ medicine for depression ■ cimetidine (medicine for ulcers) ■ heart medicine ■ medicine for glaucoma ■ aspirin, indomethacin, or phenylbutazone (medicines for arthritis) ■ medicine for diabetes ■ decongestants ■ tranquilizers ■ medicine for nausea.

SPECIAL RESTRICTIONS WHILE TAKING THIS DRUG

FOOD AND DRUG INTERACTIONS

Other Drugs	It is especially important to let your doctor know if you are taking the antihypertensive drugs reserpine or clonidine, or verapamil, nifedipine, or diltiazem (calcium blockers) since the use of these drugs with a beta-blocker may cause low blood pressure, slow heartbeat, or dizziness. Also, beta-blockers may prevent asthma medicine from working effectively. Do not take any other drugs, including over-the-counter (OTC) drugs, before checking with your doctor. OTC drugs for appetite suppression, asthma, colds, cough, hay fever, or sinus problems tend to increase blood pressure. Some medicines used for pain and/or arthritis (aspirin, indomethacin, and phenylbutazone, for example) may hamper the action of beta-blockers.
Foods and Beverages	Your doctor may prescribe a special low-salt diet, which you should follow carefully because it will help your medicine work more effectively. You may also be advised to go on a weight-reduction diet.
Alcohol	Dizziness, light-headedness, or fainting may occur if you drink alcohol while taking a beta-blocker, espe-

cially labetalol. Be careful about how much alcohol you consume.

No special restrictions on smoking.

DAILY LIVING

Driving	This drug may cause drowsiness. Be careful when driving, operating household appliances, or doing any other tasks that require alertness until you know how this drug affects you.
Exertion and Exercise	Since chest pain from exercise or exertion may be reduced or prevented by this medicine, you may be tempted to overwork yourself. Discuss with your doctor how much exercise is safe for you. Be especially careful when you exercise during hot weather or if you must stand for long periods of time, since this drug may cause side effects such as dizziness, light-headedness, and fainting.
Excessive Heat	Be careful during hot weather because of the possible side effects of dizziness, light-headedness, or fainting (especially with labetalol).
Excessive Cold	You may become more sensitive to cold temperatures while taking beta-blockers. Dress warmly—protecting your skin, fingers, and toes—and use caution during prolonged exposure to cold.
Examinations or Tests	*Check your pulse regularly.* If it is slower than your usual rate or less than 50 beats per minute, call your doctor. Many people have high blood pressure with no symptoms at all. It is important for you to keep all appointments with your doctor, even if you feel well, so that your blood pressure can be checked regularly. Periodic blood and urine tests may be required.

Other Precautions	Tell any doctor or dentist you consult that you are taking this medicine, especially if you will be undergoing any type of surgery.
	If you have diabetes, be aware that this medicine may cause your blood-sugar level to fall. It also may mask the signs of low blood sugar (such as changes in pulse rate or increased blood pressure), leaving you unaware that your blood sugar has fallen. Your doctor may want to make adjustments in the dosage of your diabetes medicine.
Helpful Hints	If your mouth or throat feels dry, chewing sugarless gum or sucking ice chips or sugarless hard candy will help. If your eyes feel dry, you may use nonmedicated or plain eyedrops for relief.
	If this medicine causes upset stomach, taking it with milk, meals, or snacks should help.

No special restriction on sun exposure.

POSSIBLE SIDE EFFECTS

Although this list of adverse effects may seem somewhat intimidating, keep in mind that some are quite rare. Of course, should these or any other problems arise while you are on medication, it is always a good idea to consult your doctor.

IF YOU DEVELOP	**WHAT TO DO**
chest pain ■ palpitations ■ irregular heartbeat ■ extremely slow heartbeat ■ swelling of face, ankles, feet, or lower legs ■ shortness of breath or coughing ■ difficulty in breathing ■ asthma or wheezing ■ restlessness, sweating, nervousness, or irritability (if you are a thyroid patient) ■ weight gain	**Urgent** Get in touch with your doctor immediately.
dizziness, light-headedness, or fainting (especially with labetalol) ■ cold hands or feet ■ slurred speech ■ confusion ■ depression ■ fever or sore	**May be serious** Check with your doctor as soon as possible.

throat ■ rash or itching ■ bleeding or bruising ■ increased sweating ■ faintness or hunger ■ pale, moist skin

nausea or vomiting ■ diarrhea or constipation ■ indigestion, gas, hiccups, or stomach cramps ■ dry eyes, mouth, or skin ■ hair loss ■ nail changes ■ inflammation of the nasal lining ■ visual disturbances ■ hearing problems or ringing in the ears ■ clumsiness ■ muscle or joint pain ■ numbness of fingers or toes ■ drowsiness ■ tiredness or weakness ■ anxiety, nervousness, or irritability ■ memory problems ■ male impotence ■ diminished sex drive ■ headache ■ hallucinations ■ nightmares ■ sleep disturbances ■ tingling or other abnormal skin sensations ■ urinary frequency

With labetalol only: taste changes

If symptoms are disturbing or persist, let your doctor know.

STORAGE INSTRUCTIONS

Store in a cool, dark place (not in a bathroom medicine cabinet).

STOPPING OR INTERRUPTING THERAPY

Since this drug does not cure high blood pressure but only controls it, you may have to take this medicine for the rest of your life. Do not stop taking it, even if you feel better. *Suddenly stopping your medicine may worsen your medical problem,* especially if you have angina. Your doctor can advise you on how to discontinue therapy gradually. *Always carry a supply of your medicine with you.* If you miss a dose, take the missed dose as soon as possible. If the next scheduled dose is within four hours (or within eight hours if you are taking atenolol, nadolol, labetalol, or once-a-day propranolol or metoprolol), skip the missed dose and resume your regular schedule. Do not take two doses at the same time.

SPECIAL CONSIDERATIONS FOR THOSE OVER SIXTY-FIVE

Although beta-blockers are quite effective in the treatment of cardiac disorders, older persons may suffer more adverse effects from these drugs, such as drowsiness, depression, nightmares, muscle or joint pain, cold hands or feet, and slow heartbeat. Doctors may start older persons on a lower dosage.

CONDITION: **HYPERTENSION**

CATEGORY: **NONDIURETICS (CENTRAL ALPHA-AGONISTS)**

GENERIC (CHEMICAL) NAME	BRAND (TRADE) NAME	DOSAGE FORMS AND STRENGTHS
Methyldopa	ALDOMET	Suspension: 250 mg per tsp Tablets: 125, 250, 500 mg

DRUG PROFILE

Methyldopa is used to treat high blood pressure. It acts to reduce the passage of impulses along certain nerve pathways; this relaxes the blood vessels and makes blood flow easier. Methyldopa is sometimes combined with other antihypertensive medicines, especially diuretics, for better control of hypertension.

BEFORE USING THIS DRUG

Let your doctor know *IF*

You have ever had allergic reactions or other problems with ■ methyldopa.

You have ever had any of the following medical problems: ■ angina (chest pain) ■ heart disease ■ kidney disease ■ liver disease ■ depression ■ Parkinson's disease ■ pheochromocytoma (adrenal gland tumor) ■ systemic lupus erythematosus ■ dizziness from other high blood pressure medicines.

You are taking any of the following medicines: ■ other medicine for high blood pressure ■ levodopa (medicine for Parkinson's disease) ■ medicine for depression (within the last two weeks) ■ tranquilizers ■ medicine for nausea.

SPECIAL RESTRICTIONS WHILE TAKING THIS DRUG

FOOD AND DRUG INTERACTIONS

Other Drugs	Do not take any other drugs, including over-the-counter (OTC) drugs, before checking with your doc-

tor. OTC drugs for appetite suppression, asthma, colds, cough, hay fever, or sinus problems tend to increase blood pressure.

Foods and Beverages	Your doctor may prescribe a special low-salt diet, which you should follow carefully because it will help your medicine work more effectively. You may also be advised to go on a weight-reduction diet.

No special restrictions on alcohol use or smoking.

DAILY LIVING

Driving	This drug may cause drowsiness. Be careful when driving, operating household appliances, or doing any other tasks that require alertness until you know how this drug affects you.
Exertion and Exercise	Use caution when exercising, exerting yourself, or standing for long periods of time because this medicine may cause you to become dizzy, light-headed, or faint. If you feel any of these symptoms coming on, sit or lie down. It is a good idea not to get up too quickly from a reclining or sitting position.
Examinations or Tests	Many people have high blood pressure with no symptoms at all. It is important for you to keep all appointments with your doctor, even if you feel well, so that your blood pressure can be checked regularly. Periodic blood and urine tests are usually required.
Other Precautions	Tell any doctor or dentist you consult that you are taking this medicine, especially if you will be undergoing any type of surgery or if you need a blood transfusion.

No special restrictions on sun exposure or exposure to excessive heat or cold.

POSSIBLE SIDE EFFECTS

Although this list of adverse effects may seem somewhat intimidating, keep in mind that some are quite rare. Of course, should these or any other problems arise while you are on medication, it is always a good idea to consult your doctor.

IF YOU DEVELOP	WHAT TO DO
fever ■ slow or fast heartbeat ■ chest pain ■ yellowing of eyes or skin ■ dark or amber-colored urine ■ dark stools	**Urgent** Get in touch with your doctor immediately.
swelling of feet or lower legs ■ weight gain ■ sleep disturbances ■ depression ■ anxiety ■ tiredness or weakness ■ severe or continuing vomiting, diarrhea, or stomach cramps ■ pale stools ■ shakiness or unusual body movements ■ sore throat ■ bleeding or bruising ■ dizziness, light-headedness, or fainting, especially when getting up from a reclining or sitting position	**May be serious** Check with your doctor as soon as possible.
drowsiness ■ dry mouth ■ headache ■ memory problems ■ inability to concentrate ■ blurred vision ■ male impotence ■ diminished sex drive ■ upset stomach ■ constipation ■ bloating or gas ■ sore or dark tongue ■ numbness or tingling in hands or feet ■ abnormal skin sensations ■ rash ■ stuffy nose ■ female breast swelling ■ male breast enlargement	If symptoms are disturbing or persist, let your doctor know.

STORAGE INSTRUCTIONS

Store in a cool, dark place (not in a bathroom medicine cabinet). If your medicine is in a liquid form, make sure that it does not freeze.

STOPPING OR INTERRUPTING THERAPY

Since this drug does not cure high blood pressure but only controls it, you may have to take this medicine for the rest of your life. Do not stop taking it, even if you feel better. If you miss a dose, take it as soon as possible. If it is almost time for your next dose, skip the missed dose and resume your regular schedule. Do not take two doses at the same time.

SPECIAL CONSIDERATIONS FOR THOSE OVER SIXTY-FIVE

The side effects of dizziness, light-headedness, memory problems, loss of sex drive, and depression occur more frequently in older people, who may also be more prone to drowsiness and tiredness when first starting this medicine or when the dosage is increased. For these reasons, a doctor may want to start with a lower dosage.

CONDITION: **HYPERTENSION**

CATEGORY: **NONDIURETICS (CENTRAL ALPHA-AGONISTS)**

GENERIC (CHEMICAL) NAME	BRAND (TRADE) NAME	DOSAGE FORMS AND STRENGTHS
Clonidine hydrochloride	CATAPRES	Patch: 0.1, 0.2, 0.3 mg/day Tablets: 0.1, 0.2, 0.3 mg

DRUG PROFILE

Clonidine is used for treatment of high blood pressure. It acts on the central nervous system to slow your heart rate and relax your blood vessels. Clonidine is sometimes used in combination with other antihypertensive medicines, especially diuretics.

BEFORE USING THIS DRUG

Let your doctor know *IF*

You have ever had allergic reactions or other problems with ■ clonidine.

You have ever had any of the following medical problems: ■ heart or blood vessel disease ■ kidney disease ■ depression ■ Raynaud's syndrome (poor circulation in the fingers and toes).

You are taking any of the following medicines: ■ diuretics, beta-blockers, or other medicines for high blood pressure ■ medicine for seizures ■ medicine for depression ■ antihistamines ■ medicine for hay fever, allergies, or colds ■ barbiturates ■ digoxin, digitoxin, or digitalis (heart medicines) ■ medicine for Parkinson's disease ■ muscle relaxants ■ narcotics or other prescription painkillers ■ sedatives ■ tranquilizers ■ sleep medicines.

SPECIAL RESTRICTIONS WHILE TAKING THIS DRUG

FOOD AND DRUG INTERACTIONS

Other Drugs	Do not take any other drugs, including over-the-counter (OTC) drugs, before checking with your doctor. OTC drugs for appetite suppression, asthma, colds, cough, hay fever, or sinus problems tend to increase blood pressure. Antihistamines, sleep medicines, tranquilizers, pain-killers, barbiturates, medicine for seizures, muscle relaxants, or anesthetics may worsen side effects of this drug such as dizziness, light-headedness, drowsiness, or faintness.
Foods and Beverages	Your doctor may prescribe a special low-salt diet, which you should follow carefully because it will help your medicine work more effectively. You may also be advised to go on a weight-reduction diet.
Alcohol	Drinking alcohol while taking this drug may worsen such side effects as dizziness, light-headedness, or fainting. Avoid alcohol unless your doctor has approved its use.

No special restrictions on smoking.

DAILY LIVING

Driving	This drug may cause drowsiness. Be careful when driving, operating household appliances, or doing any other tasks that require alertness until you know how this drug affects you.
Exertion and Exercise	Use caution when exercising, exerting yourself, or standing for long periods of time because this medicine may cause you to become dizzy, light-headed, or faint. If you feel any of these symptoms coming on, sit

or lie down. It is a good idea not to get up too quickly from a reclining or sitting position.

Excessive Heat	Use caution during hot weather, especially when you exert yourself (see above).
Examinations or Tests	Many people have high blood pressure with no symptoms at all. It is important for you to keep all appointments with your doctor, even if you feel well, so that your blood pressure can be checked regularly. Periodic eye examinations may be required.
Other Precautions	Tell any doctor or dentist you consult that you are taking this medicine, especially if you will be undergoing any type of surgery.
Helpful Hints	If your mouth or throat feels dry, chewing sugarless gum or sucking ice chips or sugarless hard candy will help. If the patch begins to loosen, apply the adhesive overlay provided. Let your doctor know if you develop a rash or other skin problems while using the patch.

No special restrictions on exposure to excessive cold.

POSSIBLE SIDE EFFECTS

Although this list of adverse effects may seem somewhat intimidating, keep in mind that some are quite rare. Of course, should these or any other problems arise while you are on medication, it is always a good idea to consult your doctor.

IF YOU DEVELOP

difficulty in breathing ■ extreme dizziness or faintness ■ slow heartbeat ■ fast heartbeat or palpitations ■ tiredness or weakness ■ continuous vomiting

WHAT TO DO

Urgent Get in touch with your doctor immediately.

After you STOP taking this medicine: anxiety
■ chest pain ■ sleeplessness ■ nervousness
■ increased salivation ■ upset stomach ■ irregular or fast heartbeat ■ shaking of hands or fingers
■ stomach cramps ■ muscle pain ■ flushing
■ headache ■ increased sweating

swelling of feet, lower legs, or any other part of the body ■ cold fingertips or toes ■ depression ■ vivid dreams or nightmares ■ nervousness ■ hallucinations ■ fever	**May be serious** Check with your doctor as soon as possible.
dizziness, light-headedness, or fainting, especially when getting up from a reclining or sitting position ■ drowsiness ■ headache ■ bone pain ■ dry mouth, throat, or nasal passages ■ dry, itching, or burning eyes ■ upset stomach ■ nausea or vomiting ■ taste changes ■ weight gain ■ constipation ■ loss of appetite ■ sexual problems ■ sleep disturbances ■ tenderness of the salivary glands (around the ear) ■ paleness ■ rash, hives, itching, change in skin color, or other skin problems (especially with patch) ■ hair loss ■ urinary retention or difficulty in urination ■ need to urinate at night	If symptoms are disturbing or persist, let your doctor know.

STORAGE INSTRUCTIONS

Store in a cool, dark place (not in a bathroom medicine cabinet).

STOPPING OR INTERRUPTING THERAPY

Always make sure you have an adequate supply of clonidine on hand, especially for weekends, holidays, or if you travel. Since this drug does not cure high blood pressure but only controls it, you may have to take this medicine for the rest of your life. Do not stop taking it, even if you feel better. If you miss a dose, take it as soon as possible. Then continue on your regular schedule. If you miss two or more doses in a row, check with your doctor right away. *Abruptly stopping this medicine can cause your blood pressure to rise rapidly, which could be dangerous to your health.* Your doctor will advise you on how to reduce your dosage gradually before stopping completely.

SPECIAL CONSIDERATIONS FOR THOSE OVER SIXTY-FIVE

The side effects of drowsiness, dizziness, and fainting are more likely to occur in older people.

CONDITION: **HYPERTENSION**

CATEGORY: **NONDIURETICS (CENTRAL ALPHA-AGONISTS)**

GENERIC (CHEMICAL) NAME	BRAND (TRADE) NAME	DOSAGE FORMS AND STRENGTHS
Guanabenz acetate	WYTENSIN	Tablets: 4, 8, 16 mg

DRUG PROFILE

Guanabenz is used for treatment of high blood pressure. It acts on the central nervous system to reduce the passage of impulses along certain nerve pathways; this relaxes the blood vessels and makes blood flow easier. Guanabenz may be used in combination with other antihypertensive medicines, especially diuretics, for better control of hypertension.

BEFORE USING THIS DRUG

Let your doctor know *IF*

You have ever had allergic reactions or other problems with ■ guanabenz.

You have ever had any of the following medical problems: ■ heart or blood vessel disease ■ kidney disease ■ liver disease.

You are taking any of the following medicines: ■ diuretics or other medicines for high blood pressure ■ medicine for seizures ■ barbiturates ■ antihistamines ■ medicine for hay fever, allergies, or colds ■ pain-killers (either prescription or over-the-counter [OTC]) ■ muscle relaxants ■ medicine for depression ■ sedatives ■ tranquilizers ■ sleep medicines.

SPECIAL RESTRICTIONS WHILE TAKING THIS DRUG

FOOD AND DRUG INTERACTIONS

Other Drugs	Do not take any other drugs, including over-the-counter (OTC) drugs, before checking with your doctor. OTC drugs for appetite suppression, asthma, colds, cough, hay fever, or sinus problems tend to increase blood pressure. Antihistamines, sleep medicines, tranquilizers, pain-killers, barbiturates, medicine for seizures, muscle relaxants, or anesthetics may worsen side effects of this drug such as dizziness, light-headedness, drowsiness, or fainting.
Foods and Beverages	Your doctor may prescribe a special low-salt diet, which you should follow carefully because it will help your medicine work more effectively. You may also be advised to go on a weight-reduction diet.
Alcohol	Drinking alcohol while taking this medicine may worsen such side effects as dizziness, light-headedness, or fainting. Avoid alcohol unless your doctor has approved its use.

No special restrictions on smoking.

DAILY LIVING

Driving	This drug often causes drowsiness. Be careful when driving, operating household appliances, or doing any other tasks that require alertness until you know how this drug affects you.
Examinations or Tests	Many people have high blood pressure with no symptoms at all. It is important for you to keep all appointments with your doctor, even if you feel well, so that your blood pressure can be checked regularly.

Other Precautions	Tell any doctor or dentist you consult that you are taking this medicine, especially if you will be undergoing any type of surgery.
Helpful Hints	If your mouth or throat feels dry, chewing sugarless gum or sucking ice chips or sugarless hard candy will help.

No special restrictions on exertion and exercise, sun exposure, or exposure to excessive heat or cold.

POSSIBLE SIDE EFFECTS

Although this list of adverse effects may seem somewhat intimidating, keep in mind that some are quite rare. Of course, should these or any other problems arise while you are on medication, it is always a good idea to consult your doctor.

IF YOU DEVELOP

severe dizziness or fainting ■ irritability ■ pinpoint pupils ■ slow heartbeat ■ tiredness or weakness ■ chest pain ■ irregular heartbeat or palpitations ■ swelling of hands and feet

After you STOP taking this medicine: anxiety ■ chest pain ■ flushing ■ headache ■ increased salivation ■ nausea or vomiting ■ shaking of hands or fingers ■ stomach cramps ■ sleep disturbances ■ increased sweating

WHAT TO DO

Urgent Get in touch with your doctor immediately.

dizziness ■ drowsiness ■ dry mouth ■ male impotence ■ headache ■ clumsiness ■ depression ■ sleep disturbances ■ blurred vision ■ difficulty in breathing ■ stuffy nose ■ ache in muscles or hands and feet ■ rash or itching ■ urinary frequency ■ male breast enlargement ■ nausea or vomiting ■ stomach pain or discomfort ■ constipation ■ taste changes

If symptoms are disturbing or persist, let your doctor know.

STORAGE INSTRUCTIONS

Store in a cool, dark place (not in a bathroom medicine cabinet).

STOPPING OR INTERRUPTING THERAPY

Since this drug does not cure high blood pressure but only controls it, you may have to take this medicine for the rest of your life. Do not stop taking it, even if you feel better. If you miss a dose, take it as soon as possible. If it is almost time for your next dose, skip the missed dose and resume your regular schedule. If you miss two or more doses in a row, check with your doctor right away. *Abruptly stopping this medicine can cause your blood pressure to rise rapidly, which could be dangerous to your health.* Your doctor wil advise you on how to reduce your dosage gradually before stopping completely.

SPECIAL CONSIDERATIONS FOR THOSE OVER SIXTY-FIVE

Dizziness or fainting is more likely to occur in older people.

CONDITION: **HYPERTENSION**

CATEGORY: **NONDIURETICS (PERIPHERAL VASODILATORS)**

GENERIC (CHEMICAL) NAME	BRAND (TRADE) NAME	DOSAGE FORMS AND STRENGTHS
Hydralazine	APRESOLINE	Tablets: 10, 25, 50, 100 mg

DRUG PROFILE

Hydralazine is used to treat high blood pressure. It acts directly on the blood vessel walls to relax them. In addition, hydralazine increases the rate and output of the heart. Hydralazine is usually used in combination with other drugs.

BEFORE USING THIS DRUG

Let your doctor know *IF*

You have ever had allergic reactions or other problems with ■ hydralazine ■ tartrazine (FD&C Yellow Dye No. 5).

You have ever had any of the following medical problems: ■ heart or blood vessel disease, including stroke ■ migraine or other severe headaches ■ rheumatic mitral valve disease ■ kidney disease ■ liver disease ■ systemic lupus erythematosus.

You are taking any of the following medicines: ■ diuretics, beta-blockers, or other medicines for high blood pressure ■ medicine for depression (within the last two weeks).

SPECIAL RESTRICTIONS WHILE TAKING THIS DRUG

FOOD AND DRUG INTERACTIONS

Other Drugs	Do not take any other drugs, including over-the-counter (OTC) drugs, before checking with your doctor. OTC drugs for appetite suppression, asthma, colds, cough, hay fever, or sinus problems tend to increase blood pressure.
Foods and Beverages	Your doctor may prescribe a special low-salt diet, which you should follow carefully because it will help your medicine work more effectively. You may also be advised to go on a weight-reduction diet.
Alcohol	Drinking alcohol while taking this medicine may worsen such side effects as dizziness, light-headedness, or fainting. Avoid alcohol unless your doctor has approved its use.

No special restrictions on smoking.

DAILY LIVING

Driving	This drug may cause dizziness, fainting, or weakness. Be careful when driving, operating household appliances, or doing any other tasks that require alertness until you know how this drug affects you.

Exertion and Exercise	Use caution when exercising, exerting yourself, or standing for long periods of time because this drug may cause you to become dizzy, light-headed, or faint. If you feel any of these symptoms coming on, sit or lie down. It is a good idea not to get up too quickly from a reclining or sitting position.
Excessive Heat	Use caution during hot weather, especially when you exert yourself (see above).
Examinations or Tests	Many people have high blood pressure with no symptoms at all. It is important for you to keep all appointments with your doctor, even if you feel well, so that your blood pressure can be checked regularly. Periodic blood tests are usually required.

No special restrictions on sun exposure or exposure to excessive cold.

POSSIBLE SIDE EFFECTS

Although this list of adverse effects may seem somewhat intimidating, keep in mind that some are quite rare. Of course, should these or any other problems arise while you are on medication, it is always a good idea to consult your doctor.

IF YOU DEVELOP	WHAT TO DO
chest pain ■ very fast heartbeat ■ severe headache ■ severe dizziness ■ weakness ■ joint pain ■ numbness, tingling, pain, or weakness of hands or feet ■ sore throat or fever ■ chills ■ rash or itching ■ swelling of lymph glands, feet, or legs ■ weight gain ■ behavior changes	**Urgent** Get in touch with your doctor immediately.
upset stomach ■ nausea or vomiting ■ headache ■ loss of appetite ■ palpitations ■ constipation or diarrhea ■ dizziness or light-headedness, especially when getting up from a reclining or sitting position ■ flushing ■ shortness of breath with	If symptoms are disturbing or persist, let your doctor know.

exercise ■ stuffy nose ■ eye irritation ■ anxiety ■ difficulty in urination ■ muscle cramps ■ increased sweating ■ tremors ■ disorientation

STORAGE INSTRUCTIONS

Store in a cool, dark place (not in a bathroom medicine cabinet).

STOPPING OR INTERRUPTING THERAPY

Since this drug does not cure high blood pressure but only controls it, you may have to take this medicine for the rest of your life. Do not stop taking it, even if you feel better. If you miss a dose, take it as soon as possible. If it is almost time for your next dose, skip the missed dose and resume your regular schedule. Do not take two doses at the same time.

SPECIAL CONSIDERATIONS FOR THOSE OVER SIXTY-FIVE

Dizziness or light-headedness occurs more frequently in older people so regular checkups may be necessary.

CONDITION: **HYPERTENSION**

CATEGORY: **NONDIURETICS (PERIPHERAL VASODILATORS)**

GENERIC (CHEMICAL) NAME	BRAND (TRADE) NAME	DOSAGE FORMS AND STRENGTHS
Minoxidil	LONITEN	Tablets: 2.5, 10 mg

DRUG PROFILE

Minoxidil is used to treat severe high blood pressure that cannot be controlled by other medicines. A diuretic and a drug to slow heart rate (such as a beta-blocker or methyldopa) are usually taken along with minoxidil. Minoxidil acts by relaxing and enlarging small blood vessels to allow easier blood flow.

BEFORE USING THIS DRUG

Let your doctor know *IF*

You have ever had allergic reactions or other problems with ■ minoxidil.

You have ever had any of the following medical problems: ■ angina (chest pain) ■ heart or blood vessel disease, especially stroke or heart attack within the last month ■ kidney disease ■ pheochromocytoma (adrenal gland tumor).

You are taking any of the following medicines: ■ diuretics or other medicines for high blood pressure (especially guanethidine) ■ nitrates (medicine for chest pain) ■ diltiazem, nifedipine, or verapamil (calcium blockers).

SPECIAL RESTRICTIONS WHILE TAKING THIS DRUG

FOOD AND DRUG INTERACTIONS

Other Drugs	Do not take any other drugs, including over-the-counter (OTC) drugs, before checking with your doctor. OTC drugs for appetite suppression, asthma, colds, cough, hay fever, or sinus problems tend to increase blood pressure. Because this medicine causes fluid and salt retention and also rapid increases in heart rate, it is always necessary to take a diuretic and a beta-blocker or methyldopa at the same time to counteract these effects.
Foods and Beverages	Your doctor may prescribe a special low-salt diet, which you should follow carefully because it will help your medicine work more effectively. You may also be advised to go on a weight-reduction diet.

No special restrictions on alcohol use or smoking.

DAILY LIVING

Examinations or Tests	Many people have high blood pressure with no symptoms at all. It is important for you to keep all appointments with your doctor, even if you feel well, so that your blood pressure can be checked regularly. Peri-

odic blood and urine tests and electrocardiograms may be required.

Your doctor may advise you to weigh yourself each morning after you get out of bed and record your weight (a weight gain of five pounds or more could indicate that the dose of your diuretic needs to be increased). Your doctor may also suggest that you monitor your blood pressure at home.

Check your own resting pulse rate regularly, and call your doctor if it increases by 20 or more beats per minute above normal.

Helpful Hints

This drug may cause an increase in hair growth on the face, back, arms, legs and scalp of both men and women. Shaving or using a hair remover may be helpful as a temporary measure. After treatment with this medicine has ended, the hair will stop growing, though it may take several months before the new hair growth disappears.

No special restrictions on driving, exertion and exercise, sun exposure, or exposure to excessive heat or cold.

POSSIBLE SIDE EFFECTS

Although this list of adverse effects may seem somewhat intimidating, keep in mind that some are quite rare. Of course, should these or any other problems arise while you are on medication, it is always a good idea to consult your doctor.

IF YOU DEVELOP

irregular or fast heartbeat ■ rapid weight gain (five pounds or more) ■ chest pain ■ shortness of breath ■ dizziness, light-headedness, or fainting ■ swelling of face, hands, ankles, or stomach

WHAT TO DO

Urgent Get in touch with your doctor immediately.

bloating ■ skin redness, itching, or rash ■ numbness, tingling, or coldness of hands, feet, or face

May be serious Check with your doctor as soon as possible.

increase in hair growth ■ female breast tenderness ■ male breast enlargement ■ headache ■ nausea	If symptoms are disturbing or persist, let your doctor know.

STORAGE INSTRUCTIONS

Store in a cool, dark place (not in a bathroom medicine cabinet).

STOPPING OR INTERRUPTING THERAPY

Since this drug does not cure high blood pressure but only controls it, you may have to take this medicine for the rest of your life. Do not stop taking it, even if you feel better. If you miss a dose, take it as soon as possible. If it is almost time for your next dose, skip the missed dose and resume your regular schedule. Do not take two doses at the same time.

SPECIAL CONSIDERATIONS FOR THOSE OVER SIXTY-FIVE

The side effects of dizziness, light-headedness, and fainting are more common in older people.

CONDITION: **HYPERTENSION**

CATEGORY: **NONDIURETICS (PERIPHERAL VASODILATORS)**

GENERIC (CHEMICAL) NAME	BRAND (TRADE) NAME	DOSAGE FORMS AND STRENGTHS
Prazosin hydrochloride	MINIPRESS	Capsules: 1, 2, 5 mg

DRUG PROFILE

Prazosin is used for treatment of high blood pressure. It acts indirectly on the blood vessel walls to relax them. Unlike hydralazine, another peripheral vasodilator, prazosin does not increase the rate or output of the heart.

BEFORE USING THIS DRUG

Let your doctor know *IF*

You have ever had allergic reactions or other problems with ■ prazosin.

You have ever had any of the following medical problems: ■ angina (chest pain) ■ heart disease ■ kidney disease.

You are taking any of the following medicines: ■ diuretics or other medicines for high blood pressure ■ aspirin, indomethacin or other medicine for arthritis.

SPECIAL RESTRICTIONS WHILE TAKING THIS DRUG

FOOD AND DRUG INTERACTIONS

Other Drugs	Do not take any other drugs, including over-the-counter (OTC) drugs, before checking with your doctor. OTC drugs for appetite suppression, asthma, colds, cough, hay fever, or sinus problems tend to increase blood pressure.
Foods and Beverages	Your doctor may prescribe a special low-salt diet, which you should follow carefully because it will help your medicine work more effectively. You may also be advised to go on a weight-reduction diet.
Alcohol	Drinking alcohol while taking this medicine may worsen such side effects as dizziness, light-headedness, or fainting. Avoid alcohol unless your doctor has approved its use.

No special restrictions on smoking.

DAILY LIVING

Driving	This drug may cause dizziness or fainting, especially during the first twenty-four hours of use. Be careful when driving, operating household appliances, or

doing any other tasks that require alertness until you know how this drug affects you.

Exertion and Exercise	Use caution when exercising, exerting yourself, or standing for long periods of time because this drug may cause you to become dizzy, light-headed, or faint. If you feel any of these symptoms coming on, sit or lie down. It is a good idea not to get up too quickly from a reclining or sitting position.
Excessive Heat	Use caution during hot weather, especially if you exert yourself (see above).
Examinations or Tests	Many people have high blood pressure with no symptoms at all. It is important for you to keep all appointments with your doctor, even if you feel well, so that your blood pressure can be checked regularly.
Other Precautions	You may feel light-headed or faint after the first dose of this drug, when there has been a significant increase in your dose, or when you start taking another antihypertensive medicine. Your doctor may suggest that you take your first dose of prazosin in his or her office.

No special restrictions on sun exposure or exposure to excessive cold.

POSSIBLE SIDE EFFECTS

Although this list of adverse effects may seem somewhat intimidating, keep in mind that some are quite rare. Of course, should these or any other problems arise while you are on medication, it is always a good idea to consult your doctor.

IF YOU DEVELOP	**WHAT TO DO**
sudden fainting ■ chest pain ■ irregular heartbeat	**Urgent** Get in touch with your doctor immediately.

dizziness or light-headedness, especially when getting up from a reclining or sitting position ■ weakness ■ shortness of breath ■ swelling of legs or feet ■ weight gain ■ difficulty in urination ■ numbness or tingling in hands or feet

May be serious Check with your doctor as soon as possible.

drowsiness ■ lack of energy ■ headache ■ upset stomach or stomach pain ■ nausea or vomiting ■ constipation ■ diarrhea ■ rash or itching ■ hair loss ■ nervousness ■ urinary frequency or urinary incontinence ■ male impotence ■ blurred vision ■ ringing in the ears ■ red eyes ■ dry mouth ■ stuffy nose ■ increased sweating ■ joint pain ■ depression

If symptoms are disturbing or persist, let your doctor know.

STORAGE INSTRUCTIONS

Store in a cool, dark place (not in a bathroom medicine cabinet).

STOPPING OR INTERRUPTING THERAPY

Since this drug does not cure high blood pressure but only controls it, you may have to take this medicine for the rest of your life. Do not stop taking it, even if you feel better. If you miss a dose, take it as soon as possible. If it is almost time for your next dose, skip the missed dose and resume your regular schedule. Do not take two doses at the same time.

SPECIAL CONSIDERATIONS FOR THOSE OVER SIXTY-FIVE

The side effects of dizziness, light-headedness, and fainting are more common in older people.

CONDITION: **HYPERTENSION**

CATEGORY: **NONDIURETICS (SYMPATHOLYTICS)**

GENERIC (CHEMICAL) NAME	BRAND (TRADE) NAME	DOSAGE FORMS AND STRENGTHS
Reserpine	SERPASIL	Tablets: 0.1, 0.25 mg
Rauwolfia serpentina	RAUDIXIN	Tablets: 50, 100 mg

DRUG PROFILE

Reserpine and rauwolfia are used to treat high blood pressure. These medicines work by inhibiting nerves that constrict blood vessels, resulting in relaxation of blood vessels and easier blood flow. A similar action on nerves in the brain results in sedative and tranquilizing effects. These medicines may be used alone or with other antihypertensive medicines.

BEFORE USING THIS DRUG

Let your doctor know *IF*

You have ever had allergic reactions or other problems with ■ rauwolfia alkaloids ■ tartrazine (FD&C Yellow Dye No. 5).

You have ever had any of the following medical problems: ■ allergies, breathing problems, or asthma ■ breast cancer ■ epilepsy ■ gallstones ■ heart disease ■ stroke ■ kidney disease ■ depression ■ Parkinson's disease ■ pheochromocytoma (adrenal gland tumor) ■ stomach ulcer ■ ulcerative colitis.

You are taking any of the following medicines: ■ diuretics, beta-blockers, or other medicine for high blood pressure ■ medicine for seizures ■ medicine for depression ■ antihistamines ■ medicine for hay fever, allergies, or colds ■ barbiturates ■ digoxin, digitoxin, or digitalis (heart medicines) ■ muscle relaxants ■ narcotics or other prescription pain-killers ■ any medicine containing phenylephrine ■ quinidine (medicine for abnormal heart rhythms) ■ sedatives ■ tranquilizers ■ sleep medicines ■ levodopa (medicine for Parkinson's disease).

You are receiving electroconvulsive therapy.

SPECIAL RESTRICTIONS WHILE TAKING THIS DRUG

FOOD AND DRUG INTERACTIONS

Other Drugs	Do not take any other drugs, including over-the-counter (OTC) drugs, before checking with your doctor. OTC drugs for appetite suppression, asthma, colds, cough, hay fever, or sinus problems tend to increase blood pressure. Antihistamines, sleep medicines, tranquilizers, pain-killers, barbiturates, medicine for seizures, muscle relaxants, or anesthetics worsen such side effects of this drug as drowsiness.
Foods and Beverages	Your doctor may prescribe a special low-salt diet, which you should follow carefully because it will help your medicine work more effectively. A weight-reduction diet may also be advised.
Alcohol	Drinking alcohol while taking this medicine may worsen such side effects as dizziness or drowsiness. Avoid alcohol unless your doctor has approved its use.

No special restrictions on smoking.

DAILY LIVING

Driving	This drug may cause drowsiness, especially when you first begin to take it or when your dose is increased. Be careful when driving, operating household appliances, or doing any other tasks that require alertness until you know how this drug affects you.
Examinations or Tests	Many people have high blood pressure with no symptoms at all. It is important for you to keep all appointments with your doctor, even if you feel well, so that your blood pressure can be checked regularly.

Other Precautions

Tell any doctor or dentist you consult that you are taking this drug, especially if you will be undergoing any type of surgery.

Helpful Hints

If your mouth or throat feels dry, chewing sugarless gum or sucking ice chips or sugarless hard candy will help. Your nose may also feel dry and stuffy; check with your doctor before using nasal decongestants.

If this medicine upsets your stomach, taking it with meals, milk, or snacks should help.

No special restrictions on exertion and exercise, sun exposure, or exposure to excessive heat or cold.

POSSIBLE SIDE EFFECTS

Although this list of adverse effects may seem somewhat intimidating, keep in mind that some are quite rare. Of course, should these or any other problems arise while you are on medication, it is always a good idea to consult your doctor.

IF YOU DEVELOP

drowsiness or faintness ■ mood changes ■ headache ■ male impotence ■ diminished sex drive ■ lack of energy or weakness ■ depression ■ sleep disturbances or nightmares ■ nervousness or anxiety ■ seizures ■ flushing or warm feeling ■ pinpoint pupils ■ very slow pulse ■ black, tarry stools ■ vomiting, with blood

After you STOP taking reserpine or rauwolfia:
dizziness or drowsiness ■ weakness ■ irregular heartbeat ■ anxiety ■ mood changes ■ sleep disturbances ■ male impotence ■ diminished sex drive

WHAT TO DO

Urgent Get in touch with your doctor immediately.

chest pain ■ irregular or slow heartbeat ■ shortness of breath ■ stiffness ■ leg pain ■ stomach cramps or pain ■ diarrhea ■ nausea or vomiting ■ shaking of hands or fingers ■ pain or difficulty in urination ■ rash or itching ■ bleeding (including nosebleed) or bruising ■ blurred vision or tearing ■ drooping eyelids

May be serious Check with your doctor as soon as possible.

upset stomach ■ dry mouth or increased salivation ■ increased appetite or loss of appetite ■ dizziness, especially when getting up from a reclining or sitting position ■ stuffy nose ■ swelling of feet or legs ■ red eyes ■ male breast enlargement ■ female breast swelling ■ hearing disturbances

If symptoms are disturbing or persist, let your doctor know.

STORAGE INSTRUCTIONS

Store in a cool, dark place (not in a bathroom medicine cabinet).

STOPPING OR INTERRUPTING THERAPY

Since this drug does not cure high blood pressure but only controls it, you may have to take this medicine for the rest of your life. Do not stop taking it, even if you feel better. If you miss a dose, skip the missed dose and resume your regular schedule. Do not take two doses at the same time.

SPECIAL CONSIDERATIONS FOR THOSE OVER SIXTY-FIVE

Side effects such as dizziness, drowsiness, and swelling from water gain are more likely to occur in older people. Also, this drug commonly causes depression, sleep disturbances, and diminished sex drive.

CONDITION: **HYPERTENSION**

CATEGORY: **NONDIURETICS (SYMPATHOLYTICS)**

GENERIC (CHEMICAL) NAME	BRAND (TRADE) NAME	DOSAGE FORMS AND STRENGTHS
Guanethidine	ISMELIN	Tablets: 10, 25 mg

DRUG PROFILE

Guanethidine is generally used for treatment of moderate or severe high blood pressure that cannot be controlled by other medicines. This medicine works by inhibiting nerves that constrict blood vessels, resulting in relaxation of blood vessels and easier blood flow. Guanethidine is usually used with other antihypertensive medicines.

BEFORE USING THIS DRUG

Let your doctor know *IF*

You have ever had allergic reactions or other problems with ■ guanethidine.

You have ever had any of the following medical problems: ■ asthma ■ diabetes ■ diarrhea ■ fever ■ heart or blood vessel disease, including heart attack or stroke ■ kidney disease ■ liver disease ■ pheochromocytoma (adrenal gland tumor) ■ stomach ulcer .

You are taking any of the following medicines: ■ diuretics or other medicines for high blood pressure ■ amphetamines ■ medicine for depression ■ barbiturates ■ digoxin, digitoxin, or digitalis (heart medicines) ■ medicine for asthma ■ medicine for diabetes ■ narcotics or other prescription pain-killers ■ weight-reduction medicine ■ tranquilizers ■ decongestants ■ levodopa (medicine for Parkinson's disease) ■ medicine for nausea.

SPECIAL RESTRICTIONS WHILE TAKING THIS DRUG

FOOD AND DRUG INTERACTIONS

Other Drugs	Do not take any other drugs, including over-the-counter (OTC) drugs, before checking with your doctor. OTC drugs for appetite suppression, asthma, colds, cough, hay fever, or sinus problems tend to increase blood pressure. Use of reserpine or rauwolfia at the same time as guanethidine may cause fainting, slow heartbeat, and depression. The blood pressure–lowering effect of guanethidine may be reduced by amphetaminelike drugs, stimulants, antidepressants, and tranquilizers.
Foods and Beverages	Your doctor may prescribe a special low-salt diet, which you should follow carefully because it will help your medicine work more effectively. A weight-reduction diet may also be advised.
Alcohol	Drinking alcohol while taking this medicine may worsen such side effects as dizziness, light-headedness, or fainting. Avoid alcohol unless your doctor has approved its use.

No special restrictions on smoking.

DAILY LIVING

Exertion and Exercise	Use caution when exercising, exerting yourself, or standing for long periods of time because this medicine may cause you to become dizzy, light-headed, or faint. If you feel any of these symptoms coming on, sit or lie down. It is a good idea not to get up too quickly from a reclining or sitting position.

Excessive Heat	Use caution during hot weather, especially if you exert yourself (see above).
Examinations or Tests	Many people have high blood pressure with no symptoms at all. It is important for you to keep all appointments with your doctor, even if you feel well, so that your blood pressure can be checked regularly.
Other Precautions	Tell any doctor or dentist you consult that you are taking this medicine, especially if you will be undergoing any type of surgery.

No special restrictions on driving, sun exposure, or exposure to excessive cold.

POSSIBLE SIDE EFFECTS

Although this list of adverse effects may seem somewhat intimidating, keep in mind that some are quite rare. Of course, should these or any other problems arise while you are on medication, it is always a good idea to consult your doctor.

IF YOU DEVELOP	WHAT TO DO
extreme dizziness, light-headedness, or fainting, especially when getting up from a reclining or sitting position	**Urgent** Get in touch with your doctor immediately.
fever ■ swelling of feet or lower legs ■ chest pain ■ shortness of breath ■ weight gain ■ headache	**May be serious** Get in touch with your doctor as soon as possible.
diarrhea or increase in bowel movements ■ depression ■ difficulty in ejaculation (in males) ■ stuffy nose ■ weakness or tiredness ■ slow heartbeat ■ blurred vision ■ drooping eyelids ■ dry mouth ■ scalp hair loss ■ muscle pain or tremors ■ nausea or vomiting ■ loss of appetite	If symptoms are disturbing or persist, let your doctor know.

■ constipation ■ need to urinate at night or other urinary problems ■ rash ■ tenderness of the salivary glands (around the ear)

STORAGE INSTRUCTIONS

Store in a cool, dark place (not in a bathroom medicine cabinet).

STOPPING OR INTERRUPTING THERAPY

Since this drug does not cure high blood pressure but only controls it, you may have to take this medicine for the rest of your life. Do not stop taking it, even if you feel better. If you miss a dose, take it as soon as possible. If it is almost time for your next dose, skip the missed dose and resume your regular schedule. Do not take two doses at the same time.

SPECIAL CONSIDERATIONS FOR THOSE OVER SIXTY-FIVE

The side effects of dizziness, light-headedness, or fainting are more likely to occur and to be more severe in older people.

CONDITION: **HYPERTENSION**

CATEGORY: **NONDIURETICS (ANGIOTENSIN-CONVERTING ENZYME INHIBITORS)**

GENERIC (CHEMICAL) NAME	BRAND (TRADE) NAME	DOSAGE FORMS AND STRENGTHS
Captopril	CAPOTEN	Tablets: 12.5, 25, 50, 100 mg
Enalapril maleate	VASOTEC	Tablets: 5, 10, 20 mg

DRUG PROFILE

Captopril and enalapril are both used to treat high blood pressure. These drugs interrupt a chain of biochemical events that lead to constriction (tightening) of the blood vessels. Blocking this process lets the blood vessels relax, lowers blood pressure, and increases the flow of blood and oxygen to the heart.

Captopril is used to treat congestive heart failure as well. Relaxing the blood vessels reduces the congestion of blood in the lungs, lessens the load on the heart, and improves the blood flow to the kidneys, facilitating the elimination of sodium and water. Long-term use of this drug improves exercise tolerance because blood flow to the muscle is increased.

BEFORE USING THIS DRUG

Let your doctor know *IF*

You have ever had allergic reactions or other problems with ■ captopril ■ enalapril.

You have ever had any of the following medical problems: ■ kidney disease ■ systemic lupus erythematosus ■ heart or blood vessel disease ■ high blood potassium levels.

You are taking any of the following medicines: ■ diuretics or other medicines for high blood pressure ■ potassium-containing medicines or supplements ■ medicine for angina ■ corticosteroids ■ aspirin, indomethacin or other medicine for arthritis

   ■ *with captopril only:* ■ medicine for cancer ■ medicine to prevent rejection of transplanted organs.

You are on a low-salt diet.

SPECIAL RESTRICTIONS WHILE TAKING THIS DRUG

FOOD AND DRUG INTERACTIONS

Other Drugs	If you are taking captopril or enalapril for high blood pressure, do not take any other drugs, including over-the-counter (OTC) drugs, before checking with your doctor. Some OTC drugs for appetite suppression, asthma, colds, cough, hay fever, or sinus problems tend to increase blood pressure. If you are taking captopril for congestive heart failure, it is especially important to let your doctor know all other drugs you are taking, especially diuretics.

Foods and Beverages

Your doctor may prescribe a special low-salt diet, which you should follow carefully because it will help your medicine work more effectively. You may also be advised to go on a weight-reduction diet. If you are taking captopril for congestive heart failure, it is especially important to discuss your sodium intake with your doctor.

These drugs may cause a build-up of the mineral potassium in your body. Let your doctor know if you are using salt substitutes because many of these products are high in potassium chloride and may increase your blood-potassium level to dangerous levels.

No special restrictions on alcohol use or smoking.

DAILY LIVING

Exertion and Exercise

These drugs increase your risk of becoming dehydrated. Be careful during strenuous exercise; make sure you drink plenty of liquids to make up for water loss by perspiration.

If you are taking captopril for congestive heart failure, avoid a sudden increase in physical activity, even if you feel better.

Sun Exposure/ Excessive Heat

Use caution during hot weather, especially when you are exercising or exerting yourself (see above). While taking captopril, your skin may become more sensitive to sunlight and more likely to develop a sunburn. It is a good idea to avoid too much sun, especially if you burn easily. Apply a sunscreen to exposed skin surfaces before going outdoors.

Examinations or Tests	Many people have high blood pressure with no symptoms at all. Whether you are being treated for heart failure or for high blood pressure, it is important for you to keep all appointments with your doctor so that your progress can be checked. Periodic blood and urine tests may be required before and during therapy.
Other Precautions	Tell any doctor or dentist you consult that you are taking this medicine, especially if you will be undergoing any type of surgery.
	If you should become sick and have severe or prolonged vomiting or diarrhea, let your doctor know, as you may be at risk of becoming dehydrated.
	If you feel light-headed while taking this medicine, especially enalapril, let your doctor know. If you actually faint, stop taking the medicine until you have checked with your doctor.
	If you are taking captopril, check with your doctor if you become ill with flulike symptoms, such as cough, fever, or body aches; lose your appetite; vomit; or have diarrhea, especially if you are also taking a diuretic. This may cause you to lose a great deal of fluid.

No special restrictions on driving or exposure to excessive cold.

POSSIBLE SIDE EFFECTS

Although this list of adverse effects may seem somewhat intimidating, keep in mind that some are quite rare. Of course, should these or any other problems arise while you are on medication, it is always a good idea to consult your doctor.

IF YOU DEVELOP	**WHAT TO DO**
sore throat or fever ■ severe dizziness or light-headedness ■ swelling of face, mouth, vocal cords, fingers, ankles, or feet ■ hoarseness *With enalapril only:* cough ■ fainting (if you faint, stop taking the drug until you have checked with your doctor)	**Urgent** Get in touch with your doctor immediately.
irregular heartbeat ■ chest pain *With captopril only:* rapid heartbeat ■ cold fingers or toes ■ flushing or paleness	**May be serious** Check with your doctor as soon as possible.
light-headedness or faintness, especially when getting up from a reclining or sitting position ■ rash or itching ■ headache ■ dizziness ■ nausea ■ increased sweating ■ sleeplessness ■ nervousness ■ drowsiness ■ tingling sensation ■ stomach pain ■ tiredness or weakness ■ diarrhea *With captopril only:* increased skin sensitivity to sunlight ■ taste changes ■ loss of appetite ■ weight loss ■ hair loss ■ constipation ■ mouth sores ■ vomiting *With enalapril only:* indigestion ■ muscle cramps ■ male impotence	If symptoms are disturbing or persist, let your doctor know.

STORAGE INSTRUCTIONS

Store in a cool, dark place (not in a bathroom medicine cabinet).

STOPPING OR INTERRUPTING THERAPY

Do not stop taking the drug prescribed for you, even if you feel better. If you are being treated for hypertension, you may have to take it for the rest of your life, as these drugs do not cure high blood pressure but only control it. If you miss a dose, take it as soon as possible. If it is almost time for your next dose, skip the missed dose and resume your regular schedule. Do not take two doses at the same time.

SPECIAL CONSIDERATIONS FOR THOSE OVER SIXTY-FIVE

None.

CONDITION: **HYPERTENSION**

CATEGORY: **CALCIUM BLOCKERS**

GENERIC (CHEMICAL) NAME	BRAND (TRADE) NAME	DOSAGE FORMS AND STRENGTHS
Verapamil	CALAN	Tablets: 80, 120 mg
	CALAN SR	Controlled-release tablets: 240 mg
	ISOPTIN	Tablets: 80, 120 mg

DRUG PROFILE

The calcium blockers are used to relieve and control angina pectoris (chest pain). Calcium is needed for muscle cells to contract; by decreasing the passage of calcium into the muscle cells, these drugs relax the blood vessels and heart muscle. This increases the supply of blood and oxygen to the heart, reduces its workload, and prevents spasms of the blood vessels of the heart. Other antianginal drugs can be used along with a calcium blocker, if necessary. Calcium blockers tend to lower blood pressure; if you are also taking an antihypertensive agent, its dosage may need to be lowered. Verapamil can also be prescribed to treat high blood pressure.

For complete information on this drug, see pages 153–156.

CONDITION: **HYPERTENSION**

CATEGORY: **DIURETIC-NONDIURETIC COMBINATIONS**

GENERIC (CHEMICAL) NAME	BRAND (TRADE) NAME	DOSAGE FORMS AND STRENGTHS
Methyldopa and hydrochlorothiazide	ALDORIL	Tablets: 250 mg methyldopa and 15 mg hydrochlorothiazide; 250 mg methyldopa and 25 mg hydrochlorothiazide; 500 mg methyldopa and 30 mg hydrochlorothiazide; 500 mg methyldopa and 50 mg hydrochlorothiazide

DRUG PROFILE

This combination of an antihypertensive agent (methyldopa) and a thiazide diuretic (hydrochlorothiazide) is used to lower high blood pressure. Methyldopa acts to reduce transmission along certain nerve pathways, resulting in the relaxation of blood vessels and easier blood flow. Hydrochlorothiazide's main action is to increase the amount of salt and water eliminated by the body through urination. (See Methyldopa on pages 62–65 and Thiazide and Thiazide-type Diuretics on pages 23–27.)

BEFORE USING THIS DRUG

Let your doctor know *IF*

You have ever had allergic reactions or other problems with ■ methyldopa or hydrochlorothiazide, alone or combined ■ any of the thiazide or thiazide-type drugs ■ sulfonamides (sulfa drugs).

You have ever had any of the following medical problems: ■ diabetes ■ chest pain ■ heart disease ■ gout ■ liver disease ■ kidney disease ■ systemic lupus erythematosus ■ depression ■ disease of the pancreas ■ Parkinson's disease ■ pheochromocytoma (adrenal gland tumor).

You are taking any of the following medicines: ■ diuretics or any other medicines for high blood pressure ■ corticosteroids or corticotropin (ACTH) ■ medicine for high cholesterol ■ medicine for diabetes ■ digoxin, digitoxin, or digitalis (heart medicines) ■ levodopa (medicine for Parkinson's disease) ■ methenamine (medicine to prevent urinary tract infections) ■ anticoagulants (blood thinners) ■ tranquilizers ■ medicine for depression ■ medicine for gout.

SPECIAL RESTRICTIONS WHILE TAKING THIS DRUG

FOOD AND DRUG INTERACTIONS

Other Drugs	Do not take any other drugs, including over-the-counter (OTC) drugs, before checking with your doctor. OTC drugs for appetite suppression, asthma, colds, cough, hay fever, or sinus problems tend to increase blood pressure.
Foods and Beverages	Your doctor may prescribe a special low-salt diet, which you should follow carefully because it will help your medicine work more effectively. You may also be advised to go on a weight-reduction diet. This drug may cause your body to lose large amounts of the mineral potassium. Your doctor may give you special instructions about eating foods or drinking beverages that have a high potassium content (such as bananas and citrus fruit juices), taking a potassium supplement, or using salt substitutes.
Alcohol	Be careful about the amount of alcohol you drink while taking this medicine. Drinking alcohol may worsen such side effects as dizziness, lightheadedness, or fainting. Avoid alcohol unless your doctor has approved its use.

No special restrictions on smoking.

DAILY LIVING

Driving	This drug may cause drowsiness. Be careful when driving, operating household appliances, or doing any other tasks that require alertness until you know how this drug affects you.
Exertion and Exercise	Use caution when exercising or exerting yourself or if you must stand for long periods of time; this drug may cause side effects such as dizziness, light-headedness, or fainting. If you feel any of these symptoms coming on, sit or lie down. It is a good idea not to get up too quickly from a reclining or sitting position.
Sun Exposure/ Excessive Heat	Your skin may become more sensitive to sunlight and heat and more likely to develop a sunburn while you are taking this medicine. It is a good idea to avoid too much sun, especially if you burn easily. Use caution during hot weather or while taking saunas or hot baths, as excessive sweating while taking this medicine may cause you to become dehydrated and to feel drowsy or faint.
Examinations or Tests	Many people have high blood pressure with no symptoms at all. It is important for you to keep all appointments with your doctor, even if you feel well, so that your blood pressure can be checked regularly.
Other Precautions	If you have diabetes, be aware that this medicine may raise blood-sugar levels. If you notice any change when testing sugar levels in your blood or urine, let your doctor know. Tell any doctor or dentist you consult that you are taking this medicine, especially if you will be undergoing any type of surgery.

No special restrictions on exposure to excessive cold.

POSSIBLE SIDE EFFECTS

Although this list of adverse effects may seem somewhat intimidating, keep in mind that some are quite rare. Of course, should these or any other problems arise while you are on medication, it is always a good idea to consult your doctor.

IF YOU DEVELOP	WHAT TO DO
fever ■ very slow or fast heartbeat ■ chest pain ■ yellowing of eyes or skin ■ dark or amber-colored urine ■ change in stool color ■ dry mouth ■ increased thirst ■ nausea or vomiting ■ diarrhea or stomach cramps ■ joint or side pain ■ irregular heartbeat ■ weak pulse ■ difficulty in breathing ■ muscle cramps or pain ■ tiredness or weakness ■ depression ■ anxiety	**Urgent** Get in touch with your doctor immediately.
rash or hives ■ sore throat ■ bleeding or bruising ■ chills ■ sleeplessness ■ nightmares or vivid dreams ■ swelling of feet or lower legs ■ shakiness or unusual body movements ■ frequent urination or need to urinate at night	**May be serious** Check with your doctor as soon as possible.
dizziness or light-headedness, especially when getting up from a reclining or sitting position ■ drowsiness ■ headache ■ memory problems ■ inability to concentrate ■ male impotence ■ diminished sex drive ■ fainting ■ increased skin sensitivity to sunlight ■ loss of appetite ■ upset stomach ■ constipation ■ bloating or gas ■ sore or dark tongue ■ numbness, tingling, pain, or weakness in hands or feet ■ female breast swelling ■ male breast enlargement ■ blurred vision	If symptoms are disturbing or persist, let your doctor know.

STORAGE INSTRUCTIONS

Store in a cool, dark place (not in a bathroom medicine cabinet).

STOPPING OR INTERRUPTING THERAPY

Since this drug does not cure high blood pressure but only controls it, you may have to take this medicine for the rest of your life. Do not stop taking it, even if you feel better. If you miss a dose, take it as soon as possible. If it is almost time for your next dose, skip the missed dose and resume your regular schedule. Do not take two doses at the same time.

SPECIAL CONSIDERATIONS FOR THOSE OVER SIXTY-FIVE

Older people are more likely to develop depression, dizziness, or light-headedness. They are also more likely to develop signs of dehydration, such as weakness or dizziness, when getting up from a reclining or sitting position. In addition, signs of potassium loss such as irregular heartbeat, weak pulse, and tiredness or weakness are more likely to develop in older people. Such people should get in touch with a doctor if they develop any of these symptoms. All doctor's appointments should be kept.

CONDITION: **HYPERTENSION**

CATEGORY: **DIURETIC-NONDIURETIC COMBINATIONS**

GENERIC (CHEMICAL) NAME	BRAND (TRADE) NAME	DOSAGE FORMS AND STRENGTHS
Reserpine, hydralazine hydrochloride, and hydrochlorothiazide	SER-AP-ES	Tablets: 0.1 mg reserpine, 25 mg hydralazine hydrochloride, and 15 mg hydrochlorothiazide

DRUG PROFILE

This combination of two different antihypertensive agents (reserpine and hydralazine) plus a thiazide diuretic (hydrochlorothiazide) is used to lower high blood pressure. Reserpine and hydralazine act together to relax the muscles of the blood vessel walls so that the blood can flow more freely. In addition, reserpine has sedative and tranquilizing effects, and hydralazine increases the rate and output of the heart. The thiazides' main action is to increase the amount of salt and water eliminated by the body through urination. (See Rauwolfia serpentina/Reserpine on pages 82–85, Hydralazine on pages 72–75, and Thiazide and Thiazide-type Diuretics on pages 23–27.)

BEFORE USING THIS DRUG

Let your doctor know *IF*

You have ever had allergic reactions or other problems with ■ hydralazine ■ thiazide diuretics ■ rauwolfia alkaloids ■ sulfonamides (sulfa drugs).

You have ever had any of the following medical problems: ■ allergies, breathing problems, or asthma ■ angina (chest pain) ■ diabetes ■ epilepsy or other seizure disorders ■ gout ■ stomach ulcer ■ ulcerative colitis ■ disease of the heart or blood vessels, including rheumatic mitral valve disease and stroke ■ systemic lupus erythematosus ■ kidney disease ■ liver disease ■ depression ■ disease of the pancreas.

You are taking any of the following medicines: ■ diuretics or other medicines for high blood pressure ■ corticosteroids or corticotropin (ACTH) ■ anticoagulants (blood thinners) ■ medicine for seizures ■ medicine for depression (within the last two weeks) ■ antihistamines ■ medicine for hay fever, allergies, or colds ■ barbiturates ■ medicine for high cholesterol ■ medicine for diabetes ■ digoxin, digitoxin, or digitalis (heart medicines) ■ medicine for asthma ■ quinidine (medicine for abnormal heart rhythms) ■ sedatives ■ tranquilizers ■ sleep medicines ■ levodopa (medicine for Parkinson's disease) ■ muscle relaxants ■ narcotics or other prescription pain-killers ■ decongestants ■ potassium-containing medicines or supplements.

SPECIAL RESTRICTIONS WHILE TAKING THIS DRUG

FOOD AND DRUG INTERACTIONS

Other Drugs	Do not take any other drugs, including over-the-counter (OTC) drugs, before checking with your doctor. OTC drugs for appetite suppression, asthma, colds, cough, hay fever, or sinus problems tend to increase blood pressure. Antihistamines, sleep medicines, tranquilizers, pain-killers, barbiturates, medicine for seizures, muscle relaxants, or anesthetics may worsen such side effects as light-headedness, drowsiness, or fainting.
Foods and Beverages	Your doctor may prescribe a special low-salt diet, which you should follow carefully because it will help your medicine work more effectively. You may also be

advised to go on a weight-reduction diet. This drug may cause your body to lose large amounts of the mineral potassium. Your doctor may give you special instructions about eating foods or drinking beverages that have a high potassium content (such as bananas and citrus fruit juices), taking a potassium supplement, or using salt substitutes.

Alcohol	Drinking alcohol while taking this medicine may worsen such side effects as dizziness and drowsiness. Avoid alcohol unless your doctor has approved its use.

No special restrictions on smoking.

DAILY LIVING

Driving	This drug may cause drowsiness. Be careful when driving, operating household appliances, or doing any other tasks that require alertness until you know how this drug affects you.
Exertion and Exercise	Use caution when exercising, exerting yourself, or standing for long periods of time because this drug may cause you to become dizzy, light-headed, or faint. If you feel any of these symptoms coming on, sit or lie down. It is a good idea not to get up too quickly from a reclining or sitting position.
Sun Exposure/ Excessive Heat	Your skin may become more sensitive to sunlight and more likely to develop a sunburn while you are taking this medicine. It is a good idea to avoid too much sun, especially if you burn easily. Apply a sunscreen to exposed skin surfaces before going outdoors. Use caution during hot weather or while taking saunas or hot baths, since excessive sweating while taking this medicine may cause you to become dehydrated and to feel drowsy or faint.

Examinations or Tests	Many people have high blood pressure with no symptoms at all. It is important for you to keep all appointments with your doctor, even if you feel well, so that your blood pressure can be checked regularly. Periodic blood and urine tests may be required.
Other Precautions	If you have diabetes, be aware that this medicine may raise blood-sugar levels. If you notice any change in the sugar levels in your blood or urine, let your doctor know.
	Tell any doctor or dentist you consult that you are taking this medicine, especially if you will be undergoing any type of surgery.
	When first starting on this type of medicine, you may feel tired and will probably experience both greater volume and frequency of urination. Until your individual pattern of urination has been established with this medicine, it may be wise to time carefully any activity that will put you out of convenient reach of a bathroom, such as bus or car travel. In addition, taking a diuretic at bedtime will probably interfere with sleep; you should discuss your dosage schedule with your doctor.
	Check with your doctor if you become ill with flulike symptoms, such as cough, fever, or body aches; lose your appetite; vomit; or have diarrhea. This may cause you to lose a great deal of fluid, making it important not to take this medicine for one or more doses.
	Following mild fluid losses, some older people are more vulnerable to symptoms of weakness or dizziness upon standing or getting up.
Helpful Hints	If your mouth or throat feels dry, chewing sugarless gum or sucking ice chips or sugarless hard candy will help. Your nose may also feel dry or stuffy; check with your doctor before using nasal decongestants.

If this medicine upsets your stomach, taking it with milk, meals, or snacks should help.

No special restrictions on exposure to excessive cold.

POSSIBLE SIDE EFFECTS

Although this list of adverse effects may seem somewhat intimidating, keep in mind that some are quite rare. Of course, should these or any other problems arise while you are on medication, it is always a good idea to consult your doctor.

IF YOU DEVELOP

general body discomfort or weakness, drowsiness, or faintness ■ headache ■ mood changes, depression, or inability to concentrate ■ anxiety or nervousness ■ disorientation ■ early-morning sleeplessness, vivid dreams, or nightmares ■ male impotence ■ diminished sex drive ■ seizures ■ dry mouth ■ flushing ■ increased thirst ■ muscle cramps or pain ■ nausea or vomiting ■ pinpoint pupils ■ changes in heart rate ■ black, tarry stools ■ vomiting, with blood ■ chest pain ■ irregular heartbeat ■ joint or side pain ■ shortness of breath ■ severe stomach pain ■ numbness, tingling, pain, or weakness in hands or feet

(If any of these side effects occurs after you STOP taking this medicine, let your doctor know immediately.)

diarrhea ■ sore throat or fever ■ rash or itching ■ stiffness ■ leg pain ■ swelling of lymph glands ■ shaking of hands and fingers ■ swelling of fingers or ankles ■ pain or difficulty in urination ■ chills ■ bleeding (including nosebleed) or bruising ■ yellowing of eyes or skin ■ blurred vision or tearing ■ drooping eyelids ■ weight gain

WHAT TO DO

Urgent Get in touch with your doctor immediately.

May be serious Check with your doctor as soon as possible.

constipation ▪ upset stomach ▪ dizziness, especially when getting up from a reclining or sitting position ▪ loss of appetite ▪ stuffy nose ▪ red eyes ▪ male breast enlargement ▪ female breast swelling ▪ hearing disturbances ▪ increased skin sensitivity to sunlight ▪ increased sweating ▪ increased salivation

If symptoms are disturbing or persist, let your doctor know.

STORAGE INSTRUCTIONS

Store in a cool, dark place (not in a bathroom medicine cabinet).

STOPPING OR INTERRUPTING THERAPY

Since this drug does not cure high blood pressure but only controls it, you may have to take this medicine for the rest of your life. Do not stop taking it, even if you feel better. If you miss a dose, take it as soon as possible. If it is almost time for your next dose, skip the missed dose and resume your regular schedule. Do not take two doses at the same time.

SPECIAL CONSIDERATIONS FOR THOSE OVER SIXTY-FIVE

Dizziness or faintness is more likely to occur in older people. Thus, doctors may require regular checkups. People over sixty-five should consult a doctor if they become ill with flulike symptoms, such as cough, fever, or body aches; lose their appetite; vomit; or have diarrhea, since they may then be more vulnerable to fluid losses.

CONDITION: **HYPERTENSION**

CATEGORY: **DIURETIC-NONDIURETIC COMBINATIONS**

GENERIC (CHEMICAL) NAME	BRAND (TRADE) NAME	DOSAGE FORMS AND STRENGTHS
Atenolol and chlorthalidone	TENORETIC	Tablets: 50 mg atenolol and 25 mg chlorthalidone; 100 mg atenolol and 25 mg chlorthalidone

DRUG PROFILE

This medicine is a combination of two kinds of drugs that lower blood pressure. By blocking certain nerve impulses, the beta-blocker atenolol relaxes blood vessels, increases the supply of blood and oxygen to the heart, and reduces the workload and pumping rate of the heart (see Beta-blockers, pages 56–61). Chlorthalidone is a thiazide diuretic that increases the amount of salt and water you eliminate through urination (see Thiazide and Thiazide-type Diuretics on pages 23–27). Other drugs that lower blood pressure may be added to this combination drug if necessary.

BEFORE USING THIS DRUG

Let your doctor know *IF*

You have ever had allergic reactions or other problems with ■ any of the thiazide or thiazide-type diuretics ■ beta-blockers ■ sulfonamides (sulfa drugs).

You have ever had any of the following medical problems: ■ allergies ■ hay fever, hives, asthma, or eczema ■ bronchitis or emphysema ■ slow heartbeat ■ diabetes ■ any heart or blood vessel disease ■ kidney disease ■ liver disease ■ thyroid disease ■ Raynaud's syndrome (poor circulation in the fingers and toes) ■ glaucoma ■ myasthenia gravis ■ hypoglycemia (low blood sugar) ■ pheochromocytoma (adrenal gland tumor) ■ gout ■ systemic lupus erythematosus ■ disease of the pancreas.

You are taking any of the following medicines: ■ any other medicines for high blood pressure ■ medicine for asthma ■ aminophylline, epinephrine, ephedrine, norepinephrine, isoproterenol, dyphylline, oxtriphylline, theophylline, or phenylephrine (vasopressor drugs) ■ diltiazem, nifedipine, or verapamil (calcium blockers) ■ medicine for depression ■ cimetidine (medicine for ulcers) ■ heart medicine ■ medicine for glaucoma ■ aspirin, indomethacin, or phenylbutazone (medicine for arthritis) ■ medicine for diabetes ■ decongestants ■ medicine for colds ■ medicine for nausea ■ tranquilizers ■ corticosteroids or corticotropin (ACTH) ■ medicine for high cholesterol ■ medicine for gout ■ lithium ■ methenamine (medicine to prevent urinary tract infections) ■ anticoagulants (blood thinners) ■ tetracycline.

SPECIAL RESTRICTIONS WHILE TAKING THIS DRUG

FOOD AND DRUG INTERACTIONS

Other Drugs	Do not take any other drugs, including over-the-counter (OTC) drugs, before checking with your doctor. OTC drugs for appetite suppression, asthma, colds, cough, hay fever, or sinus problems tend to increase blood pressure.
Foods and Beverages	Your doctor may prescribe a special low-salt diet, which you should follow carefully because it will help your medicine work more effectively. This medicine may cause your body to lose large amounts of the mineral potassium. Your doctor may give you special instructions about eating foods or drinking beverages that have a high potassium content (such as bananas and citrus fruit juices), taking a potassium supplement, or using salt substitutes.
Alcohol	Alcohol may worsen side effects of this medicine such as dizziness, light-headedness, or fainting. Be careful about how much alcohol you consume.

No special restrictions on smoking.

DAILY LIVING

Driving	This drug may cause drowsiness. Be careful when driving, operating household appliances, or doing any other tasks that require alertness until you know how this drug affects you.
Sun Exposure/Excessive Heat	Your skin may become more sensitive to sunlight and more likely to develop a sunburn while you are taking this medicine. It is a good idea to avoid too much sun,

especially if you burn easily. Apply a sunscreen to exposed skin surfaces before going outdoors. Use caution during hot weather or while taking saunas or hot baths, since excessive sweating while taking this medicine may cause you to become dehydrated and to feel drowsy or faint.

Excessive Cold

You may become more sensitive to cold temperatures while taking this medicine. Dress warmly—protecting your skin, fingers, and toes—and use caution during prolonged exposure to cold.

Examinations and Tests

Check your pulse regularly. If it is slower than your usual rate or less than fifty beats per minute, call your doctor. Many people have high blood pressure with no symptoms at all. It is important for you to keep all appointments with your doctor, even if you feel well, so that your blood pressure can be checked regularly. Periodic blood and urine tests may be required.

Other Precautions

Be sure to tell any doctor or dentist you consult that you are taking this medicine, especially if you will be undergoing any type of surgery.

If you have diabetes, be aware that this medicine may cause your blood-sugar level to fall. It may also mask the signs of low blood sugar (such as changes in pulse rate or increased blood pressure) leaving you unaware that your blood sugar has fallen. Your doctor may want to make changes in the dosage of your diabetes medicine.

When first starting on this type of medicine, you may feel tired and will probably experience both greater volume and frequency of urination. Until your individual pattern of urination has been established with this medicine, it may be wise to time carefully any activity that will put you out of convenient reach of a bathroom, such as bus or car travel. In addition, taking a diuretic at bedtime will probably interfere with sleep; you should discuss your dosage schedule with your doctor.

Check with your doctor if you become ill with flulike symptoms, such as cough, fever, or body aches; lose your appetite; vomit; or have diarrhea. This may cause you to lose a great deal of fluid, making it important not to take this drug for one or more doses.

Helpful Hints

If your mouth or throat feels dry, chewing sugarless gum or sucking ice chips or sugarless hard candy will help. If your eyes feel dry, you may use nonmedicated or plain eyedrops for relief.

No special restrictions on exertion and exercise.

POSSIBLE SIDE EFFECTS

Although this list of adverse effects may seem somewhat intimidating, keep in mind that some are quite rare. Of course, should these or any other problems arise while you are on medication, it is always a good idea to consult your doctor.

IF YOU DEVELOP

increased skin sensitivity to sunlight ■ chest pain ■ palpitations ■ irregular heartbeat ■ extremely slow heartbeat ■ swelling of face, ankles, feet, or lower legs ■ difficulty in breathing, shortness of breath, or coughing ■ asthma or wheezing ■ restlessness, sweating, nervousness, and irritability (if you are a thyroid patient) ■ weight gain ■ severe or continuing vomiting or diarrhea ■ confusion ■ depression ■ severe stomach pain or cramps ■ joint or side pain ■ weak pulse ■ decreased urination ■ dry mouth ■ increased thirst ■ muscle cramps or pain ■ weakness

WHAT TO DO

Urgent Get in touch with your doctor immediately.

dizziness, light-headedness, or confusion upon getting up from a reclining or sitting position ■ cold hands or feet ■ sore throat or fever ■ rash or hives ■ bleeding or bruising ■ yellowing of eyes or skin	**May be serious** Check with your doctor as soon as possible.
diarrhea ■ upset stomach ■ nausea or vomiting ■ loss of appetite ■ drowsiness ■ dry skin or eyes ■ numbness or tingling in fingers or toes ■ anxiety ■ male impotence ■ diminished sex drive ■ hallucinations ■ nightmares or vivid dreams ■ sleep disturbances ■ headache ■ clumsiness	If symptoms are disturbing or persist, let your doctor know.

STORAGE INSTRUCTIONS

Store in a cool, dark place (not in a bathroom medicine cabinet).

STOPPING OR INTERRUPTING THERAPY

Since this drug does not cure high blood pressure but only controls it, you may have to take this medicine for the rest of your life. Do not stop taking it, even if you feel better. If you miss a dose, take it as soon as possible. If it is almost time for your next dose, skip the missed dose and resume your regular schedule. Do not take two doses at the same time.

SPECIAL CONSIDERATIONS FOR THOSE OVER SIXTY-FIVE

Older people may be especially prone to such side effects as confusion, weakness, clumsiness, or dizziness when getting up from a reclining or sitting position, especially when first starting on this drug. Those who develop such symptoms should get in touch with a doctor, who may want to measure the amount of medicine that reaches the bloodstream.

CONDITION: **HYPERTENSION**

CATEGORY: **DIURETIC-NONDIURETIC COMBINATIONS**

GENERIC (CHEMICAL) NAME	BRAND (TRADE) NAME	DOSAGE FORMS AND STRENGTHS
Rauwolfia serpentina and bendroflumethiazide	RAUZIDE	Tablets: 50 mg rauwolfia serpentina and 4 mg bendroflumethiazide
Reserpine and hydroflumethiazide	SALUTENSIN	Tablets: 0.125 mg reserpine and 50 mg hydroflumethiazide
	SALUTENSIN-Demi	Tablets: 0.125 mg reserpine and 25 mg hydroflumethiazide
Reserpine and hydrochlorothiazide	HYDROPRES	Tablets: 0.125 mg reserpine and 25 mg hydrochlorothiazide; 0.125 mg reserpine and 50 mg hydrochlorothiazide
	SERPASIL-ESIDRIX	Tablets: 0.1 mg reserpine and 25 mg hydrochlorothiazide; 0.1 mg reserpine and 50 mg hydrochlorothiazide
Reserpine and chlorthalidone	REGROTON	Tablets: 0.25 mg reserpine and 50 mg chlorthalidone
	DEMI-REGROTON	Tablets: 0.125 mg reserpine and 25 mg chlorthalidone

Reserpine and chlorothiazide	DIUPRES	Tablets: 0.125 mg reserpine and 250 mg chlorothiazide; 0.125 mg reserpine and 500 mg chlorothiazide
Deserpidine and methychlothiazide	ENDURONYL	Tablets: 0.25 mg deserpidine and 5 mg methyclothiazide
	ENDURONYL Forte	Tablets: 0.5 mg deserpidine and 5 mg methy-clothiazide

DRUG PROFILE

This combination of an antihypertensive agent (a rauwolfia alkaloid) and a thiazide diuretic is used to lower high blood pressure. The rauwolfia alkaloids (reserpine, deserpidine, rauwolfia serpentina) cause the muscles of the blood vessels to relax, so the blood can flow more freely. The rauwolfia alkaloids also have sedative and tranquilizing effects. The thiazides' main action is to increase the amount of salt and water eliminated by the body through urination. (See Rauwolfia serpentina/ Reserpine on pages 82–85 and Thiazide and Thiazide-type Diuretics on pages 23–27.)

BEFORE USING THIS DRUG

Let your doctor know *IF*

You have ever had allergic reactions or other problems with ■ rauwolfia alkaloids ■ thiazide or thiazide-type diuretics ■ tartrazine (FD&C Yellow Dye No. 5) ■ sulfonamides (sulfa drugs).

You have ever had any of the following medical problems: ■ allergies, breathing problems, or asthma ■ diabetes ■ epilepsy ■ gallstones ■ stomach ulcer ■ ulcerative colitis ■ gout ■ disease of the heart or blood vessels, including stroke ■ kidney disease ■ liver disease ■ systemic lupus erythematosus ■ depression ■ disease of the pancreas ■ Parkinson's disease ■ breast cancer ■ pheochromocytoma (adrenal gland tumor).

You are taking any of the following medicines: ■ diuretics, beta-blockers, or other medicines for high blood pressure ■ corticosteroids or corticotropin (ACTH)

■ anticoagulants (blood thinners) ■ medicine for seizures ■ medicine for depression (within the last two weeks) ■ antihistamines ■ medicine for hay fever, allergies, or colds ■ barbiturates ■ sedatives ■ tranquilizers ■ sleep medicines ■ medicine for high cholesterol ■ medicine for diabetes ■ digoxin, digitoxin, or digitalis (heart medicines) ■ medicine for gout ■ levodopa (medicine for Parkinson's disease) ■ lithium ■ methenamine (medicine to prevent urinary tract infections) ■ muscle relaxants ■ narcotics or other prescription pain-killers ■ decongestants ■ medicine for asthma ■ quinidine (medicine for abnormal heart rhythms).

You are receiving electroconvulsive therapy.

You have ever undergone sympathectomy.

SPECIAL RESTRICTIONS WHILE TAKING THIS DRUG

FOOD AND DRUG INTERACTIONS

Other Drugs	Do not take any other drugs, including over-the-counter (OTC) drugs, before checking with your doctor. OTC drugs for appetite suppression, asthma, cough, hay fever, or sinus problems tend to increase blood pressure. Antihistamines, sleep medicines, tranquilizers, pain-killers, barbiturates, medicine for seizures, muscle relaxants, or anesthetics may worsen such side effects as dizziness, light-headedness, drowsiness, or fainting.
Foods and Beverages	Your doctor may prescribe a special low-salt diet, which you should follow carefully because it will help your medicine work more effectively. You may also be advised to go on a weight-reduction diet. This drug may cause your body to lose large amounts of the mineral potassium. Your doctor may give you special instructions about eating foods or drinking beverages that have a high potassium content (such as bananas and citrus fruit juices), taking a potassium supplement, or using salt substitutes.
Alcohol	Drinking alcohol while taking this medicine may worsen such side effects as dizziness and drowsi-

ness. Avoid alcohol unless your doctor has approved its use.

No special restrictions on smoking.

DAILY LIVING

Driving	This drug may cause drowsiness. Be careful when driving, operating household appliances, or doing any other tasks that require alertness until you know how this drug affects you.
Exertion and Exercise	Use caution when exercising or exerting yourself while taking this medicine because excessive sweating may cause you to become dehydrated and to feel dizzy, light-headed, or faint.
Sun Exposure/ Excessive Heat	Your skin may become more sensitive to sunlight and more likely to develop a sunburn while you are taking this medicine. It is a good idea to avoid too much sun, especially if you burn easily. Apply a sunscreen to exposed skin surfaces before going outdoors. Use caution during hot weather or while taking saunas or hot baths, since excessive sweating while taking this medicine may cause you to become dehydrated and to feel drowsy or faint.
Examinations or Tests	Many people have high blood pressure with no symptoms at all. It is important for you to keep all appointments with your doctor, even if you feel well, so that your blood pressure can be checked regularly. Periodic blood and urine tests may be required.
Other Precautions	Tell any doctor or dentist you consult that you are taking this medicine, especially if you will be undergoing any type of surgery.

If you have diabetes, be aware that this medicine may raise blood-sugar levels. If you notice any change when testing sugar levels in your blood or urine, let your doctor know.

When first starting on this type of medicine, you may feel tired and will probably experience both greater volume and frequency of urination. Until your individual pattern of urination has been established with this medicine, it may be wise to time carefully any activity that will put you out of convenient reach of a bathroom, such as bus or car travel. In addition, taking a diuretic at bedtime will probably interfere with sleep; you should discuss your dosage schedule with your doctor.

Check with your doctor if you become ill with flulike symptoms, such as cough, fever, or body aches; lose your appetite; vomit; or have diarrhea. This may cause you to lose a great deal of fluid, making it important not to take this drug for one or more doses.

Helpful Hints

If this medicine upsets your stomach, taking it with milk, meals, or snacks should help.

If your mouth or throat feels dry, chewing sugarless gum or sucking ice chips or sugarless hard candy will help.

No special restrictions on exposure to excessive cold.

POSSIBLE SIDE EFFECTS

Although this list of adverse effects may seem somewhat intimidating, keep in mind that some are quite rare. Of course, should these or any other problems arise while you are on medication, it is always a good idea to consult your doctor.

IF YOU DEVELOP

severe dizziness or drowsiness ■ dry mouth ■ flushing ■ increased thirst ■ muscle cramps or pain ■ nausea or vomiting ■ pinpoint pupils ■ changes in heart rate ■ weakness ■ headache ■ mood changes ■ depression ■ inability to concentrate ■ nervousness or anxiety ■ early-morning sleeplessness ■ vivid dreams or nightmares ■ male impotence ■ diminished sex drive ■ seizures ■ black, tarry stools ■ vomiting, with blood ■ shortness of breath ■ joint or side pain

After you STOP taking this medicine: dizziness, drowsiness, or fainting ■ weakness ■ male impotence ■ diminished sex drive ■ irregular heartbeat ■ mood changes ■ depression ■ inability to concentrate ■ anxiety ■ sleep disturbances

diarrhea ■ weight gain ■ chills ■ stiffness ■ shaking of hands or fingers ■ fever or sore throat ■ rash, hives, or itching ■ pain or difficulty in urination ■ stomach cramps or pain ■ bleeding (including nosebleed) or bruising ■ yellowing of eyes or skin ■ blurred vision or tearing ■ drooping eyelids

loss of appetite or increased appetite ■ increased salivation ■ upset stomach ■ stuffy nose ■ dizziness, especially when getting up from a reclining or sitting position ■ breast enlargement ■ hearing disturbances ■ increased skin sensitivity to sunlight

WHAT TO DO

Urgent Get in touch with your doctor immediately.

May be serious Check with your doctor as soon as possible.

If symptoms are disturbing or persist, let your doctor know.

STORAGE INSTRUCTIONS

Store in a cool, dark place (not in a bathroom medicine cabinet).

STOPPING OR INTERRUPTING THERAPY

Since this drug does not cure high blood pressure but only controls it, you may have to take this medicine for the rest of your life. Do not stop taking it, even if you feel better. If you miss a dose, take it as soon as possible. If it is almost time for your next dose, skip the missed dose and resume your regular schedule. Do not take two doses at the same time.

SPECIAL CONSIDERATIONS FOR THOSE OVER SIXTY-FIVE

Older people are more likely to develop dizziness, light-headedness, fainting, and weakness. Thus, doctors may require regular checkups.

CONDITION: **HYPERTENSION**

CATEGORY: **DIURETIC-NONDIURETIC COMBINATIONS**

GENERIC (CHEMICAL) NAME	BRAND (TRADE) NAME	DOSAGE FORMS AND STRENGTHS
Hydralazine and hydrochlorothiazide	APRESAZIDE	Capsules: 25 mg hydralazine and 25 mg hydrochlorothiazide; 50 mg hydralazine and 50 mg hydrochlorothiazide; 100 mg hydralazine and 50 mg hydrochloro-thiazide

DRUG PROFILE

This medicine is a combination of two kinds of drugs that lower blood pressure. Hydralazine relaxes the blood vessel walls so that the blood can flow more freely; this drug also increases the rate and output of the heart. Hydrochlorothiazide is a thiazide diuretic that increases the amount of salt and water eliminated by the body through urination. (See Hydralazine on pages 72–75 and Thiazide and Thiazide-type Diuretics on pages 23–27).

BEFORE USING THIS DRUG

Let your doctor know *IF*

You have ever had allergic reactions or other problems with ■ hydralazine ■ thiazide or thiazide-type diuretics ■ sulfonamides (sulfa drugs).

You have ever had any of the following medical problems: ■ allergies ■ asthma ■ diabetes ■ gout ■ heart or blood vessel disease, including stroke and rheumatic mitral valve disease ■ kidney disease ■ liver disease ■ systemic lupus erythematosus ■ disease of the pancreas.

You are taking any of the following medicines: ■ diuretics or other medicines for high blood pressure ■ corticosteroids or corticotropin (ACTH) ■ anticoagulants (blood thinners) ■ medicine for depression ■ medicine for high cholesterol ■ medicine for diabetes ■ digoxin, digitoxin, or digitalis (heart medicines) ■ medicine for gout ■ lithium ■ methenamine (medicine to prevent urinary tract infections) ■ barbiturates ■ muscle relaxants ■ narcotics or other prescription painkillers.

You have ever undergone sympathectomy.

SPECIAL RESTRICTIONS WHILE TAKING THIS DRUG

FOOD AND DRUG INTERACTIONS

Other Drugs	Do not take any other drugs, including over-the-counter (OTC) drugs, before checking with your doctor. OTC drugs for appetite suppression, asthma, colds, cough, hay fever, or sinus problems tend to increase blood pressure.
Foods and Beverages	Your doctor may prescribe a special low-salt diet, which you should follow carefully because it will help your medicine work more effectively. You may also be advised to go on a weight-reduction diet. This drug may cause your body to lose large amounts of the mineral potassium. Your doctor may give you special instructions about eating foods or drinking beverages that have a high potassium content (such as bananas and citrus fruit juices), taking a potassium supplement, or using salt substitutes.

Alcohol	Avoid alcohol unless your doctor has approved its use. Drinking alcohol while taking this medicine may worsen such side effects as dizziness or drowsiness.

No special restrictions on smoking.

DAILY LIVING

Driving	This drug may cause drowsiness. Be careful when driving, operating household appliances, or doing any other tasks that require alertness until you know how this drug affects you.
Exertion and Exercise	Use caution when exercising, exerting yourself, or standing for long periods of time because this medicine may cause you to become dizzy, light-headed, or faint. If you feel any of these symptoms coming on, sit or lie down. It is a good idea not to get up too quickly from a reclining or sitting position.
Sun Exposure/ Excessive Heat	Your skin may become more sensitive to sunlight and more likely to develop a sunburn while you are taking this medicine. It is a good idea to avoid too much sun, especially if you burn easily. Apply a sunscreen to exposed skin surfaces before going outdoors. Use caution during hot weather or while taking saunas or hot baths, since excessive sweating while taking this medicine may cause you to become dehydrated and to feel drowsy or faint.
Examinations or Tests	Many people have high blood pressure with no symptoms at all. It is important for you to keep all appointments with your doctor, even if you feel well, so that your blood pressure can be checked regularly. Periodic blood tests are usually required.

Other Precautions

If you have diabetes, be aware that this medicine may raise blood-sugar levels. If you notice any change when testing sugar levels in your blood or urine, let your doctor know.

When first starting on this type of medicine, you may feel tired and will probably experience both greater volume and frequency of urination. Until your individual pattern of urination has been established with this medicine, it may be wise to time carefully any activity that will put you out of convenient reach of a bathroom, such as bus or car travel. In addition, taking a diuretic at bedtime will probably interfere with sleep; you should discuss your dosage schedule with your doctor.

Check with your doctor if you become ill with flulike symptoms, such as cough, fever, or body aches; lose your appetite; vomit; or have diarrhea. This may cause you to lose a great deal of fluid, making it important not to take this medicine for one or more doses.

No special restrictions on exposure to cold.

POSSIBLE SIDE EFFECTS

Although this list of adverse effects may seem somewhat intimidating, keep in mind that some are quite rare. Of course, should these or any other problems arise while you are on medication, it is always a good idea to consult your doctor.

IF YOU DEVELOP

severe nausea or vomiting ■ dry mouth
■ increased thirst ■ irregular heartbeat ■ mood changes ■ muscle cramps or pain ■ weak pulse
■ chest pain ■ tiredness or weakness ■ joint pain
■ numbness ■ tingling, pain, or weakness in hands or feet ■ severe stomach pain or cramps
■ difficulty in breathing

WHAT TO DO

Urgent Get in touch with your doctor immediately.

chills ■ rash or itching ■ sore throat or fever ■ swollen lymph glands ■ bleeding or bruising ■ yellowing of eyes or skin ■ weight gain	**May be serious** Check with your doctor as soon as possible.
upset stomach ■ diarrhea ■ nausea or vomiting ■ loss of appetite ■ constipation ■ headache ■ changes in heart rate ■ dizziness or light-headedness, especially when getting up from a reclining or sitting position ■ increased skin sensitivity to sunlight ■ flushing ■ shortness of breath with exercise ■ stuffy nose ■ eye irritation ■ depression ■ anxiety ■ disorientation ■ difficulty in urination ■ increased sweating ■ tremors	If symptoms are disturbing or persist, let your doctor know.

STORAGE INSTRUCTIONS

Store in a cool, dark place (not in a bathroom medicine cabinet).

STOPPING OR INTERRUPTING THERAPY

Since this drug does not cure high blood pressure but only controls it, you may have to take this medicine for the rest of your life. Do not stop taking it, even if you feel better. If you miss a dose, take it as soon as possible. If it is almost time for your next dose, skip the missed dose and resume your regular schedule. Do not take two doses at the same time.

SPECIAL CONSIDERATIONS FOR THOSE OVER SIXTY-FIVE

Older people are more likely to develop dizziness; light-headedness; fainting; and signs of potassium loss, such as irregular heartbeat, weak pulse, and tiredness or weakness. Thus, doctors may require regular checkups.

CONDITION: **HYPERTENSION**

CATEGORY: **DIURETIC-NONDIURETIC COMBINATIONS**

GENERIC (CHEMICAL) NAME	BRAND (TRADE) NAME	DOSAGE FORMS AND STRENGTHS
Clonidine and chlorthalidone	COMBIPRES	Tablets: 0.1, 0.2, or 0.3 mg clonidine and 15 mg chlorthalidone

DRUG PROFILE

This combination of an antihypertensive agent (clonidine) and a thiazide diuretic (chlorthalidone) is used to lower high blood pressure. Clonidine slows the heart rate and relaxes the muscles of the blood vessels so that the blood can flow more freely. The thiazides' main action is to increase the amount of salt and water eliminated by the body through urination. (See Clonidine on pages 65–69 and Thiazide and Thiazide-type Diuretics on pages 23–27.)

BEFORE USING THIS DRUG

Let your doctor know *IF*

You have ever had allergic reactions or other problems with ■ clonidine ■ thiazide or thiazide-type diuretics ■ sulfonamides (sulfa drugs).

You have ever had any of the following medical problems: ■ diabetes ■ gout ■ heart or blood vessel disease ■ problems with your veins ■ kidney disease ■ liver disease ■ systemic lupus erythematosus ■ depression ■ disease of the pancreas ■ Raynaud's syndrome (poor circulation in the fingers and toes).

You are taking any of the following medicines: ■ diuretics or other medicines for high blood pressure, especially beta-blockers ■ corticosteroids or corticotropin (ACTH) ■ medicine for seizures ■ anticoagulants (blood thinners) ■ medicine for depression ■ lithium ■ antihistamines ■ medicine for hay fever, allergies, sinus problems, or colds ■ barbiturates ■ sedatives ■ tranquilizers ■ sleep medicines ■ medicine for gout ■ muscle relaxants ■ narcotics or other prescription pain-killers ■ methenamine or nalidixic acid (medicines to prevent urinary tract infections) ■ medicine for Parkinson's disease ■ digoxin, digitoxin, or digitalis (heart medicines) ■ medicine for arthritis ■ fenfluramine (appetite suppressant) ■ methoxsalen or trioxsalen (medicines for vitiligo and psoriasis).

SPECIAL RESTRICTIONS WHILE TAKING THIS DRUG

FOOD AND DRUG INTERACTIONS

Other Drugs	Do not take any other drugs including over-the-counter (OTC) drugs, before checking with your doctor. OTC drugs for appetite suppression, asthma, colds, cough, hay fever, or sinus problems tend to increase blood pressure. Antihistamines, sleep medicines, tranquilizers, pain-killers, barbiturates, medicine for seizures, muscle relaxants, or anesthetics may worsen side effects of this drug such as dizziness, light-headedness, drowsiness, or fainting.
Foods and Beverages	Your doctor may prescribe a special low-salt diet, which you should follow carefully because it will help your medicine work more effectively. A weight-reduction diet may also be advised.
	This drug may cause your body to lose large amounts of the mineral potassium. Your doctor may give you special instructions about eating foods or drinking beverages that have a high potassium content (such as bananas and citrus fruit juices), taking a potassium supplement, or using salt substitutes.
Alcohol	Drinking alcohol while taking this medicine may worsen such side effects as dizziness or drowsiness. Avoid alcohol unless your doctor has approved its use.

No special restrictions on smoking.

DAILY LIVING

Driving	This drug may cause drowsiness. Be careful when driving, operating household appliances, or doing any other tasks that require alertness until you know how this drug affects you.
Exertion and Exercise	Use caution when exercising, exerting yourself, or standing for long periods of time because this drug may cause you to become dizzy, light-headed, or faint. If you feel any of these symptoms coming on, sit or lie down. It is a good idea not to get up too quickly from a reclining or sitting position.
Sun Exposure/ Excessive Heat	Your skin may become more sensitive to sunlight and more likely to develop a sunburn while you are taking this medicine. It is a good idea to avoid too much sun, especially if you burn easily. Apply a sunscreen to exposed skin surfaces before going outdoors. Use caution during hot weather or while taking saunas or hot baths, since excessive sweating while taking this medicine may cause you to become dehydrated and to feel drowsy or faint.
Examinations or Tests	Many people have high blood pressure with no symptoms at all. It is important for you to keep all appointments with your doctor, even if you feel well, so that your blood pressure can be checked regularly. Periodic blood, urine, and eye tests may be required.
Other Precautions	If you have diabetes, be aware that this medicine may raise blood-sugar levels. If you notice any change when testing sugar levels in your blood or urine, let your doctor know.

Tell any doctor or dentist you consult that you are taking this medicine, especially if you will be undergoing any type of surgery. |

When first starting on this type of medicine, you may feel tired and will probably experience both greater volume and frequency of urination. Until your individual pattern of urination has been established with this medicine, it may be wise to time carefully any activity that will put you out of convenient reach of a bathroom, such as bus or car travel. In addition, taking a diuretic at bedtime will probably interfere with sleep; you should discuss your dosage schedule with your doctor.

Check with your doctor if you become ill with flulike symptoms, such as cough, fever, or body aches; lose your appetite; vomit; or have diarrhea. This may cause you to lose a great deal of fluid, making it important not to take this drug for one or more doses.

No special restrictions on exposure to excessive cold.

POSSIBLE SIDE EFFECTS

Although this list of adverse effects may seem somewhat intimidating, keep in mind that some are quite rare. Of course, should these or any other problems arise while you are on medication, it is always a good idea to consult your doctor.

IF YOU DEVELOP

difficulty in breathing ■ extreme dizziness or fainting ■ irregular or slow heartbeat ■ palpitations ■ vomiting ■ tiredness or weakness ■ depression ■ nervousness ■ severe diarrhea ■ severe stomach pain or cramps ■ dry mouth ■ increased thirst ■ mood or mental changes ■ muscle cramps or pain ■ weak pulse ■ joint or side pain ■ decreased urination ■ pain in urination

After you STOP taking this medicine: anxiety ■ chest pain ■ sleep disturbances ■ nervousness ■ flushing ■ headache ■ increased salivation ■ upset stomach ■ stomach cramps ■ irregular or

WHAT TO DO

Urgent Get in touch with your doctor immediately.

fast heartbeat ■ shaking of hands or fingers ■ increased sweating ■ muscle pain

---

swelling of feet or lower legs ■ cold fingertips or toes ■ rash or itching ■ sore throat or fever ■ bleeding or bruising ■ vivid dreams or nightmares ■ yellowing of eyes or skin ■ changes in vision ■ hallucinations	**May be serious** Check with your doctor as soon as possible.

---

constipation ■ diarrhea ■ drowsiness ■ sexual problems ■ sleep disturbances ■ dizziness, lightheadedness, or fainting, especially when getting up from a reclining or sitting position ■ upset stomach ■ nausea or vomiting ■ ear pain ■ headache ■ taste changes ■ increased skin sensitivity to sunlight ■ loss of appetite ■ weight gain ■ paleness ■ hair loss ■ dry nasal passages ■ dry, itching, or burning eyes ■ bone pain ■ tenderness of the salivary glands (around the ear) ■ urinary retention or difficulty in urination ■ need to urinate at night	If symptoms are disturbing or persist, let your doctor know.

STORAGE INSTRUCTIONS

Store in a cool, dark place (not in a bathroom medicine cabinet).

STOPPING OR INTERRUPTING THERAPY

Since this drug does not cure high blood pressure but only controls it, you may have to take this medicine for the rest of your life. *Do not stop taking it, even if you feel better.* If you miss a dose, take it as soon as possible. Then continue on your regular schedule. If you miss two doses in a row, check with your doctor right away. *Abruptly stopping this medicine can cause your blood pressure to rise rapidly, which could be dangerous to your health.* Your doctor will advise you on how to reduce your dosage gradually before stopping completely. Always make sure you have an adequate supply of this drug on hand.

SPECIAL CONSIDERATIONS FOR THOSE OVER SIXTY-FIVE

The side effects of drowsiness, dizziness, or fainting are more likely to occur in older people.

CONDITION: **HYPERTENSION**

CATEGORY: **DIURETIC-NONDIURETIC COMBINATIONS**

GENERIC (CHEMICAL) NAME	BRAND (TRADE) NAME	DOSAGE FORMS AND STRENGTHS
Guanethidine and hydrochlorothiazide	ESIMIL	Tablets: 10 mg guanethidine and 25 mg hydrochlorothiazide

DRUG PROFILE

This medicine is a combination of two kinds of drugs that lower blood pressure—an antihypertensive agent (guanethidine) and a thiazide diuretic (hydrochlorothiazide). Guanethidine causes the muscles of the blood vessels to relax so that the blood can flow more freely. The thiazides' main action is to increase the amount of salt and water eliminated by the body through urination. (See Guanethidine on pages 86–89 and Thiazide and Thiazide-type Diuretics on pages 23–27.)

BEFORE USING THIS DRUG

Let your doctor know *IF*

You have ever had allergic reactions or other problems with ■ guanethidine ■ thiazide or thiazide-type diuretics ■ sulfonamides (sulfa drugs).

You have ever had any of the following medical problems: ■ allergies ■ asthma ■ diabetes ■ diarrhea ■ fever ■ gout ■ heart or blood vessel disease, especially a recent heart attack or stroke ■ systemic lupus erythematosus ■ kidney disease ■ liver disease ■ disease of the pancreas ■ pheochromocytoma (adrenal gland tumor) ■ stomach ulcer.

You are taking any of the following medicines: ■ diuretics or any other medicines for high blood pressure ■ corticosteroids or corticotropin (ACTH) ■ amphetamines ■ anticoagulants (blood thinners) ■ medicine for depression ■ medicine for high cholesterol ■ digoxin, digitoxin, or digitalis (heart medicines) ■ dilitiazem, nifedipine, or verapamil (calcium blockers) ■ nitrates (medicine for chest pain) ■ barbiturates ■ medicine for diabetes ■ medicine for gout ■ lithium ■ tranquilizers ■ medicine for nausea ■ ephedrine (medicine for asthma or bronchitis) ■ decongestants ■ medicine for narcolepsy ■ narcotics or other prescription pain-killers ■ weight-reduction medicines ■ methenamine (medicine to prevent urinary tract infections) ■ levodopa (medicine for Parkinson's disease) ■ tetracycline.

You have ever undergone sympathectomy.

SPECIAL RESTRICTIONS WHILE TAKING THIS DRUG

FOOD AND DRUG INTERACTIONS

Other Drugs	Do not take any other drugs, including over-the-counter (OTC) drugs, before checking with your doctor. OTC drugs for appetite suppression, asthma, colds, cough, hay fever, or sinus problems tend to increase blood pressure. Use of reserpine or rauwolfia at the same time as guanethidine may cause fainting, slow heartbeat, and depression. Stimulants, antidepressants, and tranquilizers may reduce the antihypertensive effectiveness of guanethidine. Barbiturates and narcotic pain-killers may worsen the side effects of dizziness and faintness.
Foods and Beverages	Your doctor may prescribe a special low-salt diet, which you should follow carefully because it will help your medicine work more effectively. You may also be advised to go on a weight-reduction diet. This drug may cause your body to lose large amounts of the mineral potassium. Your doctor may give you special instructions about eating foods or drinking beverages that have a high potassium content (such as bananas and citrus fruit juices), taking a potassium supplement, or using salt substitutes.

Alcohol	Drinking alcohol while taking this medicine may worsen such side effects as dizziness or drowsiness. Avoid alcohol unless your doctor has approved its use.

No special restrictions on smoking.

DAILY LIVING

Exertion and Exercise	Use caution when exercising or standing for long periods of time because this drug may cause you to become dizzy, light-headed, or faint. If you feel any of these symptoms coming on, sit or lie down.
Sun Exposure/ Excessive Heat	Your skin may become more sensitive to sunlight and more likely to develop a sunburn while you are taking this medicine. It is a good idea to avoid too much sun, especially if you burn easily. Apply a sunscreen to exposed skin surfaces before going outdoors. Use caution during hot weather or while taking saunas or hot baths, since excessive sweating while taking this medicine may cause you to become dehydrated and to feel drowsy or faint.
Examinations or Tests	Many people have high blood pressure with no symptoms at all. It is important for you to keep all appointments with your doctor, even if you feel well, so that your blood pressure can be checked regularly. Periodic blood and urine tests may be required.
Other Precautions	If you have diabetes, be aware that this medicine may raise blood-sugar levels. If you notice any change when testing sugar levels in your blood or urine, let your doctor know.
	Tell any doctor or dentist you consult that you are taking this medicine, especially if you will be undergoing any type of surgery.

When first starting on this type of medicine, you may feel tired and will probably experience both greater volume and frequency of urination. Until your individual pattern of urination has been established with this medicine, it may be wise to time carefully any activity that will put you out of convenient reach of a bathroom, such as bus or car travel. In addition, taking a diuretic at bedtime will probably interfere with sleep; you should discuss your dosage schedule with your doctor.

Check with your doctor if you become ill with flulike symptoms, such as cough, fever, or body aches; lose your appetite, vomit; or have diarrhea. This may cause you to lose a great deal of fluid, making it important not to take this drug for one or more doses.

No special restrictions on driving or exposure to excessive cold.

POSSIBLE SIDE EFFECTS

Although this list of adverse effects may seem somewhat intimidating, keep in mind that some are quite rare. Of course, should these or any other problems arise while you are on medication, it is always a good idea to consult your doctor.

IF YOU DEVELOP

severe vomiting or diarrhea ■ dry mouth ■ increased thirst ■ irregular heartbeat ■ confusion ■ depression ■ muscle cramps or pain ■ weak pulse ■ tiredness or weakness ■ chest pain ■ severe stomach pain or cramps ■ joint or side pain ■ difficulty in breathing ■ decreased urination

WHAT TO DO

Urgent Get in touch with your doctor immediately.

sore throat or fever ■ headache ■ rash or hives ■ bleeding or bruising ■ yellowing of eyes or skin ■ weight gain ■ swelling of feet or lower legs

May be serious Check with your doctor as soon as possible.

diarrhea or increased bowel movements ■ dizziness, light-headedness, or fainting, especially when getting up from a reclining or sitting position ■ difficulty in ejaculation (in males) ■ stuffy nose ■ slow heartbeat ■ blurred vision ■ drooping eyelids ■ increased skin sensitivity to sunlight ■ loss of appetite ■ upset stomach ■ hair loss ■ need to urinate at night or other urinary problems ■ tenderness of the salivary glands (around the ear)

If symptoms are disturbing or persist, let your doctor know.

STORAGE INSTRUCTIONS

Store in a cool, dark place (not in a bathroom medicine cabinet).

STOPPING OR INTERRUPTING THERAPY

Since this drug does not cure high blood pressure but only controls it, you may have to take this medicine for the rest of your life. Do not stop taking it, even if you feel better. If you miss a dose, take it as soon as possible. If it is almost time for your next dose, skip the missed dose and resume your regular schedule. Do not take two doses at the same time.

SPECIAL CONSIDERATIONS FOR THOSE OVER SIXTY-FIVE

Older people are more likely to develop dizziness; light-headedness; fainting; and signs of potassium loss, such as irregular heartbeat, weak pulse, and tiredness or weakness.

CONDITION: **HYPERTENSION**

CATEGORY: **DIURETIC-NONDIURETIC COMBINATIONS**

GENERIC (CHEMICAL) NAME	BRAND (TRADE) NAME	DOSAGE FORMS AND STRENGTHS
Prazosin and polythiazide	MINIZIDE	Capsules: 1, 2, 5 mg prazosin and 0.5 mg polythiazide

DRUG PROFILE

This combination of an antihypertensive agent (prazosin) and a thiazide diuretic (polythiazide) is used to lower high blood pressure. Prazosin relaxes the muscles of the blood vessels so that the blood can flow more freely. The thiazides' main action is to increase the amount of salt and water eliminated by the body through urination. (See Prazosin on pages 78–81 and Thiazide and Thiazide-type Diuretics on pages 23–27.)

BEFORE USING THIS DRUG

Let your doctor know *IF*

You have ever had allergic reactions or other problems with ■ prazosin ■ thiazide or thiazide-type diuretics ■ sulfonamides (sulfa drugs).

You have ever had any of the following medical problems: ■ allergy ■ asthma ■ angina (chest pain) ■ diabetes ■ gout ■ heart disease ■ kidney disease ■ liver disease ■ systemic lupus erythematosus ■ disease of the pancreas.

You are taking any of the following medicines: ■ diuretics or other medicine for high blood pressure, especially beta-blockers ■ corticosteroids or corticotropin (ACTH) ■ medicine for diabetes ■ medicine for gout ■ lithium ■ muscle relaxants ■ tetracycline ■ medicine for high cholesterol ■ digoxin, digitoxin, or digitalis (heart medicines) ■ anticoagulants (blood thinners) ■ methenamine (medicine to prevent urinary tract infections).

You have ever undergone sympathectomy.

SPECIAL RESTRICTIONS WHILE TAKING THIS DRUG

FOOD AND DRUG INTERACTIONS

Other Drugs	Do not take any other drugs, including over-the-counter (OTC) drugs, before checking with your doctor. OTC drugs for appetite suppression, asthma, colds, cough, hay fever, or sinus problems tend to increase blood pressure.
	Barbiturates or narcotic pain-killers may worsen the side effect of dizziness.

Foods and Beverages	Your doctor may prescribe a special low-salt diet, which you should follow carefully because it will help your medicine work more effectively. You may also be advised to go on a weight-reduction diet. This drug may cause your body to lose large amounts of the mineral potassium. Your doctor may give you special instructions about eating foods or drinking beverages that have a high potassium content (such as bananas and citrus fruit juices), taking a potassium supplement, or using salt substitutes.
Alcohol	Drinking alcohol while you are taking this medicine may worsen such side effects as dizziness or drowsiness. Avoid alcohol unless your doctor has approved its use.

No special restrictions on smoking.

DAILY LIVING

Driving	This drug may make you dizzy. Use caution when driving, operating household appliances, or doing any other tasks that require alertness until you know how this drug affects you.
Exertion and Exercise	Use caution when exercising, exerting yourself, or standing for long periods of time because this medicine may cause you to become dizzy, light-headed, or faint. If you feel any of these symptoms coming on, sit or lie down. It is a good idea not to get up too quickly from a reclining or sitting position.
Sun Exposure/ Excessive Heat	Your skin may become more sensitive to sunlight and more likely to develop a sunburn while you are taking this medicine. It is a good idea to avoid too much sun, especially if you burn easily. Apply a sunscreen to exposed skin surfaces before going outdoors. Use caution during hot weather or while taking saunas or

hot baths, since excessive sweating while taking this medicine may cause you to become dehydrated and to feel drowsy or faint.

Examinations or Tests	Many people have high blood pressure with no symptoms at all. It is important for you to keep all appointments with your doctor, even if you feel well, so that your blood pressure can be checked regularly. Periodic blood and urine tests may be required.
Other Precautions	You may feel faint or actually lose consciousness after taking the first dose of this drug or if there has been a significant increase in your dose. Your doctor may suggest that you take your first dose in his or her office.

If you have diabetes, be aware that this medicine may raise blood-sugar levels. If you notice any change when testing sugar levels in your blood or urine, let your doctor know.

Tell any doctor or dentist you consult that you are taking this medicine, especially if you will be undergoing any type of surgery.

When first starting on this type of medicine, you may feel tired and will probably experience both greater volume and frequency of urination. Until your individual pattern of urination has been established with this medicine, it may be wise to time carefully any activity that will put you out of convenient reach of a bathroom, such as bus or car travel. In addition, taking a diuretic at bedtime will probably interfere with sleep; you should discuss your dosage schedule with your doctor.

Check with your doctor if you become ill with flulike symptoms, such as cough, fever, or body aches; lose your appetite; vomit; or have diarrhea. This may cause you to lose a great deal of fluid, making it important not to take this drug for one or more doses.

No special restrictions on exposure to excessive cold.

POSSIBLE SIDE EFFECTS

Although this list of adverse effects may seem somewhat intimidating, keep in mind that some are quite rare. Of course, should these or any other problems arise while you are on medication, it is always a good idea to consult your doctor.

IF YOU DEVELOP

severe nausea or vomiting ■ dry mouth ■ increased thirst ■ irregular heartbeat ■ palpitations ■ mood or mental changes ■ muscle cramps or pain ■ weak pulse ■ weakness ■ chest pain ■ shortness of breath

WHAT TO DO

Urgent Get in touch with your doctor immediately.

---

dizziness or light-headedness, especially when getting up from a reclining or sitting position ■ fainting ■ swelling of feet or lower legs ■ weight gain ■ difficulty in urination ■ joint, stomach, or side pain ■ numbness or tingling in hands or feet ■ rash or hives ■ sore throat or fever ■ bleeding or bruising ■ yellowing of eyes or skin

May be serious Check with your doctor as soon as possible.

---

diarrhea ■ constipation ■ vomiting ■ headache ■ loss of appetite ■ increased skin sensitivity to sunlight ■ tiredness ■ upset stomach ■ hair loss ■ nervousness ■ male impotence ■ blurred vision ■ ringing in ears ■ red eyes ■ stuffy nose ■ increased sweating

If symptoms are disturbing or persist, let your doctor know.

STORAGE INSTRUCTIONS

Store in a cool, dark place (not in a bathroom medicine cabinet).

STOPPING OR INTERRUPTING THERAPY

Since this drug does not cure high blood pressure but only controls it, you may have to take this medicine for the rest of your life. Do not stop taking it, even if you feel better. If you miss a dose, take it as soon as possible. If it is almost time for your next dose, skip the missed dose and resume your regular schedule. Do not take two doses at the same time.

SPECIAL CONSIDERATIONS FOR THOSE OVER SIXTY-FIVE

Older people are more likely to develop dizziness; light-headedness; fainting; and signs of potassium loss, such as irregular heartbeat, weak pulse, and tiredness or weakness. Thus, doctors may require regular checkups.

ANGINA

You probably saw the treatment before you even heard of the disease. A character in a movie, looking pained, furtively slips a pill under his tongue. One scene later, he is laid up in the hospital with a cardiac condition signaled by the pain of angina.

CAUSES

In real life, angina doesn't have to land you in the hospital, but the pain associated with it is all too real. Angina actually is a temporary, recurring pain or tightness in the chest, often radiating to the arms, neck, jaw, or back. It is usually caused by either a spasm or a blockage of the coronary arteries—the large blood vessels that carry oxygen to the heart—or both. As people grow older, their coronary arteries tend to accumulate fatty deposits known as plaques, which may cause narrowings in the arteries and can ultimately prevent an adequate supply of blood (and, consequently, oxygen) from reaching the heart. This lack of oxygen may cause the pain of angina. (Sometimes chest pain does not occur, even when the heart is not being supplied with enough oxygen. This condition, called silent ischemia, is more common in people with diabetes and in older people.)

About 6 percent of men and 3 percent of women over fifty have angina. Although the condition can be both frightening and debilitating, several forms of treatment are available to bring it under control. Before prescribing treatment, however, your doctor must determine what type of angina you have by learning as much as possible about your symptoms and by performing diagnostic tests.

TYPES OF ANGINA

Chest pain, although the hallmark of angina, is not its only symptom. Angina can also be associated with shortness of breath, dizziness, indigestion, and numbness in the arms and hands. In general, all these symptoms usually follow one of three patterns:

• Classic angina is brought on by physical exertion, emotional stress, or any other factor that causes the heart to work harder than usual. This most common type of angina is always caused by coronary artery disease.

• Variant angina flares up during rest or moderate, unstressful activity and appears to be caused by a spasm in a coronary artery rather than by coronary artery disease.

• Unstable angina, the most serious form of angina, occurs when a patient with classic angina begins to suffer from more serious symptoms, for example, if the attacks occur more frequently, last longer, are more severe, or occur when the patient is sedentary or asleep.

Heart attacks are more common in people with unstable angina, so this form of angina requires especially prompt treatment, often including hospitalization until the episodes are under control.

DIAGNOSIS

If you visit your doctor because of chest pain, one of the first things he or she will do is hook you up to an electrocardiogram (ECG) machine, which will record the pattern of electrical activity in your heart. This test will help determine whether you have had a heart attack or are experiencing episodes of angina. However, it is important to know that the ECG is often normal between anginal attacks, and sometimes even during an attack. In the meantime, other possible causes of angina symptoms will be ruled out. Arthritis and certain digestive disorders, for example, can mimic angina, as can muscle disorders and infections. It's important to remember that not all chest pain is a signal of heart disease.

After the initial ECG, the doctor may ask you to take an exercise stress test. In this test, you will exercise on a treadmill while hooked up to an ECG machine. If the ECG shows abnormalities, further tests may be needed.

One of these tests, a radionuclide stress evaluation, helps the doctor see where your coronary arteries may be obstructed. This test involves injecting a radioactive substance into a vein immediately following exercise, then obtaining an image of the heart with a special machine. By tracking the radioactive material through the image, the doctor can pinpoint obstructions in the arteries.

A more complicated test called a coronary angiogram can also help locate constricted areas in the arteries, as well as determine the severity of the blockage. In this procedure, the doctor injects dye into the coronary arteries through a catheter that is inserted into an artery in the leg or arm. Through electronic images of the heart, it is possible to see the movement of the dye through the arteries.

TREATMENT

Drug treatment usually begins as soon as noncardiac causes of chest pain are ruled out. For detailed information on the most common treatments for angina—the nitrates, the beta-blockers, the calcium blockers, and dipyridamole—see the charts on pages 138–159.

If your angina does not improve with drug treatment, your doctor may recommend angioplasty or bypass surgery. These procedures are commonly used to relieve angina and improve the underlying heart disease. In coronary angioplasty, the doctor passes a balloon into a coronary artery and inflates the balloon, expanding the artery. In coronary artery bypass surgery, the doctor uses a vein graft removed from a leg to bypass a blockage in a coronary artery. Both techniques have been used with success in older people.

OUTLOOK

With or without surgery, your doctor will probably recommend that, in addition to taking medicine, you try to lose any excess weight. Some people may also benefit from a medically supervised exercise program. You should also stop smoking. It is important to avoid stressful situations that may provoke attacks. Most people with angina can be effectively treated through a combination of drugs and lifestyle changes.

CONDITION: **ANGINA**

CATEGORY: **NITRATES**

GENERIC (CHEMICAL) NAME	BRAND (TRADE) NAME	DOSAGE FORMS AND STRENGTHS
Isosorbide dinitrate	DILATRATE-SR	Controlled-release capsules: 40 mg
	ISORDIL	Chewable tablets: 10 mg Controlled-release capsules: 40 mg Controlled-release tablets: 40 mg Sublingual tablets: 2.5, 5, 10 mg Tablets: 5, 10, 20, 30, 40 mg
	SORBITRATE	Chewable tablets: 5, 10 mg Controlled-release tablets: 40 mg Sublingual tablets: 2.5, 5, 10 mg Tablets: 5, 10, 20, 30, 40 mg
Nitroglycerin	NITROBID	Controlled-release capsules: 2.5, 6.5, 9 mg Ointment: 2%
	NITRODISC	Disc: 5, 10 mg per 24 hours
	NITRO-DUR	Skin patch: 2.5, 5, 7.5, 10 mg per 24 hours
	NITROL	Ointment: 2%
	NITROLINGUAL	Spray: 0.4 mg/spray
	NITROSTAT	Controlled-release capsules: 2.5, 6.5, 9 mg Ointment: 2% Sublingual tablets: 0.15, 0.3, 0.4, 0.6 mg
	TRANSDERM-NITRO	Skin patch: 2.5, 5, 10, 15 mg per 24 hours

DRUG PROFILE

Nitrates are used to treat angina pectoris (chest pain) and to prevent angina attacks. These drugs relax the blood vessels and increase the supply of blood and oxygen to the heart. At the same time, they reduce the workload and oxygen demands of the heart. The nitrates are available in a number of dosage forms. Fast-acting nitrates—sublingual (under the tongue), buccal (in the cheek or under the lip), chewable tablets, or spray—are used both to relieve an ongoing angina attack and to prevent angina. The slower-acting dosage forms (controlled-release capsules or tablets that are swallowed, skin ointments, or patches) are taken only to prevent angina. If needed, a fast-acting nitrate may be used to supplement a longer-acting one.

BEFORE USING THIS DRUG

Let your doctor know *IF*

You have ever had allergic reactions or other problems with ■ nitrates or nitrites.

You have ever had any of the following medical problems: ■ anemia ■ overactive thyroid ■ recent heart attack ■ stroke ■ head trauma (such as a blow to the head) ■ migraine or other vascular headaches ■ congestive heart failure ■ glaucoma ■ low blood pressure ■ diarrhea, loose stools, or other intestinal problems.

You are taking any of the following medicines: ■ diuretics or other medicines for high blood pressure ■ any other heart medicine, including nitrates and nitrites ■ medicine for asthma ■ medicine for colds, hay fever, or sinus problems ■ tranquilizers ■ medicine for nausea ■ appetite suppressants ■ diltiazem, nifedipine, or verapamil (calcium blockers) ■ narcotics or other prescription pain-killers.

You are often exposed to organic nitrates (e.g., you work in a plant that processes organic nitrates).

SPECIAL RESTRICTIONS WHILE TAKING THIS DRUG

FOOD AND DRUG INTERACTIONS

Other Drugs	Diuretics and other medicines for high blood pressure, calcium blockers (heart medicines), phenothiazines (tranquilizers), and narcotics and prescription pain-killers may increase the side effects of dizziness or faintness when taken with nitrates.

Foods and Beverages	Angina may be provoked by eating a meal that is too heavy.
Alcohol	Drinking alcohol while taking nitrate medicine may worsen such side effects as dizziness, light-headedness, or fainting. Avoid alcohol unless your doctor has approved its use.
Smoking	Smoking increases your chance of having an angina attack. If you smoke, try to stop or at least cut down.

DAILY LIVING

Exertion and Exercise	Use caution when exercising or if you must stand for long periods of time because this type of medicine may cause dizziness, light-headedness, or weakness. To prevent exercise-induced angina, take a chewable or sublingual tablet ten minutes before beginning exercise.
Excessive Heat	Use caution during hot weather, especially if you exert yourself, as this drug may cause dizziness, weakness, or light-headedness.
Excessive Cold	Use caution during cold weather, since excessive cold may provoke an angina attack. Your doctor may recommend that you take a chewable sublingual tablet before exposure to excessive cold.
Examinations or Tests	It is important for you to keep all appointments with your doctor, even if you feel well, so that your progress can be checked.
Other Precautions	Emotional stress may trigger an angina attack.

If you are taking nitrate tablets and notice partially dissolved tablets in your stool, let your doctor know; you may not be receiving the correct amount of your medicine.

Helpful Hints

Capsules and tablets to be swallowed. Take with a full glass of water on an empty stomach. Do not break, crush, or chew tablets or capsules.

Chewable tablets. Chew well and hold in your mouth for about two minutes. For relief of an angina attack, you may take up to three tablets over a thirty-minute period. If you still have chest pain, call your doctor or get to a hospital emergency room immediately, as you may be experiencing a heart attack.

Sublingual tablets. Do not eat, drink, or smoke while a tablet is dissolving. For relief of an angina attack, you may take up to three tablets over a fifteen-minute period. If you still have chest pain, call your doctor or get to a hospital emergency room immediately.

Buccal tablets. Allow the tablet to dissolve slowly between the cheek and gum or lower lip and gum. If you eat or drink, transfer the tablet to between the upper lip and gum. If you still feel chest pain after five minutes, call your doctor.

Ointment. Before applying a new dose, clean off any ointment remaining from the previous dose. Apply ointment in a thin, even layer to a clean area of the skin; do not massage in. To prevent irritation, apply ointment to a different area each time. Your doctor may instruct you to use an occlusive wrapping; follow instructions carefully.

Skin patch. Apply the patch to a clean, dry, hairless area of skin (not near hands or feet). If a patch becomes loose or falls off, apply a new one. If you miss a dose, apply it as soon as possible, and then go back to your regular schedule.

Spray. Sit down, if possible, holding the canister upright and the spray opening as close to the mouth as possible. Press the grooved button firmly to release the spray onto or under the tongue, and close your mouth immediately. Do not inhale for five to ten seconds and hold the vapor in your mouth for thirty to sixty seconds before swallowing. If you are taking this medicine for an attack and the chest pain persists, call your doctor or get to a hospital emergency room immediately.

For relief of angina attack. Sit down before you take your fast-acting medicine. If you feel dizzy or faint after taking the medicine, bend forward, put your head between your knees, and breathe deeply. You should feel relief from angina pain within one to five minutes.

To prevent angina attack: Factors that trigger angina include emotional stress, eating a heavy meal, smoking, and cold weather (see "Food and Drug Interactions" and "Daily Living"). If you anticipate being in a trigger situation, take a chewable or sublingual tablet five to ten minutes beforehand.

Headaches. You may experience either mild or severe headache with nitrate medicines, which should decrease in frequency and severity with continued therapy. If aspirin, acetaminophen, or ibuprofen does not control your headache, your doctor may be able to decrease your nitrate dose. If you are using an oral form, it may help to take your medicine with meals.

No special restrictions on driving or sun exposure.

POSSIBLE SIDE EFFECTS

Although this list of adverse effects may seem somewhat intimidating, keep in mind that some are quite rare. Of course, should these or any other problems arise while you are on medication, it is always a good idea to consult your doctor.

IF YOU DEVELOP	**WHAT TO DO**
collapse ■ blurred vision ■ cold sweat ■ inability to control urination or bowel movements ■ confusion (that persists even after fifteen minutes of lying down)	**Urgent** Get in touch with your doctor immediately.
rash ■ dry mouth ■ swelling of hands, feet, or ankles	**May be serious** Check with your doctor as soon as possible.
dizziness, light-headedness, or fainting, especially when getting up from a reclining or sitting position ■ headache ■ flushing of face, neck, and chest ■ upset stomach ■ nausea or vomiting ■ fast heartbeat ■ restlessness ■ weakness ■ paleness	If symptoms are disturbing or persist, let your doctor know.

STORAGE INSTRUCTIONS

Store in a cool, dark place (not in a bathroom medicine cabinet). For sublingual tablets, remove the cotton plug that comes with the bottle and keep the medicine in its original container. Pick up only the tablet you are about to take, and replace the bottle cap quickly and tightly.

Doctors generally recommend that you keep a small supply of nitroglycerin tablets with you at all times in case of an emergency. Specially designed containers are available for this purpose so that you can avoid handling the original bottle too often, since this may destroy the potency of its contents before the expiration date.

INTERRUPTING OR STOPPING THERAPY

If you are taking this medicine on a regular schedule, abruptly stopping can bring on angina attacks. Your doctor will advise you on how to reduce your dose gradually before stopping completely. If you miss a dose, take it as soon as possible unless your next scheduled dose is within two hours (chewable tablets) or six hours (controlled-release capsules or tablets). In that case, return to your regular schedule. Do not take two doses at the same time.

SPECIAL CONSIDERATIONS FOR THOSE OVER SIXTY-FIVE

The side effects of dizziness and light-headedness, especially when getting up from a reclining or sitting position, are more likely to occur in older people.

CONDITION:　**ANGINA**

CATEGORY:　**BETA-BLOCKERS**

GENERIC (CHEMICAL) NAME	BRAND (TRADE) NAME	DOSAGE FORMS AND STRENGTHS
Acebutolol	SECTRAL	Capsules: 200, 400 mg
Atenolol	TENORMIN	Tablets: 50, 100 mg
Labetalol hydrochloride	NORMODYNE TRANDATE	Tablets: 100, 200, 300 mg Tablets: 100, 200, 300 mg
Metoprolol tartrate	LOPRESSOR	Tablets: 50, 100 mg
Nadolol	CORGARD	Tablets: 40, 80, 120, 160 mg
Pindolol	VISKEN	Tablets: 5, 10 mg
Propranolol hydrochloride	INDERAL INDERAL LA	Tablets: 10, 20, 40, 60, 80, 90 mg Capsules: 80, 120, 160 mg
Timolol maleate	BLOCADREN	Tablets: 5, 10, 20 mg

DRUG PROFILE

Beta-adrenergic blocking drugs (beta-blockers) are a group of relatively new drugs that are used to control high blood pressure. By blocking certain nerve impulses, these medicines relax blood vessels, increase the supply of blood and oxygen to the heart, reduce the workload of the heart, and help the heart beat more regularly. Because of these effects, some beta-blockers are also useful for other conditions, such as angina, arrhythmias, migraine headaches, and hypertrophic subaortic stenosis (a disease of the heart muscle). They have also been found to improve a person's chance of survival for several years following a heart attack.

When used in the treatment of angina, beta-blockers prevent future attacks (they are not helpful during an acute attack of chest pain). Beta-blockers differ in the duration of action and when their peak effect occurs, and it is worthwhile to discuss with your doctor precisely how to time your doses in relation to the pattern of your attacks. If you suffer a side effect, such as depression or nightmares, with one beta-blocker, your doctor may be able to prescribe a different beta-blocker that will be equally effective. Beta-blockers may be used along with other anti-angina medicines.

For complete information on these drugs, see pages 56–61.

CONDITION: **ANGINA**

CATEGORY: **CALCIUM BLOCKERS**

GENERIC (CHEMICAL) NAME	BRAND (TRADE) NAME	DOSAGE FORMS AND STRENGTHS
Diltiazem	CARDIZEM	Tablets: 30, 60, 90, 120 mg

DRUG PROFILE

The calcium blockers are used to relieve and control angina pectoris (chest pain). Calcium is needed for muscle cells to contract; by decreasing the passage of calcium into the muscle cells, these drugs relax the blood vessels and heart muscle. This increases the supply of blood and oxygen to the heart, reduces its workload, and prevents spasms of the blood vessels of the heart. Other antianginal drugs can be used along with a calcium blocker, if necessary. Calcium blockers tend to lower blood pressure; if you are also taking an antihypertensive medicine, its dosage may need to be lowered.

BEFORE USING THIS DRUG

Let your doctor know *IF*

You have ever had allergic reactions or other problems with ■ diltiazem ■ other calcium blockers.

You have ever had any of the following medical problems: ■ other heart or blood vessel disease ■ kidney disease ■ liver disease ■ any disease of the muscles ■ low blood pressure.

You are taking any of the following medicines: ■ beta-blockers or other medicines for high blood pressure or angina ■ anticoagulants (blood thinners) ■ aspirin or aspirinlike medicine ■ sulfonamides (sulfa drugs) ■ cimetidine (medicine for ulcers) ■ digoxin, digitoxin, or digitalis (heart medicines) ■ disopyramide or quinidine (medicine for abnormal heart rhythms) ■ medicine for seizures ■ medicine for malaria.

SPECIAL RESTRICTIONS WHILE TAKING THIS DRUG

FOOD AND DRUG INTERACTIONS

Foods and Beverages	Remember that angina may be provoked by eating a meal that is too heavy.
Alcohol	Drinking alcohol while taking calcium blockers may worsen such side effects as dizziness, light-headedness, or fainting. Avoid alcohol unless your doctor has approved its use.
Smoking	Smoking increases your chance of an angina attack. If you smoke, try to stop or at least cut down.

DAILY LIVING

Exertion and Exercise	Since this medicine is taken before exercise to reduce or prevent associated chest pain, you may be tempted to become overactive. You should discuss with your doctor how much exercise is safe for you.
Sun Exposure	While taking this medicine, your eyes may become more sensitive to light; wearing dark glasses when exposed to the sun should help.

Excessive Cold	Use caution during cold weather, since excessive cold may provoke an angina attack.
Examinations or Tests	It is important for you to keep all appointments with your doctor, even if you feel well, so that your progress can be monitored and your blood pressure checked. Periodic blood and urine tests may be required.
Other Precautions	Check your pulse regularly, and call your doctor if it falls below fifty beats per minute. Tell any doctor or dentist you consult that you are taking this medicine, especially if you will be undergoing any type of surgery. Remember that emotional stress may trigger an angina attack.
Helpful Hints	For best effects, take this medicine one hour before or two hours after meals. You may have headaches after taking this medicine. Headaches usually stop with continued use of the medicine; if they do not, or if they are particularly severe, call your doctor.

No special restrictions on driving or exposure to excessive heat.

POSSIBLE SIDE EFFECTS

Although this list of adverse effects may seem somewhat intimidating, keep in mind that some are quite rare. Of course, should these or any other problems arise while you are on medication, it is always a good idea to consult your doctor.

IF YOU DEVELOP	WHAT TO DO
difficulty in breathing ■ coughing or wheezing ■ chest congestion ■ irregular or slow heartbeat ■ palpitations ■ rash, hives, or itching ■ swelling of ankles, feet, or lower legs ■ fainting ■ sore throat ■ blurred vision ■ difficulty in balance ■ fever ■ chills ■ increased sweating ■ hallucinations	**May be serious** Check with your doctor as soon as possible.
flushing or feeling of warmth ■ headache ■ dizziness or light-headedness, especially when getting up from a reclining or sitting position ■ tiredness or weakness ■ drowsiness ■ depression ■ confusion ■ sleeplessness ■ giddiness ■ anxiety ■ mood changes ■ gas ■ constipation ■ nausea or vomiting ■ stomach cramps or upset stomach ■ loss of appetite ■ diarrhea ■ heartburn ■ stuffy nose ■ increased eye sensitivity to sunlight ■ muscle cramps ■ joint stiffness or swelling ■ gum problems ■ increased urination ■ need to urinate at night	If symptoms are disturbing or persist, let your doctor know.

STORAGE INSTRUCTIONS

Store in a cool, dark place (not in a bathroom medicine cabinet).

STOPPING OR INTERRUPTING THERAPY

Take this medicine exactly as directed, even if you do not feel chest pain. Do not take more of the medicine or take it more frequently than prescribed by your doctor. Suddenly stopping your medicine may worsen your medical problem. Your doctor will advise you on how to discontinue therapy gradually before stopping completely. If you miss a dose, take it as soon as possible. If it is almost time for your next dose, skip the missed dose and resume your regular schedule. Do not take two doses at the same time.

SPECIAL CONSIDERATIONS FOR THOSE OVER SIXTY-FIVE

Dizziness, light-headedness, and fainting, especially when getting up from a reclining or sitting position, are more likely to occur in older people, who may be advised to take their first dose in a situation in which they will be able to lie down, if necessary.

Also, older people tend not to eliminate the calcium blockers as readily as young adults; thus, the drug may reach high concentrations and remain in the bloodstream for a longer time. Doctors may require regular checkups to make sure that the proper dosage is being administered and that too much drug is not accumulating in the body.

CONDITION: **ANGINA**

CATEGORY: **CALCIUM BLOCKERS**

GENERIC (CHEMICAL) NAME	BRAND (TRADE) NAME	DOSAGE FORMS AND STRENGTHS
Nifedipine	PROCARDIA	Capsules: 10, 20 mg

DRUG PROFILE

The calcium blockers are used to relieve and control angina pectoris (chest pain). Calcium is needed for muscle cells to contract; by decreasing the passage of calcium into the muscle cells, these drugs relax the blood vessels and heart muscle. This increases the supply of blood and oxygen to the heart, reduces its workload, and prevents spasms of the blood vessels of the heart. Other antianginal drugs can be used along with a calcium blocker, if necessary. Calcium blockers tend to lower blood pressure; if you are also taking an antihypertensive medicine, its dosage may need to be lowered.

BEFORE USING THIS DRUG

Let your doctor know *IF*

You have ever had allergic reactions or other problems with ■ nifedipine ■ other calcium blockers.

You have ever had any of the following medical problems: ■ other heart or blood vessel disease ■ kidney disease ■ liver disease ■ any disease of the muscles ■ low blood pressure.

You are taking any of the following medicines: ■ beta-blockers or other medicines for high blood pressure or angina ■ anticoagulants (blood thinners) ■ aspirin or aspirinlike medicine ■ sulfonamides (sulfa drugs) ■ cimetidine (medicine for ulcers) ■ quinidine (medicine for abnormal heart rhythms) ■ medicine for seizures ■ medicine for malaria.

SPECIAL RESTRICTIONS WHILE TAKING THIS DRUG

FOOD AND DRUG INTERACTIONS

Foods and Beverages	Remember that angina may be provoked by eating a meal that is too heavy.
Alcohol	Drinking alcohol while taking calcium blockers may worsen such side effects as dizziness, light-headedness, or fainting. Avoid alcohol unless your doctor has approved its use.
Smoking	Smoking increases your chance of an angina attack. If you smoke, try to stop or at least cut down.

DAILY LIVING

Exertion and Exercise	Since this medicine is taken before exercise to reduce or prevent associated chest pain, you may be tempted to become overactive. You should discuss with your doctor how much exercise is safe for you.
Sun Exposure	While taking this medicine, your eyes may become more sensitive to light; wearing dark glasses when exposed to the sun should help.
Excessive Cold	Use caution during cold weather, as excessive cold may provoke an angina attack.
Examinations or Tests	It is important for you to keep all appointments with your doctor, even if you feel well, so that your

progress can be monitored and your blood pressure checked. Periodic blood and urine tests may be required.

Other Precautions	Tell any doctor or dentist you consult that you are taking this medicine, especially if you will be undergoing any type of surgery.

Remember that emotional stress may trigger an angina attack. |
| Helpful Hints | For best effects, take this medicine one hour before or two hours after meals.

You may have headaches after taking this medicine. Headaches usually stop with continued use of the medicine; if they do not, or if they are particularly severe, call your doctor. |

No special restrictions on driving or excessive heat.

POSSIBLE SIDE EFFECTS

Although this list of adverse effects may seem somewhat intimidating, keep in mind that some are quite rare. Of course, should these or any other problems arise while you are on medication, it is always a good idea to consult your doctor.

IF YOU DEVELOP

difficulty in breathing ■ coughing or wheezing ■ chest congestion ■ irregular heartbeat or palpitations ■ rash, hives, or itching ■ swelling of ankles, feet, or lower legs ■ fainting ■ sore throat ■ blurred vision ■ difficulty in balance ■ fever ■ chills ■ increased sweating ■ hallucinations

WHAT TO DO

May be serious Check with your doctor as soon as possible.

flushing or feeling of warmth ■ headache ■ dizziness or light-headedness, especially when getting up from a reclining or sitting position ■ tiredness or weakness ■ drowsiness ■ depression ■ confusion ■ sleeplessness ■ giddiness ■ anxiety ■ mood changes ■ gas ■ constipation ■ nausea or vomiting ■ stomach cramps or upset stomach ■ loss of appetite ■ diarrhea ■ heartburn ■ stuffy nose ■ increased eye sensitivity to sunlight ■ muscle cramps ■ joint stiffness or swelling ■ gum problems ■ sexual problems

If symptoms are disturbing or persist, let your doctor know.

STORAGE INSTRUCTIONS

Store in a cool, dark place (not in a bathroom medicine cabinet).

STOPPING OR INTERRUPTING THERAPY

Take this medicine exactly as directed, even if you do not feel chest pain. Do not take more of the medicine or take it more frequently than prescribed by your doctor. Suddenly stopping your medicine may worsen your medical problem. Your doctor will advise you on how to discontinue therapy gradually before stopping completely. If you miss a dose, take it as soon as possible. If it is almost time for your next dose, skip the missed dose and resume your regular schedule. Do not take two doses at the same time.

SPECIAL CONSIDERATIONS FOR THOSE OVER SIXTY-FIVE

Dizziness, light-headedness, and fainting, especially when getting up from a reclining or sitting position, are more likely to occur in older people, who may be advised to take their first dose in a situation in which they will be able to lie down, if necessary.

Also, older people tend not to eliminate the calcium blockers as rapidly as young adults; thus, the drug may reach higher concentrations and remain in the bloodstream for a longer time. Doctors may require regular checkups to make sure that the proper dosage is being administered and that too much drug is not accumulating in the body.

CONDITION: **ANGINA**

CATEGORY: **CALCIUM BLOCKERS**

GENERIC (CHEMICAL) NAME	BRAND (TRADE) NAME	DOSAGE FORMS AND STRENGTHS
Verapamil	CALAN	Tablets: 80, 120 mg
	CALAN SR	Controlled-release tablets: 240 mg
	ISOPTIN	Tablets: 80, 120 mg

DRUG PROFILE

The calcium blockers are used to relieve and control angina pectoris (chest pain). Calcium is needed for muscle cells to contract; by decreasing the passage of calcium into the muscle cells, these drugs relax the blood vessels and heart muscle. This increases the supply of blood and oxygen to the heart, reduces its workload, and prevents spasms of the blood vessels of the heart. Other antianginal drugs can be used along with a calcium blocker, if necessary. Calcium blockers tend to lower blood pressure; if you are also taking an antihypertensive agent, its dosage may need to be lowered. Verapamil can also be prescribed to treat high blood pressure.

BEFORE USING THIS DRUG

Let your doctor know *IF*

You have ever had allergic reactions or other problems with ■ verapamil ■ other calcium blockers.

You have ever had any of the following medical problems: ■ other heart or blood vessel disease ■ kidney disease ■ liver disease ■ any disease of the muscles ■ low blood pressure.

You are taking any of the following medicines: ■ beta-blockers or other medicines for high blood pressure or angina ■ anticoagulants (blood thinners) ■ aspirin or aspirinlike medicine ■ sulfonamides (sulfa drugs) ■ cimetidine (medicine for ulcers) ■ digoxin, digitoxin, or digitalis (heart medicines) ■ disopyramide or quinidine (medicine for abnormal heart rhythms) ■ medicine for seizures ■ medicine for malaria.

SPECIAL RESTRICTIONS WHILE TAKING THIS DRUG

FOOD AND DRUG INTERACTIONS

Foods and Beverages	Remember that angina may be provoked by eating a meal that is too heavy.
Alcohol	Drinking alcohol while taking calcium blockers may worsen such side effects as dizziness, light-headedness, or fainting. Avoid alcohol unless your doctor has approved its use.
Smoking	Smoking increases your chance of an angina attack. If you smoke, try to stop or at least cut down.

DAILY LIVING

Exertion and Exercise	Since this medicine is taken before exercise to reduce or prevent associated chest pain, you may be tempted to become overactive. You should discuss with your doctor how much exercise is safe for you.
Sun Exposure	While taking this medicine, your eyes may become more sensitive to light; wearing dark glasses when exposed to the sun should help.
Excessive Cold	Use caution during cold weather, as excessive cold may provoke an angina attack.
Examinations or Tests	It is important for you to keep all appointments with your doctor, even if you feel well, so that your progress can be monitored and your blood pressure checked. Periodic blood and urine tests may be required.

Other Precautions	Check your pulse regularly, and call your doctor if it falls below fifty beats per minute.
	Tell any doctor or dentist you consult that you are taking this medicine, especially if you will be undergoing any type of surgery.
	Remember that emotional stress may trigger an angina attack.
Helpful Hints	For best effects, take this medicine one hour before or two hours after meals.
	You may have headaches after taking this medicine. Headaches usually stop with continued use of the medicine; if they do not, or if they are particularly severe, call your doctor.
	Swallow the controlled-release capsules whole—do not break, crush, or chew them.

No special restrictions on driving or exposure to excessive heat.

POSSIBLE SIDE EFFECTS

Although this list of adverse effects may seem somewhat intimidating, keep in mind that some are quite rare. Of course, should these or any other problems arise while you are on medication, it is always a good idea to consult your doctor.

IF YOU DEVELOP

difficulty in breathing ■ coughing or wheezing ■ chest congestion ■ irregular or slow heartbeat ■ palpitations ■ rash, hives, or itching ■ swelling of ankles, feet, or lower legs ■ fainting ■ sore throat or fever ■ blurred vision ■ difficulty in balance ■ chills ■ increased sweating ■ hallucinations

WHAT TO DO

May be serious Check with your doctor as soon as possible.

constipation ■ flushing or feeling of warmth ■ headache ■ dizziness or light-headedness, especially when getting up from a reclining or sitting position ■ tiredness or weakness ■ drowsiness ■ depression ■ confusion ■ sleeplessness ■ giddiness ■ anxiety ■ mood changes ■ gas ■ nausea or vomiting ■ stomach cramps or upset stomach ■ loss of appetite ■ diarrhea ■ heartburn ■ stuffy nose ■ increased eye sensitivity to sunlight ■ muscle cramps ■ joint stiffness or swelling ■ gum problems ■ sexual problems

If symptoms are disturbing or persistent, let your doctor know.

STORAGE INSTRUCTIONS

Store in a cool, dark place (not in a bathroom medicine cabinet).

STOPPING OR INTERRUPTING THERAPY

Take this medicine exactly as directed, even if you do not feel chest pain. Do not take more of the medicine or take it more frequently than prescribed by your doctor. Suddenly stopping your medicine may worsen your medical problem. Your doctor will advise you on how to discontinue therapy gradually before stopping completely. If you miss a dose, take it as soon as possible. If it is almost time for your next dose, skip the missed dose and resume your regular schedule. Do not take two doses at the same time.

SPECIAL CONSIDERATIONS FOR THOSE OVER SIXTY-FIVE

Dizziness, light-headedness, and fainting, especially when getting up from a reclining or sitting position, are more likely to occur in older people, who may be advised to take their first dose in a situation in which they will be able to lie down, if necessary. Such people may also be more susceptible to constipation as a side effect.

Also, older people tend not to eliminate the calcium blockers as readily as young adults; thus, the drug may reach higher concentrations and remain in the bloodstream for a longer time. Doctors may require checkups to make sure that the proper dosage is being administered and that too much drug is not accumulating in the body.

CONDITION: **ANGINA**

CATEGORY: **ANTIANGINAL AGENTS (MISCELLANEOUS)**

GENERIC (CHEMICAL) NAME	BRAND (TRADE) NAME	DOSAGE FORMS AND STRENGTHS
Dipyridamole	PERSANTINE	Tablets: 25, 50, 75 mg

DRUG PROFILE

Dipyridamole is used, along with another drug, to prevent angina attacks. However, the Food and Drug Administration has not approved the use of dipyridamole for angina. You should discuss its use with your doctor. Dipyridamole is also prescribed, together with an anticoagulant drug, to prevent blood clots in people who have artificial heart valves.

BEFORE USING THIS DRUG:

Let your doctor know *IF*

You have ever had allergic reactions or other problems with ■ dipyridamole.

You have ever had any of the following medical problems: ■ low blood pressure ■ congestive heart failure.

You are taking any of the following medicines: ■ medicine for high blood pressure ■ anticoagulants (blood thinners) ■ aspirin or aspirinlike medicine.

SPECIAL RESTRICTIONS

FOOD AND DRUG INTERACTIONS

Other Drugs	Diuretics and other medicine for high blood pressure may increase the effects of dizziness, light-headedness, or fainting when taken together with dipyridamole.

Foods and Beverages	Remember that angina may be provoked by eating a meal that is too heavy.
Alcohol	Drinking alcohol while taking this medicine may worsen such side effects as dizziness, light-headedness, or fainting. Avoid alcohol unless your doctor has approved its use.
Smoking	Smoking increases your chance of an angina attack. If you smoke, try to stop or at least cut down.

DAILY LIVING

Exertion and Exercise	Since this medicine reduces or prevents chest pain from exercise, you may be tempted to become over-active. You should discuss with your doctor how much exercise is safe for you.
Excessive Cold	Use caution during cold weather, as excessive cold may provoke an angina attack.
Examinations or Tests	It is important for you to keep all appointments with your doctor, even if you feel well, so that your progress can be monitored and your blood pressure checked. Periodic blood and urine tests may be required.
Other Precautions	Remember that emotional stress may trigger an angina attack. Dipyridamole is used to *prevent* angina and is not effective once an angina attack has already started. Check with your doctor if you feel you need a fast-acting drug such as nitroglycerin that will relieve the pain of an actual attack.

Helpful Hints	Swallow the tablets whole (do not chew). For best effects, take this medicine with a full glass of water at least one hour before meals.

No special restrictions on driving, sun exposure, or exposure to excessive heat.

POSSIBLE SIDE EFFECTS

Although this list of adverse effects may seem somewhat intimidating, keep in mind that some are quite rare. Of course, should these or any other problems arise while you are on medication, it is always a good idea to consult your doctor.

IF YOU DEVELOP	WHAT TO DO
chest pain or tightness	**May be serious** Check with your doctor as soon as possible.
dizziness, light-headedness, or fainting, especially when getting up from a reclining or sitting position ■ flushing ■ headache ■ nausea or vomiting ■ diarrhea ■ upset stomach or stomach cramps ■ rash ■ weakness	If symptoms are disturbing or persist, let your doctor know.

STORAGE INSTRUCTIONS

Store in a cool, dark place (not in a bathroom medicine cabinet).

STOPPING OR INTERRUPTING THERAPY

Take this medicine exactly as prescribed by your doctor. It may take two or three months before you notice beneficial effects. Do not stop taking it if you feel it is not working; check with your doctor instead. If you miss a dose, take it as soon as possible, unless it is within four hours of your next scheduled dose. In that case, skip the missed dose and resume your regular schedule. Do not take two doses at the same time.

SPECIAL CONSIDERATIONS FOR THOSE OVER SIXTY-FIVE

The side effects of light-headedness, dizziness, and fainting are more likely to occur in older people.

CONGESTIVE HEART FAILURE

Although most heart conditions are becoming less common, congestive heart failure is on the increase. The number of persons with congestive heart failure rose to two million in 1980. This condition is a particular threat to older people: it is six times more common in those sixty-five to seventy-five years of age than in those forty-five to fifty-four years of age.

CAUSES

Congestive heart failure is not actually a single disease but rather a condition that can develop from a number of underlying disorders. It occurs when the heart loses its ability to keep up with the body's demand for oxygen-rich blood. If you have congestive heart failure, it means that your heart may be pumping too weakly either to supply adequate blood to the rest of your body or to keep up with the return of oxygen-depleted blood once it has passed through the circulatory system. Or it may mean that the ability of your heart to fill with blood is impaired.

The condition may be centered in the left or the right side of the heart. Left-sided heart failure is the most common variety. It is usually caused by dysfunction of the heart muscle, heart valve disease, or circulatory obstruction in the heart. If failure in the left side of the heart goes unchecked, the right side of the heart will also be affected, as blood backs up from the left chambers to the right. Various lung diseases can also cause right-sided heart failure. In addition, certain conditions outside the cardiovascular system—such as thyroid disease, severe anemia, and severe malnutrition—can lead to congestive heart failure.

DIAGNOSIS

The symptoms of congestive heart failure vary, depending on the part of the heart that is affected. Because the condition is often marked by low cardiac output—the inability of the heart to pump sufficient blood to meet the body's needs—you may feel tired and have trouble performing even routine physical tasks. If you have left-sided heart failure, you may also find breathing difficult (this can occur when you are lying flat as well as during activity). If the heart failure has extended to the right side, you may also notice edema, which is swelling of the arms or legs (particularly the ankles) caused by fluid retention.

In severe congestive heart failure, organs other than the heart may be damaged. Left-sided heart failure can lead to a kidney disease called prerenal azotemia. Occasionally, in right-sided heart failure fluid will accumulate in the abdomen and fill the liver and intestines, causing nausea, loss of appetite, abdominal pain, and an inability to absorb nutrients.

Older people sometimes assume that the symptoms of congestive heart failure are normal changes of aging; they may think that fatigue and shortness of breath are to be expected with advancing years. Similarly, they may misinterpret abdominal discomfort resulting from fluid accumulation as a simple touch of the flu. If you have any of these symptoms and they persist, you should consult a doctor. Your doctor will look for signs of congestive heart failure such as abnormal heart sounds or lung sounds, distension of the jugular veins (important blood vessels leading from the brain to the heart), and edema of the legs.

If these signs and symptoms lead your doctor to suspect congestive heart failure, the next step will be to take an X ray of the chest to look for enlargement of the heart and fluid in the lungs, and an echocardiogram to look for evidence of underlying heart disease. An echocardiogram is an image of the heart electronically composed from sound waves bounced off the chest. One other test, a radionuclide ventriculogram (angiogram), may also be performed to determine the degree of heart failure. In this test, the doctor injects a small amount of radioactive material into a vein and films the treated blood as it moves through the heart.

Both the echocardiogram and the ventriculogram (angiogram) help determine a figure known as the heart's "ejection fraction"—the amount of blood the heart pumps out with each contraction. If you have an ejection fraction of 40 percent or less, it may mean that congestive heart failure has developed. Some people develop symptoms of congestive heart failure with normal ejection fractions, while other people with very low ejection fractions may not have any symptoms.

TREATMENT

Congestive heart failure may be the result of a treatable underlying condition, such as valvular disease. Your therapy will be aimed at both relieving the heart failure and eliminating its cause. The drugs discussed in the charts on pages 162–174, including furosemide, bumetanide, digoxin, and captopril, are the mainstays of treatment for congestive heart failure. Surgery may be recommended for treating the valve disease. Once such underlying causes are removed, congestive heart failure may no longer be a problem.

OUTLOOK

Many patients, however, will have to continue treatment even after their symptoms go away. Your doctor will probably recommend a low-salt diet to decrease your retention of fluids; in addition, you will need to have regular checkups to make sure your medicine is working properly. If you follow these recommendations, your heart condition should not unduly affect your way of life.

CONDITION: **CONGESTIVE HEART FAILURE**

CATEGORY: **LOOP DIURETICS**

GENERIC (CHEMICAL) NAME	BRAND (TRADE) NAME	DOSAGE FORMS AND STRENGTHS
Furosemide	LASIX	Solution: 10 mg per ml Tablets: 20, 40, 80 mg

DRUG PROFILE

Furosemide is a diuretic that is used to treat the edema (fluid accumulation) that may be a by-product of congestive heart failure, kidney disease, or liver disease. It is also sometimes prescribed to lower high blood pressure. Furosemide is known as a "loop" diuretic because it acts on a part of the kidney called the loop of Henle. This drug helps the kidneys eliminate excess salt and water through urination. This not only relieves edema but also decreases the volume of blood flowing through the blood vessels, which results in lower blood pressure.

BEFORE USING THIS DRUG

Let your doctor know *IF*

You have ever had allergic reactions or other problems with ■ furosemide ■ thiazide or thiazide-type diuretics ■ tartrazine (FD&C Yellow Dye No. 5) ■ aspirin ■ sulfonamides (sulfa drugs).

You have ever had any of the following medical problems: ■ diabetes ■ kidney disease ■ liver disease ■ systemic lupus erythematosus ■ gout ■ disease of the pancreas ■ heart disease ■ hearing problems ■ diarrhea.

You are taking any of the following medicines: ■ diuretics or other medicines for high blood pressure ■ corticosteroids ■ large doses of aspirin or aspirinlike medicine ■ clofibrate (medicine for high cholesterol) ■ medicine for diabetes ■ barbiturates ■ digoxin, digitoxin, or digitalis (heart medicines) ■ medicine for gout ■ medicine for arthritis, including indomethacin ■ lithium ■ narcotics or other prescription pain-killers ■ sleep medicines ■ aminoglycoside antibiotics ■ medicine for seizures ■ methenamine (medicine to prevent urinary tract infections).

You are or have recently been on a low-salt diet.

SPECIAL RESTRICTIONS WHILE TAKING THIS DRUG

FOOD AND DRUG INTERACTIONS

Other Drugs	If you are taking this medicine for high blood pressure, do not take any other drugs, including over-the-counter (OTC) drugs, before checking with your doctor. Some OTC drugs for appetite suppression, asthma, colds, cough, hay fever, or sinus problems tend to increase blood pressure.
	Your doctor will probably reduce the dose of or discontinue other medicines you may be taking for high blood pressure when you start taking furosemide.
Foods and Beverages	Your doctor may prescribe a special low-salt diet, which you should follow carefully because it will help your medicine work more effectively. You may also be advised to go on a weight-reduction diet. Continue to drink a normal amount of fluids. This drug may cause your body to lose large amounts of the mineral potassium. Your doctor may give you special instructions about eating foods or drinking beverages that have a high potassium content (such as bananas and citrus fruit juices), taking a potassium supplement, or using salt substitutes.
Alcohol	Drinking alcohol may worsen such side effects as dizziness or drowsiness. Avoid alcohol unless your doctor has approved its use.

No special restrictions on smoking.

DAILY LIVING

Exertion and Exercise	Use caution when exercising or standing for long periods of time because this medicine may cause you to become dehydrated and dizzy, light-headed, or faint.

Sun Exposure/ Excessive Heat	Your skin may become more sensitive to sunlight and more likely to develop a sunburn while you are taking this medicine. It is a good idea to avoid too much sun, especially if you burn easily. Apply a sunscreen to exposed skin surfaces before going outdoors. Use caution during hot weather or while taking saunas or hot baths, since excessive sweating while taking this medicine may cause you to become dehydrated and to feel drowsy or faint.
Examinations or Tests	Many people have high blood pressure with no symptoms at all. It is important for you to keep all appointments with your doctor, even if you feel well, so that your blood pressure can be checked regularly. Periodic blood and urine tests may be required.
Other Precautions	If you have diabetes, be aware that this medicine may raise blood-sugar levels. If you notice any change when testing sugar levels in your blood or urine, let your doctor know.
	Tell any doctor or dentist you consult that you are taking this medicine, especially if you will be undergoing any type of surgery.
	When first starting on this type of medicine, you will probably experience both greater volume and frequency of urination. Until your individual pattern of urination has been established with this medicine, it may be wise to time carefully any activity that will put you out of convenient reach of a bathroom, such as bus or car travel. In addition, taking a diuretic at bedtime will probably interfere with sleep; you should discuss your dosage schedule with your doctor.
	Check with your doctor if you become ill with flulike symptoms, such as cough, fever, or body aches; lose your appetite; vomit; or have diarrhea. This may cause you to lose a great deal of fluid, making it important not to take the diuretic for one or more doses.

Following mild fluid losses, some older people are more vulnerable to symptoms of weakness or dizziness upon standing or getting up.

Helpful Hints

If your mouth or throat feels dry, chewing sugarless gum or sucking ice chips or sugarless hard candy will help.

When you first begin to take this medicine, you may feel tired and notice that you urinate more frequently. These effects should lessen with time.

No special restrictions on driving or exposure to excessive cold.

POSSIBLE SIDE EFFECTS

Although this list of adverse effects may seem somewhat intimidating, keep in mind that some are quite rare. Of course, should these or any other problems arise while you are on medication, it is always a good idea to consult your doctor.

IF YOU DEVELOP

tiredness or weakness ■ irregular or fast heartbeat ■ confusion ■ mood or mental changes ■ numbness or tingling of fingers or toes ■ severe or continuing nausea, vomiting, or diarrhea ■ dry mouth ■ increased thirst ■ weak pulse ■ muscle cramps or pain ■ bladder spasms ■ stomach pain or cramps

WHAT TO DO

Urgent Get in touch with your doctor immediately.

joint pain ■ hearing disturbances ■ rash or hives ■ sore throat or fever ■ bleeding or bruising ■ yellowing of eyes or skin ■ swelling of hands or feet ■ blurred or yellow vision ■ headache ■ flulike symptoms, such as cough, fever, or body aches, with nausea, vomiting, and diarrhea.

May be serious Check with your doctor as soon as possible.

dizziness or light-headedness, especially when getting up from a reclining or sitting position ■ nausea or vomiting ■ upset stomach ■ loss of appetite ■ diarrhea ■ constipation ■ increased skin sensitivity to sunlight ■ increased sweating ■ restlessness

If symptoms are disturbing or persist, let your doctor know.

STORAGE INSTRUCTIONS

Store in a cool, dark place (not in a bathroom medicine cabinet). If your medicine is in a liquid form, make sure that it does not freeze.

STOPPING OR INTERRUPTING THERAPY

If you are taking furosemide for hypertension, you may have to take it for the rest of your life, as this drug does not cure high blood pressure but only controls it. Do not stop taking it, even if you feel better. If you miss a dose, take it as soon as possible. If it is almost time for your next dose, skip the missed dose and resume your regular schedule. Do not take two doses at the same time.

SPECIAL CONSIDERATIONS FOR THOSE OVER SIXTY-FIVE

The side effects of dizziness and light-headedness are more likely to occur in older people, who should be especially careful to follow doctor's instructions on how much drug to take. Too much furosemide can cause dehydration, which could have serious effects on one's health. Also, people over sixty-five who are not eating a well-balanced diet will be more prone to potassium deficiency and other problems. Such persons should check with a doctor if they become ill with flulike symptoms, such as cough, fever, or body aches; lose their appetite; vomit; or have diarrhea because they may then be more vulnerable to fluid losses.

CONDITION: **CONGESTIVE HEART FAILURE**

CATEGORY: **LOOP DIURETICS**

GENERIC (CHEMICAL) NAME	BRAND (TRADE) NAME	DOSAGE FORMS AND STRENGTHS
Bumetanide	BUMEX	Tablets: 0.5, 1 mg

DRUG PROFILE

Bumetanide is a diuretic that is used to treat edema (fluid accumulation) that may be a by-product of congestive heart failure, kidney disease, or liver disease. Bumetanide is known as a "loop" diuretic because it acts on a part of the kidney called the loop of Henle. This drug helps the kidneys eliminate excess salt and water through urination. It tends to act more quickly and for a shorter period of time than furosemide, another loop diuretic.

BEFORE USING THIS DRUG

Let your doctor know *IF*

You have ever had allergic reactions or other problems with ■ bumetanide ■ thiazide or thiazide-type diuretics ■ sulfonamides (sulfa drugs).

You have ever had any of the following medical problems: ■ diabetes ■ abnormal heart rhythms ■ gout ■ diarrhea (recent or current) ■ kidney disease ■ liver disease.

You are taking any of the following medicines: ■ other diuretics or medicines for high blood pressure ■ antibiotics ■ medicine for cancer ■ digoxin, digitoxin, or digitalis (heart medicines) ■ aspirin, indomethacin or other medicine for arthritis ■ probenecid (medicine for gout) ■ lithium ■ corticosteroids or corticotropin (ACTH) ■ medicine for malaria ■ tetracycline.

SPECIAL RESTRICTIONS WHILE TAKING THIS DRUG

FOOD AND DRUG INTERACTIONS

Foods and Beverages	This drug may cause your body to lose large amounts of the mineral potassium. Your doctor may give you special instructions about eating foods or drinking beverages that have a high potassium content (such as bananas and citrus fruit juices), taking a potassium supplement, or using salt substitutes.

No special restrictions on alcohol use or smoking.

DAILY LIVING

Exertion and Exercise	Use caution when exercising or exerting yourself, since excessive sweating while taking this medicine may cause you to become dehydrated.

Excessive Heat	Use caution during hot weather, since excessive sweating while taking this medicine may cause you to become dehydrated.

Examinations or Tests	It is important for you to keep all appointments with your doctor so that you can be checked regularly. Periodic blood and urine tests may be required.

Other Precautions

If you have diabetes, be aware that this medicine may raise blood-sugar levels. If you notice any change when testing sugar levels in your blood or urine, let your doctor know.

Tell any doctor or dentist you consult that you are taking this medicine, especially if you will be undergoing any type of surgery.

When first starting on this type of medicine you will probably experience both greater volume and frequency of urination. Until your individual pattern of urination has been established with this medicine, it may be wise to time carefully any activity that will put you out of convenient reach of a bathroom, such as bus or car travel. In addition, taking a diuretic at bedtime will probably interfere with sleep; you should discuss your dosage schedule with your doctor.

Check with your doctor if you become ill with flulike symptoms, such as cough, fever, or body aches; lose your appetite; vomit; or have diarrhea. This may cause you to lose a great deal of fluid, making it important not to take the diuretic for one or more doses.

Following mild fluid losses, some older people are more vulnerable to symptoms of weakness or dizziness upon standing or getting up.

Helpful Hints	If your mouth or throat feels dry, chewing sugarless gum or sucking ice chips or sugarless hard candy will help.

When you first begin to take this medicine, you may feel tired and notice that you urinate more frequently. These effects should lessen with time. |

No special restrictions on driving, sun exposure, or exposure to excessive cold.

POSSIBLE SIDE EFFECTS

Although this list of adverse effects may seem somewhat intimidating, keep in mind that some are quite rare. Of course, should these or any other problems arise while you are on medication, it is always a good idea to consult your doctor.

IF YOU DEVELOP	WHAT TO DO
tiredness or weakness ■ confusion ■ mood or mental changes ■ irregular heartbeat ■ tingling sensation in fingers or toes	**Urgent** Get in touch with your doctor immediately.
chest pain ■ nausea or vomiting ■ diarrhea ■ uncontrollable movements ■ dizziness ■ light-headedness ■ headache ■ loss of appetite ■ dry mouth ■ increased thirst ■ weak pulse ■ muscle cramps or pain ■ hearing disturbances ■ rash or hives ■ bleeding or bruising ■ difficulty in breathing	**May be serious** Check with your doctor as soon as possible.
stomach cramps or pain ■ upset stomach ■ male impotence ■ premature ejaculation (in males) ■ nipple tenderness ■ joint pain ■ increased sweating	If symptoms are disturbing or persist, let your doctor know.

STORAGE INSTRUCTIONS

Store in a cool, dark place (not in a bathroom medicine cabinet).

STOPPING OR INTERRUPTING THERAPY

Your doctor may prescribe a special schedule for you, whereby you take this drug on some days and do not take it on other days. Follow your doctor's instructions exactly. If you miss a dose, take it as soon as possible. If it is almost time for your next dose, skip the missed dose and resume your regular schedule. Do not take two doses at the same time.

SPECIAL CONSIDERATIONS FOR THOSE OVER SIXTY-FIVE

The side effects of dizziness and light-headedness are more likely to occur in older people. They should be especially careful to follow doctor's instructions on how much of the drug to take. Too much bumetanide can cause dehydration, which could have serious effects on one's health. People over sixty-five should check with a doctor if they become ill with flulike symptoms, such as cough, fever, or body aches; lose their appetite; vomit; or have diarrhea because they may then be more vulnerable to fluid losses.

CONDITION: **CONGESTIVE HEART FAILURE**

CATEGORY: **INOTROPIC DRUGS**

GENERIC (CHEMICAL) NAME	BRAND (TRADE) NAME	DOSAGE FORMS AND STRENGTHS
Digoxin	LANOXICAPS LANOXIN	Capsules: 0.05, 0.1, 0.2 mg Tablets: 0.125, 0.25, 0.5 mg
Digitoxin	CRYSTODIGIN	Tablets: 0.05, 0.1, 0.15, 0.2 mg

DRUG PROFILE

The cardiac glycosides, extracted from the leaves of the digitalis plant (foxglove), are used to treat heart failure or abnormal heart rhythms. These medicines, called inotropic drugs, act directly on the heart to increase the force and efficiency of each heartbeat and control the rhythm of the beats. This improves blood circulation, helps the body rid itself of excess fluid, and results in easier breathing and greater overall strength.

BEFORE USING THIS DRUG

Let your doctor know *IF*

You have ever had allergic reactions or other problems with ■ digoxin ■ digitoxin ■ any other digitalis medicines.

You have ever had any of the following medical problems: ■ any heart disease ■ heart attack ■ rheumatic fever ■ asthma or other lung disease ■ high or low calcium blood levels ■ low potassium or magnesium blood levels ■ kidney disease ■ liver disease ■ thyroid disease ■ prolonged diarrhea ■ congestive heart failure.

You are taking any of the following medicines: ■ diuretics or other medicines for high blood pressure ■ antacids ■ antibiotics ■ medicine for cancer ■ medicine for asthma or hay fever ■ beta-blockers ■ cholestyramine (medicine for high cholesterol) ■ medicine for cough or cold ■ appetite suppressants ■ decongestants ■ medicine for diarrhea ■ laxatives ■ medicine for stomach pain or cramps ■ medicine for ulcers ■ medicine for glaucoma ■ aspirin or aspirinlike medicine ■ medicine for nausea.

You have taken any of the following within the last two weeks: digitalis, quinidine, or other heart medicines ■ corticosteroids or corticotropin (ACTH) ■ nifedipine, verapamil, diltiazem (calcium blockers) ■ sleep medicines ■ tranquilizers ■ medicine for seizures ■ potassium-containing medicines or supplements ■ medicine for thyroid disorders.

SPECIAL RESTRICTIONS WHILE TAKING THIS DRUG

FOOD AND DRUG INTERACTIONS

Other Drugs	Do not take any other drugs, including over-the-counter (OTC) drugs, before checking with your doctor. Some OTC drugs, such as those used for appetite suppression, asthma, colds, cough, hay fever, diarrhea, constipation, and acid indigestion, may react adversely with the cardiac glycosides. Taking digoxin

with quinidine or verapamil may result in dangerously high blood levels of digoxin. It is especially important to let your doctor know if you are taking either of these drugs.

Foods and Beverages	Tell your doctor if you are on a high-fiber diet. In general, try to maintain a well-balanced diet. If these drugs are taken with a meal high in bran fiber, absorption of medicine into the body may be reduced.
	If you are deficient in potassium or magnesium (as may occur if you are taking a diuretic or not eating properly), these drugs may not work correctly. Ask your doctor for diet suggestions.
Smoking	Nicotine may precipitate abnormal heart rhythms. If you smoke, try to stop or at least cut down.

No special restrictions on alcohol use.

DAILY LIVING

Examinations or Tests	It is important for you to keep all appointments with your doctor, even if you feel well, so that your progress can be checked. Periodic blood and urine tests may be required.
	While you are taking digitalis, you should check your pulse regularly and tell your doctor if you notice any changes in rhythm, rate, or force.
Other Precautions	Tell any doctor or dentist you consult that you are taking this medicine, especially if you will be undergoing any type of surgery.
	The effective level of this medicine is very close to the toxic level; you should immediately report any signs of overdose (listed below as ''Urgent'').

Helpful Hints

During the first one to two days of therapy, you may urinate more frequently than usual. This effect should disappear as you continue to take your medicine.

No special restrictions on driving, exertion and exercise, sun exposure, or exposure to excessive heat or cold.

POSSIBLE SIDE EFFECTS

Although this list of adverse effects may seem somewhat intimidating, keep in mind that some are quite rare. Of course, should these or any other problems arise while you are on medication, it is always a good idea to consult your doctor.

IF YOU DEVELOP

loss of appetite ■ stomach pain ■ nausea or vomiting ■ diarrhea ■ mouth watering ■ difficulty in swallowing ■ hiccups ■ bloating ■ irregular heartbeat ■ headache ■ tiredness or weakness ■ drowsiness ■ general feeling of unwellness ■ dizziness ■ fainting ■ excitement, restlessness, or nervousness ■ sleeplessness ■ euphoria ■ irritability ■ seizures ■ pain around the face or any other pain ■ tremors ■ memory problems ■ personality changes ■ nightmares ■ delirium ■ depression ■ confusion ■ hallucinations ■ blurred vision ■ changes in color vision or other visual disturbances ■ increased eye sensitivity to light

WHAT TO DO

Urgent Get in touch with your doctor immediately.

rash, hives, itching, or other skin problems

May be serious Check with your doctor as soon as possible.

female breast tenderness ■ male breast enlargement

If symptoms are disturbing or persist, let your doctor know.

STORAGE INSTRUCTIONS

Store in a cool, dark place (not in a bathroom medicine cabinet).

STOPPING OR INTERRUPING THERAPY

It is important to continue taking this medicine, even if you feel well. Suddenly stopping this medicine may seriously worsen your medical condition; follow your doctor's instructions carefully. If you miss a dose of this medicine, skip the missed dose and resume your regular schedule. Do not take two doses at the same time. If you miss doses for two or more days, check with your doctor.

SPECIAL CONSIDERATIONS FOR THOSE OVER SIXTY-FIVE

Older people may be more sensitive to the side effects of this drug and may accumulate toxic blood levels of the drug at lower doses. Such people should get in touch with a doctor if they develop any of the symptoms listed under ''Possible Side Effects.''

CONDITION: **CONGESTIVE HEART FAILURE**

CATEGORY: **ANGIOTENSIN-CONVERTING ENZYME INHIBITORS**

GENERIC (CHEMICAL) NAME	BRAND (TRADE) NAME	DOSAGE FORMS AND STRENGTHS
Captopril	CAPOTEN	Tablets: 12.5, 25, 50, 100 mg

DRUG PROFILE

Captopril is used to treat high blood pressure. These drugs interrupt a chain of biochemical events that lead to constriction (tightening) of the blood vessels. Blocking this process lets the blood vessels relax, lowers blood pressure, and increases the flow of blood and oxygen to the heart.

Captopril is used to treat congestive heart failure as well. Relaxing the blood vessels reduces the congestion of blood in the lungs, lessens the load on the heart, and improves the blood flow to the kidneys, facilitating the elimination of sodium and water. Long-term use of this drug improves exercise tolerance because blood flow to the heart muscle is increased.

For complete information on this drug, see pages 89–93.

ABNORMAL HEART RHYTHMS

A steady, measured beat is one of the hallmarks of a healthy heart. This rhythm is the result of a finely tuned electrical current that originates in the sinus node, a group of pacemaker cells in the heart's upper right side. The current then darts through the atrium, the heart's upper chamber, toward the atrioventricular node, a group of conductor cells located between the heart's upper and lower chambers. Finally, the impulse travels to the ventricle, the lower chamber of the heart.

If you've been told you have an arrhythmia, the term for abnormal heart rhythms, this indicates that the heart's circuitry has been thrown awry. This can happen as the result of heart diseases and other illnesses, or effects of medicines and nonmedicinal drugs such as caffeine, alcohol, and tobacco. Arrhythmias are most common among older people, with some forms affecting more than 10 percent of the over-sixty-five population.

CAUSES

Different types of disruptions cause different disorders in the heart's rhythm. If the sinus node malfunctions, the resulting pattern of arrhythmias is known as the sick sinus syndrome. This syndrome can cause an abnormally slow rate (fewer than sixty beats per minute) or both an abnormally fast rate (over one hundred beats per minute) and an abnormally slow heart rate.

Another possible disruption known as heart block occurs when the conduction system malfunctions. Though heart block itself sometimes does not create noticeable problems, it can lead to a loss of conduction to the ventricles. When this happens, the upper and lower heart chambers no longer contract in the pattern needed to prevent serious symptoms of arrhythmias.

Occasionally, the electrical impulse begins outside the heart's normal conduction system, producing another type of arrhythmia. If the impulse begins in the atrium, the resulting arrythmia is called premature atrial contraction; if it begins in the ventricle, it is called premature ventricular contraction. You may have heard your doctor refer to these arrhythmias as PACs and PVCs. (Occasional PACs or PVCs are common among people over sixty-five, often without noticeable symptoms.)

Sometimes, the conduction system becomes disorganized and the electrical current travels in circles. If this malfunction occurs in the atrium, it is called atrial fibrillation, or flutter; in the ventricle, it is called ventricular tachycardia, or ventricular fibrillation.

DIAGNOSIS

The symptoms of arrythmias stem from two factors: the regularity of contractions and the heart rate. When contractions are irregular, you experience a sensation of missed beats, irregular pulse, or palpitations. With a fast heart rate, you may feel dizzy, light-headed, or short of breath or notice a feeling of fullness and fluttering in the chest. With a slow heart rate, you may actually faint.

Most serious arrhythmias are detected through an electrocardiogram (ECG), a device that graphs the pattern of electrical activity in your heart over a period of several minutes. In some instances, the ECG will not show evidence of an arrhythmia, even though symptoms point to one. Therefore, the doctor may want you to wear a Holter monitor for an extended period as you go about your daily activities. The Holter monitor records the heart's electrical activity for up to twenty-four hours. While you wear the monitor, your doctor may want you to write down your heart signs and symptoms as well as your activities. Your record will be compared with that of the Holter monitor so your doctor can see any changes in heart rhythm that occurred when you were experiencing symptoms.

TREATMENT

When an abnormally slow heart rate develops from sick sinus syndrome or heart block, the doctor may recommend a pacemaker, an electronic device implanted beneath the skin near the heart or elsewhere in the chest. The pacemaker will supply the current that is lacking in people with these conditions. In rare instances, surgery is required for frequent PVCs to remove the tissue that is generating an abnormal current.

The drugs discussed in the charts on pages 177–193—including quinidine, digoxin, procainamide, disopyramide, tocainide, and mexiletine—are used both to correct abnormal heart rhythms and to prevent their occurrence. In some instances, the doctor will want to check a drug's effectiveness by having you wear a Holter monitor during treatment.

OUTLOOK

Many people with arrhythmias may need to continue their medicine indefinitely. To make the medicine more effective, you should avoid stimulants such as caffeine, as well as alcohol and tobacco. Finally, you should have regular checkups to make sure that the medicine is working properly.

CONDITION: **ABNORMAL HEART RHYTHMS**

CATEGORY: **ANTIARRHYTHMICS**

GENERIC (CHEMICAL) NAME	BRAND (TRADE) NAME	DOSAGE FORMS AND STRENGTHS
Quinidine gluconate	QUINAGLUTE	Controlled-release tablets: 324 mg
Quinidine sulfate	QUINIDEX	Controlled-release tablets: 300 mg Tablets: 100, 200, 300 mg

This drug is available under a variety of brand names.

DRUG PROFILE

This drug helps normalize irregular heartbeats and also slows down the heart if it is beating too rapidly. Quinidine works directly on the heart itself, as well as on the nerves that lead to the heart muscles.

BEFORE USING THIS DRUG

Let your doctor know *IF*

You have ever had allergic reactions or other problems with ■ quinidine ■ quinine.

You have ever had any of the following medical problems: ■ asthma or other lung disease ■ high or low blood pressure ■ congestive heart failure or other heart problems ■ liver disease ■ kidney disease ■ muscle weakness ■ myasthenia gravis ■ thyroid disorder ■ blood disease ■ recent infection ■ psoriasis.

You are taking any of the following medicines: ■ other medicine for abnormal heart rhythms ■ medicine for seizures ■ medicine for Parkinson's disease ■ medicine for urinary retention ■ medicine for ulcers or irritable bowel syndrome ■ anticoagulants (blood thinners) ■ digoxin, digitoxin, or digitalis (heart medicines) ■ diuretics ■ antacids ■ Bicitra, Polycitra (medicine to make the urine less acidic) ■ tranquilizers ■ sinus medicines ■ medicine for nausea ■ muscle relaxants ■ medicine for myasthenia gravis ■ medicine for glaucoma ■ antibiotics ■ sleep medicines ■ potassium-containing medicines or supplements.

SPECIAL RESTRICTIONS WHILE TAKING THIS DRUG

FOOD AND DRUG INTERACTIONS

Other Drugs	Use of this drug with digoxin may result in dangerously high blood levels of digoxin. It is especially important to let your doctor know if you are taking digoxin.
Alcohol	Drinking alcohol while taking this medicine may worsen such side effects as drowsiness, light-headedness, or dizziness. Avoid alcohol unless your doctor has approved its use.
Smoking	Smoking may aggravate cardiac arrhythmias. If you smoke, try to stop or at least cut down.

No special restrictions on foods and beverages.

DAILY LIVING

Examinations or Tests	It is important for you to keep all appointments with your doctor so that your progress and reactions to therapy can be checked. Periodic electrocardiograms and blood tests may be required.
Other Precautions	Tell any doctor or dentist you consult that you are taking this medicine, especially if you will be undergoing any type of surgery.
	Occasionally, patients experience blurred vision or loss of consciousness with their first dose. If this happens, contact your doctor immediately.

Helpful Hints	Quinidine is usually taken on an empty stomach—one hour before or two hours after meals—with a full glass of water. However, if this medicine upsets your stomach, ask your doctor if you may take it with food or milk. Swallow the controlled-release capsules whole—do not break, crush, or chew them.

No special restrictions on exertion and exercise, driving, sun exposure, or exposure to excessive heat or cold.

POSSIBLE SIDE EFFECTS

Although this list of adverse effects may seem somewhat intimidating, keep in mind that some are quite rare. Of course, should these or any other problems arise while you are on medication, it is always a good idea to consult your doctor.

IF YOU DEVELOP	WHAT TO DO
difficulty in breathing ■ visual disturbances ■ dizziness ■ headache ■ ringing in the ears ■ hearing loss ■ faintness or light-headedness ■ fever ■ rash ■ bleeding or bruising ■ very fast heartbeat ■ tremors ■ nausea or vomiting ■ blurred vision or fainting after the first dose	**Urgent** Get in touch with your doctor immediately.
nervousness ■ excitement ■ confusion ■ personality changes ■ cold sweat ■ delirium ■ yellowing of eyes or skin ■ diarrhea	**May be serious** Check with your doctor as soon as possible.
bitter taste ■ loss of appetite ■ stomach pain or cramps ■ flushed skin with itching ■ joint pain ■ increased eye sensitivity to light	If symptoms are disturbing or persist, let your doctor know.

STORAGE INSTRUCTIONS

Store in a cool, dark place (not in a bathroom medicine cabinet).

STOPPING OR INTERRUPTING THERAPY

Take this drug exactly as instructed. Check with your doctor on what to do should you miss a dose.

SPECIAL CONSIDERATIONS FOR THOSE OVER SIXTY-FIVE

Older people sometimes metabolize quinidine more slowly, which may allow the drug to reach higher concentrations and accumulate in the body. Doctors will adjust the dosage accordingly.

CONDITION: **ABNORMAL HEART RHYTHMS**

CATEGORY: **ANTIARRHYTHMICS**

GENERIC (CHEMICAL) NAME	BRAND (TRADE) NAME	DOSAGE FORMS AND STRENGTHS
Disopyramide phosphate	NORPACE NORPACE CR	Capsules: 100, 150 mg Controlled-release capsules: 100, 150 mg

DRUG PROFILE

This drug helps normalize irregular heartbeats and also slows down the heart if it is beating too rapidly. Disopyramide works directly on the heart itself, as well as on the nerves that lead to the heart muscles.

BEFORE USING THIS DRUG

Let your doctor know *IF*

You have ever had allergic reactions or other problems with ■ disopyramide.

You have ever had any of the following medical problems: ■ congestive heart failure or any other heart problems ■ low blood pressure ■ diabetes ■ hypoglycemia (low blood sugar) ■ high or low potassium blood levels ■ urinary retention ■ enlarged prostate ■ glaucoma or a family history of glaucoma ■ liver disease ■ kidney disease ■ myasthenia gravis ■ malnutrition.

You are taking any of the following medicines: ■ other medicine for abnormal heart rhythms ■ anticoagulants (blood thinners) ■ medicine for diabetes ■ medicine for high blood pressure, including beta-blockers ■ medicine for angina or other heart problems ■ sleep medicines ■ medicine for seizures ■ potassium-containing medicines or supplements ■ rifampin (medicine for tuberculosis) ■ medicine for glaucoma.

SPECIAL RESTRICTIONS WHILE TAKING THIS DRUG

FOOD AND DRUG INTERACTIONS

Other Drugs	Do not take any other drugs, including over-the-counter (OTC) drugs, before checking with your doctor. OTC drugs for appetite suppression, coughs, colds, asthma, allergies, or sinus problems may aggravate your heart problems.
Foods and Beverages	Your doctor may give you special instructions about eating foods or drinking beverages that have a high potassium content (such as bananas and citrus fruit juices), taking a potassium supplement, or using salt substitutes.
Alcohol	Drinking alcohol while taking this medicine may worsen such side effects as hypoglycemia (low blood sugar) or dizziness. Avoid alcohol unless your doctor has approved its use.
Smoking	Smoking may aggravate cardiac arrhythmias. If you smoke, try to stop or at least cut down.

DAILY LIVING

Driving	This drug may cause drowsiness. Be careful when driving, operating household appliances, or doing any other tasks that require alertness until you know how this drug affects you.

Exertion and Exercise	This medicine may cause you to sweat less than normally. Sweating is your body's natural way of cooling down, and not sweating enough can be dangerous. Use caution not to become overheated when you exercise or exert yourself.
Excessive Heat	Use caution during hot weather, especially if you exert yourself (see above).
Examinations or Tests	It is important for you to keep all appointments with your doctor, even if you feel well, so that your progress can be checked. Periodic blood or urine tests may be required.
Other Precautions	If you experience symptoms of low blood sugar (see list of symptoms in "Possible Side Effects"), eat or drink something containing sugar and contact your doctor immediately.
Helpful Hints	For best results, take this medicine on an empty stomach—either one hour before or two hours after meals.
	Swallow the controlled-release capsules whole—do not break, crush, or chew them.
	If your mouth or throat feels dry, chewing sugarless gum or sucking ice chips or sugarless hard candy will help. Your nose may also feel dry or stuffy; check with your doctor before using nasal decongestants.

No special restrictions on sun exposure or exposure to excessive cold.

POSSIBLE SIDE EFFECTS

Although this list of adverse effects may seem somewhat intimidating, keep in mind that some are quite rare. Of course, should these or any other problems arise while you are on medication, it is always a good idea to consult your doctor.

IF YOU DEVELOP

shortness of breath ■ urinary retention

WHAT TO DO

Urgent Get in touch with your doctor immediately.

---

urinary urgency or frequency ■ chest pain ■ dizziness, light-headedness, or fainting, especially when getting up from a reclining or sitting position ■ confusion ■ depression ■ muscle weakness ■ swelling of feet or lower legs ■ numbness or tingling ■ irregular heartbeat ■ rapid weight gain ■ eye pain ■ sore throat or fever ■ yellowing of eyes or skin ■ nausea or vomiting ■ diarrhea ■ stomach pain ■ rash, itching, or other skin problems ■ personality changes ■ tiredness ■ headache ■ general feeling of unwellness

Signs of low blood sugar: anxiety; chills; pale skin; headache; hunger; nausea; shakiness; increased sweating; tiredness

May be serious Check with your doctor as soon as possible.

---

dry mouth, eyes, nose, and throat ■ bloating or gas ■ blurred vision ■ constipation ■ loss of appetite ■ male impotence ■ sleep disturbances ■ male breast enlargement ■ aches and pains

If symptoms are disturbing or persist, let your doctor know.

STORAGE INSTRUCTIONS

Store in a cool, dark place (not in a bathroom medicine cabinet).

STOPPING OR INTERRUPTING THERAPY

It is very important to continue taking this medicine, even if you feel better. Suddenly stopping this medicine may seriously worsen your medical condition. Follow your doctor's instructions carefully. If you miss a dose of this medicine, take it as soon as possible unless your next regular dose will be within the next four hours. If so, skip the missed dose and resume your regular schedule. Do not take two doses at the same time.

SPECIAL CONSIDERATIONS FOR THOSE OVER SIXTY-FIVE

Dizziness and light-headedness are more likely to occur in older people. The side effects of constipation, blurred vision, and urinary retention can also be particularly troublesome. In addition, this drug lessens the effectiveness of glaucoma treatment.

CONDITION: **ABNORMAL HEART RHYTHMS**

CATEGORY: **ANTIARRHYTHMICS**

GENERIC (CHEMICAL) NAME	BRAND (TRADE) NAME	DOSAGE FORMS AND STRENGTHS
Procainamide hydrochloride	PROCAN SR	Controlled-release tablets: 250, 500, 750, 1,000 mg
	PRONESTYL	Capsules: 250, 375, 500 mg
	PRONESTYL SR	Controlled-release tablets: 500 mg

DRUG PROFILE

This drug helps normalize irregular heartbeats and also slows down the heart if it is beating too rapidly. Procainamide works directly on the heart itself, as well as on the nerves that lead to the heart muscles.

BEFORE USING THIS DRUG

Let your doctor know *IF*

You have ever had allergic reactions or other problems with ■ procainamide ■ procaine or any other "caine-type" medicines ■ aspirin ■ tartrazine (FD&C Yellow Dye No. 5) (contained in Pronestyl tablets).

You have ever had any of the following medical problems: ■ any heart disease ■ asthma ■ kidney disease ■ liver disease ■ systemic lupus erythematosus ■ high or low blood-potassium levels ■ high blood pressure ■ myasthenia gravis.

You are taking any of the following medicines: ■ other medicine for heart disease, including medicine for abnormal heart rhythms ■ antibiotics ■ medicine for high blood pressure ■ medicine for myasthenia gravis ■ medicine for ulcers ■ medicine for Parkinson's disease ■ medicine for urinary retention ■ medicine for irritable bowel syndrome.

SPECIAL RESTRICTIONS WHILE TAKING THIS DRUG

FOOD AND DRUG INTERACTIONS

Alcohol	Drinking alcohol while taking this medicine may worsen such side effects as drowsiness, light-headedness, or dizziness. Avoid alcohol unless your doctor has approved its use.
Smoking	Smoking may aggravate cardiac arrhythmias. If you smoke, try to stop or at least cut down.

No special restrictions on foods and beverages.

DAILY LIVING

Driving	This drug may cause light-headedness or dizziness. Be careful when driving, operating household appliances, or doing any other tasks that require alertness until you know how this drug affects you.
Examinations or Tests	It is important for you to keep all appointments with your doctor, even if you feel well, so that your progress can be checked. Periodic blood and urine tests may be required.
Other Precautions	Tell any doctor or dentist you consult that you are taking this medicine, especially if you will be undergoing any type of surgery.
Helpful Hints	For best results, take this medicine at the exact intervals indicated, on an empty stomach—either one

hour before or two hours after meals. However, if this drug upsets your stomach, ask your doctor if you can take it with food or milk.

Swallow the controlled-release capsules whole—do not break, crush, or chew them. Do not be concerned if you notice the remains of the controlled-release tablets in your stool; your body has already absorbed the medicine that was in the tablet.

No special restrictions on exertion and exercise, sun exposure, or exposure to heat or cold.

POSSIBLE SIDE EFFECTS

Although this list of adverse effects may seem somewhat intimidating, keep in mind that some are quite rare. Of course, should these or any other problems arise while you are on medication, it is always a good idea to consult your doctor.

IF YOU DEVELOP	WHAT TO DO
severe dizziness or fainting ■ seizures ■ irregular or fast heartbeat	**Urgent** Get in touch with your doctor immediately.
fever or chills ■ general feeling of unwellness ■ decreased urination ■ drowsiness ■ nausea or vomiting ■ rash, hives, or itching ■ joint pain or swelling ■ pain or difficulty in breathing ■ confusion ■ depression ■ personality changes ■ hallucinations ■ sore mouth, gums, or throat ■ bleeding or bruising ■ tiredness or weakness ■ muscle pain ■ headache	**May be serious** Check with your doctor as soon as possible.
diarrhea ■ stomach pain ■ bitter taste ■ loss of appetite ■ dizziness or light-headedness	If symptoms are disturbing or persist, let your doctor know.

STORAGE INSTRUCTIONS

Store in a cool, dark place (not in a bathroom medicine cabinet).

STOPPING OR INTERRUPTING THERAPY

It is very important to continue taking this medicine exactly as prescribed, even if you feel well. Suddenly stopping this medicine may seriously worsen your medical condition. Your doctor will advise you on how to reduce the dosage gradually when you no longer need this drug. If you miss a dose, take it as soon as possible, unless it is within two hours (regular dosage forms) or four hours (controlled-release dosage forms) of your next scheduled dose. In that case, skip the missed dose and resume your regular schedule. Do not take two doses at the same time.

SPECIAL CONSIDERATIONS FOR THOSE OVER SIXTY-FIVE

The side effects of dizziness, light-headedness, and fainting are more likely to occur in older people, who should take care to avoid falling.

CONDITION: **ABNORMAL HEART RHYTHMS**

CATEGORY: **ANTIARRHYTHMICS**

GENERIC (CHEMICAL) NAME	BRAND (TRADE) NAME	DOSAGE FORMS AND STRENGTHS
Mexiletine hydrochloride	MEXITIL	Capsules: 150, 200, 250 mg

DRUG PROFILE

This drug helps normalize irregular heartbeats and also slows down the heart if it is beating too rapidly. Mexiletine acts directly on the heart itself.

BEFORE USING THIS DRUG

Let your doctor know *IF*

You have ever had allergic reactions or other problems with ■ mexiletine.

You have ever had any of the following medical problems: ■ liver disease ■ heart disease.

You are taking any of the following medicines: ■ other medicine for abnormal heart rhythms ■ medicine to make the urine more acidic ■ narcotic or other prescription pain-killers ■ phenobarbital ■ cimetidine (medicine for ulcers) ■ magnesium aluminum hydroxide (antacid) ■ metoclopramide (medicine for nausea or vomiting) ■ phenytoin (medicine for seizures) ■ rifampin (antibiotic) ■ any medicine containing atropine.

SPECIAL RESTRICTIONS WHILE TAKING THIS DRUG

FOOD AND DRUG INTERACTIONS

Smoking	Smoking may aggravate cardiac arrhythmias. If you smoke, try to stop or at least cut down.

No special restrictions on other drugs, food and beverages, or alcohol use.

DAILY LIVING

Exertion and Exercise	Physical exertion may worsen some kinds of arrhythmias. Ask your doctor to recommend a safe exercise program.
Examinations or Tests	It is important for you to keep all appointments with your doctor, even if you feel well, so that your progress can be checked. Periodic tests and electrocardiograms may be required.
Helpful Hints	Take this medicine with food, milk, or an antacid to reduce upset stomach.

No special restrictions on driving, sun exposure, or exposure to excessive heat or cold.

POSSIBLE SIDE EFFECTS

Although the list of adverse effects may seem somewhat intimidating, keep in mind that some are quite rare. Of course, should these or any other problems arise while you are on medication, it is always a good idea to consult your doctor.

IF YOU DEVELOP	**WHAT TO DO**

IF YOU DEVELOP

irregular heartbeat ■ seizures ■ chest pain ■ fainting ■ difficulty in breathing ■ coma

WHAT TO DO

Urgent Get in touch with your doctor immediately.

---

chills, fever, or sore throat ■ bleeding or bruising ■ tremors ■ difficulty in coordination ■ tiredness or weakness ■ drowsiness ■ swelling of hands or feet ■ hot flashes ■ nervousness ■ confusion ■ difficulty in speech ■ numbness or tingling in hands or feet ■ ringing in ears ■ depression ■ memory problems ■ hallucinations ■ behavior or mood changes ■ blurred vision or other visual disturbances ■ decreased urination ■ rash ■ painful joints ■ hoarseness ■ taste changes ■ general feeling of unwellness

May be serious Check with your doctor as soon as possible.

---

upset stomach ■ heartburn ■ nausea or vomiting ■ diarrhea ■ constipation ■ stomach pain or discomfort ■ change in appetite ■ difficulty in swallowing ■ hiccups ■ dizziness or light-headedness ■ sleep disturbances ■ headache ■ male impotence ■ diminished sex drive ■ dry mouth or other mouth changes ■ dry skin ■ increased sweating ■ hair loss

If symptoms are disturbing or persist, let your doctor know.

STORAGE INSTRUCTIONS

Store in a cool, dark place (not in a bathroom medicine cabinet).

STOPPING OR INTERRUPTING THERAPY

Take this drug exactly as instructed. Check with your doctor on what to do should you miss a dose.

SPECIAL CONSIDERATIONS FOR THOSE OVER SIXTY-FIVE

Older people may be more susceptible to such side effects as drowsiness, dizziness, and light-headedness. They should get in touch with their doctor if they develop any of these symptoms.

CONDITION: **ABNORMAL HEART RHYTHMS**

CATEGORY: **ANTIARRHYTHMICS**

GENERIC (CHEMICAL) NAME	BRAND (TRADE) NAME	DOSAGE FORMS AND STRENGTHS
Tocainide hydrochloride	TONOCARD	Tablets: 400, 600 mg

DRUG PROFILE

This drug helps normalize irregular heartbeats and also slows down the heart if it is beating too rapidly. Tocainide acts directly on the heart itself.

BEFORE USING THIS DRUG

Let your doctor know *IF*

You have ever had allergic reactions or other problems with ■ tocainide ■ local anesthetics, such as lidocaine.

You have ever had any of the following medical problems: ■ heart disease, including congestive heart failure ■ high blood pressure ■ kidney disease ■ liver disease.

You are taking any of the following medicines: ■ other medicine for abnormal heart rhythms ■ acebutolol, atenolol, metoprolol, nadolol, pindolol, propranolol, or timolol (beta-blockers) ■ anticoagulants (blood thinners) ■ diuretics ■ digoxin, digitoxin, or digitalis (heart medicines).

SPECIAL RESTRICTIONS WHILE TAKING THIS DRUG

FOOD AND DRUG INTERACTIONS

Smoking	Smoking may aggravate cardiac arrhythmias. If you smoke, try to stop or at least cut down.

No special restrictions on other drugs, foods and beverages, or alcohol use.

DAILY LIVING

Driving	This drug may cause dizziness, light-headedness, or loss of alertness. Be careful when driving, operating household appliances, or doing any other tasks that require alertness until you know how this drug affects you.
Examinations and Tests	It is important for you to keep all appointments with your doctor, even if you feel well, so that your progress can be checked. Periodic blood tests, especially during the first three months of therapy, and electrocardiograms may be required.
Other Precautions	Tell any doctor or dentist you consult that you are taking this drug, especially if you will be undergoing any type of surgery.
Helpful Hints	Taking this drug with meals or a snack may help prevent the side effects of nausea, dizziness, and light-headedness.

No special restrictions on exertion and exercise, sun exposure, or exposure to excessive heat or cold.

POSSIBLE SIDE EFFECTS

Although this list of adverse effects may seem somewhat intimidating, keep in mind that some are quite rare. Of course, should these or any other problems arise while you are on medication, it is always a good idea to consult your doctor.

IF YOU DEVELOP

severe dizziness or fainting ■ seizures ■ irregular or fast heartbeat ■ chest pain ■ coma ■ convulsions ■ confusion ■ disorientation ■ hallucinations ■ difficulty in breathing ■ coughing or wheezing ■ bleeding or bruising ■ fever, chills, or sore throat

WHAT TO DO

Urgent Get in touch with your doctor immediately.

---

slow heartbeat ■ swelling of hands or feet ■ tremors ■ shakiness ■ loss of coordination ■ clumsiness ■ difficulty in balance ■ disturbances in walking ■ anxiety ■ double vision or other visual disturbances ■ ringing in ears, earache, or other ear problems ■ tiredness ■ drowsiness ■ depression ■ behavior changes ■ changes in taste or smell ■ inability to concentrate or memory problems ■ speech problems ■ sleeplessness ■ increased thirst ■ muscle weakness ■ muscle twitch or spasm ■ rash, itching, or other skin problems ■ muscle or joint pain ■ chilliness ■ clammy skin ■ night sweats ■ hot flashes ■ increased urination ■ urinary retention ■ general feeling of unwellness ■ strange taste in mouth ■ neck pain ■ unusual paleness or flushing ■ pressure on shoulder ■ yawning ■ yellowing of eyes or skin ■ numbness, tingling, pain, or cold in fingers or toes.

May be serious Check with your doctor as soon as possible.

---

light-headedness or dizziness ■ leg cramps ■ nervousness ■ agitation ■ headache ■ blurred vision nausea or vomiting ■ diarrhea ■ loss of appetite ■ indigestion ■ stomach pain ■ constipation ■ difficulty in swallowing ■ dry mouth ■ hiccups ■ hair loss

If symptoms are disturbing or persist, let your doctor know.

STORAGE INSTRUCTIONS

Store in a cool, dark place (not in a bathroom medicine cabinet).

STOPPING OR INTERRUPTING THERAPY

Take this drug exactly as instructed. Check with your doctor on what to do should you miss a dose.

SPECIAL CONSIDERATIONS FOR THOSE OVER SIXTY-FIVE

Older people may be more susceptible to such side effects as drowsiness, dizziness, and light-headedness.

TRANSIENT ISCHEMIC ATTACKS

Most doctors view transient ischemic attacks (TIAs) not as an illness but as a warning. These short episodes of blurred vision, slurred speech, or dizziness are signals that a person may be heading for a serious stroke. Fortunately, it is a warning that can be heeded with good medical care.

CAUSES

TIAs are not uncommon; it is estimated that up to 10 percent of people over the age of sixty-five experience these attacks. Often called ministrokes, TIAs result from a temporary reduction in the blood supply to specific portions of the brain. Several different contributing factors may be involved, the most common of which is blockage of a blood vessel due to atherosclerosis—the buildup of fatty deposits on the blood vessel walls. Small blood clots or clumps of platelets (blood cells that are instrumental in clotting) may also lead to TIAs. Undetected or uncontrolled high blood pressure may be another important underlying cause (see guide to hypertension on pages 20–22).

DIAGNOSIS

In addition to the symptoms noted above, TIAs may cause temporary blindness, confusion, numbness or paralysis in the arms or legs, and twitching, or difficulty in performing routine tasks. These problems may last anywhere from a few seconds to up to twenty-four hours; in most people they clear in less than an hour. Unlike true strokes, TIAs do not leave residual problems, such as continued paralysis or weakness in the limbs or brain damage.

The symptoms themselves are the best clues that doctors have in diagnosing TIAs. The type and frequency of these episodes provide important information and may even pinpoint the areas of the brain that are affected.

TREATMENT

Once a firm diagnosis of a TIA is made, your doctor can choose from a range of medical or surgical treatment options (See drug charts on pages 196–200). Anticoagulant drugs are often prescribed to prevent the formation of clots in the blood vessels that feed the brain. These drugs will not dissolve existing blood clots, but they can limit their growth and help prevent new ones.

If you're taking anticoagulant drugs, your doctor will order a test called prothrombin time or protime to see how long it takes for your blood to clot. The results will help determine how much of the drug you can take safely.

Aspirin is another drug that is often used to prevent TIAs. Recent studies have found that aspirin interferes with platelet function and may therefore help to forestall or even dissolve some blood clots.

The most common type of surgery for TIAs involves removal of fatty deposits from the carotid arteries, which are located on the sides of the neck and are the major blood vessels carrying blood to the brain. Another, newer operation shifts the position of smaller blood vessels. While both of these operations usually ease the symptoms of TIAs, more time and study are needed before doctors can be sure that they are effective in preventing a later stroke.

OUTLOOK

Although experiencing TIAs may be frightening, they actually serve a positive function—they signal that a stroke may be impending and that medical help should be sought. If you follow your doctor's treatment plan carefully, there's a good chance that these ministrokes will become part of your medical past—and that a full-blown stroke will *not* await you in the future.

CONDITION: **TRANSIENT ISCHEMIC ATTACKS**

CATEGORY: **ANTICOAGULANTS**

GENERIC (CHEMICAL) NAME	BRAND (TRADE) NAME	DOSAGE FORMS AND STRENGTHS
Warfarin	COUMADIN	Tablets: 2, 2.5, 5, 7.5, 10 mg
	PANWARFIN	Tablets: 2, 2.5, 5, 7.5, 10 mg

DRUG PROFILE

Warfarin is an anticoagulant—a drug that slows the clotting of the blood and prevents harmful clots from forming and blocking the blood vessels. This type of drug interferes with the action of vitamin K, which is involved in the production of four different clotting factors. An anticoagulant is often used to treat certain heart and blood vessel conditions that make a person more likely to develop blood clots. This medicine cannot dissolve a blood clot that has already formed but can prevent an existing clot from getting larger.

BEFORE USING THIS DRUG

Let your doctor know *IF*

You have ever had allergic reactions or other problems with ■ anticoagulants ■ tartrazine (FD&C Yellow Dye No. 5) (contained in Panwarfin 7.5 mg tablets).

Any member of your family has had problems taking anticoagulant drugs.

You have ever had any of the following medical problems: ■ any heart or blood vessel disease, including stroke or transient ischemic attacks ■severe allergies ■ asthma or other lung disease ■ diabetes ■ kidney disease ■ liver disease ■ high blood pressure ■ high cholesterol ■ congestive heart failure ■ infectious disease, such as hepatitis ■ seizures ■ ulcers ■ bleeding problems ■ any fall or blow to body or head ■ recent fever lasting longer than a few days ■ malnutrition or vitamin deficiency ■ jaundice ■ severe or continuing diarrhea ■ recent medical or dental surgery ■ gallbladder disease ■ collagen disorders ■ swelling of hands, feet, or ankles ■ thyroid disease ■ arthritis ■ mental illness ■ alcoholism ■ cancer.

You are taking any of the following medicines: ■ any other medicine for heart or blood vessel disease ■ aspirin ■ medicine for arthritis ■ medicine for gout ■ narcotic or other prescription pain-killers ■ medicine for fungal infection ■ antibiotic ■ medicine for seizures ■ sleep medicines ■ thyroid hormones ■ male or female hormones ■ medicine for high cholesterol ■ medicine for high blood pressure ■ vitamins C, E, or K ■ corticosteroids or corticotropin (ACTH) ■ medicine for ulcers ■ tranquilizers ■ muscle relaxants ■ medicine for diabetes ■ medicine for tuberculosis or malaria ■ medicine for abnormal heart rhythms ■ medicine for cancer ■ antacids ■ medicine for nausea ■ medicine for colds or sinus problems ■ medicine for depression or other mental illness ■ vaccines ■ mineral oil ■ oxolinic acid (medicine for urinary tract infections) ■ any other medicine, including over-the-counter (OTC) drugs.

You are on a weight-reduction diet.

You are undergoing radiation therapy.

SPECIAL RESTRICTIONS WHILE TAKING THIS DRUG

FOOD AND DRUG INTERACTIONS

Other Drugs	Many drugs affect or are affected by warfarin. Tell your doctor *all* other medicines you are taking, including over-the-counter (OTC) drugs, before starting treatment with warfarin or any other anticoagulant. In addition, *do not stop* taking any other medicines before checking with your doctor.
Foods and Beverages	Eat a well-balanced diet; check with your doctor before going on any weight-reduction diet. Do not begin taking vitamins or other supplements without checking with your doctor. Vitamin K may interfere with the action of warfarin. Do not eat large amounts of foods that contain vitamin K (fish, liver, onions, spinach, kale, cauliflower, and cabbage).
Alcohol	Alcohol interferes with the effectiveness of warfarin. Do not drink regularly while taking this medicine. If you do drink, do not have more than one or two drinks at a time.

No special restrictions on smoking.

DAILY LIVING

Exertion and Exercise	Because bleeding, either external or internal, may be dangerous while you are taking this medicine, try to avoid sports or activities (such as moving heavy objects) that may cause injury.
Excessive Heat	Hot weather may make this medicine less effective.
Examinations or Tests	It is very important for you to keep all appointments with your doctor, even if you feel well, so that your progress can be checked. Periodic blood and urine tests may be required.
Other Precautions	Wear protective gloves when working in a situation in which you may cut or injure yourself. When you brush your teeth, use a soft toothbrush; floss gently. When shaving, use an electric shaver instead of a blade. If you do suffer a cut or injury, call your doctor immediately. Continue these precautions after stopping therapy, as it will take about five days before clotting returns to normal.

No special restrictions on driving, sun exposure, or exposure to excessive cold.

POSSIBLE SIDE EFFECTS

Although this list of adverse effects may seem somewhat intimidating, keep in mind that some are quite rare. Of course, should these or any other problems arise while you are on medication, it is always a good idea to consult your doctor.

IF YOU DEVELOP	**WHAT TO DO**
sore throat, fever, or chills ■ sores in mouth or throat ■ any change in urination ■ weight gain ■ swelling of feet or lower legs ■ tiredness ■ yellowing of eyes or skin ■ pain or color changes (to blue or purple) in toes ■ heavy bleeding or oozing from cuts or wounds ■ nosebleeds ■ bleeding from gums after brushing teeth ■ bruises or other skin marks ■ vomiting or coughing blood or material that looks like coffee grounds ■ bloody or black, tarry stools ■ constipation ■ blood in urine ■ pain or swelling of abdomen, back, joints, or stomach ■ severe headache ■ dizziness	**Urgent** Get in touch with your doctor immediately.
diarrhea ■ nausea or vomiting ■ rash, hives, or itching	**May be serious** Check with your doctor as soon as possible.
bloating or gas ■ visual problems ■ loss of appetite ■ hair loss	If symptoms are disturbing or persist, let your doctor know.

STORAGE INSTRUCTIONS

Store in a cool, dark place (not in a bathroom medicine cabinet).

STOPPING OR INTERRUPTING THERAPY

Take this medicine for exactly the time prescribed. Do not stop taking it abruptly; your doctor will advise you on how to gradually reduce your dosage. When you stop taking this medicine, it usually takes about five days before your clotting ability returns to normal. If you miss a dose of this medicine, take it as soon as possible. If it is almost time for your next dose, skip the missed dose and resume your regular schedule. Do not take two doses at the same time.

SPECIAL CONSIDERATIONS FOR THOSE OVER SIXTY-FIVE

None.

CONDITION: **TRANSIENT ISCHEMIC ATTACKS**

CATEGORY: **ANTIPLATELET DRUGS**

GENERIC (CHEMICAL) NAME	BRAND (TRADE) NAME	DOSAGE FORMS AND STRENGTHS
Aspirin and other salicylate drugs		

Aspirin and other salicylate drugs are available over the counter under a variety of brand names, dosage forms, and strengths. Some of these preparations have a special coating or contain ingredients (buffers) to help protect the lining of the stomach against possible irritation. Because of the importance of salicylate drugs in the treatment of chronic pain, even though they are most often nonprescription drugs, they are included in this book for reader reference.

DRUG PROFILE

Aspirin and other drugs in the salicylate family are used to relieve pain, inflammation, and fever. Large doses are used to treat symptoms of arthritis and rheumatism such as swelling, stiffness, and joint pain. Aspirin and other salicylates are thought to control pain and swelling by blocking the production of naturally occurring triggers of pain and inflammation, called prostaglandins. These drugs relieve fever by resetting the body's thermostat to its normal temperature.

Because aspirin helps prevent the blood cells from clumping together, it is also sometimes prescribed to reduce the risk of recurrent ministrokes (transient ischemic attacks, or TIAs) and stroke. The benefits of aspirin in ministrokes have to date been proven only in men—but not in women. Aspirin may also help prevent another heart attack in people who have survived a heart attack or who have the extremely severe type of chest pain known as unstable angina. Aspirin is also sometimes prescribed to prevent blood clots in people who are susceptible to this problem.

For complete information on these drugs, see pages 379–383.

HYPERLIPIDEMIA

Hyperlipidemia is usually a silent problem. For most people, the first indication is a blood test showing high levels of cholesterol or triglycerides— fatty substances known as lipids. If you have a family history of either coronary artery disease or premature atherosclerosis, your doctor will probably want to order such a blood test.

CAUSES

Our bodies need small amounts of cholesterol in order to make certain hormones and to keep the nerve fibers healthy. But if there is too much cholesterol in the blood, it tends to accumulate on the walls of the blood vessels. This can lead to atherosclerosis, the narrowing of vital blood vessels that is a major cause of heart attacks and strokes.

Some triglycerides are burned for energy, while the remainder are stored as body fat. For many years, doctors believed that an excess of triglycerides in the blood could lead to heart disease, but today they are not so sure. What is known, however, is that a very high level of triglycerides can cause stomach pain and inflammation of the pancreas (acute pancreatitis).

DIAGNOSIS

When your doctor told you that you had hyperlipidemia, he or she probably mentioned some numbers. Lipids are measured in milligrams (mg) per deciliter (dl) of blood (for example, 200

mg/dl). This is often shortened to 200 mg or simply given as a number (for example, 200). Blood tests not only measure triglycerides and total cholesterol but fractions or types of cholesterol as well. This is important information, since each type of cholesterol plays a different role in the body and may require a different treatment.

A blood test for lipids will give your doctor four numbers: one expresses the triglyceride level and the others stand for three types of cholesterol:

- LDL (low-density lipoprotein) cholesterol. This is the so-called bad cholesterol that seems to be a culprit in the development of atherosclerosis and is associated with a high risk of heart disease.
- HDL (high-density lipoprotein) cholesterol. This is the "good" cholesterol; it helps clear lipids from the bloodstream and appears to protect against heart disease.
- VLDL (very low-density lipoprotein) cholesterol. An excess of this type of cholesterol in the blood is linked to high triglyceride levels and also contributes to the production of LDL cholesterol.

Ideally, your HDL level should be one-fourth of your total blood cholesterol. Thus, if your total cholesterol count is 200 mg, your HDL level should be at least 50.

Normally, your body manufactures all the cholesterol it needs. Additional cholesterol comes from dietary sources, such as red meat, egg yolk, butter, lard, whole milk, and hard cheese. However, the body's ability to clear cholesterol from the blood varies widely from one individual to another. For this reason, some people who conscientiously follow a low-cholesterol diet may still have high blood-cholesterol levels, while others who are not so careful about what they eat may maintain relatively low cholesterol counts.

High triglyceride levels are usually related to lifestyle habits. A rich, high-calorie diet can send triglyceride levels soaring; so can large amounts of alcohol, being overweight, cigarette smoking, and a lack of physical activity. In addition, chronic illnesses, such as diabetes and kidney disease, and certain drugs, such as beta-blockers and thiazide diuretics, may cause a problem with triglycerides.

TREATMENT

According to the American Heart Association (AHA), the ideal total cholesterol level for adults is under 200 mg. When cholesterol levels exceed 220, the AHA recommends a change in diet. This means reducing your intake of the above-mentioned foods, which are high in cholesterol and saturated fat, and replacing them with skinless poultry, veal, seafood, margarine, vegetable oils, and skimmed or low-fat milk products. Certain types of fiber found in apples, carrots, soybeans, dried beans and peas, and oatmeal are believed to lower cholesterol levels. Fish oils, especially those from "fatty" fish like salmon, trout, and mackerel, also seem to have a cholesterol-lowering effect. Regular, moderate exercise (like a daily walk-

ing program) is often recommended as an accompaniment to dietary changes. Although exercise by itself will not lower total cholesterol, it does seem to boost the levels of HDL ("good") cholesterol in the blood.

When a blood test reports a cholesterol level of 265 or more, diet and exercise changes may not be enough. At this point, your doctor may choose to prescribe one or more drugs to bring your cholesterol levels down. A number of factors may influence this decision. If, for example, you are overweight, smoke cigarettes, or have high blood pressure or a family history of early heart disease, the doctor may be more likely to start you on lipid-lowering drugs right away. Gender may also play a role. Since men face a higher risk of developing heart disease than women, doctors tend to treat elevated cholesterol levels more aggressively in men.

Triglyceride levels seem to rise naturally as we grow older. However, if they exceed 200 mg, it may be time for diet or drug therapy. As a first step, doctors sometimes suggest a low-fat diet. If, after a trial period of several weeks, your triglyceride level stays high, medicine may be necessary to bring it under control. In cases in which the triglyceride count is abnormally high (over 300) or is causing severe stomach pain, doctors often start off by prescribing medicine.

OUTLOOK

Drugs that lower triglyceride and cholesterol levels will not completely cure the problem, but they do help to interrupt the body's manufacture and storage of excess lipids. Don't expect immediate results. It usually takes several weeks of regular use before these drugs have a noticeable effect, and the prescription may have to be continued for months or even years to get cholesterol or triglycerides down to healthy levels. At that point, your doctor may taper off the drugs to see if diet and other changes (increased exercise, stopping smoking, losing weight) will keep your lipid levels under control. For some people, it may be necessary to continue the medicine indefinitely. (See charts on pages 204–216.)

To lower particularly high or stubborn lipid levels, your doctor may prescribe two or more of these drugs together. Such combinations may also be used when both triglyceride and LDL cholesterol levels are high.

In people whose high triglyceride levels are causing severe stomach pain, drug treatment will probably produce welcome relief within a few days. However, treatment for hyperlipidemia will not make an obvious difference in the way most people feel from day to day. But in the following months, their blood tests may well show a gradual decline in lipid levels. And, as the cholesterol count falls, so does the risk of heart disease. A recent, major study sponsored by the National Institutes of Health demonstrated that for every 1 percent reduction in blood cholesterol levels, there was a 2 percent decrease in the risk of heart attack. Other studies indicate that a combination of the lipid-lowering drug cholestyramine and dietary modification may slow or possibly even reverse the process of atherosclerosis—an encouraging sign that effective treatment of hyperlipidemia can help prevent heart disease and stroke.

In addition to the drugs described in the charts in this chapter, a new drug called lovastatin (Mevacor) shows promise as an effective, safe, and convenient cholesterol-lowering agent. As of this writing, lovastatin has just been approved for use by the Food and Drug Administration, and you might want to ask your doctor about the drug's benefits and risks.

CONDITION: **HYPERLIPIDEMIA**

CATEGORY: **LIPID-LOWERING AGENTS**

GENERIC (CHEMICAL) NAME	BRAND (TRADE) NAME	DOSAGE FORMS AND STRENGTHS
Clofibrate	ATROMID-S	Capsules: 500 mg

DRUG PROFILE

Clofibrate lowers excess amounts of triglycerides (fatty substances) in the blood. This may help guard against atherosclerosis ("hardening" of the arteries caused by deposits of fat) and lower your risk of developing heart disease.

BEFORE USING THIS DRUG

Let your doctor know *IF*

You have ever had allergic reactions or other problems with ■ clofibrate.

You have ever had any of the following medical problems: ■ gallstones ■ heart disease ■ kidney disease ■ liver disease, including jaundice ■ stomach or intestinal ulcer ■ underactive thyroid ■ diabetes ■ angina (chest pain).

You are taking any of the following medicines: ■ cholestyramine (medicine for high cholesterol) ■ anticoagulants (blood thinners) ■ furosemide (diuretic).

This drug may increase your risk for tumors, liver disease, inflammation of the pancreas, and gallstones. Be sure to discuss these possible risks with your doctor before taking clofibrate.

SPECIAL RESTRICTIONS WHILE TAKING THIS DRUG

FOOD AND DRUG INTERACTIONS

Other Drugs	It is especially important to let your doctor know if you are taking an anticoagulant (blood thinner) because clofibrate can exaggerate the effect of the anticoagulant.

Foods and Beverages	Your doctor may prescribe a special diet for you that is low in fats and/or cholesterol, which you should follow carefully. If you are overweight, a weight-reduction diet may be recommended.
Alcohol	Alcohol may be a cause of high cholesterol. Your doctor will probably suggest that you reduce your intake of alcoholic beverages.

No special restrictions on smoking.

DAILY LIVING

Examinations or Tests	It is important for you to keep all appointments with your doctor, even if you feel well, so that your progress can be checked. Periodic blood tests may be required.
Helpful Hints	To lessen the chance of upset stomach, take this medicine with or immediately after a meal.

No special restrictions on driving, exertion and exercise, sun exposure, or exposure to excessive heat or cold.

POSSIBLE SIDE EFFECTS

Although this list of adverse effects may seem somewhat intimidating, keep in mind that some are quite rare. Of course, should these or any other problems arise while you are on medication, it is always a good idea to consult your doctor.

IF YOU DEVELOP

chest pain ■ irregular heartbeat ■ severe stomach pain with nausea and vomiting ■ shortness of breath

WHAT TO DO

Urgent Get in touch with your doctor immediately.

blood in urine ■ decreased urination ■ swelling of feet or lower legs ■ fever, chills, or sore throat	**May be serious** Check with your doctor as soon as possible.
diarrhea ■ nausea or vomiting ■ increased appetite or weight gain ■ sores in the mouth or on the lips ■ stomach pain ■ gas or bloating ■ heartburn ■ aching or cramped muscles ■ tiredness or weakness ■ male impotence ■ diminished sex drive ■ headache ■ dizziness ■ drowsiness ■ male breast tenderness ■ rash, hives, or itching ■ dry skin or hair ■ hair loss ■ pain or difficulty in urination	If symptoms are disturbing or persist, let your doctor know.

STORAGE INSTRUCTIONS

Store in a cool, dark place (not in a bathroom medicine cabinet).

STOPPING OR INTERRUPTING THERAPY

Take this medicine exactly as directed by your doctor and do not stop taking it without checking with your doctor. If you miss a dose, take it as soon as possible; if it is almost time for your next dose, skip the missed dose and resume your regular schedule. Do not take two doses at the same time.

SPECIAL CONSIDERATIONS FOR THOSE OVER SIXTY-FIVE

Older people may be more troubled by such side effects as nausea. They should let their doctors know if such problems are particularly bothersome.

CONDITIONS: **HYPERLIPIDEMIA**

CATEGORY: **LIPID-LOWERING AGENTS**

GENERIC (CHEMICAL) NAME	BRAND (TRADE) NAME	DOSAGE FORMS AND STRENGTHS
Gemfibrozil	LOPID	Capsules: 300 mg

DRUG PROFILE

Gemfibrozil is used to lower high levels of triglycerides (fatty substances) in the blood. Lowering these substances is important because the buildup of these substances along the walls of the blood vessels can lead to such serious conditions as angina, heart attack, or stroke.

BEFORE USING THIS DRUG

Let your doctor know *IF*

You have ever had allergic reactions or other problems with ■ gemfibrozil.

You have ever had any of the following medical problems: ■ gallbladder disease, including gallstones ■ heart disease ■ kidney disease ■ liver disease ■ underactive thyroid ■ diabetes.

You are taking: ■ anticoagulants (blood thinners).

This drug may increase your risk for tumors, liver disease, inflammation of the pancreas, and gallstones. Be sure to discuss these possible risks with your doctor before taking gemfibrozil.

SPECIAL RESTRICTIONS WHILE TAKING THIS DRUG

FOOD AND DRUG INTERACTIONS

Other Drugs	It is especially important to let your doctor know if you are taking an anticoagulant (blood thinner), because gemfibrozil can exaggerate the effect of the anticoagulant.
Foods and Beverages	Your doctor may suggest a diet low in fats and/or cholesterol. If you are overweight, a weight-reduction diet may be recommended.
Alcohol	Alcohol may be a cause of high cholesterol. Your doctor will probably suggest that you reduce your intake of alcoholic beverages.

No special restrictions on smoking.

DAILY LIVING

Exertion or Exercise	To get the maximum benefit from this medicine, follow both a proper diet and a regular exercise program.
Examinations or Tests	It is important for you to keep all appointments with your doctor, even if you feel well, so that your progress can be checked. Periodic blood tests may be required.
Other Precautions	Although there have been no reports of major problems from gemfibrozil, this drug is very similar to clofibrate, which has been found to increase the risk of gallstones (see clofibrate chart, pages 204–206). If you have diabetes, be aware that this medicine may raise blood-sugar levels. If you notice any change when testing sugar levels in your blood or urine, let your doctor know.

No special restrictions on driving, sun exposure, or exposure to excessive heat or cold.

POSSIBLE SIDE EFFECTS

Although this list of adverse effects may seem somewhat intimidating, keep in mind that some are quite rare. Of course, should these or any other problems arise while you are on medication, it is always a good idea to consult your doctor.

IF YOU DEVELOP	**WHAT TO DO**
fever, chills, or sore throat ■ severe stomach pain with nausea and vomiting ■ irregular heartbeat	**Urgent** Get in touch with your doctor immediately.

diarrhea ■ nausea and vomiting ■ stomach pain ■ gas ■ heartburn ■ rash, hives, or itching ■ muscle or bone pain ■ blurred vision ■ headache ■ dizziness

May be serious Check with your doctor as soon as possible.

STORAGE INSTRUCTIONS

Store in a cool, dark place (not in a bathroom medicine cabinet).

STOPPING OR INTERRUPTING THERAPY

If you miss a dose of this medicine, take it as soon as possible. If it is almost time for your next dose, skip the missed dose and resume your regular schedule. Do not take two doses at the same time.

SPECIAL CONSIDERATIONS FOR THOSE OVER SIXTY-FIVE

None.

CONDITION: **HYPERLIPIDEMIA**

CATEGORY: **LIPID-LOWERING AGENTS**

GENERIC (CHEMICAL) NAME	BRAND (TRADE) NAME	DOSAGE FORMS AND STRENGTHS
Probucol	LORELCO	Tablets: 250 mg

DRUG PROFILE

Probucol is used to treat high levels of cholesterol in the blood. Lowering high cholesterol is important because the buildup of cholesterol along the walls of the blood vessels can lead to such serious conditions as angina, heart attack, or stroke.

BEFORE USING THIS DRUG

Let your doctor know *IF*

You have ever had allergic reactions or other problems with ■ probucol.

You have ever had any of the following medical problems: ■ gallbladder disease or gallstones ■ heart disease, especially heart attack or abnormal heart rhythms ■ liver disease ■ underactive thyroid ■ diabetes.

You are taking: ■ clofibrate (medicine for high cholesterol).

SPECIAL RESTRICTIONS WHILE TAKING THIS DRUG

FOOD AND DRUG INTERACTIONS

Foods and Beverages	Your doctor may suggest a diet low in fats and/or cholesterol. If you are overweight, a weight-reduction diet may be recommended.
Alcohol	Alcohol may be a cause of high cholesterol. Your doctor will probably suggest that you reduce your intake of alcoholic beverages.

No special restrictions on other drugs or smoking.

DAILY LIVING

Exertion and Exercise	To get the maximum benefit from this medicine, follow both a proper diet and a regular exercise program.
Examinations or Tests	It is important for you to keep all appointments with your doctor, even if you feel well, so that your progress can be checked. Periodic blood tests may be required. Your doctor may also want to take an electrocardiogram before and during therapy.
Other Precautions	Occasionally, there may be a reaction at the beginning of therapy that consists of fainting or dizziness, irregular heartbeat, nausea, vomiting, and sometimes chest pain as well. If this should occur, call your doctor at once.

Helpful Hints	This medicine works best when taken with meals.

No special restrictions on driving, sun exposure, or exposure to excessive heat or cold.

POSSIBLE SIDE EFFECTS

Although this list of adverse effects may seem somewhat intimidating, keep in mind that some are quite rare. Of course, should these or any other problems arise while you are on medication, it is always a good idea to consult your doctor.

IF YOU DEVELOP	WHAT TO DO
When beginning therapy: fainting ■ dizziness ■ irregular heartbeat ■ nausea or vomiting ■ chest pain	**Urgent** Get in touch with your doctor immediately.
swelling of face, hands, feet, or inside of mouth ■ irregular heartbeat ■ chest pain ■ fainting ■ dizziness	**May be serious:** Check with your doctor as soon as possible.
diarrhea or loose stools ■ nausea or vomiting ■ indigestion ■ stomach pain ■ gas ■ headache ■ numbness or tingling in fingers, toes, or face ■ diminished sense of taste or smell ■ blurred vision ■ tearing ■ red or itching eyes ■ ringing in the ears ■ increased or decreased appetite ■ sleeplessness ■ rash or hives ■ need to urinate at night ■ male sexual problems ■ increased sweating or foul-smelling sweat	If symptoms are disturbing or persist, let your doctor know.

STORAGE INSTRUCTIONS

Store in a cool, dark place (not in a bathroom medicine cabinet).

STOPPING OR INTERRUPTING THERAPY

Because this medicine only controls and does not cure high cholesterol, you may have to take it for a long period of time. Suddenly stopping this medicine may raise your cholesterol level. Your doctor will advise you on how to gradually decrease your medicine when you no longer need it. If you miss a dose, take it as soon as possible. If it is almost time for your next dose, skip the missed dose and resume your regular schedule. Do not take two doses at the same time.

SPECIAL CONSIDERATIONS FOR THOSE OVER SIXTY-FIVE

None.

CONDITION: **HYPERLIPIDEMIA**

CATEGORY: **LIPID-LOWERING AGENTS**

GENERIC (CHEMICAL) NAME	BRAND (TRADE) NAME	DOSAGE FORMS AND STRENGTHS
Cholestyramine	QUESTRAN	Powder: 4 g of anhydrous cholestyramine resin in 9 g of powder per packet or scoopful

DRUG PROFILE

Cholestyramine is used to lower blood levels of cholesterol. Lowering high cholesterol is important because the buildup of cholesterol along the walls of the blood vessels can lead to such serious conditions as angina, heart attack, or stroke. Cholestyramine is also used to relieve severe itching caused by high levels of bile acids in the blood of people whose bile ducts are obstructed. This drug is not actually absorbed into the body but works by remaining in the digestive tract and attacking certain substances in the intestine.

BEFORE USING THIS DRUG

Let your doctor know *IF*

You have ever had allergic reactions or other problems with ■ cholestyramine ■ tartrazine (FD&C Yellow Dye No. 5) ■ aspirin.

You have ever had any of the following medical problems: ■ heart or blood vessel disease ■ liver disease ■ bleeding problems ■ gallstones ■ obstruction of the gallbladder or bile ducts ■ kidney disease ■ stomach ulcer ■ constipation ■ hemorrhoids ■ underactive thyroid ■ diabetes ■ osteoporosis.

You are taking any of the following medicines: ■ anticoagulants (blood thinners) digoxin, digitoxin, or digitalis (heart medicines) ■ thyroid medicine ■ vitamins ■ medicine for arthritis or gout ■ diuretics ■ tetracycline ■ penicillin ■ medicine for seizures ■ sleep medicines ■ medicine for gallstones.

SPECIAL RESTRICTIONS WHILE TAKING THIS DRUG

FOOD AND DRUG INTERACTIONS

Other Drugs	Do not take other medicine at the same time you take cholestyramine. Other drugs should be taken one hour before or four to six hours after taking a dose of cholestyramine.
	Cholestyramine interferes with a number of other drugs (see above). In addition, if you have been taking both cholestyramine and digitalis and suddenly stop taking cholestyramine, concentrations of digitalis in the blood can rise to dangerous levels.
Foods and Beverages	Your doctor may suggest a diet low in fats and/or cholesterol. If you are overweight, a weight-reduction diet may be recommended.
	It is important to drink plenty of fluids while taking this medicine. This drug may interfere with your absorption of certain vitamins. If you develop a vitamin deficiency, your doctor may give you special vitamin supplements.

No special restrictions on smoking or alcohol use.

DAILY LIVING

Exertion and Exercise	To get the most benefit from this medicine, follow both a proper diet and a regular exercise program.

Examinations or Tests	It is important for you to keep all appointments with your doctor, even if you feel well, so that your progress can be checked. Periodic blood tests are usually required.

Helpful Hints	Do not take the powder in dry form. Mix one scoopful or packetful with at least two to six fluid ounces of water, fruit juice, milk, or any other noncarbonated beverage. Let the powder sit, without stirring, for a minute or two, and then stir until it is completely mixed; it will not dissolve. After drinking, add a little more liquid to the glass and drink it to make sure you have swallowed all the medicine.
	Mild constipation is a common side effect of this drug and can usually be relieved by laxatives or stool softeners. Let your doctor know if constipation continues or is severe.

No special restrictions on driving, sun exposure, or exposure to excessive heat or cold.

POSSIBLE SIDE EFFECTS

Although this list of adverse effects may seem somewhat intimidating, keep in mind that some are quite rare. Of course, should these or any other problems arise while you are on medication, it is always a good idea to consult your doctor.

IF YOU DEVELOP	WHAT TO DO
black, tarry stools ■ severe stomach pain with nausea and vomiting	**Urgent** Get in touch with your doctor immediately.
constipation ■ weight loss ■ aggravation of hemorrhoids	**May be serious** Check with your doctor as soon as possible.

heartburn ■ indigestion ■ diarrhea ■ nausea or vomiting ■ loss of appetite ■ stomach pain ■ belching, bloating, or gas ■ rash or soreness of skin, tongue, or anal tissues

If symptoms are disturbing or persist, let your doctor know.

STORAGE INSTRUCTIONS

Store in a cool, dark place (not in a bathroom medicine cabinet).

STOPPING OR INTERRUPTING THERAPY

Because this medicine controls but does not cure high cholesterol, you may have to take it for an extended period of time. If you miss a dose, take it as soon as possible. If it is almost time for your next dose, skip the missed dose and resume your regular dosing schedule. Do not take two doses at the same time.

SPECIAL CONSIDERATIONS FOR THOSE OVER SIXTY-FIVE

Older people may be more prone to the side effect of constipation. Also, this drug may worsen osteoporosis because it causes loss of calcium, an important component of bone.

CONDITION: **HYPERLIPIDEMIA**

CATEGORY: **LIPID-LOWERING AGENTS**

GENERIC (CHEMICAL) NAME	BRAND (TRADE) NAME	DOSAGE FORMS AND STRENGTHS
Niacin	NICOBID	Controlled-release capsules: 125, 250, 500 mg

This drug is available both by prescripton and over the counter under a variety of brand names and dosage forms.

DRUG PROFILE

Niacin helps the body break down food so that it can be used for energy. This type of supplement is used to prevent or treat niacin deficiency, or pellagra. Niacin is also used to lower blood levels of fats and cholesterol.

For complete information on this drug, see pages 547 .

INTERMITTENT CLAUDICATION

Intermittent claudication, which literally means "limping that comes and goes," is the name of a condition that affects the legs. Cramping leg pain during walking or exercise or very tired legs are its most common symptoms. It is usually the first sign of chronic peripheral atherosclerotic disease, a type of atherosclerosis—or "hardening of the arteries"—that affects the arteries in the legs and arms.

CAUSES

In atherosclerosis, a fatty plaque partially or completely blocks the artery. The amount of blood that can get through a partially blocked artery may be sufficient at rest, but an active muscle demands more circulating blood than a resting one; if no more blood can pass through the artery, intermittent claudication results.

People who smoke; are obese; or have diabetes, hypertension, or high blood-cholesterol levels face the greatest risk for developing intermittent claudication. This condition affects men almost twice as often as women and becomes increasingly common with age. In fact, one out of every one hundred people between the ages of sixty-five and seventy-four has intermittent claudication.

DIAGNOSIS

The pain associated with intermittent claudication is usually in the calf, but some people have pain in the foot, thigh, hip, buttock, or even the lower back. Usually one leg is involved. The symptom is quite consistent, occurring after the same amount of exercise each time. Some people suffer from weakness and fatigue rather than pain. Relief comes two to five minutes after stopping the activity.

If the blockage in the artery worsens, intermittent claudication progresses to leg pain even at rest. In this advanced stage, other symptoms that you may develop include numbness, burning, changes in skin color (to pale or red), loss of hair on the leg, bluish nails, and ulcers. Permanent damage to the leg, including gangrene, can occur.

To find out if you have this condition, your doctor will probably use a blood pressure cuff to check your ankle pulse; this pulse is faint or even absent in intermittent claudication. Doppler ultrasound may be used to measure blood flow. This measurement is taken by moving a transducer over the skin to direct sound waves into the blood vessels. The sonic echoes reflected back measure the amount of blood flow with great accuracy, in addition to locating the blockage.

If you haven't had a physical examination in some time, your doctor may decide to test for diseases that can contribute to intermittent claudication. Your examination might then include a glucose tolerance test for diabetes and a blood test for elevated cholesterol.

TREATMENT

There are several different drugs that can be prescribed to treat intermittent claudication. For detailed information on these drugs, see the charts on pages 219–225.

Surgery is seldom necessary for mild or moderate intermittent claudication. However, if the condition worsens and becomes advanced, a graft to bypass the blockage (arterial bypass surgery) may be done.

The most important part of treatment involves steps—both literally and otherwise—you can take on your own. Walking is ideal for anyone who has intermittent claudication. It should be done every day for at least thirty to sixty minutes. When discomfort occurs, stop and wait until it subsides; then continue walking. Although exercise may set off an attack, regular exercise will actually help develop new blood vessels and improve your tolerance.

Tobacco in all forms must be avoided because it aggravates this condition. Diabetes, elevated cholesterol, and high blood pressure should be carefully controlled by diet and by any drugs that are prescribed. If you are overweight, ask your doctor to recommend a diet and an exercise program. Weight loss can make a big difference in how much exertion you can tolerate.

Give your feet tender, loving care. Reduced circulation may have made your feet less sensitive, so a daily inspection for injuries is mandatory. Your shoes should fit correctly, and your feet should be kept clean and dry. Clip your toenails regularly, cutting straight across and taking care not to injure your toes. Because even minor injuries pose the danger of infection, seek the services of a podiatrist for treatment of corns, calluses, and ingrown toenails.

OUTLOOK

A diagnosis of intermittent claudication may be the first indication that you have atherosclerosis. Although atherosclerosis cannot be cured, the chances of further complications can be reduced. Most of the success in controlling peripheral atherosclerotic disease will come from your own efforts. By working with your doctor and taking the prescribed medicines, you may find that you are living a healthier life than before.

CONDITION: **INTERMITTENT CLAUDICATION**

CATEGORY: **HEMORHEOLOGIC DRUGS**

GENERIC (CHEMICAL) NAME	BRAND (TRADE) NAME	DOSAGE FORMS AND STRENGTHS
Pentoxifylline	TRENTAL	Controlled-release tablets: 400 mg

DRUG PROFILE

Pentoxifylline is used to treat intermittent claudication. It is a hemorheologic drug, which means that it works by making the red blood cells more flexible. This allows the blood to flow more easily, especially through the smaller blood vessels in the limbs.

BEFORE USING THIS DRUG

Let your doctor know *IF*

You have ever had allergic reactions or other problems with ■ pentoxifylline ■ caffeine ■ aminophylline, oxtriphylline, or theophylline (medicine for asthma).

You have ever had any of the following medical problems: ■ high or low blood pressure ■ angina (chest pain) ■ abnormal heart rhythm ■ stroke or other disease of the blood vessels ■ heart disease ■ kidney disease.

You are taking any of the following medicines: ■ medicine for high blood pressure ■ anticoagulants (blood thinners).

SPECIAL RESTRICTIONS WHILE TAKING THIS DRUG

FOOD AND DRUG INTERACTIONS

Smoking	Smoking may worsen your medical condition. If you smoke, try to stop or at least cut down.

No special restrictions on other drugs, foods and beverages, or alcohol use.

DAILY LIVING

Examinations or Tests	It is important for you to keep all appointments with your doctor so that your progress can be checked.
Helpful Hints	To avoid upset stomach, take this medicine with meals or a snack.
	Swallow the controlled-release tablets whole—do not break, chew, or crush them.

No special restrictions on driving, exertion and exercise, sun exposure, or exposure to excessive heat or cold.

POSSIBLE SIDE EFFECTS

Although this list of adverse effects may seem somewhat intimidating, keep in mind that some are quite rare. Of course, should these or any other problems arise while you are on medication, it is always a good idea to consult your doctor.

IF YOU DEVELOP	WHAT TO DO
drowsiness ■ flushing ■ fainting ■ excitement ■ fever ■ seizures ■ chest pain	**Urgent** Get in touch with your doctor immediately.
irregular or fast heartbeat ■ nervousness ■ agitation ■ sleeplessness	**May be serious** Check with your doctor as soon as possible.
dizziness ■ headache ■ tremors ■ nausea or vomiting ■ upset stomach ■ belching ■ bloating or gas	If symptoms are disturbing or persist, let your doctor know.

STORAGE INSTRUCTIONS

Store in a cool, dark place (not in a bathroom medicine cabinet).

STOPPING OR INTERRUPTING THERAPY

It may take several weeks before you feel any beneficial effects from this medicine. Do not stop taking this drug without checking with your doctor. If you miss a dose, take it as soon as possible. If it is almost time for your next dose, skip the missed dose and resume your regular schedule. Do not take two doses at the same time.

SPECIAL CONSIDERATIONS FOR THOSE OVER SIXTY-FIVE

None.

CONDITION: **INTERMITTENT CLAUDICATION**

CATEGORY: **PERIPHERAL VASODILATORS**

GENERIC (CHEMICAL) NAME	BRAND (TRADE) NAME	DOSAGE FORMS AND STRENGTHS
Nylidrin hydrochloride	ARLIDIN	Tablets: 6, 12 mg

DRUG PROFILE

Nylidrin plays a supporting role in the treatment of conditions caused by poor circulation, such as diabetic vascular disease, Raynaud's syndrome, phlebitis, frostbite, inner ear disturbances, cerebral vascular disease, and atherosclerosis. The National Academy of Sciences, the National Research Council, and the Food and Drug Administration have classified this drug as "possibly" effective and recommended that it be reevaluated. You should discuss its use with your doctor.

BEFORE USING THIS DRUG

Let your doctor know *IF*

You have ever had allergic reactions of other problems with ■ nylidrin.

You have ever had any of the following medical problems: ■ angina (chest pain)
■ heart disease, including recent heart attack ■ fast heartbeat ■ stomach ulcer
■ overactive thyroid.

SPECIAL RESTRICTIONS WHILE TAKING THIS DRUG

FOOD AND DRUG INTERACTIONS

Smoking	Smoking may reduce the beneficial effects of this drug. If you smoke, try to stop or at least cut down.

No special restrictions on other drugs, foods and beverages, or alcohol use.

DAILY LIVING

Helpful Hints	Because this drug can cause fast or pounding heartbeat, do not take your last dose just before bedtime, since it may disturb your sleep. Discuss with your doctor the best dosage schedule for you.

No special restrictions on exertion and exercise, sun exposure, or exposure to excessive heat or cold.

POSSIBLE SIDE EFFECTS

Although this list of adverse effects may seem somewhat intimidating, keep in mind that some are quite rare. Of course, should these or any other problems arise while you are on medication, it is always a good idea to consult your doctor.

IF YOU DEVELOP	WHAT TO DO
chest pain ■ decreased urination or inability to urinate ■ fever ■ blurred vision ■ metallic taste	**Urgent** Get in touch with your doctor immediately.
irregular or fast heartbeat ■ dizziness, faintness, or light-headedness, especially when getting up from a reclining or sitting position ■ tiredness or weakness	**May be serious** Check with your doctor as soon as possible.

| nausea or vomiting ■ headache ■ tremors ■ nervousness ■ flushing ■ chilliness | If symptoms are disturbing or persist, let your doctor know. |

STORAGE INSTRUCTIONS

Store in a cool, dark place (not in a bathroom medicine cabinet).

STOPPING OR INTERRUPTING THERAPY

Do not stop taking this medicine, even if you see no difference in your condition, without consulting your doctor. If you miss a dose of this medicine, take it as soon as possible. If it is almost time for your next dose, skip the missed dose and resume your regular schedule. Do not take two doses at the same time.

SPECIAL CONSIDERATIONS FOR THOSE OVER SIXTY-FIVE

None.

CONDITION: **INTERMITTENT CLAUDICATION**

CATEGORY: **PERIPHERAL VASODILATORS**

GENERIC (CHEMICAL) NAME	BRAND (TRADE) NAME	DOSAGE FORMS AND STRENGTHS
Cyclandelate	CYCLOSPASMOL	Capsules: 200, 400 mg

DRUG PROFILE

Cyclandelate plays a supporting role in the treatment of conditions caused by poor circulation, such as diabetic vascular disease, Raynaud's syndrome, phlebitis, intermittent claudication, night leg cramps, and atherosclerosis. The National Academy of Sciences, the National Research Council, and the Food and Drug Administration have classified this drug as "possibly" effective and recommended that it be reevaluated. You should discuss its use with your doctor.

BEFORE USING THIS DRUG

Let your doctor know *IF*

You have ever had allergic reactions or other problems with ■ cyclandelate.

You have ever had any of the following medical problems: ■ angina (chest pain) ■ recent heart attack or stroke ■ glaucoma ■ bleeding problems.

SPECIAL RESTRICTIONS WHILE TAKING THIS DRUG

FOOD AND DRUG INTERACTIONS

Smoking	Smoking may reduce the benefits of this drug. If you smoke, try to stop or at least cut down.

No special restrictions on other drugs, foods and beverages, or alcohol use.

DAILY LIVING

Precautions	This drug may cause dizziness; use caution when getting up from a reclining or sitting position or when climbing stairs, and let your doctor know if the dizziness becomes a problem. You also may experience flushing, headache, weakness, or fast heartbeat, especially during the first few weeks of therapy.
Helpful Hints	If this medicine upsets your stomach, taking it with milk, meals, snacks, or an antacid should help.

No special restrictions on driving, exertion and exercise, sun exposure, or exposure to excessive heat or cold.

POSSIBLE SIDE EFFECTS

Although this list of adverse effects may seem somewhat intimidating, keep in mind that some are quite rare. Of course, should these or any other problems arise while you are on medication, it is always a good idea to consult your doctor.

IF YOU DEVELOP

fast heartbeat ■ dizziness, especially when getting up from a reclining or sitting position ■ tiredness or weakness ■ headache ■ flushing ■ tingling in face, fingers, or toes ■ increased sweating ■ gas ■ heartburn ■ nausea ■ stomach pain or discomfort

WHAT TO DO

If symptoms are disturbing or persist, let your doctor know.

STORAGE INSTRUCTIONS

Store in a cool, dark place (not in a bathroom medicine cabinet).

STOPPING OR INTERRUPTING THERAPY

It may take several weeks before you feel any beneficial effects from this medicine. Do not stop taking this medicine without checking with your doctor. If you miss a dose, take it as soon as possible. If it is almost time for your next dose, skip the missed dose and resume your regular schedule. Do not take two doses at the same time.

SPECIAL CONSIDERATIONS FOR THOSE OVER SIXTY-FIVE

Older people may be more prone to the side effect of dizziness, especially when getting up from a reclining or sitting position.

Chapter 2
Disorders of the Brain and Nervous System

MEMORY DISORDERS

Perhaps the greatest fear many of us have about growing older is that we will lose part of ourselves—our memory. We forget a name, and we are convinced we are on a one-way road to "senility." But occasional forgetfulness is not a sign of mental decline. Nor is "senility" an inevitable part of growing older.

Severe memory loss, however, does occur in some older people. It may be coupled with confusion and other changes in personality and behavior. There are a number of causes for this, many of which respond to prompt treatment. (These reversible conditions include, for example, a minor head injury, a high fever, vitamin deficiency, or an adverse reaction to a drug.) In other instances, treatment can help to reduce symptoms but not restore lost brain function. Therefore, it is important to find out the source of the symptoms.

CAUSES

Alzheimer's Disease The most common cause of memory loss that is as yet incurable is Alzheimer's disease, a condition that afflicts less than 7 percent of the population aged sixty-five and older. The severe intellectual impairments it produces—serious confusion, memory lapses, and loss of recognition of family and friends—stem from abnormal changes in the cerebral cortex (the outer layer of the brain), as well as from deeper structures in the brain. A number of theories have been advanced as to the underlying cause of Alzheimer's, but none has yet been confirmed.

The first sign of Alzheimer's disease is usually the inability to recall recent events. These memory lapses are minor at first, and are generally blamed on physical illness or emotional upsets. Eventually, these memory lapses and the failure to recognize friends and family interfere with work and social life. Personality changes, trouble with language, and difficulty with routines of daily living, such as brushing teeth, are other early symptoms.

As the disease progresses, victims of Alzheimer's disease lose the ability to handle finances and to carry out such routine tasks as marketing or traveling to familiar places. Frequently they develop crying spells and admit to a sense of shame about their memory problems. The disease may develop gradually, with these earlier stages lasting many years.

With further progression, people with Alzheimer's reach the point at which they can no longer dress or bathe themselves without help. They may become agitated, and delusions set in. Symptoms may accelerate so rapidly that home care is no longer possible. In the final stages of the disease, individuals can no longer care for themselves at all. They lose the ability to speak intelligibly and become bedridden.

Cerebral Atherosclerosis A less common cause of mental impairment in older people is multi-infarct dementia. In this condition, a series of minor strokes results in widespread death of brain tissue and the progressive loss of mental functioning.

Emotional Problems Memory loss sometimes accompanies such emotional problems as depression (including loss of self-esteem) and anxiety. These problems may be mistakenly confused with irreversible brain disease, and a depressed individual labeled "senile." This will lead to inappropriate treatment.

DIAGNOSIS

To rule out the possibility of a treatable disease, people with severe memory loss and mental confusion should have an extensive workup, including thorough physical, psychological, and neurological evaluations. Laboratory studies of the blood and computed axial tomography (CAT) scans of the brain are particularly important in differentiating Alzheimer's disease from other conditions causing similar symptoms. However, it should be emphasized that there is not a single definitive test for Alzheimer's disease. Scientists have recently identified a genetic marker for Alzheimer's disease, and it is possible that this discovery may eventually provide the basis for a diagnostic test.

If other disorders are ruled out, the diagnosis of Alzheimer's disease can be made on the basis of the person's current symptoms, laboratory data, and the way in which the illness has progressed. A relative or close friend may be called in to help piece together past events, giving the doctor an accurate picture of the person's medical history.

Testing does not come to an end once the diagnosis is made. Many doctors perform periodic neurological examinations and psychological tests to evaluate the progress of the disease and its response to therapy.

TREATMENT

Serious memory loss is sometimes treated by cerebral vasodilators, such as ergoloid mesylates, isoxsuprine, and papaverine. These medicines act by relaxing and enlarging the blood vessels in the brain, allowing more oxygen to reach the brain. The efficacy of these drugs, however, has not been established; the Food and Drug Administration considers isoxsuprine and papaverine to be lacking in substantial evidence of effectiveness. More information on these products appears in the drug charts on pages 231–239.

So far, there is no known cure or prevention for Alzheimer's disease. However, some of the troubling symptoms can be alleviated through proper medical care. Antidepressant medicines help control the depression seen in the early stages of the illness, and tranquilizers can lessen the agitation and anxiety associated with more advanced stages. Appropriate medicine can also help improve sleeping patterns. Some researchers are testing drugs that raise brain levels of the chemical acetylcholine in an effort to make up for the deficiency of that nerve signal transmitter, which is characteristic of Alzheimer's disease patients.

OUTLOOK

Family members and friends can provide a great deal of help for people who have multi-infarct dementia and those who have Alzheimer's disease. It's important to keep activities as close to normal as possible and to encourage physical activities and social contacts. Memory aids—such as calendars, lists of chores, and written reminders of safety measures—often help in the early stages. Although people with these illnesses may not be able to undertake shopping trips, or go to movies, go on hikes, or go to ball games or other athletic activities alone, they can still participate in them with a friend or family member as company.

Victims of Alzheimer's disease are often cared for at home during the early stages. When this becomes impossible, a day-care center may answer the need for supervised care. During later stages, however, a full-time care facility usually becomes necessary.

Self-help and support groups for relatives of people with Alzheimer's disease and similar illnesses are forming throughout the country. These groups are an important source of information and a place to share experiences with others. For the location of a group in your area, contact the Alzheimer's Disease and Related Disorders Association, 360 North Michigan Avenue, Chicago, IL 60601.

CONDITION: **MEMORY DISORDERS, ALZHEIMER'S DISEASE, AND CEREBRAL ATHEROSCLEROSIS**

CATEGORY: **CEREBRAL VASODILATORS**

GENERIC (CHEMICAL) NAME	BRAND (TRADE) NAME	DOSAGE FORMS AND STRENGTHS
Ergoloid mesylates	HYDERGINE	Liquid: 1 mg per ml Oral tablets: 1 mg Sublingual tablets: 0.5 or 1 mg
	HYDERGINE LC	Capsules: 1 mg

DRUG PROFILE

Ergoloid mesylates are used to improve mental function by enhancing the circulation of blood to the brain. This medicine is used to treat changes in mood and memory as well as depression.

BEFORE USING THIS DRUG

Let your doctor know *IF*

You have ever had allergic reactions or other problems with ■ ergoloid mesylates ■ ergotamine.

You have ever had any of the following medical problems: ■ mental illness ■ slow pulse ■ low blood pressure ■ liver disease.

You are taking any of the following medicines: ■ ergotamine or methysergide (medicine for migraine headaches) ■ medicine for depression or other mental illness.

SPECIAL RESTRICTIONS WHILE TAKING THIS DRUG

FOOD AND DRUG INTERACTIONS

Other Drugs	Do not take any other drugs, including over-the-counter (OTC) drugs, before checking with your doctor.

| Smoking | Smoking may reduce the beneficial effects of this drug. Let your doctor know if you smoke. |

No special restrictions on foods and beverages or alcohol use.

DAILY LIVING

Excessive Cold	Avoid exposure to long periods of cold, since this medicine may interfere with your body's ability to adjust to cold temperatures.
Examinations or Tests	It is important for you to keep all appointments with your doctor so that your progress can be checked.
Other Precautions	Take this medicine exactly as directed by your doctor; do not take more of it or take it for a longer time than prescribed.
Helpful Hints	The sublingual tablets should not be chewed or swallowed; instead, dissolve them under your tongue. Do not eat, drink, or smoke while taking them.

No special restrictions on driving, exertion and exercise, sun exposure, or exposure to excessive heat.

POSSIBLE SIDE EFFECTS

Although this list of adverse effects may seem somewhat intimidating, keep in mind that some are quite rare. Of course, should these or any other problems arise while you are on medication, it is always a good idea to consult your doctor.

IF YOU DEVELOP

nausea or vomiting ■ stomach cramps ■ loss of appetite ■ dizziness or light-headedness, especially when getting up from a reclining or sitting position ■ drowsiness ■ slow pulse ■ blurred vision ■ headache ■ flushing ■ stuffy nose ■ runny nose ■ rash

With sublingual tablets: soreness under the tongue

WHAT TO DO

If symptoms are disturbing or persist, let your doctor know.

STORAGE INSTRUCTIONS

Store in a cool, dark place (not in a bathroom medicine cabinet). If your medicine is in a liquid form, make sure that it does not freeze.

STOPPING OR INTERRUPTING THERAPY

Some people do not show improvement with this medicine; let your doctor know if your symptoms have not improved after several weeks. If you miss a dose, take it as soon as possible. If it is almost time for your next dose, skip the missed dose and resume your regular schedule. Do not take two doses at the same time.

SPECIAL CONSIDERATIONS FOR THOSE OVER SIXTY-FIVE

None.

CONDITION: **MEMORY DISORDERS, ALZHEIMER'S DISEASE, AND CEREBRAL ATHEROSCLEROSIS**

CATEGORY: **CEREBRAL VASODILATORS**

GENERIC (CHEMICAL) NAME	BRAND (TRADE) NAME	DOSAGE FORMS AND STRENGTHS
Isoxsuprine hydrochloride	VASODILAN	Tablets: 10, 20 mg

DRUG PROFILE

Isoxsuprine is prescribed for problems that are caused by poor circulation of blood to the head (cerebral vascular insufficiency) and to the extremities, such as the tip of the nose (Buerger's disease, Raynaud's syndrome). It is also prescribed for arteriosclerosis obliterans, a condition in which some of the arteries in the body narrow so much that blood cannot pass through them. The Food and Drug Administration has recently ruled that this drug lacks substantial evidence of effectiveness. You should discuss with your doctor why you are being treated with it and what you can expect from therapy with this drug.

BEFORE USING THIS DRUG

Let your doctor know *IF*

You have ever had allergic reactions or other problems with ■ isoxsuprine.

You have ever had any of the following medical problems: ■ hardening of the arteries ■ recent heart attack or stroke ■ angina (chest pain) ■ bleeding problems ■ glaucoma.

SPECIAL RESTRICTIONS WHILE TAKING THIS DRUG

FOOD AND DRUG INTERACTIONS

Other Drugs	Do not take any other drugs, including over-the-counter (OTC) drugs, before checking with your doctor.
Smoking	Smoking may reduce the beneficial effects of this drug. Let your doctor know if you smoke.

No special restrictions on foods and beverages or alcohol use.

DAILY LIVING

Driving	This drug may cause dizziness or light-headedness. Be careful when driving, operating household appliances, or doing any other tasks that require alertness until you know how this drug affects you.

Examinations or Tests	It is important for you to keep all appointments with your doctor so that your progress can be checked.
Helpful Hints	If this drug upsets your stomach, taking it with meals, milk, snacks, or an antacid should help.
	Dizziness or light-headedness may occur, especially when you get up from a reclining or sitting position. Getting up slowly may help prevent this.

No special restrictions on exertion and exercise, sun exposure, or exposure to excessive heat or cold.

POSSIBLE SIDE EFFECTS

Although this list of adverse effects may seem somewhat intimidating, keep in mind that some are quite rare. Of course, should these or any other problems arise while you are on medication, it is always a good idea to consult your doctor.

IF YOU DEVELOP	WHAT TO DO
chest pain ■ irregular or fast heartbeat	**Urgent** Get in touch with your doctor immediately.
rash ■ dizziness or fainting, especially when getting up from a reclining or sitting position ■ tremors ■ nervousness ■ weakness ■ flushing	**May be serious** Check with your doctor as soon as possible.
nausea or vomiting ■ stomach discomfort	If symptoms are disturbing or persist, let your doctor know.

STORAGE INSTRUCTIONS

Store in a cool, dark place (not in a bathroom medicine cabinet).

STOPPING OR INTERRUPTING THERAPY

If you miss a dose of this medicine, take it as soon as possible. If it is almost time for your next dose, skip the missed dose and resume your regular schedule. Do not take two doses at the same time.

SPECIAL CONSIDERATIONS FOR THOSE OVER SIXTY-FIVE

None.

CONDITION: **MEMORY DISORDERS, ALZHEIMER'S DISEASE, AND CEREBRAL ATHEROSCLEROSIS**

CATEGORY: **CEREBRAL VASODILATORS**

GENERIC (CHEMICAL) NAME	BRAND (TRADE) NAME	DOSAGE FORMS AND STRENGTHS
Papaverine hydrochloride	PAVABID	Controlled-release capsules: 150 mg
	PAVABID HP	Capsules: 300 mg

DRUG PROFILE

Papaverine is used to treat conditions that are caused by poor circulation of blood to the head (cerebral vascular insufficiency), limbs (peripheral vascular insufficiency), and heart (angina). This drug works by relaxing and enlarging the blood vessels. The Food and Drug Administration has recently ruled that this drug lacks substantial evidence of effectiveness. You should discuss with your doctor why you are being treated with it and what you can expect from therapy with this drug.

BEFORE USING THIS DRUG

Let your doctor know *IF*

You have ever had allergic reactions or other problems with ■ papaverine.

You have ever had any of the following medical problems: ■ angina (chest pain)
■ heart or blood vessel disease, including recent heart attack or stroke
■ glaucoma.

You are taking any of the following medicines: ■ levodopa (medicine for Parkinson's disease) ■ narcotics or other prescription pain-killers ■ sleep medicines
■ medicine for seizures.

SPECIAL RESTRICTIONS WHILE TAKING THIS DRUG

FOOD AND DRUG INTERACTIONS

Other Drugs	Do not take any other drugs, including over-the-counter (OTC) drugs, before checking with your doctor.
Alcohol	The action of this medicine may be affected by alcohol. Avoid alcohol unless your doctor has approved its use.
Smoking	Smoking may reduce the beneficial effects of this drug. Let your doctor know if you smoke.

No special restrictions on foods and beverages.

DAILY LIVING

Driving	This drug may cause dizziness or light-headedness. Be careful when driving, operating household appliances, or doing any other tasks that require alertness until you know how this drug affects you.
Examinations or Tests	It is important for you to keep all appointments with your doctor so that your progress can be checked.

Helpful Hints

If this drug upsets your stomach, taking it with meals, milk, snacks, or antacids should help.

Do not crush or chew the capsules; instead, swallow them whole. If the capsule is too large for you, you can mix the contents with a spoonful of jam and swallow it without chewing.

If your mouth or throat feels dry, chewing sugarless gum or sucking ice chips or sugarless hard candy will help.

No special restrictions on exertion or exercise, sun exposure, or exposure to excessive heat or cold.

POSSIBLE SIDE EFFECTS

Although this list of adverse effects may seem somewhat intimidating, keep in mind that some are quite rare. Of course, should these or any other problems arise while you are on medication, it is always a good idea to consult your doctor.

IF YOU DEVELOP

blurred or double vision ■ drowsiness ■ weakness ■ rash or itching ■ depression ■ yellowing of eyes or skin

WHAT TO DO

May be serious Check with your doctor as soon as possible.

deep breathing ■ dizziness, especially when getting up from a reclining or sitting position ■ headache ■ nausea or vomiting ■ loss of appetite ■ constipation ■ diarrhea ■ stomach discomfort ■ general feeling of unwellness ■ flushing ■ increased sweating ■ dry mouth or throat

If symptoms are disturbing or persist, let your doctor know.

STORAGE INSTRUCTIONS

Store in a cool, dark place (not in a bathroom medicine cabinet).

STOPPING OR INTERRUPTING THERAPY

This medicine may take a while to produce noticeable results. Do not stop taking it, even if you see no difference in your condition, without consulting your doctor. If you miss a dose, take it as soon as possible. If it is almost time for your next dose, skip the missed dose and resume your regular schedule. Do not take two doses at the same time.

SPECIAL CONSIDERATIONS FOR THOSE OVER SIXTY-FIVE

None.

VERTIGO

The sensation of vertigo is an uncomfortable one—the feeling that you are spinning or that the room is whirling around you, or that you are about to fall down. At the same time, you might become nauseated or even vomit.

An attack of vertigo can last for only a few seconds or go on for hours. It can affect people at any age and for many reasons. Finding and treating the cause in older people can be particularly difficult if other medical problems are present.

CAUSES

You may have heard that your sense of balance, or equilibrium, is maintained by structures in your inner ear in an area behind your eardrum. Therefore, a disease or disturbance in your inner ear could be the reason for your vertigo. This is thought to be what happens in people who suffer from motion sickness—the swaying of the vehicle disrupts the equilibrium center of the inner ear, causing the sensation of dizziness.

But other organs and systems also play a part. For instance, you may feel dizzy if you cannot see clearly, or if things are moving too fast for your eyes to keep up with them. Glaucoma, in which there is too much pressure inside the eye, can cause dizziness too. (See pages 814–815 for a detailed discussion of glaucoma.)

You may also feel dizzy if you have low blood pressure or if your heart is not pumping enough blood to your brain. Your body normally sends messages to your brain about balance and position; dizziness can occur when arthritis or a neck injury causes pressure on the nerves that transmit those messages or when certain diseases damage the nerves.

DIAGNOSIS

To help determine the underlying reason for your vertigo, your doctor will ask you when your dizzy spells occur, what seems to bring them on, how long they last, and what other symptoms accompany them. A thorough medical history may also provide a clue to your problem. You may wonder about questions regarding your consumption of coffee, aspirin, alcohol, and cigarettes. The reason for such questions is that all of these ordinary things can cause dizziness.

Vertigo is sometimes caused by a sudden drop in blood pressure, which often happens in older people when they stand up. Therefore, your doctor will probably check your pressure when you are lying down, when you sit up, and again when you stand. At the same time, the doctor will be checking your pulse to see whether your heart rate changes the way it should as you move.

The way your eyes move when you get dizzy can also suggest some causes, so your doctor might observe your eyes as you turn your head sharply from side to side. You may be asked to walk in heel-to-toe fashion, with your eyes open and with your eyes closed, as another part of the exam.

After all this activity, you may be referred to a specialist for further evaluation, or the source of your problem may be apparent and quite simply managed. For example, you might have a buildup of wax in your outer ear, which is pressing against your eardrum and causing problems in your inner ear. Or the cause of the vertigo could be an infection that is treatable with antibiotics.

If your dizzy spells only occur when you move your head—and nothing else seems to be wrong with you—your doctor might say you have "benign positional vertigo." This is a temporary condition that will eventually go away by itself without causing any damage. It is the most frequent cause of dizziness in adults.

TREATMENT

For some people, just knowing that the vertigo is not a sign of a serious problem is enough to make the episodes bearable. Others may need drugs to relieve their symptoms. If you fall into this category, your doctor may prescribe certain antihistamines, described in detail in the drug charts on pages 242–244, to control the nausea, vomiting, and dizziness caused by a benign disturbance in the inner ear.

If your doctor finds that your vertigo is caused by a problem of the heart or circulatory system, a reaction to other medicine, or a visual or neurological disturbance, treatment will focus on the underlying problem.

OUTLOOK

Vertigo is a serious symptom and should be paid attention to. However, that whirling, giddy, or unsteady feeling does not have to keep you from enjoying life. Even if the medical evaluation of your vertigo takes time—and perhaps visits to more than one doctor—quick symptomatic relief might be available through prescription medicine. Then, with correct diagnosis and treatment of the underlying problem, you may find that you can once again get on with your daily activities.

CONDITION: **VERTIGO**

CATEGORY: **ANTIHISTAMINES**

GENERIC (CHEMICAL) NAME	BRAND (TRADE) NAME	DOSAGE FORMS AND STRENGTHS
Meclizine hydrochloride	ANTIVERT	Chewable tablets: 25 mg Tablets: 12.5, 25, 50 mg

DRUG PROFILE

Meclizine, which belongs to the category of drugs called antihistamines, is used to prevent the nausea, vomiting, and dizziness that are associated with motion sickness. This medicine also is used to treat dizziness resulting from inner-ear disturbances. Meclizine works by reducing the sensitivity of the nerves in the inner ear that control balance; it also blocks the nerve pathways to the part of the brain that controls vomiting.

BEFORE USING THIS DRUG

Let your doctor know *IF*

You have ever had allergic reactions or other problems with ■ meclizine ■ other antihistamines.

You have ever had any of the following medical problems: ■ asthma or other lung disease ■ enlarged prostate ■ urinary problems, including difficulty in urination ■ glaucoma ■ epilepsy or other seizure disorders ■ intestinal blockage ■ stomach ulcer.

You are taking any of the following medicines: ■ medicine for nausea ■ antihistamines ■ medicine for Parkinson's disease ■ tranquilizers ■ medicine for depression ■ cimetidine or ranitidine (medicine for ulcers) ■ medicine for stomach pain or cramps ■ medicine for spasmodic conditions of the digestive or urinary tract ■ medicine for asthma or bronchitis.

SPECIAL RESTRICTIONS WHILE TAKING THIS DRUG

FOOD AND DRUG INTERACTIONS

Other Drugs	Do not take any other drugs, including over-the-counter (OTC) drugs, before checking with your doctor. This drug increases the effects of drugs that depress the central nervous system—such as antihistamines; medicine for hay fever, allergies, or colds; sleep medicines; tranquilizers; medicine for depression; narcotics or other prescription pain-killers; muscle relaxants; and medicine for seizures. This drug may mask ringing in the ears caused by aspirin. Let your doctor know if you are taking aspirin or aspirin-like medicine.
Alcohol	Drinking alcohol while taking this medicine may increase the risk of such side effects as dizziness, light-headedness, or drowsiness. Avoid alcohol unless your doctor has approved its use.

No special restrictions on foods and beverages or smoking.

DAILY LIVING

Driving	This drug may cause drowsiness or blurred vision. Be careful when driving, operating household appliances, or doing any other tasks that require alertness until you know how this drug affects you.
Other Precautions	Because this drug controls nausea and vomiting, it can mask some of the symptoms of appendicitis. If you develop sharp pains in your stomach or lower abdomen, be sure to let your doctor know at once.

If you are going to be tested for allergies, let the doctor in charge know that you are taking this drug, since it affects the results of allergy tests. |

Helpful Hints	If this drug upsets your stomach, taking it with meals, milk, snacks, or water should help.
	If your mouth or throat feels dry, chewing sugarless gum or sucking ice chips or sugarless hard candy will help.

No special restrictions on exertion and exercise, sun exposure, or exposure to excessive heat or cold.

POSSIBLE SIDE EFFECTS

Although this list of adverse effects may seem somewhat intimidating, keep in mind that some are quite rare. Of course, should these or any other problems arise while you are on medication, it is always a good idea to consult your doctor.

IF YOU DEVELOP

drowsiness ■ tiredness ■ irregular or fast heart-beat ■ headache ■ blurred vision ■ nervousness or restlessness ■ sleep disturbances ■ loss of appetite ■ upset stomach ■ dry mouth, nose, or throat ■ pain or difficulty in urination ■ rash

WHAT TO DO

If symptoms are disturbing or persist, let your doctor know.

STORAGE INSTRUCTIONS

Store in a cool, dark place (not in a bathroom medicine cabinet).

STOPPING OR INTERRUPTING THERAPY

If you are taking this medicine regularly and you miss a dose, take it as soon as possible. If it is almost time for your next dose, skip the missed dose and resume your regular schedule. Do not take two doses at the same time.

SPECIAL CONSIDERATIONS FOR THOSE OVER SIXTY-FIVE

None.

PARKINSON'S DISEASE

Parkinson's disease occurs in one out of every one hundred individuals over the age of sixty-five. It begins so gradually and its early symptoms are so mild that many people do not even suspect they have it. They might just feel more tired than usual or notice a slight, occasional tremor in a finger, which may gradually affect the hand and arm as well. Or the first sign might be stiffness of a hand or leg, a slouching posture, or difficulty in rising from a chair. A family member or friend might be the first to observe that the person is slowing down, limping a little, or talking in a monotonous tone of voice.

As Parkinson's disease advances, it may cause some difficulty in walking or keeping one's balance. Some people with parkinsonism may find that they have trouble swallowing or that they sweat excessively or urinate slowly. Oddly enough, the handwriting of a person with parkinsonism may get smaller and smaller over the course of time.

CAUSES

At the root of Parkinson's disease is a deficiency of dopamine, which is an important chemical messenger in the brain and nervous system. Not enough dopamine means a slowdown in the transmission of messages from the nerve cells in the brain to the nerve cells in the muscles of the arms, legs, and face. Therefore, a person with Parkinson's disease cannot always control his or her movements.

EXERCISE, PHYSICAL THERAPY, AND COPING

Keeping active is especially important for people with Parkinson's disease, to keep already rigid muscles in the arms and legs from growing stiffer. Your doctor may recommend stretching exercises to keep your muscles flexible as well as exercises to improve your balance. If your symptoms are interfering with your daily routine, your doctor may refer you to a physical therapist for help in planning strategies for overcoming these practical problems. Some helpful tips are outlined below.

Walking
• Wear leather-soled shoes rather than rubber or crepe soles, which grip the floor and can cause you to fall forward.
• Try consciously to take steps as large as possible, raising your toes up when you step forward and hitting the ground on your heel.
• Keep your feet nine to fifteen inches apart and your posture straight, arms swinging at your sides. Practice swinging your right arm with your left leg and your left arm with your right leg.
• Look straight ahead, not at the floor.
• In cases of "freezing," relax back on your heels, toes raised. To start moving again, tap the leg that you want to move or shift your weight from side to side in a rocking motion.

Getting in or out of a Chair
• To sit down, approach slowly with your back to the chair. When you reach the chair, bend forward and sit down slowly.
• To get up, put your feet under the chair, if possible. Rock forward once or twice in preparation; then bend forward and push up vigorously with your arms.
If your favorite chair is too soft and too low to the floor, raise the back legs with blocks.
If you need assistance in getting up, ask someone to help by pushing you from the back, not pulling you up by the arms. Sometimes, a slight touch is all that is necessary.

Getting out of Bed
• Rock into a sitting position by placing your arms over your head and swinging them forward and moving your legs toward the side of the bed. If you need further assistance, tie a knotted rope to the foot of the bed for use in pulling yourself up. You may want to raise the head of the bed by placing blocks under the legs.

Getting Dressed
• Avoid clothes that fasten up the back or have very small buttons.
• Practice buttoning and unbuttoning garments while watching television or listening to the radio. Another exercise to help straighten stiff fingers is to bounce a large ball with your open hand. Toss the ball against a wall or to another person.
• For help in putting on shoes, use a shoehorn. If your shoes have laces, try elastic or extra-long laces, or avoid laces entirely by wearing loafers or sneakers that have a Velcro closing.

TREATMENT
Although Parkinson's disease cannot be cured, medication can dramatically relieve the symptoms, often for years. The most important drug used to treat parkinsonism is levodopa (see chart on pages 248–251), which improves the supply of dopamine in the brain. Sometimes doctors also prescribe other drugs to boost the effectiveness of levodopa or as alternatives if levodopa's effectiveness seems to be wearing off (see charts on pages 252–263 for more details on these drugs).

OUTLOOK
Continuing your normal daily activities and thinking positively are especially important for people with parkinsonism. Although you'll probably have to make some changes in your life to cope with the symptoms, most likely you'll be able to continue your usual activities. Hobbies that involve the use of the fingers (such as sewing or playing cards) are particularly useful to keep the hands and fingers from stiffening. Your doctor can help you make other decisions about adapting to parkinsonism, such as whether you should continue driving a car. Good sources of information and support include the following:
• The American Parkinson's Disease Association, 116 John Street, New York, NY 10038, (212) 732-9550
• The Parkinson's Disease Foundation, Columbia-Presbyterian Medical

Center, 640 West 168th Street, New York, NY 10032, (212) 923-4700
• The National Parkinson's Foundation, 111 Park Place, New York, NY 10007, (212) 374-1741 and 1501 Northwest Ninth Avenue, Miami, FL 33136, (800) 327-4545

• The United Parkinson's Foundation, 220 South State Street, Chicago, IL 60604, (312) 922-9734
• PEP-USA (Parkinson's Educational Program), 1800 Park Newport, #302, Newport Beach, CA 92660, (714) 640-0218

CONDITION: **PARKINSON'S DISEASE**

CATEGORY: **ANTIPARKINSON AGENTS**

GENERIC (CHEMICAL) NAME	BRAND (TRADE) NAME	DOSAGE FORMS AND STRENGTHS
Levodopa	DOPAR	Capsules: 100, 250, 500 mg
	LARODOPA	Capsules: 100, 250, 500 mg Tablets: 100, 250, 500 mg
Levodopa and carbidopa	SINEMET	Tablets: 10 mg carbidopa and 100 mg levodopa; 25 mg carbidopa and 100 mg levodopa; 25 mg carbidopa and 250 mg levodopa

DRUG PROFILE

Levodopa or the combination of levodopa and carbidopa helps to improve muscle control in Parkinson's disease. Many experts think that the rigidity, shaking, and difficulty initiating movement characteristic of Parkinson's disease result from a deficiency of a chemical called dopamine in the brain. Levodopa is converted to dopamine in the brain, thereby helping restore the chemical balance that regulates the nervous system. Carbidopa helps more levodopa reach the brain.

BEFORE USING THIS DRUG

Let your doctor know *IF*

You have ever had allergic reactions or other problems with ■ levodopa ■ the combination of levodopa and carbidopa ■ aspirin.

■ *with Dopar only:* ■ tartrazine (FD&C Yellow Dye No. 5).

You have ever had any of the following medical problems: ■ epilepsy or other seizure disorders ■ diabetes ■ asthma or other lung disease ■ glaucoma ■ heart or blood vessel disease ■ abnormal heart rhythms ■ hormone disturbances ■ kidney disease ■ liver disease ■ mental illness ■ skin cancer ■ stomach ulcer.

You are taking any of the following medicines: ■ other medicine for Parkinson's disease ■ amantadine (medicine for flu) ■ antacids ■ amphetamines ■ phenytoin (medicine for seizures) ■ medicine for high blood pressure ■ medicine for stomach pain or cramps ■ medicine for spasmodic conditions of the digestive or urinary tract ■ appetite suppressants ■ medicine for asthma or bronchitis ■ vitamin B_6 ■ tranquilizers ■ sinus medicines ■ antihistamines ■ medicine for nausea ■ medicine for depression (within the last two weeks) ■ muscle relaxants ■ sleep medicines ■ furazolidone (antibiotic) ■ papaverine (medicine for poor blood circulation) ■ methyldopa or clonidine (medicine for high blood pressure).

SPECIAL RESTRICTIONS WHILE TAKING THIS DRUG

FOOD AND DRUG INTERACTIONS

Other Drugs	Vitamin B_6 reduces the effects of levodopa (this does not occur with the combination of levodopa and carbidopa). If you are taking levodopa alone, do not take any vitamin supplement containing B_6 unless prescribed by your doctor.
Foods and Beverages	If you are taking levodopa alone, see the above warning regarding vitamin B_6. Foods with a high vitamin B_6 content, such as bacon, beef liver, pork, beans, peas, tuna, oatmeal, and avocados, should be eaten only in limited quantities.

No special restrictions on alcohol use or smoking.

DAILY LIVING

Driving	This drug may cause drowsiness or loss of alertness. Be careful when driving, operating household appliances, or doing any other tasks that require alertness until you know how this drug affects you.

Exertion and Exercise	As your symptoms improve, be sure not to overdo physical activity. Let yourself gradually get used to your improving balance and coordination.
Examinations or Tests	It is important for you to keep all appointments with your doctor, even if your symptoms improve, so that your progress can be checked. Periodic blood and urine tests may be required.
Other Precautions	If you have diabetes, you may find that this medicine affects the results of urine tests for ketones or sugar; ask your doctor what kind of tests you should use. Tell any doctor or dentist you consult that you are taking this medicine, especially if you will be undergoing any type of surgery.
Helpful Hints	If this drug upsets your stomach, taking it with solid, protein-rich foods should help. Dizziness or light-headedness may occur, especially when getting up from a reclining or sitting position. Getting up slowly may help prevent this.

No special restrictions on sun exposure or exposure to excessive heat or cold.

POSSIBLE SIDE EFFECTS

Although this list of adverse effects may seem somewhat intimidating, keep in mind that some are quite rare. Of course, should these or any other problems arise while you are on medication, it is always a good idea to consult your doctor.

IF YOU DEVELOP	WHAT TO DO
breathing changes ■ hoarseness ■ blurred or double vision ■ changes in pupil size ■ spasm or closing of eyelids or any other eye problems	**May be serious** Check with your doctor as soon as possible.

■ tiredness or weakness ■ unusual, uncontrollable movements of the body ■ clumsiness ■ disturbances in walking ■ slowing of movement
■ increased hand tremors ■ irregular heartbeat
■ dizziness or light-headedness, especially when
getting up from a reclining or sitting position ■ difficulty in urination ■ nausea or vomiting ■ stomach pain ■ hallucinations ■ delusions ■ agitation
■ paranoia (unreasonable fears) ■ depression

runny nose ■ anxiety, confusion, or nervousness
■ inability to concentrate ■ memory problems
■ restlessness ■ drowsiness ■ general feeling of
unwellness ■ headache ■ sleeplessness ■ nightmares ■ increased sweating ■ urinary frequency
or incontinence ■ numbness ■ rash ■ hot flashes
■ vaginal bleeding ■ weight gain or loss ■ painful
or persistent male erection ■ pain or swelling of
hands or feet ■ hair loss ■ grinding of teeth ■ constipation ■ diarrhea ■ dark urine or sweat ■ dry
mouth ■ loss of appetite ■ flushing ■ muscle
twitching ■ gas ■ hiccups ■ bitter taste or taste
changes ■ difficulty in swallowing ■ burning feeling in tongue ■ difficulty in opening mouth

If symptoms are disturbing
or persist, let your doctor
know.

STORAGE INSTRUCTIONS

Store in a cool, dark place (not in a bathroom medicine cabinet).

STOPPING OR INTERRUPTING THERAPY

Take this medicine exactly as directed by your doctor; do not stop taking it, even if
your symptoms have not improved. In some people, it takes several weeks or even
months before effects of this medicine are seen. If you miss a dose, take it as soon
as possible. If it is within two hours of your next dose, skip the missed dose and
resume your regular schedule. Do not take two doses at the same time.

SPECIAL CONSIDERATIONS FOR THOSE OVER SIXTY-FIVE

Older people may be especially sensitive to the side effects of this medicine. For
those who have osteoporosis, it is particularly important not to overdo physical
activity and to take special care to avoid falling.

CONDITION: **PARKINSON'S DISEASE**

CATEGORY: **ANTIPARKINSON AGENTS**

GENERIC (CHEMICAL) NAME	BRAND (TRADE) NAME	DOSAGE FORMS AND STRENGTHS
Amantadine hydrochloride	SYMMETREL	Capsules: 100 mg Syrup: 50 mg per tsp

DRUG PROFILE

Amantadine is used to treat Parkinson's disease and other movement disorders. Many experts think that the rigidity, shaking, and walking disturbances associated with these conditions result from a deficiency of a chemical called dopamine in the brain. Amantadine makes more dopamine available to the brain, thereby helping restore the chemical balance that regulates the nervous system. This drug is sometimes used along with levodopa or other antiparkinson medicine.

BEFORE USING THIS DRUG

Let your doctor know *IF*

You have ever had allergic reactions or other problems with ■ amantadine.

You have ever had any of the following medical problems: ■ heart disease, including congestive heart failure ■ circulation problems ■ blood vessel disease of the brain ■ low blood pressure ■ swelling of feet or ankles ■ epilepsy or other seizure disorders ■ mental illness ■ kidney disease ■ liver disease ■ stomach or intestinal ulcers ■ recurring eczema.

You are taking any of the following medicines: ■ carbidopa and/or levodopa (other medicine for Parkinson's disease) ■ amphetamines ■ diet pills ■ medicine for depression ■ tranquilizers ■ medicine for nausea ■ sleep medicines ■ antihistamines ■ medicine for asthma, hay fever, allergies, or breathing problems ■ cough medicine ■ sinus medicine ■ medicine for diarrhea ■ medicine for stomach spasms or cramps ■ medicine for narcolepsy.

SPECIAL RESTRICTIONS WHILE TAKING THIS DRUG

FOOD AND DRUG INTERACTIONS

Other Drugs	Do not take any other drugs, including over-the-counter (OTC) drugs, before checking with your doctor. OTC drugs for appetite suppression, asthma, colds, cough, hay fever, or sinus problems should be avoided since these products can aggravate the stimulant effects of amantadine.
Alcohol	Drinking alcohol while taking this medicine may increase the risk of such side effects as dizziness, light-headedness, fainting, confusion, and circulation problems. Avoid alcohol unless your doctor has approved its use.

No special restrictions on foods and beverages or smoking.

DAILY LIVING

Driving	This drug may cause dizziness, light-headedness, or fainting. Be careful when driving, operating household appliances, or doing any other tasks that require alertness until you know how this drug affects you.
Exertion and Exercise	As your symptoms improve, be sure not to overdo physical activity. Let yourself gradually get used to your improving balance and coordination.
Examinations or Tests	It is important for you to keep all appointments with your doctor, even if your symptoms improve, so that your progress and reactions to this medicine can be checked.

Helpful Hints	If you have been taking this medicine for a while and feel that it is not working as well as it has in the past, let your doctor know.
	If your mouth or throat feels dry, chewing sugarless gum or sucking ice chips or sugarless hard candy will help.
	Dizziness or light-headedness may occur, especially when you get up from a reclining or sitting position. Getting up slowly may help prevent this.

No special restrictions on sun exposure or exposure to excessive heat or cold.

POSSIBLE SIDE EFFECTS

Although this list of adverse effects may seem somewhat intimidating, keep in mind that some are quite rare. Of course, should these or any other problems arise while you are on medication, it is always a good idea to consult your doctor.

IF YOU DEVELOP	WHAT TO DO
confusion ■ hallucinations ■ slurred speech ■ fainting ■ difficulty in urination ■ sore throat or fever ■ depression ■ shakiness ■ clumsiness ■ uncontrollable facial movements ■ eye rolling ■ swelling of feet or lower legs ■ shortness of breath ■ difficulty in breathing ■ rapid weight gain ■ convulsions ■ sleeplessness or other sleep disturbances ■ feeling of drunkenness or detachment	**May be serious** Check with your doctor as soon as possible.
dizziness or light-headedness, especially when getting up from a reclining or sitting position ■ nervousness ■ drowsiness ■ anxiety ■ inability to concentrate ■ memory problems ■ irritability ■ headache ■ tiredness or weakness ■ loss of appetite ■ nausea or vomiting ■ constipation ■ dry mouth, nose, or throat ■ purplish red,	If symptoms are disturbing or persist, let your doctor know.

netlike, blotchy spots on skin ■ other rash
■ blurred vision or other visual disturbances
■ increased skin sensitivity to sunlight

STORAGE INSTRUCTIONS

Store in a cool, dark place (not in a bathroom medicine cabinet). If your medicine is in a liquid form, make sure that it does not freeze.

STOPPING OR INTERRUPTING THERAPY

It may take up to two weeks before you feel the helpful effects of this medicine. Do not stop taking it without consulting your doctor. Stopping this medicine suddenly may seriously worsen your medical condition. If you miss a dose, take it as soon as possible. If it is within four hours of your next scheduled dose, skip the missed dose and resume your regular schedule. Do not take two doses at the same time.

SPECIAL CONSIDERATIONS FOR THOSE OVER SIXTY-FIVE

Older people are more likely to experience such side effects as dizziness, confusion, and difficulty in urination. For those who have osteoporosis, it is particularly important not to overdo physical activity and to take special care to avoid falling.

CONDITION: **PARKINSON'S DISEASE**

CATEGORY: **ANTIPARKINSON AGENTS**

GENERIC (CHEMICAL) NAME	BRAND (TRADE) NAME	DOSAGE FORMS AND STRENGTHS
Benztropine mesylate	COGENTIN	Tablets: 0.5, 1, 2 mg
Biperiden	AKINETON	Tablets: 2 mg
Trihexyphenidyl hydrochloride	ARTANE	Controlled-release capsules: 5 mg Elixir: 2 mg per tsp Tablets: 2, 5 mg

DRUG PROFILE

These medicines are used to treat Parkinson's disease, as well as other movement disorders. They reduce rigidity, shakiness, and disturbances in walking. These drugs are often used along with levodopa or other antiparkinson medicines.

BEFORE USING THIS DRUG

Let your doctor know *IF*

You have ever had allergic reactions or other problems with ■ benztropine ■ biperiden ■ trihexyphenidyl ■ other medicine for Parkinson's disease or movement disorders ■ any other medicine.

You have ever had any of the following medical problems: ■ heart or blood vessel disease, including congestive heart failure, abnormal heart rhythms, hardening of the arteries, or high blood pressure ■ stomach ulcer ■ hiatal hernia ■ esophageal reflux ■ intestinal blockage ■ diarrhea ■ ulcerative colitis or other digestive disorders ■ kidney disease ■ liver disease ■ myasthenia gravis ■ uncontrolled movements of hands, mouth, or tongue ■ difficulty in urination ■ enlarged prostate ■ glaucoma ■ overactive thyroid ■ recent fever ■ bleeding problems ■ mental illness.

You are taking any of the following medicines: ■ other medicine for Parkinson's disease ■ medicine for depression (within the last two weeks) ■ medicine for seizures ■ antihistamines ■ medicine for hay fever, allergies, or colds ■ barbiturates ■ narcotics or other prescription pain-killers ■ sedatives ■ tranquilizers ■ sleep medicines ■ muscle relaxants ■ medicine for stomach spasms or cramps ■ medicine for diarrhea ■ antacids ■ medicine for nausea ■ medicine for abnormal heart rhythms ■ medicine for high blood pressure ■ medicine or vaccine for flu.

SPECIAL RESTRICTIONS WHILE TAKING THIS DRUG

FOOD AND DRUG INTERACTIONS

Other Drugs	Do not take any other drugs, including over-the-counter (OTC) drugs, before checking with your doctor. This medicine increases the effect of drugs that depress the central nervous system—such as antihistamines; medicine for hay fever, allergies, or colds; sleep medicines; tranquilizers; narcotics or other prescription pain-killers; muscle relaxants; medicine for

seizures—and worsens such side effects as dizziness, light-headedness, or drowsiness. Do not take antacids or medicine for diarrhea within one hour of taking benztropine, biperiden, or trihexyphenidyl.

Alcohol	Drinking alcohol while taking this medicine may increase the risk of such side effects as dizziness, light-headedness, or drowsiness. Avoid alcohol unless your doctor has approved its use.

No special restrictions on foods and beverages or smoking.

DAILY LIVING

Driving	This drug may cause dizziness, light-headedness, or blurred vision. Be careful when driving, operating household appliances, or doing any other tasks that require alertness until you know how this drug affects you.
Exertion and Exercise	This drug may cause you to sweat less than normally. Sweating is your body's natural way of cooling down, and not sweating enough can be dangerous. Use caution not to become overheated when you exert yourself.
Sun Exposure	Your eyes may become more sensitive to sunlight or other bright light while you are on this medicine. It is a good idea to avoid too much sun exposure. If your eyes become more sensitive to bright light, wearing dark glasses should lessen discomfort.
Excessive Heat	See "Exertion and Exercise"; use caution during hot weather, since overexertion may result in heat stroke. Avoid extremely hot baths or saunas. Also, check with your doctor if you develop a fever for any reason.

Examinations or Tests	It is important for you to keep all appointments with your doctor so that your progress and reactions to this drug can be checked. You may have to have your eyes checked before and during therapy with this medicine.
Other Precautions	Tell any doctor or dentist you consult that you are taking this medicine, especially if you will be undergoing any type of surgery.
Helpful Hints	If your mouth or throat feels dry, chewing sugarless gum or sucking ice chips or sugarless hard candy will help.

Swallow the controlled-release capsules whole—do not break, crush, or chew them. |

No special restrictions on exposure to excessive cold.

POSSIBLE SIDE EFFECTS

Although this list of adverse effects may seem somewhat intimidating, keep in mind that some are quite rare. Of course, should these or any other problems arise while you are on medication, it is always a good idea to consult your doctor.

IF YOU DEVELOP

seizures ■ clumsiness or unsteadiness ■ severe drowsiness ■ severe dryness of mouth, nose, or throat ■ hallucinations ■ delirium ■ mood or mental changes ■ shortness of breath ■ difficulty in breathing ■ sleeplessness ■ irregular or fast heartbeat ■ warm skin or flushing ■ dry skin ■ fever

WHAT TO DO

Urgent Get in touch with your doctor immediately.

confusion ■ disorientation ■ agitation ■ personality changes ■ rash ■ blood in urine ■ depression ■ constipation ■ diarrhea ■ nausea or vomiting ■ bloating ■ stomach pain

May be serious Check with your doctor as soon as possible.

weakness or inability to move certain muscles ■ blurred vision ■ increased skin sensitivity to sunlight ■ increased eye sensitivity to light ■ pupil changes ■ restlessness ■ dry or sore mouth, nose, or throat ■ decreased sweating ■ pain or difficulty in urination ■ headache ■ dizziness or light-headedness, especially when getting up from a reclining or sitting position ■ nervousness or excitement ■ muscle cramps ■ numbness or weakness in hands or feet

If symptoms are disturbing or persist, let your doctor know.

STORAGE INSTRUCTIONS

Store in a cool, dark place (not in a bathroom medicine cabinet). If your medicine is in a liquid form, make sure that it does not freeze.

STOPPING OR INTERRUPTING THERAPY

Follow your doctor's instructions carefully on how to take this medicine. Stopping this medicine suddenly may worsen your medical condition. Your doctor will advise you on how to reduce your dosage gradually before stopping completely. If you miss a dose of this medicine, take it as soon as possible. If it is within two hours of your next dose, skip the missed dose and resume your regular schedule. Do not take two doses at the same time.

SPECIAL CONSIDERATIONS FOR THOSE OVER SIXTY-FIVE

Older people may be more susceptible to such side effects as mental changes and confusion, disorientation, agitation, excitement, hallucinations, and difficulty in urination. Thus, doctors may require regular checkups.

CONDITION: **PARKINSON'S DISEASE**

CATEGORY: **ANTIPARKINSON AGENTS**

GENERIC (CHEMICAL) NAME	BRAND (TRADE) NAME	DOSAGE FORMS AND STRENGTHS
Bromocriptine mesylate	PARLODEL	Capsules: 5 mg Tablets: 2.5 mg

DRUG PROFILE

Bromocriptine belongs to a family of drugs called ergot alkaloids. It is used to treat Parkinson's disease and is often given along with levodopa. Many experts think that the rigidity, shakiness, and disturbances in walking associated with Parkinson's disease result from a deficiency of a chemical called dopamine in the brain. Bromocriptine makes dopamine more available to the brain, thereby helping restore the chemical balance that regulates the nervous system. Bromocriptine may also be used to treat a variety of other medical problems, including tumors of the pituitary gland or pituitary hormone disturbances.

BEFORE USING THIS DRUG

Let your doctor know *IF*

You have ever had allergic reactions or other problems with ■ bromocriptine ■ any other ergot medicines (ergoloid mesylates, ergotamine, or methysergide).

You have ever had any of the following medical problems: ■ heart attack ■ abnormal heart rhythms ■ liver disease ■ kidney disease ■ mental illness ■ low blood pressure ■ migraine headaches.

You are taking any of the following medicines: ■ other medicine for Parkinson's disease ■ diuretics or other medicines for high blood pressure ■ hormones ■ medicine for nausea ■ medicine for depression or other mental illness ■ tranquilizers.

SPECIAL RESTRICTIONS WHILE TAKING THIS DRUG

FOOD AND DRUG INTERACTIONS

Other Drugs	Diuretics and medicine for high blood pressure may increase the risk of such side effects as dizziness and fainting while you are taking this medicine.
Alcohol	This medicine increases the effect of alcohol, a central nervous system depressant. Avoid alcohol unless your doctor has approved its use.

No special restrictions on foods and beverages or smoking.

DAILY LIVING

Driving	This drug may cause dizziness, light-headedness, or confusion. Be careful when driving, operating household appliances, or doing any other tasks that require alertness until you know how this drug affects you.
Examinations or Tests	It is important for you to keep all appointments with your doctor so that your progress and reactions to therapy can be checked. Periodic blood and urine tests may be required.
Helpful Hints	If this drug upsets your stomach, taking it with milk, meals, or snacks should help.

No special restrictions on exertion and exercise, sun exposure, or exposure to excessive heat or cold.

POSSIBLE SIDE EFFECTS

Although this list of adverse effects may seem somewhat intimidating, keep in mind that some are quite rare. Of course, should these or any other problems arise while you are on medication, it is always a good idea to consult your doctor.

IF YOU DEVELOP	WHAT TO DO
black, tarry stools ■ vomiting, with blood ■ seizures ■ weakness ■ irregular or fast heartbeat ■ chest pain	**Urgent** Get in touch with your doctor immediately.
dizziness or light-headedness, especially when getting up from a reclining or sitting position ■ fainting ■ confusion ■ behavior changes ■ hallucinations ■ uncontrollable movements of the face, tongue, arms, hands, head, or upper body ■ shortness of breath ■ swollen feet or ankles ■ clumsiness ■ pain, heat, or redness in feet or hands	**May be serious** Check with your doctor as soon as possible.
drowsiness or tiredness ■ headache (including migraine) ■ constipation ■ diarrhea ■ urinary frequency ■ urinary retention or incontinence ■ loss of appetite ■ stomach pain or cramps ■ indigestion ■ nausea or vomiting ■ dry mouth ■ metallic taste ■ difficulty in swallowing ■ stuffy nose ■ leg cramps ■ tingling or pain in fingers or toes, especially when exposed to cold ■ depression ■ sleeplessness ■ nightmares ■ nervousness ■ burning eyes or other eye problems ■ double vision or other visual disturbances ■ rash or hives ■ mottled skin	If symptoms are disturbing or persist, let your doctor know.

STORAGE INSTRUCTIONS

Store in a cool, dark place (not in a bathroom medicine cabinet).

STOPPING OR INTERRUPTING THERAPY

It may take several weeks before you feel the helpful effects of this medicine. Do not stop taking it without consulting your doctor. Stopping this medicine suddenly may worsen your medical condition. If you miss a dose, take it as soon as possible. If it is within four hours of your next scheduled dose, skip the missed dose and resume your regular schedule. Do not take two doses at the same time.

SPECIAL CONSIDERATIONS FOR THOSE OVER SIXTY-FIVE

Older people may be more susceptible to such side effects as confusion, hallucinations, and uncontrollable movements.

EPILEPSY

When we think about epilepsy, most of us see the image of a person losing consciousness, falling down, and jerking all over. That *is* what happens during a grand mal seizure. But in some people with epilepsy—a condition in which episodes of abnormal activity in some brain cells cause uncontrolled activity in the body—the seizure is just a twitching of one hand or foot. In others, the seizure consists of a feeling that one side of the body is numb or prickling. Or it is expressed as repeated behavior that has no purpose, like lip-smacking or hand-clapping. Sometimes epilepsy appears as just a few seconds of blinking or a vacant stare.

CAUSES

Brain cells, known as neurons, produce tiny electric charges that can be monitored through electrodes placed on the head. In epilepsy, the neurons periodically misfire. If the misfiring occurs in the part of the brain that controls vision, the seizure will consist of a hallucination. If it occurs in the part that directs the fingers, the fingers will twitch. Sometimes the abnormal electricity in one part of the brain sets off abnormal discharges elsewhere in the brain, sending several parts of the body into abnormal motion.

In most cases, the reason for the epilepsy is unknown. In others, it can be traced to an injury to the brain caused by oxygen deprivation, a blow to the head, a tumor, or a stroke. Most new cases of epilepsy show up in babies and young children, but brain injury can occur at any age. People who have never had a seizure before can suddenly develop the disorder when they are past fifty, sixty, or even eighty.

DIAGNOSIS

Your doctor will begin by taking a medical history and doing a physical exam. You will also be questioned about the circumstances in which the seizure occurred and whether it was preceded by an aura—a strange sensation that comes right before some types of seizures (and also before some migraine headaches). An aura may be just an ill-defined feeling, or something more specific such as visual disturbances or the impression of hearing peculiar sounds. If anyone was with you when the aura occurred, you should bring that person along to talk to the doctor, since you might not be able to recall much about the event.

Because epilepsy is marked by abnormal electrical activity in the brain, electroencephalogram (EEG) examinations are an important part of the diagnostic procedure. In addition to helping identify the cause of the seizure, they aid in selecting appropriate drug treatments. However, as valuable as the EEG is, it has certain limitations. Some people with epilepsy only have abnormal brain waves during the actual seizure; the rest of the time, their charts show regular patterns. Other people, who do not have epilepsy at all, sometimes produce abnormal tracings. Your doctor might, therefore, want you to have several EEGs to see whether the pattern is the same at different times of the day or after different kinds of stimulation.

Your doctor might also want you to have a computed axial tomography (CAT) scan, which provides a detailed image of the inside of your brain, or a positron emission tomography (PET) scan, which is an even newer method of detecting and mapping your brain's activity. Like the EEG, these tests are painless and noninvasive; there is no radiation to be concerned about, nor any physical probing inside your brain.

TREATMENT

If it's found that you do have epilepsy, these diagnostic tests should give your doctor a fairly good idea of the type it is and the location of the neurons that set it off. He or she can therefore prescribe the medicine that has the best chance of bringing your disorder entirely under control. If the first-choice drug does not work for you, or if it causes severe adverse reactions, the doctor can juggle drugs and doses until you get the relief you need. For information on anticonvulsant medicines, see the charts on pages 266–277. In those few cases in which medicine does not help, doctors and patients can explore the possibility of surgical removal of the part of the brain that is causing the problem. If the seizures always arise in a single area in the brain, surgery may provide a permanent cure.

OUTLOOK

Most people with epilepsy have to cope with it for the rest of their lives, though it can usually be controlled with drugs. There is no evidence that it gets either better or worse as a person gets older. But diagnostic and treatment techniques *are* getting better, giving hope of a more normal life, without the constant fear of seizures.

CONDITION: **EPILEPSY AND SEIZURES**

CATEGORY: **ANTICONVULSANTS**

GENERIC (CHEMICAL) NAME	BRAND (TRADE) NAME	DOSAGE FORMS AND STRENGTHS
Phenytoin	DILANTIN	Capsules: 30,100 mg Suspension: 125 mg per tsp Tablets: 50 mg

DRUG PROFILE

Phenytoin is used to treat epilepsy and other types of seizure disorders. It prevents seizures or makes them occur less often by dampening the overactive nerve impulses in the brain.

BEFORE USING THIS DRUG

Let your doctor know *IF*

You have ever had any allergic reactions or other problems with ■ phenytoin ■ other medicine for seizures.

You have ever had any of the following medical problems: ■ diabetes ■ high blood sugar ■ liver disease ■ kidney disease ■ alcoholism ■ blood disease ■ bone disease.

You are taking any of the following medicines: ■ any other medicine for seizures ■ Antabuse (used in treatment of alcoholism) ■ barbiturates ■ tranquilizers ■ sleep medicines ■ muscle relaxants ■ medicine for depression ■ phenyl-butazone or oxyphenbutazone (medicine for arthritis) ■ vitamin B_9 (folic acid) ■ vitamin D (calcifediol) ■ antibiotics ■ cimetidine (medicine for ulcers) ■ anticoagulants (blood thinners) ■ corticosteroids ■ medicine for diabetes ■ medicine for tuberculosis ■ digoxin, digitoxin, or digitalis (heart medicines) ■ hormones ■ propoxyphene (prescription pain-killer) ■ medicine for nausea ■ quinidine (medicine for abnormal heart rhythms) ■ any medicine containing alcohol.

SPECIAL RESTRICTIONS WHILE TAKING THIS DRUG

FOOD AND DRUG INTERACTIONS

Other Drugs	Do not take any other drugs, including over-the-counter (OTC) drugs, before checking with your doctor. A number of drugs affect the way phenytoin works, and your doctor may want to adjust the dose of phenytoin or of the other drugs you may be taking. Also, do not switch to another brand or dosage form (e.g., tablets to capsules) without consulting your doctor, since different forms of this medicine are absorbed by the body in different ways, and your dosage may have to be adjusted.
Foods and Beverages	Because this drug may cause folic acid deficiency, be sure to eat a well-rounded diet containing plenty of B vitamins. Your doctor may recommend that you take a multivitamin.
Alcohol	Drinking alcohol while taking this medicine may increase the risk of drowsiness and reduce the effects of the drug. Avoid alcohol unless your doctor has approved its use.

No special restrictions on smoking.

DAILY LIVING

Driving	This drug may cause drowsiness or loss of alertness. Be careful when driving, operating household appliances, or doing any other tasks that require alertness until you know how this drug affects you.
Examinations or Tests	It is important for you to keep all appointments for blood tests so that your progress and side effects can be checked.

Other Precautions	If you have diabetes, be aware that this medicine may affect blood-sugar levels. If you notice any change when testing sugar levels in your blood or urine, let your doctor know.

Tell any doctor or dentist you consult that you are taking this medicine, especially if you will be undergoing any type of surgery. |
| Helpful Hints | If this medicine upsets your stomach, taking it with meals, snacks, or water should help.

This medicine may cause your gums to become red and swollen. Practicing good oral hygiene (flossing and brushing carefully) can minimize this effect. |

No special restrictions on exertion and exercise, sun exposure, or exposure to excessive heat or cold.

POSSIBLE SIDE EFFECTS

Although this list of adverse effects may seem somewhat intimidating, keep in mind that some are quite rare. Of course, should these or any other problems arise while you are on medication, it is always a good idea to consult your doctor.

IF YOU DEVELOP

uncontrollable eye movements ■ crossed eyes or any other eye problems ■ blurred or double vision ■ rash ■ sore throat or fever ■ dark urine or gray stools ■ yellowing of eyes or skin ■ severe headache ■ swelling of the tip of the penis ■ enlarged lymph glands ■ stomach pain ■ bleeding or bruising ■ hallucinations ■ confusion ■ memory loss ■ severe dizziness or drowsiness ■ slurred speech ■ clumsiness ■ staggering walk ■ sleeplessness ■ behavior or personality changes ■ depression ■ pain in urination ■ urinary frequency ■ swelling of feet or hands ■ uncontrollable muscle movements

WHAT TO DO

Urgent Get in touch with your doctor immediately.

irritability ■ restlessness ■ red, swollen gums ■ constipation ■ upset stomach ■ nausea or vomiting ■ diarrhea ■ loss of taste ■ difficulty in swallowing ■ loss of appetite ■ weight loss ■ acne ■ dizziness ■ drowsiness ■ hair growth ■ headache ■ muscle twitching ■ red eyes ■ stuffy nose

If symptoms are disturbing or persist, let your doctor know.

STORAGE INSTRUCTIONS

Store in a cool, dark place (not in a bathroom medicine cabinet). If your medicine is in a liquid form, make sure that it does not freeze.

STOPPING OR INTERRUPTING THERAPY

Since this drug does not cure your condition but only controls it, you may have to take this medicine for the rest of your life. Do not stop taking this medicine unless instructed to do so by your doctor. Suddenly stopping this medicine could trigger seizures; your doctor will advise you on how to reduce your dosage gradually before stopping completely. If you take phenytoin once a day and you miss a dose, take it as soon as possible and resume your regular schedule. If you do not remember until the following day, skip the missed dose and resume your regular schedule. If you take phenytoin several times a day and you miss a dose, take the missed dose as soon as possible. If your next dose is within four hours, skip the missed dose and resume your regular schedule. If you miss your dose for two or more days, check with your doctor.

SPECIAL CONSIDERATIONS FOR THOSE OVER SIXTY-FIVE

Older people may be more prone to such side effects as clumsiness and red, swollen gums. Also, the body's absorption of calcium may be lowered, leading to osteomalacia (softening of the bones), a condition to which this age group may be susceptible.

CONDITION: **EPILEPSY AND SEIZURES**

CATEGORY: **ANTICONVULSANTS**

GENERIC (CHEMICAL) NAME	BRAND (TRADE) NAME	DOSAGE FORMS AND STRENGTHS
Primidone	MYSOLINE	Suspension: 250 mg per tsp Tablets: 50, 250 mg

DRUG PROFILE

Primidone is used to treat epilepsy. It prevents seizures or makes them occur less often by dampening the overactive nerve impulses in the brain. Primidone can be used alone or with other medicine for more effective seizure control.

BEFORE USING THIS DRUG

Let your doctor know *IF*

You have ever had allergic reactions or other problems with ■ primidone ■ barbiturates.

You have ever had any of the following medical problems: ■ asthma or other lung disease ■ kidney disease ■ liver disease ■ porphyria.

You are taking any of the following medicines: ■ other medicine for seizures ■ corticosteroids ■ anticoagulants (blood thinners) ■ antihistamines ■ medicine for hay fever, allergies, or colds ■ barbiturates ■ narcotics or other prescription pain-killers ■ tranquilizers ■ sleep medicines ■ medicine for fungal infection ■ doxycycline ■ muscle relaxants ■ quinidine (medicine for abnormal heart rhythms) ■ any medicine containing alcohol.

SPECIAL RESTRICTIONS WHILE TAKING THIS DRUG

FOOD AND DRUG INTERACTIONS

Other Drugs	This medicine increases the effects of drugs that depress the central nervous system—such as antihistamines; medicine for hay fever, allergies, or colds; sleep medicines; tranquilizers; narcotics or other prescription pain-killers; muscle relaxants; and other medicine for seizures.
Alcohol	Drinking alcohol may increase the effects of this medicine or cause dangerously high levels of this medicine in your body. Avoid alcohol unless your doctor has approved its use.

No special restrictions on foods and beverages or smoking.

DAILY LIVING

Driving	This drug may cause dizziness, light-headedness, or drowsiness. Be careful when driving, operating household appliances, or doing any other tasks that require alertness until you know how this drug affects you.
Examinations or Tests	It is important for you to keep all appointments with your doctor so that your progress and any side effects can be checked. Periodic blood tests may be required.
Other Precautions	Tell any doctor or dentist you consult that you are taking this drug, especially if you will be undergoing any type of surgery.

No special restrictions on exertion and exercise, sun exposure, or exposure to excessive heat or cold.

POSSIBLE SIDE EFFECTS

Although this list of adverse effects may seem somewhat intimidating, keep in mind that some are quite rare. Of course, should these or any other problems arise while you are on medication, it is always a good idea to consult your doctor.

IF YOU DEVELOP	WHAT TO DO
yellowing of eyes or skin ■ dark urine ■ pale stools ■ discoloration of skin	**Urgent** Get in touch with your doctor immediately.
wheezing or tightness in chest ■ extreme excitement ■ tiredness or weakness ■ rash or hives ■ swelling or twitching of eyelids ■ double vision ■ confusion ■ difficulty in breathing ■ emotional disturbances ■ mental changes, including depression ■ difficulty in swallowing ■ sore throat or fever ■ bleeding (including nosebleed) or bruising ■ swelling of the legs ■ speech difficulties ■ swelling of the tip of the penis ■ urinary problems	**May be serious** Check with your doctor as soon as possible.
clumsiness or unsteadiness ■ drowsiness ■ dizziness or light-headedness ■ male impotence ■ headache ■ loss of appetite ■ nausea or vomiting ■ upset stomach ■ constipation ■ diarrhea ■ loss of taste ■ hair loss ■ stuffy nose ■ red, itching eyes	If symptoms are disturbing or persist, let your doctor know.

STORAGE INSTRUCTIONS

Store in a cool, dark place (not in a bathroom medicine cabinet). If your medicine is in a liquid form, make sure that it does not freeze.

STOPPING OR INTERRUPTING THERAPY

It may be several weeks before you feel the beneficial effects of this drug. Do not suddenly stop taking this medicine, as this may trigger seizures. Your doctor will advise you on how to stop gradually and safely when you no longer need this medicine. If you miss a dose, take it as soon as possible. If it is within an hour of your next dose, skip the missed dose and resume your regular schedule. Do not take two doses at the same time.

SPECIAL CONSIDERATIONS FOR THOSE OVER SIXTY-FIVE

Older people may be more prone to such side effects as dizziness, drowsiness, excitement, confusion, and depression.

CONDITION: **EPILEPSY AND SEIZURES**

CATEGORY: **ANTICONVULSANTS**

GENERIC (CHEMICAL) NAME	BRAND (TRADE) NAME	DOSAGE FORMS AND STRENGTHS
Carbamazepine	TEGRETOL	Chewable tablets: 100 mg Tablets: 200 mg

DRUG PROFILE

This drug is used to treat certain types of epilepsy. It prevents seizures or makes them occur less often by dampening the overactive nerve impulses in the brain. Carbamazepine is also used to treat trigeminal neuralgia (tic douloureux), which is a type of facial pain.

BEFORE USING THIS DRUG

Let your doctor know *IF*

You have ever had allergic reactions or other problems with ■ carbamazepine ■ tricyclic antidepressants (medicine for depression).

You have ever had any of the following medical problems: ■ heart or blood vessel disease, including thrombophlebitis, congestive heart failure, high or low blood pressure, or heart attack ■ kidney disease ■ liver disease ■ blood disease ■ bone marrow depression ■ anemia ■ alcoholism ■ mental illness ■ diabetes ■ urinary problems ■ systemic lupus erythematosus ■ glaucoma.

You are taking any of the following medicines: ■ other medicines for seizures ■ medicine for depression (within the last two weeks) ■ anticoagulants (blood thinners) ■ barbiturates ■ tranquilizers ■ sleep medicines ■ muscle relaxants ■ narcotics and other prescription pain-killers ■ antibiotics ■ cimetidine (medicine for ulcers) ■ medicine for abnormal heart rhythms ■ tetracyclines.

Any drug you have taken has ever affected your blood.

SPECIAL RESTRICTIONS WHILE TAKING THIS DRUG

FOOD AND DRUG INTERACTIONS

Other Drugs	Do not take any other drugs, including over-the-counter (OTC) drugs, before checking with your doctor. This drug affects the way many other drugs work, and your doctor may want to adjust the dose of carbamazepine or of the other drugs you may be taking.
Alcohol	Avoid alcohol unless your doctor has approved its use.

No special restrictions on foods and beverages or smoking.

DAILY LIVING

Driving	This drug may cause dizziness, light-headedness, or blurred vision. Be careful when driving, operating household appliances, or doing any other tasks that require alertness until you know how this drug affects you.
Sun Exposure	Your skin may become more sensitive to sunlight and more likely to develop a sunburn while taking this

medicine. It is a good idea to apply a sunscreen to exposed skin surfaces before going outdoors.

Excessive Heat	Use caution during hot weather since overexertion may result in heat stroke. Avoid extremely hot baths and saunas.
Examinations or Tests	It is important for you to keep all appointments with your doctor so that your progress can be checked. Your dosage may have to be adjusted from time to time. Periodic blood and urine tests, as well as eye examinations, are usually required before and during therapy.
Other Precautions	Tell any doctor or dentist you consult that you are taking this medicine, especially if you will be undergoing any type of surgery or any kind of tests. If you have diabetes, be aware that this drug may cause false urine-sugar tests. Discuss with your doctor what kind of home tests you should use.
Helpful Hints	If this medicine upsets your stomach, taking it with milk, meals, or snacks should help. If your mouth or throat feels dry, chewing sugarless gum or sucking ice chips or sugarless hard candy will help.

No special restrictions on exertion and exercise or exposure to excessive cold.

POSSIBLE SIDE EFFECTS

Although this list of adverse effects may seem somewhat intimidating, keep in mind that some are quite rare. Of course, should these or any other problems arise while you are on medication, it is always a good idea to consult your doctor.

IF YOU DEVELOP	WHAT TO DO
mouth sores ■ sore throat or fever ■ bleeding or bruising ■ chills ■ extreme tiredness or weakness	**Extremely Urgent: Stop taking this drug and get in touch with your doctor immediately.**
fainting ■ collapse ■ stuffy nose ■ red, irritated eyes ■ swelling of the tip of the penis ■ swelling of lower legs or feet ■ pain, tenderness, or bluish color in legs or feet ■ dark urine ■ pale stools ■ yellowing of eyes or skin ■ seizures ■ irregular or fast heartbeat ■ severe dizziness or drowsiness ■ shortness of breath ■ irregular or shallow breathing ■ tremors ■ pain or difficulty in urination ■ rash, hives, or itching	**Urgent** Get in touch with your doctor immediately.
blurred or double vision ■ confusion ■ chest pain ■ slow or pounding heartbeat ■ back and forth eye movements or other eye problems ■ uncontrollable body movements ■ spasms ■ numbness, tingling, pain, or weakness in hands or feet ■ speech difficulties ■ swollen glands ■ restlessness and nervousness ■ depression ■ hallucinations ■ ringing in ears ■ increased sensitivity to sound ■ flushing ■ dilated pupils ■ urinary frequency ■ decreased urination ■ nausea or vomiting ■ stomach pain or discomfort ■ loss of appetite ■ diarrhea ■ constipation	**May be serious** Check with your doctor as soon as possible.
clumsiness or unsteadiness ■ light-headedness or dizziness ■ drowsiness ■ dry mouth or throat ■ tongue irritation ■ joint or muscle aches ■ leg cramps ■ headache ■ increased skin sensitivity to sunlight ■ changes in skin color ■ hair loss ■ male impotence ■ increased sweating ■ difficulty in swallowing	If symptoms are disturbing or persist, let your doctor know.

STORAGE INSTRUCTIONS

Store in a cool, dark place (not in a bathroom medicine cabinet).

STOPPING OR INTERRUPTING THERAPY

Do not stop taking this drug unless instructed to do so by your doctor. If you miss a dose, take it as soon as possible. If it is almost time for your next dose, skip the missed dose and resume your regular schedule. Do not take two doses at the same time. If you miss two or more doses in the same day, consult your doctor.

SPECIAL CONSIDERATIONS FOR THOSE OVER SIXTY-FIVE

Older people may be more susceptible to such side effects as confusion, nervousness, and restlessness.

CONDITION: **EPILEPSY AND SEIZURES**

CATEGORY: **BENZODIAZEPINES**

GENERIC (CHEMICAL) NAME	BRAND (TRADE) NAME	DOSAGE FORMS AND STRENGTHS
Clonazepam	KLONOPIN	Tablets: 0.5, 1, 2 mg

DRUG PROFILE

Benzodiazepines are used to treat a number of conditions, including anxiety, insomnia, muscle spasm, and seizures. Exactly how these drugs work is a matter of some debate. However, what they all seem to have in common is that they reduce nerve cell activity in those areas of the central nervous system (CNS) and peripheral nervous system (PNS) thought to be responsible for the experience of anxiety and muscular tension. Low doses are usually prescribed for older people.

For complete information on this drug, see pages 478–483.

HEADACHES

Headaches strike people of any age and either sex and occur at least once a month in 90 percent of the U.S. population. For most of these people, headaches are a fleeting discomfort caused by fatigue, hunger, or stress and are quickly relieved by aspirin or acetaminophen, fresh air, rest, or perhaps a gentle massage. But for others, headaches are a relentless fact of life that cannot be easily banished or easily borne.

The majority of headaches can be classified into three categories: organic headaches, muscle contraction (or tension) headaches, and vascular headaches.

ORGANIC HEADACHES

Although organic headaches are the least common type, they may indicate a serious disorder, such as high blood pressure or, rarely, a brain tumor. They should be considered a warning sign, and merit immediate medical attention. See a doctor if your headaches are sudden, severe, or progressive; are accompanied by confusion or loss of consciousness; recur in one area, such as an eye or temple; are accompanied by fever and stiff neck; or frequently awaken you from a sound sleep.

One variety of organic headache (actually a facial pain) that occurs more commonly in women than in men is caused by trigeminal neuralgia, often referred to as *tic douloureux*. This condition, a painful inflammation of the nerves in the cheek, most often begins between the ages of thirty and sixty. An attack of this disorder consists of repetitive painful jabs; this lasts one or more hours, and commonly occurs at night. Attacks may go on for several months, and then ease up for a year or more. This condition is generally treated with medicine. See pages 273–277 for a description of the drug most commonly used to relieve the distress of tic douloureux. In some cases, medical therapy eventually loses its effectiveness, and surgical techniques are used quite successfully to treat this condition.

TENSION HEADACHES

Muscle contraction, or tension, headaches are the most common type of headache. They often result from physical or emotional stress, which causes head and neck muscles to contract and feel tender. Poor posture or prolonged sitting may also lead to this type of headache. The steady, dull pain of a tension headache localizes in the forehead, back of the neck, or temples; sometimes the pain seems to wrap itself around the head like a steel band. Sufferers can often find quick relief from the tension through massage, heat, or a hot shower. Practicing relaxation techniques—such as meditation, yoga, or biofeedback—can often work magically. Also, aspirin or acetaminophen may effectively relieve the pain. For severe muscle tension headaches, slightly more potent drugs may be prescribed.

VASCULAR HEADACHES

Vascular headaches occur when blood vessels in the brain either constrict or dilate, forcing the blood to pulse, and causing the throbbing sensation characteristic of these headaches. Hangovers, hunger, and certain substances in food (such as monosodium glutamate, often used in Chinese cooking, and tyramine, found in red wine, certain shellfish and cheeses, and other foods), account for many of these headaches.

Migraine Headaches Migraine headaches, a frightening form of vascular headache caused by blood vessel dilation, are excruciating and may incapacitate their victims for days at a time. Migraines usually start on one side of the head and remain there during the length of the attack. The intense throbbing is often accompanied by nausea, loss of appetite, and even vomiting. Two types of migraine headaches exist. The common variety has few or no warning symptoms and can occur two or three times a week if the patient is unduly stressed. The classic migraine headache, on the other hand, gives an unmistakable ten-to thirty-minute warning of its onset, with sensations known as auras—the victim may see flashing lights, zigzagging lines, or areas of total darkness. When the aura fades, the pain begins and can last from an hour or two to twenty-four or seventy-two hours.

Migraine headaches appear to run in families and to be associated with hard-driving, perfectionist personalities. Migraine therapy begins with pinpointing the headache's triggering factor—whether stress, fatigue, certain foods, flickering lights, or cigarette smoke, for example—and then attacking the condition with pharmacological, environmental, or psychological treatments. Biofeedback training has been effective in treating some cases of chronic migraine. Drug treatments are available that can either prevent a migraine from developing or stop it in its earliest stages. See the drug charts on pages 284–291 for a description of these agents.

Cluster Headaches Cluster headaches, also caused by vascular irregularities, strike suddenly; recur repeatedly for a certain period (usually two to twelve weeks); and then disappear—only to return for another period of "clustered" pain. More common in men than in women, these headaches are associated with intense pain and have been known to cause some sufferers to bang their heads against a wall. Because it's important for therapy to begin early in an attack, drugs are often administered by injection or suppository to enable them to enter the bloodstream rapidly.

OUTLOOK

Although certain types of headaches merit prompt attention from a doctor, the vast majority are not symptoms of serious medical problems. Usually they can be controlled by the use of simple drugs and by changes in everyday habits.

CONDITION: **HEADACHE**

CATEGORY: **ANALGESIC-BARBITURATE COMBINATIONS**

GENERIC (CHEMICAL) NAME	BRAND (TRADE) NAME	DOSAGE FORMS AND STRENGTHS
Butalbital, aspirin, and caffeine	FIORINAL	Capsules: 50 mg butalbital, 325 mg aspirin, and 40 mg caffeine Tablets: 50 mg butalbital, 325 mg aspirin, and 40 mg caffeine

DRUG PROFILE

The combination of butalbital (a barbiturate), aspirin, and caffeine is used to treat tension (muscle contraction) headaches. Aspirin blocks the production of naturally occurring triggers of pain and inflammation called prostaglandins. Butalbital produces a calming effect, and caffeine strengthens the action of aspirin.

BEFORE USING THIS DRUG

Let your doctor know *IF*

You have ever had allergic reactions or other problems with ■ any barbiturates ■ aspirin or any other salicylates ■ indomethacin ■ ibuprofen ■ caffeine ■ mefanic acid ■ phenylbutazone ■ sodium benzoate ■ tartrazine (FD&C Yellow Dye No. 5).

You have ever had any of the following medical problems: ■ hay fever ■ asthma or other lung disease ■ ulcers, gastritis, or any other digestive disorders ■ liver disease ■ kidney disease ■ systemic lupus erythematosus ■ glucose-6-phosphate dehydrogenase (G-6-PD) deficiency ■ vitamin K deficiency ■ pyruvate kinase deficiency ■ nasal polyps ■ chronic hives ■ chronic stuffy nose ■ rheumatic fever ■ heart or blood vessel disease ■ any bleeding disorder ■ recent oral surgery ■ diabetes ■ porphyria ■ mental illness ■ glaucoma ■ anemia ■ overactive thyroid ■ high or low blood pressure ■ drug abuse, including alcoholism.

You are taking any of the following medicines: ■ aspirin or aspirinlike medicine ■ medicine for arthritis or gout ■ anticoagulants (blood thinners) ■ corticosteroids ■ antacids ■ any medicine containing alcohol ■ nadolol, propranolol, timolol, metoprolol, atenolol, pindolol, or labetalol (beta-blockers) ■ medicine for high blood pressure ■ medicine for seizures ■ medicine for diabetes ■ methotrexate (medicine for cancer or severe psoriasis) ■ procarbazine (medicine for cancer) ■ other medicine for cancer ■ nitrates (medicine for chest pain) ■ medicine to make the urine more alkaline or more acidic ■ isoniazid (medicine for tuberculosis) ■ medicine for colds, cough, or hay fever ■ antihistamines ■ tranquilizers ■ sleep medicines ■ appetite suppressants ■ muscle relaxants ■ narcotics or other prescription pain-killers ■ barbiturates ■ medicine for depression ■ male hormones ■ thyroid hormones ■ digoxin, digitoxin, or digitalis (heart medicines) ■ phenytoin (medicine for seizures) ■ quinidine (medicine for abnormal heart rhythms) ■ theophylline (medicine for asthma) ■ penicillin, chloramphenicol, doxycycline, griseofulvin, or metronidazole (antibiotics) ■ vitamin D or K.

SPECIAL RESTRICTIONS WHILE TAKING THIS DRUG

FOOD AND DRUG INTERACTIONS

Other Drugs	Do not take any other drugs, including over-the-counter (OTC) drugs, before checking with your doctor. This medicine increases the effects of drugs that depress the central nervous system—such as antihistamines; medicine for hay fever, allergies, or colds; sleep medicines; tranquilizers; narcotics or other prescription pain-killers; muscle relaxants; and medicine for seizures. It is a good idea not to take other medicines that contain salicylates (even medicines that are applied to the skin). Check the labels of OTC products, such as special shampoos, lotions, and creams, to see if they contain aspirin, salicylic acid, or other salicylate drugs.
Foods and Beverages	Because this drug contains caffeine, you should probably limit your intake of caffeine-containing foods and beverages.

Alcohol	Avoid alcohol while taking this medicine; this combination can be dangerous, as well as irritating to the stomach.

No special restrictions on smoking.

DAILY LIVING

Driving	This drug may cause dizziness or loss of alertness. Be careful when driving, operating household appliances, or doing any other tasks that require alertness until you know how this drug affects you.
Examinations or Tests	It is important for you to keep all appointments with your doctor so that your progress can be checked. Ask your doctor every couple of months if you need to keep taking this medicine.
Other Precautions	Take this medicine exactly as prescribed by your doctor; taking it more often or for a longer period of time than prescribed may make it habit forming. If you suspect that this medicine is not working, do not increase the dose without first checking with your doctor.

If you accidentally take an overdose of this medicine, go to an emergency room immediately.

Also, let your doctor know if you notice a buzzing or ringing sound in your ears, since this may be a sign that you are taking too much of this medicine.

Tell any doctor or dentist you consult that you are taking this drug, especially if you will be undergoing any type of surgery.

If you have diabetes, be aware that false urine-sugar tests may occur while you are taking this drug. Check with your doctor before increasing the dose of any diabetes medicine you may be taking.

Helpful Hints   If this drug upsets your stomach, taking it with meals, milk, or water should help.

No special restrictions on exertion and exercise, sun exposure, or exposure to excessive heat or cold.

POSSIBLE SIDE EFFECTS

Although this list of adverse effects may seem somewhat intimidating, keep in mind that some are quite rare. Of course, should these or any other problems arise while you are on medication, it is always a good idea to consult your doctor.

IF YOU DEVELOP

cold, clammy skin ■ very slow or fast heartbeat ■ dizziness ■ drowsiness ■ light-headedness ■ confusion ■ slurred speech ■ chest pain ■ wheezing or other difficulty in breathing ■ loss of balance ■ fever ■ severe or continuing headache ■ swelling of the tip of the penis ■ pain in urination ■ blood in urine ■ decreased urination ■ seizures ■ diarrhea ■ extreme excitement or nervousness ■ hallucinations ■ talkativeness or incoherence ■ personality changes ■ tremors ■ severe or continuing nausea or vomiting ■ continuing stomach pain ■ increased sweating ■ increased thirst ■ visual disturbances ■ uncontrollable flapping movements of the hands ■ watery eyes ■ fainting

WHAT TO DO

Urgent Get in touch with your doctor immediately.

bleeding lip sores or other mouth sores ■ bleeding (including nosebleed) or bruising ■ muscle or joint pain, or any other pain ■ scaly, red skin ■ rash or hives ■ swollen eyes, face, or lips ■ red, itching eyes ■ stuffy nose ■ depression ■ agitation ■ extreme tiredness ■ yellowing of eyes or skin

May be serious Check with your doctor as soon as possible.

clumsiness ■ "hangover" feeling ■ anxiety ■ constipation ■ nausea or vomiting ■ nightmares ■ sleeplessness ■ irritability	If symptoms are disturbing or persist, let your doctor know.

STORAGE INSTRUCTIONS

Store in a cool, dark place (not in a bathroom medicine cabinet). If you notice a vinegarlike odor coming from the bottle, this means that the drug is breaking down and should be discarded.

STOPPING OR INTERRUPTING THERAPY

Take this medicine exactly as prescribed by your doctor. If you are taking this medicine on a regular schedule and you miss a dose, take it as soon as possible. If it is almost time for your next dose, skip the missed dose and resume your regular schedule.

SPECIAL CONSIDERATIONS FOR THOSE OVER SIXTY-FIVE

Older people may be especially prone to such side effects as difficulty in breathing, digestive upset, urinary problems, excitement, depression, and confusion.

CONDITION: **MIGRAINE HEADACHE**

CATEGORY: **ERGOT ALKALOIDS**

GENERIC (CHEMICAL) NAME	BRAND (TRADE) NAME	DOSAGE FORMS AND STRENGTHS
Ergotamine tartrate	ERGOMAR	Sublingual tablets: 2 mg
	ERGOSTAT	Sublingual tablets: 2 mg
	MEDIHALER ERGOTAMINE	Aerosol spray: 9 mg per ml

Ergotamine tartrate and caffeine	CAFERGOT	Capsules: 1 mg ergotamine tartrate and 100 mg caffeine
		Rectal suppositories: 2 mg ergotamine and 100 mg caffeine
	WIGRAINE	Tablets: 1 mg ergotamine tartrate and 100 mg caffeine
		Rectal suppositories: 2 mg ergotamine and 100 mg caffeine

DRUG PROFILE

Ergotamine is used to treat migraine headaches. By narrowing the blood vessels in the head, this drug relieves the pain of migraine (which results from an expansion of the blood vessels in the head). Some ergotamine preparations also contain caffeine, which, in addition to narrowing the blood vessels in the head, speeds up the absorption of ergotamine.

BEFORE USING THIS DRUG

Let your doctor know *IF*

You have ever had allergic reactions or other problems with ■ ergot alkaloids ■ caffeine.

You have ever had any of the following medical problems: ■ angina (chest pain) ■ phlebitis, hardening of the arteries, or Raynaud's syndrome (poor circulation in the fingers and toes) ■ high blood pressure ■ liver disease ■ kidney disease ■ sepsis or other infections ■ peptic ulcer ■ malnutrition.

■ *with aerosol form of drug only:* ■ asthma.

You are taking any of the following medicines: ■ methysergide ■ timolol, nadolol, atenolol, propranolol, metoprolol, pindolol, acebutolol, or labetolol (beta-blockers).

SPECIAL RESTRICTIONS WHILE TAKING THIS DRUG

FOOD AND DRUG INTERACTIONS

Alcohol	Avoid alcohol, which can aggravate headache.
Smoking	Nicotine aggravates the narrowing of the blood vessels of the arms and legs that may occur with this drug. If you smoke, try to stop or at least cut down.

No special restrictions on other drugs or foods and beverages.

DAILY LIVING

Excessive Cold	Avoid exposure to excessive cold, which aggravates the narrowing of the blood vessels in the arms and legs that may occur with this drug.
Examinations or Tests	If you need to take this drug frequently, your doctor may wish to examine you regularly to make sure that the drug is not causing harmful narrowing of the blood vessels in your arms and legs.
Other Precautions	Be careful not to exceed the dose your doctor recommends. Let your doctor know if you develop an infection while taking this medicine.
Helpful Hints	This medicine works best if you take it at the first sign of a headache. Once you have taken your medicine, lie down and relax in a quiet, darkened room. If you have been storing the suppository form of this medicine in a warm place, it may be too soft to use. Put it in the refrigerator for half an hour or run cold water over the wrapped suppository before use.

No special restrictions on driving, exertion and exercise, sun exposure, or exposure to excessive heat.

POSSIBLE SIDE EFFECTS

Although this list of adverse effects may seem somewhat intimidating, keep in mind that some are quite rare. Of course, should these or any other problems arise while you are on medication, it is always a good idea to consult your doctor.

IF YOU DEVELOP	WHAT TO DO
seizures ■ coma ■ severe loss of alertness ■ fainting ■ chest pain ■ stomach pain or bloating ■ extreme thirst ■ red or purple blisters on the hands or feet	**Urgent** Get in touch with your doctor immediately.
weak pulse ■ slow or fast heartbeat ■ weakness ■ muscle pain ■ numbness, coldness, or paleness of the arms or legs ■ swelling of the feet or legs ■ itching ■ arm, leg, or back pain ■ confusion ■ blurred vision *After you STOP taking this medicine:* headache	**May be serious** Check with your doctor as soon as possible.
nausea or vomiting ■ drowsiness ■ sleep disturbances ■ diarrhea ■ dizziness	If symptoms are disturbing or persist, let your doctor know.

STORAGE INSTRUCTIONS

Store in a cool, dark place (not in a bathroom medicine cabinet). Suppositories should be stored in the refrigerator.

STOPPING OR INTERRUPTING THERAPY

If you have been taking this medicine frequently for a prolonged period, you should not suddenly stop taking it. Discuss with your doctor how to stop gradually to avoid unpleasant aftereffects.

SPECIAL CONSIDERATIONS FOR THOSE OVER SIXTY-FIVE

Older people may be more sensitive to the tendency of this drug to narrow the blood vessels of the arms and legs. Older people who have narrowed coronary arteries may also be more vulnerable to chest pain while taking this medicine.

CONDITION: **MIGRAINE HEADACHE**

CATEGORY: **ERGOT ALKALOIDS**

GENERIC (CHEMICAL) NAME	BRAND (TRADE) NAME	DOSAGE FORMS AND STRENGTHS
Methysergide	SANSERT	Tablets: 2 mg

DRUG PROFILE

Methysergide is used to prevent frequent or severe vascular headaches including migraine and cluster headaches. This drug cannot stop a vascular headache attack once it has started. Methysergide acts by narrowing the blood vessels in the head. (The head pain of migraine results from an expansion of those blood vessels.)

BEFORE USING THIS DRUG

Let your doctor know *IF*

You have ever had allergic reactions or other problems with ■ methysergide ■ ergot alkaloids ■ tartrazine (FD&C Yellow Dye No. 5).

You have ever had any of the following medical problems: ■ angina (chest pain) ■ hardening of the arteries ■ valvular or other heart or blood vessel disease ■ high blood pressure ■ asthma or other lung disease ■ liver disease ■ kidney disease ■ serious infection ■ rheumatoid arthritis ■ systemic lupus erythematosus ■ scleroderma ■ fibrotic diseases, including heart murmurs ■ peripheral vascular disease, including phlebitis and cellulitis.

You are taking any of the following medicines: ■ ergotamine or medicines containing ergotamine ■ acebutolol, atenolol, metoprolol, nadolol, pindolol, propranolol, or timolol (beta-blockers).

SPECIAL RESTRICTIONS WHILE TAKING THIS DRUG

FOOD AND DRUG INTERACTIONS

Alcohol	Avoid alcohol, which can aggravate headache.

No special restrictions on other drugs, foods and beverages, or smoking.

DAILY LIVING

Driving	This drug may cause drowsiness, light-headedness, and dizziness, and may also affect mental alertness and physical coordination. Be careful when driving, operating household appliances, or doing any other tasks that require alertness until you know how this drug affects you.
Excessive Cold	Try to avoid exposure to very cold temperatures while taking this medicine, since cold may increase the chance of negative side effects.
Examinations or Tests	It is important for you to keep all appointments with your doctor so that your progress can be checked.
Other Precautions	Do not take more than three tablets a day to prevent a migraine or four tablets a day to prevent cluster headaches. If the amount of medicine prescribed does not seem to be working, do not increase your intake without first checking with your doctor. Taking this medicine more often or for a longer period of time than prescribed by your doctor makes you more prone to developing side effects.
	If you develop edema (swelling due to water retention), consult your doctor, who may reduce your dosage of this drug or prescribe a diuretic. Limiting your salt intake may also help correct this problem.

Helpful Hints

This medicine may cause weight gain. Your doctor may suggest that you reduce your caloric intake.

This medicine may upset your stomach; your doctor may advise you to take it with meals.

No special restrictions on exertion and exercise, sun exposure, or exposure to excessive heat.

POSSIBLE SIDE EFFECTS

Although this list of adverse effects may seem somewhat intimidating, keep in mind that some are quite rare. Of course, should these or any other problems arise while you are on medication, it is always a good idea to consult your doctor.

IF YOU DEVELOP

chest pain ■ shortness of breath ■ swelling of hands, legs, or ankles ■ pale or cold hands or feet ■ loss of weight or appetite ■ fever ■ pain or cramps in flank, groin, leg, or lower back ■ numbness or coldness in fingers, toes, or face ■ weakness in legs ■ pain or difficulty in urination ■ decreased urination ■ severe dizziness ■ general feeling of unwellness ■ fatigue

WHAT TO DO

Urgent Get in touch with your doctor immediately.

itching ■ weak pulse ■ visual disturbances ■ changes in heart rate ■ feelings of excitement or unreality ■ cloudy thinking ■ hallucinations ■ nightmares ■ "high" feeling ■ restlessness ■ nervousness ■ confusion ■ hypersensitivity ■ muscle or joint pain ■ clumsiness

May be serious Check with your doctor as soon as possible.

dizziness or light-headedness, especially when getting up from a reclining or sitting position ■ drowsiness ■ sleeplessness ■ diarrhea ■ nausea, vomiting, or stomach pain ■ heartburn ■ constipation ■ depression ■ sleep disturbances ■ hair loss ■ flushing ■ weight gain ■ spots on the skin

If symptoms are disturbing or persist, let your doctor know.

STORAGE INSTRUCTIONS

Store in a cool, dark place (not in a bathroom medicine cabinet).

STOPPING OR INTERRUPTING THERAPY

If you miss a dose of this medicine, skip the missed dose, and resume your regular schedule. Do not take two doses at the same time. If you have been taking this medicine for several weeks, do not suddenly stop taking it without consulting your doctor. You may be advised to stop taking it gradually to avoid unpleasant side effects. Your doctor will probably not want you to take this medicine for more than six months at a time; if the doctor does suggest a rest from this medicine (usually about three to four weeks), follow instructions carefully. Let your doctor know if your headaches return after you have stopped taking this medicine.

SPECIAL CONSIDERATIONS FOR THOSE OVER SIXTY-FIVE

Older people, especially those with blood vessel problems, are more likely to experience side effects with this medicine.

CONDITION: **MIGRAINE HEADACHE**

CATEGORY: **BETA-BLOCKERS**

GENERIC (CHEMICAL) NAME	BRAND (TRADE) NAME	DOSAGE FORMS AND STRENGTHS
Propranolol hydrochloride	INDERAL	Tablets: 10, 20, 40, 60, 80, 90 mg
	INDERAL LA	Capsules: 80, 120, 160 mg

DRUG PROFILE

Beta-adrenergic blocking drugs (beta-blockers) are a group of relatively new drugs that are used to control high blood pressure. By blocking certain nerve impulses, these medicines relax blood vessels, increase the supply of blood and oxygen to the heart, reduce the workload of the heart, and help the heart beat more regularly. Because of these effects, some beta-blockers are also useful for other conditions, such as angina, arrhythmias, migraine headaches, and hypertrophic subaortic stenosis (a disease of the heart muscle). They have also been found to improve a person's chance of survival for several years following a heart attack.

For complete information on this drug, see pages 56–61.

Chapter 3
Disorders of the Digestive System

PEPTIC ULCERS

Ulcers are small, craterlike sores that develop in the lining of the stomach (gastric ulcers) or the duodenum (duodenal ulcers), the first section of the small intestine. The term *peptic ulcer* is sometimes used to describe both types of ulcer. Learning how your ulcer may have developed and understanding what irritates it will help you work with your doctor to establish an effective treatment plan.

CAUSES

Peptic ulcers occur only in those regions of the digestive system that come in contact with digestive juices secreted by the stomach. These juices include stomach acid (hydrochloric acid) and a protein-digesting enzyme called pepsin. Many people with duodenal ulcers manufacture an excess of digestive juices. In contrast, many people with gastric ulcers have less stomach acid than would be expected. Scientists believe, therefore, that poor resistance of the protective mucous lining of the stomach and duodenum may be an important factor leading to the development of a peptic ulcer.

Duodenal ulcers are more common than gastric ulcers. It is estimated that the duodenal variety affects 10 percent of the male population at any one time (men are affected three times more frequently than women). People in their forties and fifties are the most likely to be affected. Gastric ulcers are about equally common in men and women, and they generally strike an older population. Peak incidence is in the fifties and sixties.

DIAGNOSIS

The symptoms of ulcer disease are less specific in people over fifty, and the beginnings of the ulcer may be harder to pinpoint. The most common symptom of duodenal ulcer is pain. The pain, which is usually felt in the middle of the upper abdomen, between the breastbone and the navel, varies from a hunger pang to a continuous gnawing or burning sensation. It usually occurs two or three hours after eating, when the stomach is empty, and is usually relieved by antacids or eating. Other common symptoms include a bloated feeling after you eat and weight gain due to the tendency to overeat to relieve the pain.

Symptoms of a gastric ulcer are similar to those of a duodenal ulcer but tend to be less predictable. Again, there is pain, which may be felt in the same place as that of a duodenal ulcer or slightly higher. The pain sometimes occurs when the stomach is full, leading to a loss of appetite and weight loss. Other signs of a gastric ulcer include indigestion and occasionally even heartburn. Both duodenal and gastric ulcers can cause such serious complications as gastrointestinal bleeding, perforation (erosion of the ulcer all the way through the wall of the stomach or the duodenum), or obstruction of the digestive tract.

If you develop suspicious symptoms, your doctor will order some diagnostic tests. An X-ray film called an upper gastrointestinal series (or UGI) may be done. In this test, the person swallows a barium suspension, a thick, chalky liquid, which allows the radiologist to see the shape of the stomach and small intestine and to identify the ulcer. Another diagnostic procedure that may be done is known as endoscopy. Using a gastroscope—a flexible fiberoptic tube with a light at one end inserted through the mouth— the doctor can see the ulcer crater, photograph it for further study, and take tissue samples (biopsy) for study under the microscope. (Occasionally, what appears on X-ray film examination to be a benign stomach ulcer may actually be a cancerous growth.)

TREATMENT

Several different types of drugs are available today for treating ulcers. A common treatment plan includes liquid antacids, which neutralize stomach acid, in addition to one of the following four medicines: cimetidine, ranitidine, famotidine, or sucralfate. These drugs are effective in healing and controlling symptoms of peptic ulcer disease. For more detailed information, see the charts on pages 297–307.

Your doctor may prescribe other medicines according to your specific needs. Rarely, drugs that prevent or relieve spasm—most often used for treating irritable bowel syndrome (see page 333)—are used in the treatment of peptic ulcers to suppress nighttime acid secretion. However, most doctors do not recommend antispasmodics for older people because they can cause such potentially serious side effects as difficulty in swallowing and urinating, as well as constipation.

Antacids (available under many brand names) reduce the amount of acid in the upper digestive tract by neutralizing (buffering) it. Liquid antacids are generally more effective than tablets. Many doctors prescribe antacids to be taken one to three hours after meals and at bedtime (food acts as a buffer in the hour following a meal).

In most people, medicine will heal ulcers. But surgery is sometimes necessary, particularly if an ulcer complication occurs. The operation may entail removing portions of the lower part of the stomach that secrete acid and the acid-stimulating hormone gastrin. Most people get along well following surgery—but it is only performed if medicine does not work or if a sudden serious complication develops.

There are things you can do—or not do—to help your ulcer heal. Smoking cigarettes has consistently been found to slow the healing of an ulcer, so you'd be wise to stop. Avoidance of aspirin and other antiarthritis drugs and alcohol is also advisable and important. As for your diet, consuming a lot of milk and cream is no longer considered an ulcer cure-all. Instead, the main dietary rule is to eat regular, nutritious meals. Avoid any foods that seem to bother you. Although the role of stress and anxiety in ulcer disease is not clear, it's a good idea to try to relax, avoid irritating situations, and work off tensions by exercising (at a level recommended by your doctor).

OUTLOOK

If you follow your doctor's recommendations, the chances are excellent that your ulcer will heal within a month or two. You may experience flare-ups from time to time, or you may go for years without feeling even a twinge of pain. Even though ulcer disease may recur periodically, it's a controllable problem that probably will not make too much of a change in your daily routine.

CONDITION: **PEPTIC ULCERS**

CATEGORY: **ANTIULCER AGENTS**

GENERIC (CHEMICAL) NAME	BRAND (TRADE) NAME	DOSAGE FORMS AND STRENGTHS
Cimetidine	TAGAMET	Liquid: 300 mg per tsp Tablets: 200, 300, 400, 800 mg

DRUG PROFILE

Cimetidine, which blocks the release of stomach acid, is used to heal duodenal (intestinal) and gastric (stomach) ulcers. It is also used to prevent the recurrence of ulcers. This drug may also be prescribed for other conditions in which the stomach produces excess acid.

BEFORE USING THIS DRUG

Let your doctor know *IF*

You have ever had allergic reactions or other problems with ■ cimetidine, ranitidine, or famotidine.

You have ever had any of the following medical problems: ■ kidney disease ■ liver disease.

You are taking any of the following medicines: ■ other ulcer medicine ■ aspirin or other medicine for arthritis ■ anticoagulants (blood thinners) ■ diazepam or chlordiazepoxide (tranquilizers) ■ medicine for seizures ■ medicine for high blood pressure ■ theophylline (medicine for asthma) ■ antacids ■ medicines with enteric coating.

SPECIAL RESTRICTIONS WHILE TAKING THIS DRUG

FOOD AND DRUG INTERACTIONS

Other Drugs	Your doctor may advise you to avoid certain drugs, such as aspirin and any other medicine for arthritis and pain, that may aggravate your symptoms. However, if it is critical that you take this medicine, your doctor may instruct you to take cimetidine along with it. Allow at least one hour between the time you take this drug and the time you take an antacid.
Foods and Beverages	Your doctor may advise you to avoid certain foods and beverages (coffee, cola drinks, cocoa, chocolate) known to irritate the ulcer. If you are taking several doses of this medicine a day, you will probably be instructed to take them at meals and at bedtime.
Alcohol	Avoid alcohol, which can irritate an ulcer.
Smoking	Cigarette smoking irritates the stomach lining and can decrease the benefits of this drug. If you smoke, try to stop or at least cut down.

DAILY LIVING

Examinations or Tests	Your doctor may want to perform an endoscopy after a period of treatment in order to monitor the healing process, particularly if you have a gastric ulcer.
Other Precautions	If the pain continues or worsens after several days of treatment, contact your doctor immediately.

No special restrictions on driving, exertion and exercise, sun exposure, or exposure to excessive heat or cold.

POSSIBLE SIDE EFFECTS

Although this list of adverse effects may seem somewhat intimidating, keep in mind that some are quite rare. Of course, should these or any other problems arise while you are on medication, it is always a good idea to consult your doctor.

IF YOU DEVELOP	WHAT TO DO
confusion ■ depression ■ agitation ■ tiredness or weakness ■ drowsiness ■ bleeding or bruising ■ sore throat or fever ■ joint or muscle pain ■ rash or hives	**May be serious** Check with your doctor as soon as possible.
diarrhea ■ dizziness ■ headache ■ sore or enlarged breasts in men ■ male impotence ■ hair loss	If symptoms are disturbing or persist, let your doctor know.

STORAGE INSTRUCTIONS

Store in a cool, dark place (not in a bathroom medicine cabinet). If your medicine is in a liquid form, make sure that it does not freeze.

STOPPING OR INTERRUPTING THERAPY

Take this drug for the full length of time prescribed (usually six to eight weeks), even if you feel better, unless otherwise directed by your doctor. If you miss a dose, take it as soon as possible. If it is almost time for your next dose, skip the missed dose and resume your regular schedule. Do not take two doses at the same time.

SPECIAL CONSIDERATIONS FOR THOSE OVER SIXTY-FIVE

Those older people who have reduced kidney function may require a reduction in dosage.

CONDITION: **PEPTIC ULCERS**

CATEGORY: **ANTIULCER AGENTS**

GENERIC (CHEMICAL) NAME	BRAND (TRADE) NAME	DOSAGE FORMS AND STRENGTHS
Ranitidine	ZANTAC	Tablets: 150, 300 mg

DRUG PROFILE

Ranitidine, which blocks the release of stomach acid, is used to treat active duodenal (intestinal) and gastric (stomach) ulcers. It may also be prescribed for gastrointestinal reflux and for other conditions in which the stomach produces excess acid.

BEFORE USING THIS DRUG

Let your doctor know *IF*

You have ever had allergic reactions or other problems with ■ ranitidine, cimetidine, or famotidine.

You have ever had any of the following medical problems: ■ kidney disease ■ liver disease.

You are taking any of the following medicines: ■ antacids ■ medicine for asthma ■ medicine for high blood pressure ■ heart medicine ■ anticoagulants (blood thinners) ■ tranquilizers ■ muscle relaxants ■ acetaminophen ■ aspirin or other medicine for arthritis ■ medicines with enteric coating.

SPECIAL RESTRICTIONS WHILE TAKING THIS DRUG

FOOD AND DRUG INTERACTIONS

Other Drugs	Your doctor may advise you to avoid certain drugs, such as aspirin and any other medicine for arthritis and pain, that may aggravate your symptoms. However, if it is critical that you take this medicine, your doctor may instruct you to take ranitidine along with it.

Allow at least an hour between the time you take this drug and the time you take an antacid.

Foods and Beverages	Your doctor may advise you to avoid certain foods and beverages (coffee, cola drinks, cocoa, chocolate) known to irritate an ulcer.
Alcohol	Avoid alcohol, which can irritate an ulcer.
Smoking	Cigarette smoking irritates the stomach lining and can decrease the benefits of this drug. If you smoke, try to stop or at least cut down.

DAILY LIVING

Examinations or Tests	Your doctor may want to perform an endoscopy after a period of treatment in order to monitor the healing process, especially if you have a gastric ulcer.
Other Precautions	If the pain continues or worsens after several days of treatment, contact your doctor immediately.

No special restrictions on driving, exertion and exercise, sun exposure, or exposure to excessive heat or cold.

POSSIBLE SIDE EFFECTS

Although this list of adverse effects may seem somewhat intimidating, keep in mind that some are quite rare. Of course, should these or any other problems arise while you are on medication, it is always a good idea to consult your doctor.

IF YOU DEVELOP

confusion ■ depression ■ agitation ■ irregular or fast heartbeat ■ male impotence ■ general feeling of unwellness ■ breast swelling in men ■ difficulty in breathing ■ yellowing of eyes or skin

WHAT TO DO

May be serious Check with your doctor as soon as possible.

constipation ■ dizziness ■ headache ■ nausea ■ rash ■ stomach pain

If symptoms are disturbing or persist, let your doctor know.

STORAGE INSTRUCTIONS

Store in a cool, dark place (not in a bathroom medicine cabinet).

STOPPING OR INTERRUPTING THERAPY

This drug should be taken without interruption for the full length of time prescribed by your doctor (usually about four weeks), even once you begin to feel better. If you miss a dose, take it as soon as possible. If it is almost time for your next dose, skip the missed dose and resume your regular schedule. Do not take two doses at the same time.

SPECIAL CONSIDERATIONS FOR THOSE OVER SIXTY-FIVE

Those older people who have reduced kidney function may require a reduction in dosage.

CONDITION: **PEPTIC ULCERS**

CATEGORY: **ANTIULCER AGENTS**

GENERIC (CHEMICAL) NAME	BRAND (TRADE) NAME	DOSAGE FORMS AND STRENGTHS
Famotidine	PEPCID	Powder: 40 mg per tsp Tablets: 20, 40 mg

DRUG PROFILE

Famotidine, which blocks the release of stomach acid, is used to treat active duodenal (intestinal) and gastric (stomach) ulcers. It may also be prescribed for other conditions in which the stomach produces excess acid.

BEFORE USING THIS DRUG

Let your doctor know *IF*

You have ever had allergic reactions or other problems with ■ famotidine, cimetidine, or ranitidine.

You have ever had any of the following medical problems: ■ kidney disease ■ liver disease.

You are taking any of the following medicines: ■ medicines with enteric coating.

SPECIAL RESTRICTIONS WHILE TAKING THIS DRUG

FOOD AND DRUG INTERACTIONS

Other Drugs	Your doctor may advise you to avoid certain drugs, such as aspirin and any other medicine for arthritis and pain, that may aggravate your symptoms. However, if it is critical that you take this medicine, your doctor may instruct you to take famotidine along with it.
	Allow at least an hour between the time you take this drug and the time you take an antacid.
Foods and Beverages	Your doctor may advise you to avoid certain foods and beverages (coffee, cola drinks, cocoa, chocolate) known to irritate an ulcer.
Alcohol	Alcohol should be avoided because it irritates an ulcer.
Smoking	Cigarette smoking irritates the stomach lining and can decrease the benefits of this drug. If you smoke, try to stop or at least cut down.

DAILY LIVING

Examinations or Tests	Your doctor may want to perform an endoscopy after a period of treatment in order to monitor the healing process.
Other Precautions	If the pain continues or worsens after several days of treatment, contact your doctor immediately.

No special restrictions on driving, exertion and exercise, sun exposure, or exposure to excessive heat or cold.

POSSIBLE SIDE EFFECTS

Although this list of adverse effects may seem somewhat intimidating, keep in mind that some are quite rare. Of course, should these or any other problems arise while you are on medication, it is always a good idea to consult your doctor.

IF YOU DEVELOP	WHAT TO DO
confusion ■ irregular or fast heartbeat ■ difficulty in breathing	**May be serious** Check with your doctor as soon as possible.
diarrhea ■ constipation ■ dizziness ■ headache ■ nausea or vomiting ■ rash or other skin problems ■ stomach discomfort	If symptoms are disturbing or persist, let your doctor know.

STORAGE INSTRUCTIONS

Store in a cool, dark place (not in a bathroom medicine cabinet).

STOPPING OR INTERRUPTING THERAPY

Famotidine should be taken without interruption for the full length of time prescribed by your doctor (usually about four weeks for an active ulcer), even after you begin to feel better. If you miss a dose, take it as soon as possible. If it is almost time for your next dose, skip the missed dose and resume your regular schedule. Do not take two doses at the same time.

SPECIAL CONSIDERATIONS FOR THOSE OVER SIXTY-FIVE

Those older people who have reduced kidney function may require a reduction in dosage.

CONDITION: **PEPTIC ULCERS**

CATEGORY: **ANTIULCER AGENTS**

GENERIC (CHEMICAL) NAME	BRAND (TRADE) NAME	DOSAGE FORMS AND STRENGTHS
Sucralfate	CARAFATE	Tablets: 1 g

DRUG PROFILE

Sucralfate is used to treat duodenal (intestinal) ulcers. This drug forms a protective coating over the ulcer, which gives the duodenal lining time to heal.

BEFORE USING THIS DRUG

Let your doctor know *IF*

You have ever had allergic reactions or other problems with ■ sucralfate.

You have ever had the following medical problem: ■ constipation.

You are taking any of the following medicines: ■ other medicine for ulcers ■ antacids ■ tetracycline ■ phenytoin (medicine for seizures) ■ digoxin, digitoxin, or digitalis (heart medicines).

SPECIAL RESTRICTIONS WHILE TAKING THIS DRUG

FOOD AND DRUG INTERACTIONS

Other Drugs	Antacids should be taken at least thirty minutes before or after taking your dose of sucralfate. If these medicines are taken close together, sucralfate will not be as effective.

Foods and Beverages	Your doctor may advise you to avoid certain foods and beverages (coffee, cola drinks, cocoa, chocolate) known to irritate an ulcer.
Alcohol	Avoid alcohol, which can irritate an ulcer.
Smoking	Ulcers generally heal faster if you do not smoke. Cigarette smoking irritates the stomach lining and can decrease the benefits of this drug. If you are being treated for an ulcer and you smoke, try to stop or at least cut down.

DAILY LIVING

Helpful Hints	Take this medicine on an empty stomach, one hour before meals and at bedtime, unless instructed otherwise by your doctor. Do not chew tablets; instead, swallow them with water for best results.

No special restrictions on driving, exertion and exercise, sun exposure, or exposure to excessive heat or cold.

POSSIBLE SIDE EFFECTS

Although this list of adverse effects may seem somewhat intimidating, keep in mind that some are quite rare. Of course, should these or any other problems arise while you are on medication, it is always a good idea to consult your doctor.

IF YOU DEVELOP	WHAT TO DO
dizziness ■ drowsiness ■ dry mouth ■ constipation ■ nausea ■ stomach discomfort ■ back pain ■ rash or itching	If symptoms are disturbing or persist, let your doctor know.

STORAGE INSTRUCTIONS

Store in a cool, dark place (not in a bathroom medicine cabinet).

STOPPING OR INTERRUPTING THERAPY

This drug should be taken without interruption for the full length of time prescribed by your doctor (usually four to eight weeks), even if your symptoms disappear. If you miss a dose, take it as soon as possible. If it is less than one hour before a meal, skip the missed dose and resume your regular schedule. Do not take two doses at the same time.

SPECIAL CONSIDERATIONS FOR THOSE OVER SIXTY-FIVE

Older people may be more prone to constipation with this drug.

CONDITION: **PEPTIC ULCERS**

CATEGORY: **ANTIULCER AGENTS**

GENERIC (CHEMICAL) NAME	BRAND (TRADE) NAME	DOSAGE FORMS AND STRENGTHS
Propantheline bromide	PRO-BANTHINE	Tablets: 7.5, 15 mg

DRUG PROFILE

Propantheline is used along with other drugs to treat peptic ulcers. This drug works by reducing the amount of acid produced by the stomach.

BEFORE USING THIS DRUG

Let your doctor know *IF*

You have ever had allergic reactions or other problems with ■ propantheline.

You have ever had any of the following medical problems: ■ digestive problems, including colitis or severe diarrhea ■ asthma or other lung disease ■ difficulty in urination or other urinary problems ■ enlarged prostate ■ glaucoma ■ heart or circulatory problems ■ abnormal heart rhythms ■ hiatal hernia ■ high blood pressure ■ kidney disease ■ liver disease ■ myasthenia gravis ■ overactive thyroid.

You are taking any of the following medicines: ■ other medicine for ulcers ■ antacids or medicine for stomach spasms and cramps ■ medicine for diarrhea ■ medicine for Parkinson's disease ■ tranquilizers ■ medicine for nausea ■ medicine for seizures ■ antihistamines ■ medicine for hay fever, coughs, or colds ■ narcotics or other prescription pain-killers ■ sleep medicines ■ medicine for depression ■ digoxin, digitoxin, or digitalis (heart medicines) ■ medicine for abnormal heart rhythms ■ potassium-containing medicines or supplements ■ acetaminophen ■ medicine for fungal infections ■ timolol, nadolol, propranolol, metoprolol, atenolol, or pindolol (beta-blockers) ■ thiazide diuretics ■ nitrofurantoin (medicine for urinary tract infections) ■ corticosteroids.

SPECIAL RESTRICTIONS WHILE TAKING THIS DRUG

FOOD AND DRUG INTERACTIONS

Other Drugs	Do not take any other drugs, including over-the-counter (OTC) drugs, before checking with your doctor. This drug may affect how fast your body absorbs other drugs; it also increases the effect of drugs that depress the central nervous system, such as antihistamines; medicine for hay fever, allergies, or colds; sleep medicines; tranquilizers; narcotics or other prescription pain-killers; muscle relaxants; and medicine for seizures.
	Allow one to two hours between the time you take this drug and the time you take an antacid.
Alcohol	This medicine increases the effect of alcohol, a central nervous system depressant. Avoid alcohol unless your doctor has approved its use.

No special restrictions on foods and beverages or smoking.

DAILY LIVING

Driving	This drug may cause dizziness, drowsiness, or blurred vision. Be careful when driving, operating household appliances, or doing any other tasks that

require alertness until you know how this drug affects you.

Exertion and Exercise	This drug may cause you to sweat less. Sweating is your body's natural way of cooling down, and not sweating enough can be dangerous. Use caution not to become overheated when you exercise or exert yourself.
Excessive Heat	See above; use caution during hot weather, since overexertion may result in heat stroke. Avoid extremely hot baths or saunas. Also, check with your doctor if you develop a fever for any reason.
Other Precautions	Tell any doctor or dentist you consult that you are taking this drug, especially if you will be undergoing any type of surgery. Take this medicine exactly as prescribed by your doctor; taking it more often or for a longer period of time than prescribed makes you more prone to developing side effects.
Helpful Hints	If your mouth or throat feels dry, chewing sugarless gum or sucking ice chips or sugarless hard candy should help. This medicine is generally taken one half to one hour before meals.

No special restrictions on sun exposure or exposure to excessive cold.

POSSIBLE SIDE EFFECTS

Although this list of adverse effects may seem somewhat intimidating, keep in mind that some are quite rare. Of course, should these or any other problems arise while you are on medication, it is always a good idea to consult your doctor.

IF YOU DEVELOP	WHAT TO DO
fever ■ delirium ■ confusion ■ nervousness ■ rash or hives ■ irregular or fast heartbeat	**Urgent** Get in touch with your doctor immediately.
constipation ■ difficulty in urination ■ eye pain ■ flushing ■ restlessness ■ excitement ■ behavior changes	**May be serious** Check with your doctor as soon as possible.
bloating ■ nausea or vomiting ■ dry mouth ■ dizziness ■ headache ■ blurred vision ■ changes in pupil size ■ increased eye sensitivity to light ■ drowsiness ■ weakness ■ decreased sweating ■ loss of taste ■ male impotence ■ sleeplessness	If symptoms are disturbing or persist, let your doctor know.

STORAGE INSTRUCTIONS

Store in a cool, dark place (not in a bathroom medicine cabinet).

STOPPING OR INTERRUPTING THERAPY

If you miss a dose, take it as soon as possible. If it is almost time for your next dose, skip the missed dose and resume your regular schedule. Do not take two doses at the same time.

SPECIAL CONSIDERATIONS FOR THOSE OVER SIXTY-FIVE

Older people may be more prone to such side effects as confusion, excitement, difficulty in urination, blurred vision, and constipation. For this reason, a doctor may want to start treatment with a lower dosage and check the person frequently.

INDIGESTION

You may have noticed that you're just not enjoying mealtimes as much as you used to. This may have nothing to do with the quality of the cuisine but everything to do with the digestive ailments you've been experiencing during or soon after eating. Some people can't get through a meal without feeling gnawing pains in the abdomen. Others get that gassy feeling, even if baked beans weren't on the menu. Still others make it through the meal all right, only to experience a burning chest pain and a sour taste in the mouth. Indigestion is the culprit that can turn mealtime into a medley of digestive complaints. Indigestion is not a precise medical term; it is used to refer to a whole spectrum of abdominal aches, pains, twinges, and discomforts that can detract from your dining pleasure.

Most conditions that cause indigestion are harmless, and you can ease your distress through some self-help measures outlined here. If these measures don't work, consult your doctor for advice. Less frequently, there may be something more serious behind your mealtime miseries, and you should be alert to those symptoms that signal a more urgent need for a medical consultation.

HEARTBURN

Perhaps one of the most universal symptoms of indigestion is heartburn, which occurs when food, stomach acid, and digestive enzymes back up from the stomach into the esophagus. In addition to a temporary burning pain behind the breastbone, there is often an acidic aftertaste and sometimes belching, bloating, nausea, and vomiting. Known medically as gastroesophageal reflux, heartburn is usually caused by a weakness in the lower esophagus; this allows stomach acid and other irritating substances to flow up into the esophagus. In other instances, heartburn occurs because digested food is not emptied efficiently from the stomach into the intestines. The longer the food stays in the stomach, the more opportunity there is for it to back up into the esophagus. (It used to be thought that hiatal hernias cause heartburn, but it is now known that the majority of normal people past the age of fifty have a hiatal hernia—a condition in which part of the stomach slides up through the diaphragm into the chest cavity. This condition by itself does not cause heartburn.)

Useful self-help measures to combat heartburn include the shedding of some extra pounds if you're overweight; the avoidance of lifting, bending, and lying down after eating; and wearing clothes that do not bind the waist and abdomen. You may find that not eating for two to three hours before bedtime and elevating the head of your bed six inches or so will prevent your discomfort. (The head of the bed itself should be raised. It is not advised to simply prop up your head with an extra, fluffy pillow.) You may also find that altering your diet by staying away from foods that weaken the lower esophagus (such as fatty foods, chocolate, alcohol, and peppermint) and avoiding foods that irritate the lining of the esophagus (such as acidic fruit juice and spicy tomato drinks) might help relieve the symptoms of heartburn.

Over-the-counter (OTC) antacids can provide quick, short-term relief, curbing the pain within ten minutes or so. If the pain persists past that time, it's a clue that the burning sensation is not heartburn at all but a more severe condition. In either case, it is prudent to check with your doctor.

Another common remedy to relieve heartburn is a combination of antacids and an ingredient called alginic acid (Gaviscon). This compound acts to form a foam barrier that floats on top of the stomach contents and prevents reflux from occurring. Your doctor may be able to prescribe a medicine for heartburn, such as metoclopramide (see page 315).

Not every symptom that occurs under the rib cage signals gastroesophageal reflux. If food seems to stick in your throat when you try to swallow, or if your symptoms of heartburn don't go away with the treatment outlined here, your doctor may order some diagnostic tests to rule out other diagnoses (such as peptic ulcer) or complications of the heartburn (such as esophageal scarring or ulcer). During the early phase of evaluation, an upper gastrointestinal series may be performed, which is a special X-ray test that shows the esophagus, stomach, and duodenum. In many cases, additional tests such as endoscopy are needed.

INTESTINAL GAS

It can be painful. Even worse, it can be embarrassing. However, unless it occurs at a socially inappropriate moment, it is usually harmless. And perhaps the best news about gas—a problem familiar to all of us—is that it is often preventable.

Technically known as flatus, gas is shapeless and usually odorless matter that is produced in the digestive system. Gas may cause distress in the upper or lower digestive tract. Upper gas, which lodges in the stomach, is usually caused by swallowing too much air while talking, eating, drinking, or simply chewing. The faster these actions are performed, the more air is swallowed, and the more gas results. The other type, lower gas, is formed in the large intestine by the action of bacteria on undigested food particles.

Upper gas—with its accompanying belching—can be combated by changing some everyday habits. You'll swallow less air if you don't chew gum, don't use a straw to drink, and don't talk a lot while you eat. If you're in the habit of taking effervescent OTC medicines, you may be making matters worse, not better. The added carbonation in these products increases the amount of swallowed air—and the amount of belching.

What you consume also affects the amount of gas passed rectally, and beans are not the only culprit. Milk, cabbage, broccoli, brussels sprouts, and onions are also gassy, as are carbonated drinks and coffee. You may find that you've been particularly gassy while dieting. This is because many artificial sweeteners are non-digestible carbohydrates; the bacteria in the lower bowel act upon these sugars, resulting in the production of rectal gas.

What you *should* do, in the way of diet, is eat slowly and moderately and include whole grains, root vegetables, and raw fruits on your daily menu. These foods will help you move your bowels freely and will prevent the entrapment of gas. Exercise is also important. The abdominal muscles overlying the intestines help reduce feelings of distention and bloating, but with increasing age, decreasing physical activity, or both, these muscles become lax. Doing such exercises as sit-ups will tighten these muscles and reduce your bloated feeling after meals.

You may find that some OTC medicines, such as those containing simethicone, will relieve your discomfort. Activated charcoal has also been marketed as an antiflatulent. Most people, however, find that diet modification is the most effective way to relieve the pain, and embarrassment, of too much gas.

If your gas pain continues despite your best efforts, you should check with your doctor. Gas pains can be quite sharp and usually occur in the left or right upper abdomen under the ribs or in the back. Persistent abdominal pains may mean that an obstruction is blocking the normal passage of gas out of the rectum or that something other than gas is causing your symptoms.

PANCREATITIS

Indigestion can also be caused by other conditions, such as irritable bowel syndrome (see page 333), gallbladder disease (see pages 370–371), or peptic ulcer (see pages 294–296). Still another possible cause is pancreatitis, which is an inflammation of the pancreas gland. This disorder usually results either from the lodging of a gallstone in the pancreatic ducts or excessive intake of alcohol over a long period of time. The major symptom of pancreatitis is severe pain above and around the navel; there may also be nausea, vomiting, fever, and chills. Pancreatitis can be a serious disease, but most people who have it recover completely. It is important to get medical help at once if you develop the above symptoms. Some people develop chronic pancreatitis and suffer from indigestion between their attacks of pain. The damaged pancreas can no longer manufacture certain enzymes required for digestion or produce insulin to control the blood sugar levels. In these cases, doctors may prescribe pancrelipase (see pages 330–332), or other agents with pancreatic enzymes (see pages 327–329). These medicines—combinations of enzymes that are naturally produced by the pancreas—help the body digest food properly.

Occasionally, some people with chronic pancreatitis undergo surgery to remove the damaged pancreatic tissue or sever the nerves that carry the pain. If a significant portion of the pancreas is removed, insulin injections and medicines containing pancreatic enzymes may be necessary.

OUTLOOK

Indigestion is a common digestive disorder that has many causes. Dietary modification and some simple self-help measures are generally sufficient to relieve the pain and other symptoms. Over-the-counter medications may also play a role in easing your distress. But sometimes this is not enough. If your symptoms persist, if an unexplained new symptom develops, or if you have any of these additional symptoms (loss of appetite, weight loss, back pain along with abdominal distress, change in bowel habits, or bleeding from the digestive tract), consult your doctor. Indigestion can be more than it seems.

CONDITION: **HEARTBURN**

CATEGORY: **PROMOTILITY DRUGS**

GENERIC (CHEMICAL) NAME	BRAND (TRADE) NAME	DOSAGE FORMS AND STRENGTHS
Metoclopramide	REGLAN	Syrup: 5 mg per tsp Tablets: 10 mg

DRUG PROFILE

Metoclopramide is used to relieve symptoms such as nausea, vomiting, loss of appetite, and continued feeling of fullness after eating. The drug, called a promotility agent, acts by increasing the contractions of the stomach and intestines, thus quickening the pace at which food empties from the stomach and moves through the intestines. It is also prescribed for gastroesophageal reflux (heartburn), diabetic gastroparesis (a condition in which the stomach loses its ability to contract), and prevention of nausea associated with chemotherapy.

For complete information on this drug, see pages 366–369.

CONDITION: **INDIGESTION**

CATEGORY: **ANTISPASMODICS**

GENERIC (CHEMICAL) NAME	BRAND (TRADE) NAME	DOSAGE FORMS AND STRENGTHS
Chlordiazepoxide hydrochloride and clidinium bromide	LIBRAX	Capsules: 5 mg chlordiazepoxide and 2.5 mg clidinium

DRUG PROFILE

Chlordiazepoxide/clidinium is a combination drug used to treat peptic ulcers and irritable bowel syndrome (spastic colon). It relaxes the digestive system, reduces stomach acid, and provides a sedative effect.

BEFORE USING THIS DRUG

Let your doctor know *IF*

You have ever had allergic reactions or other problems with ■ chlordiazepoxide or any other benzodiazepines ■ clidinium.

You have ever had any of the following medical problems: ■ difficulty in urination ■ asthma or other lung disease ■ glaucoma ■ enlarged prostate ■ kidney disease ■ liver disease ■ depression or severe mental illness ■ intestinal blockage ■ myasthenia gravis ■ drug or alcohol addiction ■ constipation.

You are taking any of the following medicines: ■ medicine for spasmodic conditions of the intestinal or urinary tract ■ tranquilizers ■ medicine for diarrhea ■ medicine for Parkinson's disease ■ medicine for seizures ■ antihistamines ■ barbiturates ■ muscle relaxants ■ narcotics or other prescription pain-killers ■ sleep medicines ■ medicine for depression.

SPECIAL RESTRICTIONS WHILE TAKING THIS DRUG

FOOD AND DRUG INTERACTIONS

Other Drugs	Do not take any other drugs, including over-the-counter (OTC) drugs, before checking with your doctor. This medicine increases the effect of drugs that depress the central nervous system, such as antihistamines; medicine for hay fever, allergies, or colds; sleep medicines; tranquilizers; narcotics or other prescription pain-killers; muscle relaxants; and medicine for seizures.
	If you are taking any medicine for diarrhea, allow at least one hour between the time you take that medicine and the time you take chlordiazepoxide/clidinium.

Foods and Beverages	If you are being treated for an ulcer, your doctor may advise you to avoid certain foods and beverages (coffee, cola drinks, cocoa, chocolate) known to irritate an ulcer.
Alcohol	This medicine increases the effect of alcohol, a central nervous system depressant. Avoid alcohol unless your doctor has approved its use.
Smoking	Ulcers generally heal faster if you do not smoke. If you are being treated for an ulcer and you smoke, try to stop or at least cut down.

DAILY LIVING

Driving	This medicine may cause dizziness or drowsiness. Be careful when driving, operating household appliances, or doing any other tasks that require alertness until you know how this drug affects you.
Exertion and Exercise	This drug may cause you to sweat less than normally. Sweating is your body's natural way of cooling down, and not sweating enough can be dangerous. Use caution not to become overheated when you exercise or exert yourself.
Excessive Heat	See above; use caution during hot weather, since overexertion may result in heat stroke. Avoid extremely hot baths or saunas. Also, check with your doctor if you develop a fever for any reason.
Other Precautions	Take this medicine exactly as prescribed by your doctor; taking it more often or for a longer period of time than prescribed may make it habit forming.

Helpful Hints	If your mouth or throat feels dry, chewing sugarless gum or sucking ice chips or sugarless hard candy will help.
	Take this medicine before meals and at bedtime unless instructed otherwise by your doctor.

No special restrictions on sun exposure or exposure to excessive cold.

POSSIBLE SIDE EFFECTS

Although this list of adverse effects may seem somewhat intimidating, keep in mind that some are quite rare. Of course, should these or any other problems arise while you are on medication, it is always a good idea to consult your doctor.

IF YOU DEVELOP	WHAT TO DO
confusion ■ difficulty in urination ■ severe drowsiness ■ fast heartbeat ■ flushing ■ skin dryness ■ fainting ■ rash ■ shortness of breath	**Urgent** Get in touch with your doctor immediately.
constipation ■ severely dry mouth, nose, or throat ■ blurred vision ■ depression ■ excitement ■ agitation ■ nervousness ■ irritability ■ clumsiness ■ tiredness or weakness ■ sleep disturbances ■ mood changes	**May be serious** Check with your doctor as soon as possible.
dizziness ■ drowsiness ■ nausea ■ dry mouth ■ headache ■ vivid dreams ■ decreased or increased sweating ■ increased or diminished sex drive	If symptoms are disturbing or persist, let your doctor know.

STORAGE INSTRUCTIONS

Store in a cool, dark place (not in a bathroom medicine cabinet).

STOPPING OR INTERRUPTING THERAPY

Do not stop taking this medicine abruptly without consulting your doctor. If you miss a dose take it as soon as possible. If it is almost time for your next dose, skip the missed dose and resume your regular schedule. Do not take two doses at the same time. If you have been taking this medicine for a long period of time, or in large doses, your doctor will probably want you to gradually reduce the amount rather than stop abruptly.

SPECIAL CONSIDERATIONS FOR THOSE OVER SIXTY-FIVE

Older people may be more sensitive to this medicine and may be particularly prone to confusion, agitation, drowsiness, excitement, difficulty in urination, or blurred vision.

CONDITION: **INDIGESTION**

CATEGORY: **ANTISPASMODICS**

GENERIC (CHEMICAL) NAME	BRAND (TRADE) NAME	DOSAGE FORMS AND STRENGTHS
Dicyclomine	BENTYL	Capsules: 10 mg Syrup: 10 mg per tsp Tablets: 20 mg

This drug is available under many other brand names as well.

DRUG PROFILE

Dicyclomine is used to treat irritable bowel syndrome (spastic colon). It reduces the production of stomach acid and relieves intestinal spasms. It is not known exactly how this drug works.

BEFORE USING THIS DRUG

Let your doctor know *IF*

You have ever had allergic reactions or other problems with ■ dicyclomine.

You have ever had any of the following medical problems: ■ digestive problems, including severe diarrhea ■ difficulty in urination or other urinary problems ■ enlarged prostate ■ glaucoma ■ heart disease, including abnormal heart rhythms or fast heartbeat ■ kidney disease ■ liver disease ■ overactive thyroid ■ myasthenia gravis ■ asthma or other lung disease.

You are taking any of the following medicines: ■ medicine for stomach spasms or cramps ■ medicine for Parkinson's disease ■ medicine for diarrhea ■ tranquilizers ■ medicine for nausea ■ narcotics or other prescription pain-killers ■ sleep medicines ■ medicine for depression ■ medicine for abnormal heart rhythms.

SPECIAL RESTRICTIONS WHILE TAKING THIS DRUG

FOOD AND DRUG INTERACTIONS

Other Drugs	Do not take any other drugs, including over-the-counter (OTC) drugs, before checking with your doctor. This drug may increase the effect of drugs that depress the central nervous system, such as antihistamines; medicine for hay fever, allergies, or colds; sleep medicines; tranquilizers; narcotics or other prescription pain-killers; muscle relaxants; and medicine for seizures. Allow at least one hour between the time you take this drug and the time you take an antacid.
Foods and Beverages	If you are being treated for an ulcer, your doctor may advise you to avoid certain foods and beverages (coffee, cola drinks, cocoa, chocolate) known to irritate an ulcer.
Alcohol	This medicine increases the effect of alcohol, a central nervous system depressant. Avoid alcohol unless your doctor has approved its use.
Smoking	Ulcers generally heal faster if you do not smoke. If you are being treated for an ulcer and you smoke, try to stop or at least cut down.

DAILY LIVING

Driving	This medicine may cause dizziness or drowsiness. Be careful when driving, operating household appliances, or doing any other tasks that require alertness until you know how this drug affects you.
Exertion and Exercise	This medicine may cause you to sweat less than normally. Sweating is your body's natural way of cooling down, and not sweating enough can be dangerous. Use caution when you exercise or exert yourself.
Excessive Heat	See above; use caution during hot weather, as over-exertion may result in heat stroke. Avoid extremely hot baths and saunas. Also, check with your doctor if you develop a fever for any reason.
Other Precautions	Take this medicine exactly as prescribed by your doctor; taking it more often or for a longer period of time than prescribed makes you more prone to developing side effects.
	Be sure to let your doctor know if you develop constipation.
	Tell any doctor or dentist you consult that you are taking this medicine, especially if you will be undergoing any type of surgery.
Helpful Hints	Take this medicine before meals and at bedtime, unless otherwise instructed by your doctor.

No special restrictions on exposure to excessive cold.

POSSIBLE SIDE EFFECTS

Although this list of adverse effects may seem somewhat intimidating, keep in mind that some are quite rare. Of course, should these or any other problems arise while you are on medication, it is always a good idea to consult your doctor.

IF YOU DEVELOP	WHAT TO DO
constipation ■ difficulty in urination ■ rash ■ irregular or fast heartbeat ■ flushing ■ eye pain	**May be serious** Check with your doctor as soon as possible.
bloating ■ nausea or vomiting ■ dry mouth ■ dizziness ■ headache ■ blurred vision ■ changes in pupil size ■ increased eye sensitivity to light ■ confusion ■ male impotence ■ drowsiness ■ weakness ■ nervousness ■ excitement ■ decreased sweating ■ loss of taste	If symptoms are disturbing or persist, let your doctor know.

STORAGE INSTRUCTIONS

Store in a cool, dark place (not in a bathroom medicine cabinet). If your medicine is in a liquid form, make sure that it does not freeze.

STOPPING OR INTERRUPTING THERAPY

This medicine should be taken exactly as prescribed by your doctor. If you miss a dose, take it as soon as possible. If it is almost time for your next dose, skip the missed dose and resume your regular schedule. Do not take two doses at the same time.

SPECIAL CONSIDERATIONS FOR THOSE OVER SIXTY-FIVE

Older people may be more prone to the side effects of constipation, confusion, and excitement. For this reason, doctors may wish to check their progress frequently.

CONDITION: **INDIGESTION**

CATEGORY: **ANTISPASMODICS**

GENERIC (CHEMICAL) NAME	BRAND (TRADE) NAME	DOSAGE FORMS AND STRENGTHS
Belladonna alkaloids (atropine, scopolamine, hyoscyamine, and hyoscine) and barbiturates (phenobarbital)	DONNATAL	Capsules: 16.2 mg phenobarbital, 0.1037 mg hyoscyamine, 0.0194 mg atropine, and 0.0065 mg hyoscine
		Controlled-release tablets: 48.6 mg phenobarbital, 0.3111 mg hyoscyamine, 0.0582 mg atropine, and 0.0195 mg hyoscine
		Elixir: 16.2 mg phenobarbital, 0.1037 mg hyoscyamine, 0.0194 mg atropine, and 0.0065 mg hyoscine per tsp
		No. 2 Tablets: 32.4 mg phenobarbital, 0.1037 mg hyoscyamine, 0.0194 mg atropine, and 0.0065 mg hyoscine
		Tablets: 16.2 mg phenobarbital, 0.1037 mg hyoscyamine, 0.0194 mg atropine, and 0.0065 mg hyoscine
	KINESED	Chewable tablets: 16 mg phenobarbital, 0.1 mg hyoscyamine, 0.02 mg atropine, and 0.007 mg scopolamine

This combination drug is available under a variety of other brand names as well.

DRUG PROFILE

The combination of belladonna alkaloids and a barbiturate is used to relieve stomach and intestinal cramping and spasms. It is used along with other drugs to treat irritable bowel syndrome and intestinal infections. Belladonna prevents muscular contraction and excessive acid secretion in the stomach and intestines, while phenobarbital acts on the brain to provide a calming effect.

BEFORE USING THIS DRUG

Let your doctor know *IF*

You have ever had allergic reactions or other problems with ■ belladonna alkaloids, such as atropine, hyoscyamine, or scopolamine ■ barbiturates.

You have ever had any of the following medical problems: ■ digestive problems, including colitis or severe diarrhea ■ asthma or other lung disease ■ difficulty in urination or other urinary problems ■ enlarged prostate ■ glaucoma ■ heart disease, including abnormal heart rhythms or fast heartbeat ■ kidney disease ■ liver disease ■ overactive thyroid ■ myasthenia gravis ■ porphyria.

You are taking any of the following medicines: ■ medicine for stomach spasm or cramps ■ medicine for Parkinson's disease ■ medicine for diarrhea ■ tranquilizers ■ medicine for nausea ■ medicine for seizures ■ antihistamines ■ narcotics or other prescription pain-killers ■ sleep medicines ■ medicine for depression ■ medicine for abnormal heart rhythms ■ digoxin, digitoxin, or digitalis (heart medicines).

SPECIAL RESTRICTIONS WHILE TAKING THIS DRUG

FOOD AND DRUG INTERACTIONS

Other Drugs	Do not take any other drugs, including over-the-counter (OTC) drugs, before checking with your doctor. This medicine increases the effect of drugs that depress the central nervous system, such as antihistamines; medicine for hay fever, allergies, or colds; sleep medicines; tranquilizers; narcotics or other prescription pain-killers; muscle relaxants; and medicine for seizures.
	Allow at least one hour between the time you take this drug and the time you take an antacid or medicine for diarrhea.

Alcohol	This medicine increases the effect of alcohol, a central nervous system depressant. Avoid alcohol unless your doctor has approved its use.

No special restrictions on foods and beverages or smoking.

DAILY LIVING

Driving	This medicine may cause dizziness, drowsiness, or blurred vision. Be careful when driving, operating household appliances, or doing any other tasks that require alertness until you know how this drug affects you.
Exertion and Exercise	This drug may cause you to sweat less than normally. Sweating is your body's natural way of cooling down, and not sweating enough can be dangerous. Use caution not to become overheated when you exercise or exert yourself.
Excessive Heat	See above; use caution during hot weather, since overexertion may result in heat stroke. Avoid extremely hot baths or saunas. Getting up from a reclining or sitting position may cause you to become dizzy. Also, check with your doctor if you develop any kind of fever.
Other Precautions	Be sure to let your doctor know if you develop constipation.
Helpful Hints	If your mouth or throat feels dry, chewing sugarless gum or sucking ice chips or sugarless hard candy will help.

No special restrictions on sun exposure or exposure to excessive cold.

POSSIBLE SIDE EFFECTS

Although this list of adverse effects may seem somewhat intimidating, keep in mind that some are quite rare. Of course, should these or any other problems arise while you are on medication, it is always a good idea to consult your doctor.

IF YOU DEVELOP

continual blurred vision ■ seizures ■ confusion ■ severe drowsiness ■ hallucinations ■ difficulty in breathing ■ slurred speech ■ fast heartbeat ■ palpitations ■ flushing ■ fever ■ rash or hives ■ difficulty in urination

After you STOP taking this medicine: delirium ■ seizures

WHAT TO DO

Urgent Get in touch with your doctor immediately.

---

eye pain ■ changes in pupil size ■ sore throat ■ nervousness ■ excitement ■ sleeplessness ■ restlessness ■ irritability

May be serious Check with your doctor as soon as possible.

---

constipation ■ decreased sweating ■ dizziness ■ drowsiness ■ dry mouth, nose, throat, or skin ■ increased eye sensitivity to light ■ loss of taste ■ bloating ■ nausea or vomiting ■ headache ■ male impotence

If symptoms are disturbing or persist, let your doctor know.

STORAGE INSTRUCTIONS

Store in a cool, dark place (not in a bathroom medicine cabinet). If your medicine is in a liquid form, make sure that it does not freeze.

STOPPING OR INTERRUPTING THERAPY

This medicine should be taken without interruption for the length of time prescribed by your doctor. If you miss a dose, take it as soon as possible. If it is almost time for your next dose, skip the missed dose and resume your regular schedule. Do not take two doses at the same time.

SPECIAL CONSIDERATIONS FOR THOSE OVER SIXTY-FIVE

Older people may be more sensitive to this drug combination and more likely to experience such side effects as confusion, constipation, difficulty in urination, drowsiness, nervousness, irritability, and restlessness, even with small doses.

CONDITION: **INDIGESTION**

CATEGORY: **DIGESTANTS**

GENERIC (CHEMICAL) NAME	BRAND (TRADE) NAME	DOSAGE FORMS AND STRENGTHS
Pancreatic enzyme and digestant combinations	DONNAZYME	Tablets: 300 mg pancreatin, 150 mg pepsin, 150 mg bile salts, 0.0518 mg hyoscyamine, 0.0097 mg atropine, 0.0033 mg scopolamine, 8.1 mg phenobarbital

DRUG PROFILE

These preparations of enzymes normally produced by the pancreas are used to treat miscellaneous digestive disorders. Some of these preparations also contain drugs that relax the digestive system.

BEFORE USING THIS DRUG

Let your doctor know *IF*

You have ever had allergic reactions or other problems with ■ belladonna alkaloids such as atropine, hyoscyamine, or scopolamine ■ barbiturates ■ pancrelipase or pancreatin ■ pork products ■ beef products.

You have ever had any of the following medical problems: ■ asthma or other lung disease ■ digestive problems, including severe diarrhea ■ difficulty in urination or other urinary problems ■ enlarged prostate ■ glaucoma ■ heart disease, including abnormal heart rhythms or fast heartbeat ■ kidney disease ■ liver disease ■ overactive thyroid ■ myasthenia gravis.

You are taking any of the following medicines: ■ medicine for stomach spasm or cramps ■ medicine for Parkinson's disease ■ medicine for diarrhea ■ tranquilizers ■ medicine for nausea ■ medicine for seizures ■ antihistamines ■ narcotics or other prescription pain-killers ■ sleep medicines ■ medicine for depression ■ medicine for abnormal heart rhythms ■ digoxin, digitoxin, or digitalis (heart medicines).

SPECIAL RESTRICTIONS WHILE TAKING THIS DRUG

FOOD AND DRUG INTERACTIONS

Other Drugs	Do not take any other drugs, including over-the-counter (OTC) drugs, before checking with your doctor. This medicine increases the effect of drugs that depress the central nervous system, such as antihistamines; medicine for hay fever, allergies, or colds; sleep medicines; tranquilizers; narcotics or other prescription pain-killers; muscle relaxants; and medicine for seizures. Allow at least one hour between the time you take this drug and the time you take an antacid or medicine for diarrhea.
Alcohol	This medicine increases the effect of alcohol, a central nervous system depressant. Avoid alcohol unless your doctor has approved its use.

No special restrictions on foods and beverages, smoking, driving, exertion and exercise, sun exposure, or exposure to excessive heat or cold.

POSSIBLE SIDE EFFECTS

Although this list of adverse effects may seem somewhat intimidating, keep in mind that some are quite rare. Of course, should these or any other problems arise while you are on medication, it is always a good idea to consult your doctor.

IF YOU DEVELOP

blood in urine ■ joint pain ■ difficulty in breathing ■ stuffy nose ■ continual blurred vision ■ convulsions ■ confusion ■ severe drowsiness ■ hallucinations ■ slurred speech ■ fast heartbeat ■ palpitations ■ flushing ■ fever ■ voice changes ■ restlessness ■ clumsiness ■ staggering

WHAT TO DO

Urgent Get in touch with your doctor immediately.

---

rash or hives ■ diarrhea ■ nausea or vomiting ■ stomach cramps or pain ■ sore throat ■ eye pain ■ changes in pupil size ■ bleeding or bruising ■ yellowing of eyes or skin ■ difficulty in urination ■ nervousness ■ excitement ■ agitation ■ irritability ■ sleeplessness

May be serious Check with your doctor as soon as possible.

---

constipation ■ decreased sweating ■ dizziness ■ drowsiness ■ dry mouth, nose, throat, or skin ■ increased eye sensitivity to light ■ loss of taste ■ bloating ■ headache ■ male impotence ■ aching muscles or bones

If symptoms are disturbing or persist, let your doctor know.

STORAGE INSTRUCTIONS

Store in a cool, dark place (not in a bathroom medicine cabinet).

STOPPING OR INTERRUPTING THERAPY

This medicine should be taken without interruption for the full length of time prescribed by your doctor. If you miss a dose, take it as soon as possible. If it is almost time for your next dose, skip the missed dose and resume your regular schedule. Do not take two doses at the same time.

SPECIAL CONSIDERATIONS FOR THOSE OVER SIXTY-FIVE

Older people may be more sensitive to this medicine and more likely to experience such side effects as confusion, difficulty in urination, drowsiness, nervousness, agitation, irritability, and restlessness.

CONDITION: **INDIGESTION**

CATEGORY: **DIGESTANTS**

GENERIC (CHEMICAL) NAME	BRAND (TRADE) NAME	DOSAGE FORMS AND STRENGTHS
Pancrelipase	COTAZYM	Capsules: 8,000 units lipase, 30,000 units protease, and 30,000 units amylase
	COTAZYM-S	Capsules: 5,000 units lipase, 20,000 units protease, and 20,000 units amylase
	ILOZYME	Tablets: 11,000 units lipase, $\geq$ 30,000 units protease, and $\geq$ 30,000 units amylase
	PANCREASE	Capsules: $\geq$ 4,000 units lipase, 20,000 units amylase, and 25,000 units protease
	VIOKASE	Powder: 16,800 units lipase, 70,000 units protease, and 70,000 units amylase per 1/4 tsp Tablets: 8,000 units lipase, 30,000 units protease, and 30,000 units amylase

DRUG PROFILE

Pancrelipase, a combination of enzymes that are naturally produced by the pancreas, helps the body digest food properly. It is prescribed for people who have insufficient amounts of these enzymes as a result of inflammation of the pancreas (pancreatitis) or have had their pancreas surgically removed (pancreatectomy).

BEFORE USING THIS DRUG

Let your doctor know *IF*

You have ever had allergic reactions or other problems with ■ pancrelipase ■ pancreatin ■ pork products.

SPECIAL RESTRICTIONS WHILE TAKING THIS DRUG

FOOD AND DRUG INTERACTIONS

Foods and Beverages	Your doctor will probably prescribe a special diet to follow while taking this medicine.

No special restrictions on other drugs, alcohol use, or smoking.

DAILY LIVING

Helpful Hints	Avoid touching or inhaling the powder form of this drug, because it can be quite irritating.

No special restrictions on driving, exertion and exercise, sun exposure, or exposure to excessive heat or cold.

POSSIBLE SIDE EFFECTS

Although this list of adverse effects may seem somewhat intimidating, keep in mind that some are quite rare. Of course, should these or any other problems arise while you are on medication, it is always a good idea to consult your doctor.

IF YOU DEVELOP

blood in urine ■ joint pain ■ swollen feet or legs ■ difficulty in breathing ■ stuffy nose

WHAT TO DO

Urgent Get in touch with your doctor immediately.

rash ■ diarrhea ■ nausea ■ stomach cramps or pain

May be serious Check with your doctor as soon as possible.

STORAGE INSTRUCTIONS

Store in a cool, dark place (not in a bathroom medicine cabinet).

STOPPING OR INTERRUPTING THERAPY

This medicine should be taken without interruption for the full length of time prescribed by your doctor. If you miss a dose, take it as soon as possible. If it is almost time for your next dose, skip the missed dose and resume your regular schedule. Do not take two doses at the same time.

SPECIAL CONSIDERATIONS FOR THOSE OVER SIXTY-FIVE

None.

DIARRHEA

You may have found yourself, of late, making more trips to the bathroom than you would like. Your friends may be constantly complaining of constipation, but you sometimes experience the opposite—frequent and loose bowel movements. This is a problem that can be treated in different ways, depending on its cause. Sometimes it's just a matter of drinking fluids to avoid dehydration until the disorder resolves itself. In other cases there's more that you—and your doctor—can do to alleviate your distress.

IRRITABLE BOWEL SYNDROME

Diarrhea may be a symptom of a disorder known as irritable bowel syndrome, or IBS. This syndrome is one of the most common digestive disorders seen in medical practice. Also referred to as spastic colon, mucous colitis, and irritable colon, it occurs twice as frequently in women as in men and can strike any age group.

IBS occurs when the contractions of the colon—which are usually gentle and rhythmic—become irregular and poorly coordinated. When this happens, the fecal material does not proceed normally along the five-foot length of the colon toward the rectum. Instead, it is either expelled too soon from the colon or retained too long.

The most common symptom of IBS is pain, which usually worsens soon after eating. It typically occurs in the lower left side of the abdomen but may occur on the right side or higher up. Other common symptoms of irritable

bowel syndrome include bloating, heartburn, belching, gas, and loss of appetite. And, of course, there is the disturbance in bowel function that may produce diarrhea, constipation, or alternating bouts of each.

It's important that you inform your doctor of any change in your normal bowel habits or the appearance of blood in your stools. If your doctor diagnoses IBS, there's a lot you can do to keep the condition under control. By adding fiber to your diet, avoiding fats, and exercising and strengthening the abdominal muscles (enabling them to better handle the gas problem accompanying IBS), you will go a long way toward freeing yourself of the disabling symptoms of this digestive disorder. It's also a good idea to avoid emotionally charged situations that produce anxiety; anxiety and tension seem to trigger the diarrhea and constipation of IBS. Your doctor may suggest you take medicine to treat the problem. The medicines available for people with IBS are discussed on pages 315–327.

INFECTIOUS GASTROENTERITIS

This is the term for poisoning or invasion of the intestines by bacteria or viruses that produce the symptoms of an upset stomach. You may experience a mild attack of nausea followed by diarrhea, or you may feel severely ill, with recurrent attacks of watery diarrhea, abdominal cramps, fever, and extreme weakness.

Severe cases of gastroenteritis can

be particularly dangerous to older people with chronic illnesses because diarrhea can cause dehydration—the loss of body fluid without adequate replacement. It is important that an older person continually replace these lost fluids and take in some sugar along with liquids (drinking juice or sweetened tea will help the intestine to absorb water and salt). Other things you should do during an attack are stay at home, rest, and eat only when you are hungry.

Some over-the-counter medicines may help relieve the diarrhea once the nausea and vomiting have subsided. But don't take aspirin or other pain-killers because they may worsen the condition. If you don't feel better after two or three days or if there's any blood, mucus, or pus in your stool, consult your doctor. He or she will question you about your symptoms and may send a sample of your bowel movements to a laboratory for analysis to establish or confirm a diagnosis. Depending on the findings, you may receive a prescription for an anti-spasmodic drug, a drug that slows down bowel activity, or an antibiotic. Those prescription medicines are discussed on pages 315–327.

TRAVELER'S DIARRHEA

Traveler's diarrhea is a type of gastroenteritis that usually lasts about three to five days—just long enough to have ruined many a vacation. Known also as "turista" and "Montezuma's revenge," it is noted mainly for the watery diarrhea it produces. The high-risk areas for contracting this ailment are developing countries in Latin America, Africa, the Mediterranean areas, and the Middle and Far East.

It used to be thought that traveler's diarrhea is caused by a general change in the bacteria inhabiting the intestines or by eating spicy, unfamiliar foods. But its most frequent cause is actually a bacterium called *Escherichia coli*, or *E. coli*. If you consume food or water (or ice) contaminated by this organism, your small intestine may become infected. A likely result is not only diarrhea but also abdominal cramps, nausea, vomiting, and a low fever.

Wise dietary precautions to take while traveling include the avoidance of raw meats, raw seafood, raw vegetables, and unpeeled raw fruits. Stick to such drinks as bottled carbonated beverages without ice, beer, wine, hot coffee, and hot tea. Only drink water that's been bottled or treated with chlorine or iodine.

If you're careful, you'll lower your chances of developing traveler's diarrhea, but you can't eliminate them altogether. If you do find yourself laid low by this condition, try to avoid dehydration and stay out of the sun as much as possible. You may find that resting in bed lessens the abdominal cramping. Generally, if you experience one to three loose stools a day and feel well otherwise, no treatment is required. If you have three to five loose stools a day and feel well otherwise, two tablespoons of bismuth subsalicylate (Pepto-Bismol) every half hour for up to eight doses should help clear up your symptoms. If you are experiencing six or more loose stools a day, and if you have a fever or there is blood in the stools, you should check with a doctor.

Antidiarrheal medicine should be used sparingly, if at all. In some cases, a doctor may prescribe one of the drugs discussed on pages 336–341.

TREATMENT

Although the conditions described in this section are often managed without medicine, your doctor may find it appropriate to put you on medicine to relieve your discomfort. A variety of medicines are available to help your gastrointestinal system function more normally.

OUTLOOK

An attack of infectious gastroenteritis or traveler's diarrhea is generally a passing phenomenon. If you take effective measures to prevent dehydration, you should be none the worse for it. If the diarrhea is prolonged, however, or if there is fever or severe and persistent pain in the abdomen, check with a doctor; a more serious abdominal disorder may be the cause of your symptoms.

Irritable bowel syndrome, in contrast, may be a recurrent problem. Doctors are now able to control many of its unpleasant symptoms, enabling you to lead a normal life. As you pay more attention to your diet and your need for exercise and try to avoid stressful situations, you may even feel healthier than ever.

CONDITION: **DIARRHEA**

CATEGORY: **ANTIDIARRHEAL AGENTS**

GENERIC (CHEMICAL) NAME	BRAND (TRADE) NAME	DOSAGE FORMS AND STRENGTHS
Diphenoxylate and atropine sulfate	LOMOTIL	Liquid: 2.5 mg diphenoxylate and 0.025 mg atropine per tsp Tablets: 2.5 mg diphenoxylate and 0.025 mg atropine

DRUG PROFILE

This drug is used along with other therapy to treat severe diarrhea and intestinal cramping. Diphenoxylate is thought to reduce the movements of the stomach and intestines.

BEFORE USING THIS DRUG

Let your doctor know *IF*

You have ever had allergic reactions or other problems with ■ diphenoxylate ■ atropine.

You have ever had any of the following medical problems: ■ severe colitis ■ severe bleeding ■ kidney disease ■ liver disease ■ drug addiction ■ fever (at present) ■ rectal bleeding.

You are taking any of the following medicines: ■ other medicine for diarrhea ■ antacids ■ medicine for stomach spasms or cramps ■ medicine for Parkinson's disease ■ medicine for nausea ■ tranquilizers ■ medicine for seizures ■ antihistamines ■ narcotics or other prescription pain-killers ■ sleep medicines ■ medicine for depression ■ medicine for abnormal heart rhythms ■ digoxin, digitoxin, or digitalis (heart medicines) ■ acetaminophen ■ antibiotics.

You have recently traveled to a foreign country.

SPECIAL RESTRICTIONS WHILE TAKING THIS DRUG

FOOD AND DRUG INTERACTIONS

Other Drugs	Do not take any other drugs, including over-the-counter (OTC) drugs, before checking with your doctor. This medicine increases the effect of drugs that depress the central nervous system, such as antihistamines; medicine for hay fever, allergies, or colds; sleep medicines; tranquilizers; narcotics or other prescription pain-killers; muscle relaxants; and medicine for seizures.
Alcohol	This medicine increases the effect of alcohol, a central nervous system depressant. Avoid alcohol unless your doctor has approved its use.

No special restrictions on foods and beverages or smoking.

DAILY LIVING

Driving	This medicine may cause dizziness, drowsiness, or blurred vision. Be careful when driving, operating household appliances, or doing any other tasks that require alertness until you know how this drug affects you.
Other Precautions	Take this medicine exactly as prescribed by your doctor; taking it more often or for a longer period of time than prescribed may make it habit forming.

Let your doctor know if your diarrhea does not stop within a few days, or if you develop a fever or rectal bleeding.

Tell any doctor or dentist you consult that you are taking this drug, especially if you will be undergoing any type of surgery. |

No special restrictions on exertion and exercise, sun exposure, or exposure to excessive heat or cold.

POSSIBLE SIDE EFFECTS

Although this list of adverse effects may seem somewhat intimidating, keep in mind that some are quite rare. Of course, should these or any other problems arise while you are on medication, it is always a good idea to consult your doctor.

IF YOU DEVELOP	WHAT TO DO
blurred vision ■ severe drowsiness ■ severely dry mouth ■ difficulty in breathing ■ fast heartbeat ■ flushing ■ severe bloating ■ constipation ■ severe nausea or vomiting ■ stomach pain ■ fever ■ changes in pupil size ■ rectal bleeding ■ difficulty in urination ■ swelling of face, hands, or feet ■ rash, hives, or itching	**Urgent** Get in touch with your doctor immediately.
dizziness ■ drowsiness ■ headache ■ depression ■ feeling of euphoria ■ weakness ■ general feeling of unwellness ■ numbness in hands or feet ■ dry mouth, throat, nose, or skin ■ increased thirst ■ swollen gums ■ nausea or vomiting ■ stomach discomfort or bloating ■ loss of appetite ■ restlessness ■ sleeplessness	**May be serious** Check with your doctor as soon as possible.

STORAGE INSTRUCTIONS

Store in a cool, dark place (not in a bathroom medicine cabinet). If your medicine is in a liquid form, make sure that it does not freeze.

STOPPING OR INTERRUPTING THERAPY

If you miss a dose, take it as soon as possible. If it is almost time for your next dose, skip the missed dose and resume your regular schedule. Do not take two doses at the same time.

SPECIAL CONSIDERATIONS FOR THOSE OVER SIXTY-FIVE

Older people may be more prone to constipation with this drug.

CONDITION: **DIARRHEA**

CATEGORY: **ANTIDIARRHEAL AGENTS**

GENERIC (CHEMICAL) NAME	BRAND (TRADE) NAME	DOSAGE FORMS AND STRENGTHS
Loperamide hydrochloride	IMODIUM	Capsules: 2 mg Liquid: 1 mg per tsp

DRUG PROFILE

Loperamide is used to treat mild acute (short-term) diarrhea as well as chronic (long-term) diarrhea resulting from intestinal resection, irritable bowel syndrome, or incontinence.

BEFORE USING THIS DRUG

Let your doctor know *IF*

You have ever had allergic reactions or other problems with ■ loperamide.

You have ever had any of the following medical problems: ■ colitis ■ liver disease ■ fever (at present) ■ rectal bleeding.

You are taking any of the following medicines: ■ antibiotics ■ diphenoxylate and atropine sulfate (Lomotil).

SPECIAL RESTRICTIONS WHILE TAKING THIS DRUG

FOOD AND DRUG INTERACTIONS

Foods and Beverages	Your doctor may suggest changes in your diet. Tell your doctor if you find that certain foods or beverages cause a diarrheal attack.

No special restrictions on other drugs, alcohol use, or smoking.

DAILY LIVING

Examinations or Tests	If you are taking this drug on a long-term basis, your doctor may want to check your progress periodically.
Other Precautions	Let your doctor know if your diarrhea does not stop within a few days or if you develop a fever or rectal bleeding.

No special restrictions on driving, exertion and exercise, sun exposure, or exposure to excessive heat or cold.

POSSIBLE SIDE EFFECTS

Although this list of adverse side effects may seem somewhat intimidating, keep in mind that some are quite rare. Of course, should these or any other problems arise while you are on medication, it is always a good idea to consult your doctor.

IF YOU DEVELOP	WHAT TO DO
rectal bleeding	**Urgent** Get in touch with your doctor immediately.
bloating ■ constipation ■ dizziness ■ drowsiness ■ tiredness ■ dry mouth ■ fever ■ nausea or vomiting ■ rash ■ stomach pain or discomfort	**May be serious** Check with your doctor as soon as possible.

STORAGE INSTRUCTIONS

Store in a cool, dark place (not in a bathroom medicine cabinet). If your medicine is in a liquid form, make sure that it does not freeze.

STOPPING OR INTERRUPTING THERAPY

Take this drug exactly as prescribed by your doctor. If you miss a dose, take it as soon as possible. If it is almost time for your next dose, skip the missed dose and resume your regular schedule. Do not take two doses at the same time.

SPECIAL CONSIDERATIONS FOR THOSE OVER SIXTY-FIVE

Older people may be more prone to constipation with this drug.

INFLAMMATORY BOWEL DISEASE

Among the most serious and least understood of all the problems of the digestive tract, inflammatory bowel disease is really two diseases—ulcerative colitis and Crohn's disease. More than two million Americans suffer from the disabling effects of these diseases, and each year one-hundred thousand new cases are diagnosed.

You may have heard that these disorders are "young people's" diseases, but about 10 to 20 percent of cases occur in individuals over the age of fifty. So, if you've just been told you have ulcerative colitis or Crohn's disease, you are certainly not alone in your age group.

CAUSES

Just what *are* ulcerative colitis and Crohn's disease? Ulcerative colitis is a chronic disorder characterized by inflammation and sores on the inner lining of the large intestine, or colon. It does not involve the small intestine. Crohn's disease typically affects the ileum, the lower portion of the small intestine, and/or the colon. This disorder causes the intestinal wall to become inflamed and deeply scarred. In severe cases, small openings (fistulas) develop in the intestinal wall, and infected contents may leak out.

Ulcerative colitis and Crohn's disease are grouped together under the same name (inflammatory bowel disease) because of their similarities and because the causes of both disorders are unknown. But there are several telling differences between the two conditions. For example, the presence of fistulas occurs only in Crohn's disease. In Crohn's disease, the rectum frequently is normal, and there are often "skip areas" in the colon—patches of normal-appearing intestine interspersed with the areas of disease. In chronic ulcerative colitis, by contrast, the rectum is always affected, and inflammation in the colon is continuous.

Crohn's disease expresses itself somewhat differently in older people than in their younger couterparts, as it is more likely to affect the colon in this older population. Crohn's disease of the colon alone may have a better outlook than the form of the disease that affects the small intestine.

DIAGNOSIS

Ulcerative colitis usually begins gradually. However, an initial attack or a flare-up may occur suddenly, giving no preliminary warning. The most common symptom is bloody diarrhea. Severe cases may involve painful abdominal cramps, fever, loss of appetite, anemia, and frequent loose stools containing blood and pus. Some people with ulcerative colitis experience such serious complications as hemorrhage or distention and rupture of the bowel. In most people, the pattern of the disease is a cyclical one of alternating flare-ups and periods of improvement.

The typical symptoms of Crohn's disease are also diarrhea, abdominal pain, low-grade fever, poor appetite, and gradual weight loss. Sometimes this disease is confused with ulcerative colitis because of the similarity of symptoms. People with Crohn's disease are less likely to have blood in their stool. Many people with Crohn's disease develop a noncancerous mass in their right lower abdomen that may be painful to the touch. In advanced Crohn's disease, the drainage of nutrients from the damaged intestinal wall may lead to malnutrition.

Many doctors are unaware of the occurrence of inflammatory bowel disease in older people and may attribute bowel symptoms to other conditions, such as diverticular disease of the colon or cancer. This will lead to a delay in diagnosis. But inflammatory bowel disease can be distinguished from other problems that affect the intestines through a careful history of your symptoms, a thorough physical examination, and appropriate diagnostic tests.

The initial diagnostic test done is often a sigmoidoscopy. This is a simple procedure performed in the doctor's office in which a fiberoptic tube with a light at one end is passed through the anus to inspect the rectum and lower part of the colon. Looking through the viewing end, the doctor can see the lining of the rectum and lower colon quite clearly. A specimen of tissue may also be obtained (biopsy) that can be studied under the microscope to help the doctor make a diagnosis.

If the symptoms seem to point to Crohn's disease and the disease appears to be higher up in your bowel, the doctor may decide to perform a similar procedure known as a colonoscopy. Your doctor may also request that you have an upper gastrointestinal or small bowel series and a barium-enema X-ray examination to find out the extent of the disease. For these tests, a radiopaque dye is swallowed or introduced into the rectum through a short enema tube. The dye passes through the entire small or large intestine, and the features of the bowels can be seen on the developed X rays.

TREATMENT

As yet, there is no drug known to cure inflammatory bowel disease, but various medicines can effectively relieve symptoms and keep them in check. For more information on the available medicines for this disorder, see the drug charts on pages 345–351.

Your doctor may decide that surgery is necessary if medicine can no longer control the symptoms of your illness, if your intestines become blocked, or if your ulcerative colitis is considered likely to progress to cancer. (People who have had colitis involving the entire colon for ten years or more are at an increased risk of developing colon cancer.) Surgery for ulcerative colitis entails removing all or most of the colon. Surgery for Crohn's disease is usually less extensive; only the most severely affected portions of the intestine are removed.

OUTLOOK

Inflammatory bowel disease is a potentially serious intestinal disorder that can affect young and old alike.

Fortunately, the great majority of cases can be kept under control with medicine and, sometimes, surgery.

While this can be an emotionally trying illness, the support of family and friends can be enormously helpful to you in coping with this disease and in dealing with recovery from any necessary surgery. In the case of ulcerative colitis, a complete cure through surgery is possible. Otherwise, inflammatory bowel disease is a remittent illness. During the months or even years that it stays dormant, you can lead a normal life in every way.

FOR MORE INFORMATION

A good source for further information on inflammatory bowel disease is the National Foundation for Ileitis and Colitis, Inc., which has chapters located in many states. For the location of the chapter nearest you, contact the national office at 295 Madison Avenue, New York, NY 10017; (212) 685-3440. You can also obtain a free pamphlet, *Inflammatory Bowel Disease*, by writing to the Gastrointestinal Research Foundation, University of Chicago Medical Center, 5841 S. Maryland Avenue, Chicago, IL 60637.

CONDITION: **INFLAMMATORY BOWEL DISEASE**

CATEGORY: **SULFONAMIDES**

GENERIC (CHEMICAL) NAME	BRAND (TRADE) NAME	DOSAGE FORMS AND STRENGTHS
Sulfasalazine	AZULFIDINE	Coated tablets: 500 mg Suspension: 250 mg per tsp Tablets: 500 mg

DRUG PROFILE

Sulfasalazine is used to treat inflammatory bowel disease—ulcerative colitis and Crohn's disease. This sulfa drug primarily acts to relieve inflammation within the colon.

BEFORE USING THIS DRUG

Let your doctor know *IF*

You have ever had allergic reactions or other problems with ■ sulfonamides (sulfa drugs) ■ thiazide diuretics ■ medicine for diabetes ■ aspirin or other salicylate drugs.

You have ever had any of the following medical problems: ■ glucose-6-phosphate dehydrogenase (G-6-PD) deficiency ■ porphyria ■ kidney disease ■ liver disease ■ blood disease ■ asthma or severe allergies ■ intestinal blockage ■ urinary tract blockage.

You are taking any of the following medicines: ■ other sulfa drugs ■ any drugs you take by mouth containing para-aminobenzoic acid (PABA) ■ phenytoin (medicine for seizures) ■ digoxin, digitoxin, or digitalis (heart medicines) ■ sulfinpyrazone or probenicid (medicines for gout) ■ aspirin, aspirinlike medicine, or other medicine for pain and inflammation ■ methotrexate (medicine for cancer and severe psoriasis) ■ anticoagulants (blood thinners) ■ folic acid ■ medicine for diabetes ■ medicine for depression ■ antibiotics for urinary tract infections.

SPECIAL RESTRICTIONS WHILE TAKING THIS DRUG

FOOD AND DRUG INTERACTIONS

No special restrictions on other drugs, foods and beverages, alcohol use, or smoking.

DAILY LIVING

Sun Exposure	Your skin may become more sensitive to sunlight and more likely to sunburn while taking this medicine. It is a good idea to apply a sunscreen to exposed skin surfaces before going outdoors.
Examinations or Tests	It is important for you to keep all appointments with your doctor so that your progress can be checked. Blood or urine tests may be required.
Other Precautions	Tell any doctor or dentist you consult that you are taking this medicine, especially if you will be undergoing any type of surgery or diagnostic testing.
	If you have diabetes, be aware that this drug may affect urine-sugar and ketone tests. Check with your doctor to see if you should use a different type of test.
	Let your doctor know if you are taking the coated tablets and you notice whole tablets in your stool; you may be unable to digest this dosage form.
Helpful Hints	If this medicine upsets your stomach, taking it with meals should help.
	For maximum benefit, take this drug on an empty stomach (one hour before or two hours after meals). Be sure to drink four to six glasses of water a day while taking this drug.

No special restrictions on driving, exertion and exercise, or exposure to excessive heat or cold.

POSSIBLE SIDE EFFECTS

Although this list of adverse effects may seem somewhat intimidating, keep in mind that some are quite rare. Of course, should these or any other problems arise while you are on medication, it is always a good idea to consult your doctor.

IF YOU DEVELOP	WHAT TO DO
seizures ■ bluish tinge to skin ■ rash ■ difficulty in breathing ■ sore throat or fever ■ swollen tongue or vocal cords	**Urgent** Get in touch with your doctor immediately.
numbness, tingling, or pain in hands or feet ■ paleness ■ chills ■ bleeding or bruising ■ hives, itching, or other skin problems ■ severe headache ■ mouth sores ■ red, itching eyes with runny nose ■ swelling around eyes, neck, or ears ■ swelling of the tip of the penis ■ joint pain ■ yellowing of eyes or skin ■ stomach pain ■ blood in urine ■ decreased or increased urination ■ amber color to urine or skin ■ pain or burning in urination ■ low-back pain ■ clumsiness ■ depression ■ confusion ■ hallucinations ■ behavior changes ■ tiredness or weakness ■ ringing or buzzing sound in ears or other hearing problems	**May be serious** Check with your doctor as soon as possible.
upset stomach ■ nausea or vomiting ■ increased skin sensitivity to sunlight ■ headache ■ dizziness ■ drowsiness ■ restlessness ■ sleeplessness ■ loss of appetite ■ diarrhea ■ diarrhea, with blood ■ anxiety	If symptoms are disturbing or persist, let your doctor know.

STORAGE INSTRUCTIONS

Store in a cool, dark place (not in a bathroom medicine cabinet). If your medicine is in a liquid form, make sure that it does not freeze.

STOPPING OR INTERRUPTING THERAPY

If you miss a dose, take it as soon as possible. If it is almost time for your next dose, skip the missed dose and resume your regular schedule. Do not take two doses at the same time.

SPECIAL CONSIDERATIONS FOR THOSE OVER SIXTY-FIVE

None.

CONDITION: **INFLAMMATORY BOWEL DISEASE**

CATEGORY: **CORTICOSTEROIDS**

GENERIC (CHEMICAL) NAME	BRAND (TRADE) NAME	DOSAGE FORMS AND STRENGTHS
Hydrocortisone	CORTENEMA	Suspension: 100 mg

This drug is available under other brand names as well.

DRUG PROFILE

Hydrocortisone enema is used to treat ulcerative colitis. It reduces swelling and provides relief for the inflamed colon.

BEFORE USING THIS DRUG

Let your doctor know *IF*

You have ever had allergic reactions or other problems with ■ corticosteroids ■ any other drugs.

You have ever had any of the following medical problems: ■ rectal infection or bleeding ■ pain, burning, itching, or blisters in the rectal area ■ colitis or diverticulitis ■ diabetes ■ bone disease, such as osteoporosis ■ fungal infection ■ herpes eye infection ■ high blood pressure ■ kidney disease ■ liver disease ■ myasthenia gravis ■ peptic ulcer ■ stomach cramps ■ tuberculosis ■ underactive thyroid ■ mental illness ■ seizures.

You are taking any of the following medicines: ■ antibiotics ■ diuretics or medicine for high blood pressure ■ medicine for inflammation, such as arthritis (including aspirin) ■ insulin or other medicine for diabetes ■ anticoagulants (blood thinners) ■ medicine for seizures ■ estrogens.

You have recently had a vaccination.

SPECIAL RESTRICTIONS WHILE TAKING THIS DRUG

FOOD AND DRUG INTERACTIONS

Other Drugs	Corticosteroids interact with many other drugs. Tell your doctor if you are taking any of the drugs listed above.
Foods and Beverages	Your doctor will probably suggest some changes in your diet to avoid aggravating your inflammatory bowel condition. A low-salt, high-potassium diet may also be recommended to counterbalance some corticosteroid side effects, such as fluid retention.

No special restrictions on alcohol use or smoking.

DAILY LIVING

Examinations or Tests	Your doctor may perform a sigmoidoscopy (examination of the colon with a lighted instrument) to check whether your condition is responding to treatment.

Other Precautions	Tell your doctor if you develop burning, itching, or pain in the rectum during treatment with this medicine.
	Tell any doctor or dentist you consult that you are taking this medicine, especially if you are going to have a vaccination or immunization or if you will be undergoing any type of surgery or allergy skin tests.
	If you have diabetes, be aware that this medicine may raise blood-sugar levels. If you notice any change when testing sugar levels in your blood or urine, let your doctor know.
Helpful Hints	When using a hydrocortisone enema, it is best to retain the fluid for at least one hour (preferably overnight) for maximum benefit. The medicine comes with complete instructions for use.

No special restrictions on driving, exertion and exercise, sun exposure, or exposure to excessive heat or cold.

POSSIBLE SIDE EFFECTS

Although this list of adverse effects may seem somewhat intimidating, keep in mind that some are quite rare. Of course, should these or any other problems arise while you are on medication, it is always a good idea to consult your doctor.

IF YOU DEVELOP	WHAT TO DO
severe abdominal pain	**Urgent** Get in touch with your doctor immediately.
rash, hives, or other skin changes ■ blood in stools ■ bloating ■ diarrhea ■ constipation ■ stomach pain	**May be serious** Check with your doctor as soon as possible.

STORAGE INSTRUCTIONS

Store in a cool, dark place (not in a bathroom medicine cabinet). Make sure that your medicine does not freeze.

STOPPING OR INTERRUPTING THERAPY

Do not stop using this medicine without consulting your doctor. If you miss a dose, take it as soon as possible. If it is almost time for your next dose, skip the missed dose and resume your regular schedule.

SPECIAL CONSIDERATIONS FOR THOSE OVER SIXTY-FIVE

Long-term use of corticosteroids by mouth may cause gradual bone loss, which can be serious in older people, particularly women, who are vulnerable to osteoporosis. However, corticosteroid enemas are usually used only for a limited time.

CONDITION: **INFLAMMATORY BOWEL DISEASE**

CATEGORY: **CORTICOSTEROIDS**

GENERIC (CHEMICAL) NAME	BRAND (TRADE) NAME	DOSAGE FORMS AND STRENGTHS
Prednisone	DELTASONE	Tablets: 2.5, 5, 10, 20, 50 mg

DRUG PROFILE

Oral corticosteroids (also known as steroids) are used to treat a wide variety of inflammatory diseases, such as arthritis, and other rheumatic disorders, such as lupus. They are also used in conjunction with immunosuppressive agents to prevent reactions from kidney and heart transplants. Although these multifaceted drugs do not cure the underlying disease, they suppress the redness, swelling, and heat that signal inflammation.

For complete information on this drug, see pages 439–443.

NAUSEA AND VOMITING

When your body tries to get rid of irritating or disease-causing substances in the digestive tract, nausea and vomiting may occur. These substances can be viruses or bacteria that have lodged in your intestine or things you've eaten that for one reason or another don't agree with you.

Or you might become nauseated during an attack of vertigo, or dizziness, which can result from a disturbance in the balance-maintaining structures of the inner ear or from a distortion of vision. Nausea and vomiting are also symptoms of motion sickness, which makes some people miserable when they take a cruise or even just ride in a car; for unknown reasons, some people are more prone to motion sickness than others. And sometimes emotional stress can make you feel that you want to throw up.

Persistent nausea can be a sign of liver inflammation or gallbladder disease. Also, if you suffer nausea after starting on a new medicine, it may be an adverse effect of that medicine.

As unpleasant as they are, nausea and vomiting are usually mild and self-limiting; that is, you feel bad and throw up a few times, but then you feel better in a day or two. However, nausea and vomiting can also be symptoms of serious disease, or they can lead to a dangerous loss of fluids or an imbalance of vital body chemicals. This is a special problem for older people who are chronically ill or who rely on daily medicines to preserve their well-being. If you are in either of these categories, an attack of vomiting should be a signal for you to call your doctor right away.

CAUSES

Infectious gastroenteritis is the general term for infections in the stomach and intestine. Cramps, diarrhea, and loss of appetite may accompany the nausea and vomiting. You can get gastroenteritis if you eat improperly cooked or refrigerated food in which bacteria have been multiplying; it can happen when the normal bacteria in your own body are upset or unbalanced by another illness; and it can also be the result of a contagious viral infection that we generally refer to as stomach or intestinal flu.

Similar symptoms occur with *gastritis*, an inflammation of the stomach lining, which can be caused by a viral infection but is more often the result of smoking, drinking, using too much aspirin or other anti-inflammatory drugs, overeating, or eating something that you're allergic to or that's too spicy or acidic for you.

In addition, a number of other conditions can cause the symptoms of nausea and vomiting, including pancreatitis (inflammation of the pancreas), gallstones, cholecystitis (inflammation of the gallbladder), gastritis, gastric obstruction, ulcers, certain types of cancer, and some diseases of the central nervous system.

TREATMENT AND OUTLOOK

Most cases of gastroenteritis and gastritis clear up if you just take it easy for a day or two, staying in bed if you can. You will probably not want to eat anything, but you should make an effort to take in fluids like water, weak tea, or fruit juice. If you have recognized a particular food or behavior that has caused your problem, you should abstain from it even after you feel better; if you think one of your medicines is causing the difficulty, talk to your doctor before discontinuing its use.

You should also ask your doctor for help if your symptoms seem unusually severe, if they persist for more than a couple of days, or if they recur several times in a week. And you should get immediate medical attention if your nausea and vomiting are accompanied by any of the following:

• Severe pain in your abdomen that does not go away when you throw up; this might be a sign of appendicitis, inflammation of the pancreas, or gallbladder disease.

• Pain in one eye and blurred vision; these are symptoms of acute glaucoma.

• The appearance of blood or black particles ("coffee grounds") in your vomit; this is a sign of internal bleeding.

• A feeling that you are parched or dried out, along with infrequent urination; these are signs of dehydration.

Also, if you had received a blow to the head within twenty-four hours of the time you started feeling nauseated, see a doctor to find out if any brain injury has occurred.

Drugs are available that will relieve nausea and stop the vomiting, but your doctor may want to examine you before prescribing to be sure you do not have something that requires some other kind of treatment. Medicines that will prevent motion sickness and its accompanying symptoms are also available, so if you suspect or know that you are subject to that disorder, check with your doctor before you set out on your next trip. For more information on the available medicines for nausea and vomiting, see the drug charts on pages 354–369.

CONDITION: **NAUSEA AND VOMITING**

CATEGORY: **ANTIHISTAMINES**

GENERIC (CHEMICAL) NAME	BRAND (TRADE) NAME	DOSAGE FORMS AND STRENGTHS
Meclizine hydrochloride	ANTIVERT	Chewable tablets: 25 mg Tablets: 12.5, 25, 50 mg

DRUG PROFILE

Meclizine, which belongs to the category of drugs called antihistamines, is used to prevent the nausea, vomiting, and dizziness that are associated with motion sickness. This medicine also is used to treat dizziness resulting from inner-ear disturbances. Meclizine works by reducing the sensitivity of the nerves in the inner ear that control balance; it also blocks the nerve pathways to the part of the brain that controls vomiting.

For complete information on this drug, see pages 242–244.

CONDITION: **NAUSEA AND VOMITING**

CATEGORY: **ANTINAUSEANTS**

GENERIC (CHEMICAL) NAME	BRAND (TRADE) NAME	DOSAGE FORMS AND STRENGTHS
Dimenhydrinate	DRAMAMINE	Liquid: 12.5 mg per 4 ml Tablets: 50 mg

This drug is available by prescription and over the counter under many other brand names as well.

DRUG PROFILE

Dimenhydrinate, which belongs to the category of drugs called antihistamines, is used to prevent nausea, vomiting, and dizziness associated with motion sickness. This drug works by reducing the sensitivity of the nerves in the inner ear that control balance. It also blocks the nerve pathways to the part of the brain that controls vomiting.

BEFORE USING THIS DRUG

Let your doctor know *IF*

You have ever had allergic reactions or other problems with ■ dimenhydrinate ■ other antihistamines.

You have ever had any of the following medical problems: ■ asthma or other lung disease ■ enlarged prostate ■ difficulty in urination or other urinary problems ■ glaucoma ■ irregular or fast heartbeat.

You are taking any of the following medicines: ■ medicine for Parkinson's disease ■ medicine for seizures ■ aspirin or aspirinlike medicine ■ medicine for cancer ■ antibiotics ■ digoxin, digitoxin, or digitalis (heart medicines) ■ medicine for abnormal heart rhythms ■ barbiturates ■ muscle relaxants ■ antihistamines ■ narcotics or other prescription pain-killers ■ sleep medicines ■ tranquilizers ■ medicine for depression ■ medicine for high blood pressure ■ appetite suppressants.

SPECIAL RESTRICTIONS WHILE TAKING THIS DRUG

FOOD AND DRUG INTERACTIONS

Other Drugs	Do not take any other drugs, including over-the-counter (OTC) drugs, before checking with your doctor. This medicine increases the effect of drugs that depress the central nervous system such as antihistamines; medicine for hay fever, allergies, or colds; sleep medicines; tranquilizers; narcotics or other prescription pain-killers; muscle relaxants; and medicine for seizures. This drug may mask ringing in the ears caused by aspirin. Let your doctor know if you are taking aspirin or aspirinlike medicine.

Alcohol	This medicine increases the effect of alcohol, a central nervous system depressant. Avoid alcohol unless your doctor has approved its use.

No special restrictions on foods and beverages or smoking.

DAILY LIVING

Driving	This medicine may cause dizziness, drowsiness, weakness, or blurred vision. Be careful when driving, operating household appliances, or doing any other tasks that require alertness until you know how this drug affects you.
Other Precautions	This drug, because it controls nausea and vomiting, can mask some of the symptoms of appendicitis. If you have sharp stomach or lower abdominal pain, be sure to let your doctor know at once.
	If you are going to be tested for allergies, tell the doctor in charge that you are taking this drug, since it affects the results of allergy tests.
Helpful Hints	Taking this drug with food, milk, or water will lessen the chance of upset stomach. For maximum benefit, take it one to two hours before traveling.
	If your mouth or throat feels dry, chewing sugarless gum or sucking ice chips or sugarless hard candy will help.

No special restrictions on exertion and exercise, sun exposure, or exposure to excessive heat or cold.

POSSIBLE SIDE EFFECTS

Although this list of adverse effects may seem somewhat intimidating, keep in mind that some are quite rare. Of course, should these or any other problems arise while you are on medication, it is always a good idea to consult your doctor.

IF YOU DEVELOP

seizures ■ unsteadiness or clumsiness ■ severe drowsiness ■ fainting ■ flushing ■ hallucinations ■ difficulty in breathing ■ dilation of pupils ■ insomnia ■ confusion ■ difficulty in speaking or swallowing ■ nervousness ■ irritability ■ restlessness ■ excitement or other mood changes ■ weakness ■ tremors ■ tightness of chest

WHAT TO DO

Urgent Get in touch with your doctor immediately.

---

tiredness ■ palpitations

May be serious Check with your doctor as soon as possible.

---

drowsiness ■ dizziness ■ thickened phlegm ■ blurred vision or other visual disturbances ■ pain or difficulty in urination ■ urinary frequency ■ dry mouth, throat, or nose ■ increased skin sensitivity to sunlight ■ nightmares ■ rash ■ fast heartbeat ■ loss of appetite ■ upset stomach ■ constipation ■ diarrhea ■ nausea or vomiting ■ male sexual problems ■ chills ■ increased sweating ■ ringing in the ears or other hearing problems

If symptoms are disturbing or persist, let your doctor know.

STORAGE INSTRUCTIONS

Store in a cool, dark place (not in a bathroom medicine cabinet). If your medicine is in a liquid form, make sure that it does not freeze.

STOPPING OR INTERRUPTING THERAPY

This medicine should be taken without interruption for the full length of time prescribed by your doctor. If you miss a dose, take it as soon as possible. If it is almost time for your next dose, skip the missed dose and resume your regular schedule. Do not take two doses at the same time.

SPECIAL CONSIDERATIONS FOR THOSE OVER SIXTY-FIVE

Older people taking this medicine may be more prone to develop confusion, pain or difficulty in urination, dizziness, drowsiness, fainting, or dry mouth. Nightmares, restlessness, and irritability are also more apt to occur in those over sixty-five.

CONDITION: **NAUSEA AND VOMITING (MOTION SICKNESS)**

CATEGORY: **ANTINAUSEANTS**

GENERIC (CHEMICAL) NAME	BRAND (TRADE) NAME	DOSAGE FORMS AND STRENGTHS
Scopolamine	TRANSDERM-SCOP	Patch: 1.5 mg

DRUG PROFILE

Scopolamine is used to prevent the dizziness, nausea, and vomiting associated with motion sickness. The medicine is contained in a disc-like patch, which is placed behind the ear and worn for up to three days. The active ingredient is slowly released from the patch and absorbed through the skin.

BEFORE USING THIS DRUG

Let your doctor know *IF*

You have ever had allergic reactions or other problems with ■ scopolamine ■ atropine ■ belladonna ■ hyoscyamine.

You have ever had any of the following medical problems: ■ severe bleeding problems ■ colitis ■ severe dry mouth ■ enlarged prostate ■ glaucoma ■ heart disease ■ high blood pressure ■ hiatal hernia ■ intestinal blockage or other intestinal problems ■ kidney disease ■ liver disease ■ asthma or other lung disease ■ myasthenia gravis ■ urinary blockage or other urinary problems.

You are taking any of the following medicines: ■ medicine for depression ■ antihistamines ■ medicine for hay fever, allergies, or colds ■ muscle relaxants ■ narcotics or other prescription pain-killers ■ tranquilizers ■ sleep medicines ■ medicine for seizures.

SPECIAL RESTRICTIONS WHILE TAKING THIS DRUG

FOOD AND DRUG INTERACTIONS

Other Drugs	Do not take any other drugs, including over-the-counter (OTC) drugs, before checking with your doctor. This medicine increases the effect of drugs that depress the central nervous system, such as antihistamines; medicine for hay fever, allergies, or colds; sleep medicines; tranquilizers; narcotics or other prescription pain-killers; muscle relaxants; and medicine for seizures.
Alcohol	This medicine increases the effect of alcohol, a central nervous system depressant. Avoid alcohol unless your doctor has approved its use.

No special restrictions on foods and beverages or smoking.

DAILY LIVING

Driving	This drug may cause blurred vision or drowsiness. Be careful when driving, operating household appliances, or doing any other tasks that require alertness until you know how this drug affects you.
Exertion and Exercise	This drug may cause you to sweat less than normally. Sweating is your body's natural way of cooling down, and not sweating enough can be dangerous. Use caution not to become overheated when you exercise or exert yourself.
Sun Exposure	This medicine may make your eyes unusually sensitive to sunlight; sunglasses may help relieve this problem.

Excessive Heat	See "Exertion and Exercise"; use caution during hot weather, since overexertion may result in heat stroke. Avoid extremely hot baths or saunas.
Other Precautions	Tell any doctor or dentist you consult that you are taking this medicine, especially if you will be undergoing any type of surgery.
	Before using this medicine, read the directions for use carefully. Wash and dry your hands thoroughly before and after handling a patch to avoid accidentally getting some of the medicine in your eye. Apply the patch to the hairless area of the skin behind the ear; be sure you do not place it over any skin that has been irritated or cut.
Helpful Hints	Plan to wear a patch for at least four hours before you will need it. Although you can swim or bathe with a patch on, try to keep the patch as dry as possible so it will not fall off. If the patch does loosen, remove it and replace it with a new one.
	If your mouth or throat feels dry, chewing sugarless gum or sucking ice chips or sugarless hard candy will help.

No special restrictions on exposure to excessive cold.

POSSIBLE SIDE EFFECTS

Although this list of adverse effects may seem somewhat intimidating, keep in mind that some are quite rare. Of course should these or any other problems arise while you are on medication, it is always a good idea to consult your doctor.

IF YOU DEVELOP	**WHAT TO DO**

clumsiness ■ confusion ■ dizziness ■ severe drowsiness ■ seizures ■ slurred speech ■ extremely dry mouth, nose, or throat ■ fever ■ hallucinations ■ shortness of breath ■ difficulty in breathing ■ extreme excitement, nervousness, restlessness, or anxiety ■ fast heartbeat ■ extremely dry or warm skin ■ flushing

Urgent Get in touch with your doctor immediately.

---

eye pain ■ rash or hives

May be serious Get in touch with your doctor as soon as possible.

---

constipation ■ dry mouth, nose, throat, or skin ■ difficulty in swallowing ■ decreased sweating ■ increased eye sensitivity to sunlight ■ blurred vision ■ drowsiness ■ weakness ■ headache ■ problems with urination ■ bloating ■ nausea or vomiting ■ unusual euphoria ■ memory problems ■ sleep disturbances

After you STOP taking this medicine: increased eye sensitivity to sunlight ■ anxiety ■ irritability ■ sleep disturbances or nightmares

If symptoms are disturbing or persist, let your doctor know.

STORAGE INSTRUCTIONS

Store in a cool, dark place (not in a bathroom medicine cabinet).

STOPPING OR INTERRUPTING THERAPY

A patch can be worn for up to three days. If you still need this medicine, remove the old patch before putting on a new one. Never wear two patches at the same time.

SPECIAL CONSIDERATIONS FOR THOSE OVER SIXTY-FIVE

Older people may be more prone to such side effects as confusion, drowsiness, nervousness, constipation, problems with urination, and dry mouth, nose, throat, or skin.

CONDITION: **NAUSEA AND VOMITING**

CATEGORY: **PHENOTHIAZINES**

GENERIC (CHEMICAL) NAME	BRAND (TRADE) NAME	DOSAGE FORMS AND STRENGTHS
Prochlorperazine	COMPAZINE	Controlled-release capsules: 10, 15, 30 mg Rectal suppositories: 2.5, 5, 25 mg Syrup: 5 mg per tsp Tablets: 5, 10, 25 mg
Thiethylperazine maleate	TORECAN	Rectal suppositories: 10 mg Tablets: 10 mg

DRUG PROFILE

Phenothiazines are used to treat a variety of emotional disorders, including very severe anxiety, agitation, depression, and sleep disturbances. Some phenothiazines (prochlorperazine, thiethylperazine, and thorazine) are also used to treat nausea and vomiting. These drugs are thought to work by inhibiting the action of dopamine, a chemical messenger, in the part of the brain that is the seat of the emotions as well as in the zone of the brain that controls nausea and vomiting.

For complete information on these drugs, see pages 499–505.

CONDITION: **NAUSEA AND VOMITING**

CATEGORY: **ANTICHOLINERGIC DRUGS**

GENERIC (CHEMICAL) NAME	BRAND (TRADE) NAME	DOSAGE FORMS AND STRENGTHS
Trimethobenzamide hydrochloride	TIGAN	Capsules: 100, 250 mg Rectal suppositories: 200 mg

DRUG PROFILE

Trimethobenzamide is used to treat nausea and vomiting. Although it is not known exactly how this drug works, it is thought to affect the nerve pathways in the part of the brain that controls vomiting.

BEFORE USING THIS DRUG

Let your doctor know *IF*

You have ever had allergic reactions or other problems with ■ trimethobenzamide ■ benzocaine or other local anesthetics.

You have ever had any of the following medical problems: ■ intestinal problems ■ encephalitis or any other brain disease.

You are taking any of the following medicines: ■ other medicine for nausea ■ aspirin ■ medicine for convulsions ■ antihistamines ■ barbiturates ■ narcotics or other prescription pain-killers ■ tranquilizers ■ sleep medicines ■ medicine for depression ■ medicine for stomach pain or cramps.

You currently have a fever.

SPECIAL RESTRICTIONS WHILE TAKING THIS DRUG

FOOD AND DRUG INTERACTIONS

Other Drugs	Do not take any other drugs, including over-the-counter (OTC) drugs, before checking with your doctor. This medicine increases the effect of drugs that depress the central nervous system, such as antihistamines; medicine for hay fever, allergies, or colds; sleep medicines; tranquilizers; narcotics and other prescription pain-killers; muscle relaxants; and medicine for seizures. Because this drug prevents nausea and vomiting, it may mask the overdosage symptoms of other drugs you may be taking. This drug may also mask ringing in the ears caused by aspirin.
Alcohol	This medicine increases the effect of alcohol, a central nervous system depressant. Avoid alcohol unless your doctor has approved its use.

No special restrictions on foods and beverages or smoking.

DAILY LIVING

Driving	This medicine may cause dizziness, drowsiness, or blurred vision. Use caution when driving, operating household appliances, or doing any other tasks that require alertness until you know how this drug affects you.
Other Precautions	This medicine, because it controls nausea and vomiting, can mask some of the symptoms of appendicitis. If you have sharp stomach or lower abdominal pain, be sure to let your doctor know at once.

Helpful Hints   If you have been storing the suppository form of this medicine in a warm place, it may be too soft to use. Put it in the refrigerator for half an hour or run cold water over the wrapped suppository before use.

No special restrictions on exertion and exercise, sun exposure, or exposure to excessive heat or cold.

POSSIBLE SIDE EFFECTS

Although this list of adverse effects may seem somewhat intimidating, keep in mind that some are quite rare. Of course, should these or any other problems arise while you are on medication, it is always a good idea to consult your doctor.

IF YOU DEVELOP	WHAT TO DO
seizures	**Urgent** Get in touch with your doctor immediately.
depression ■ confusion ■ shakiness or tremors ■ sore throat or fever ■ tiredness ■ increased nausea or severe vomiting ■ yellowing of eyes or skin	**May be serious** Check with your doctor as soon as possible.
drowsiness ■ blurred vision ■ diarrhea ■ dizziness ■ headache ■ muscle cramps	If symptoms are disturbing or persist, let your doctor know.

STORAGE INSTRUCTIONS

Store in a cool, dark place (not in a bathroom medicine cabinet). Suppositories should be stored in the refrigerator.

STOPPING OR INTERRUPTING THERAPY

Trimethobenzamide should be taken without interruption for the full length of time prescribed by your doctor. If you miss a dose, take it as soon as possible. If it is almost time for your next dose, skip the missed dose and resume your regular schedule. Do not take two doses at the same time.

SPECIAL CONSIDERATIONS FOR THOSE OVER SIXTY-FIVE

Older people with fever and/or dehydration may be more susceptible to the adverse effects of this drug.

CONDITION: **NAUSEA AND VOMITING**

CATEGORY: **PROMOTILITY DRUGS**

GENERIC (CHEMICAL) NAME	BRAND (TRADE) NAME	DOSAGE FORMS AND STRENGTHS
Metoclopramide	REGLAN	Syrup: 5 mg per tsp Tablets: 10 mg

DRUG PROFILE

Metoclopramide is used to relieve symptoms such as nausea, vomiting, loss of appetite, and continued feeling of fullness after eating. The drug, called a promotility agent, acts by increasing the contractions of the stomach and intestines, thus quickening the pace at which food empties from the stomach and moves through the intestines. It is also prescribed for gastroesophageal reflux (heartburn), diabetic gastroparesis (a condition in which the stomach loses its ability to contract), and prevention of nausea associated with chemotherapy.

BEFORE USING THIS DRUG

Let your doctor know *IF*

You have ever had allergic reactions or other problems with ■ metoclopramide ■ procaine ■ procainamide (medicine for abnormal heart rhythms).

You have ever had any of the following medical problems: ■ stomach surgery ■ intestinal or stomach bleeding ■ epilepsy or other seizure disorders ■ intestinal blockage or adhesions ■ kidney disease ■ liver disease ■ Parkinson's disease ■ pheochromocytoma (adrenal gland tumor).

You are taking any of the following medicines: ■ other medicine for nausea and vomiting ■ medicine for Parkinson's disease ■ tranquilizers ■ medicine for seizures ■ antihistamines ■ barbiturates ■ narcotics or other prescription painkillers ■ sleep medicines ■ medicine for depression ■ insulin (medicine for diabetes) ■ sodium bicarbonate (baking soda) ■ medicine for intestinal spasms.

SPECIAL RESTRICTIONS WHILE TAKING THIS DRUG

FOOD AND DRUG INTERACTIONS

Other Drugs	Do not take any other drugs, including over-the-counter (OTC) drugs, before checking with your doctor. This medicine increases the effect of drugs that depress the central nervous system, such as antihistamines; medicine for hay fever, allergies, or colds; sleep medicines; tranquilizers; narcotics or other prescription pain-killers; muscle relaxants; and medicine for seizures.
Alcohol	This medicine increases the effect of alcohol, a central nervous system depressant. Avoid alcohol unless your doctor has approved its use.

No special restrictions on foods and beverages or smoking.

DAILY LIVING

Driving	This medicine may cause dizziness, drowsiness, or blurred vision. Be careful when driving, operating household appliances, or doing any other tasks that require alertness until you know how this drug affects you.
Other Precautions	Tell any doctor or dentist you consult that you are taking this drug, especially if you will be undergoing any type of surgery.
	If you have diabetes, you may need to adjust the timing or amount of insulin dosages, since this medicine hastens the body's passage of food through the intestine and the rise of sugar levels in the bloodstream.

Helpful Hints	If this medicine upsets your stomach, ask your doctor if you can take it with food.

No special restrictions on exertion and exercise, sun exposure, or exposure to excessive heat or cold.

POSSIBLE SIDE EFFECTS

Although this list of adverse effects may seem somewhat intimidating, keep in mind that some are quite rare. Of course, should these or any other problems arise while you are on medication, it is always a good idea to consult your doctor.

IF YOU DEVELOP	WHAT TO DO
confusion ■ severe drowsiness ■ muscle spasms ■ shuffling walk ■ uncontrollable movements of hands, face, tongue, jaw, or mouth ■ other uncontrollable muscle changes ■ change in facial expression ■ slurred speech ■ trembling or shaking of hands ■ tongue inflammation ■ swelling of eye area ■ seizures ■ hallucinations ■ difficulty in breathing ■ mood changes ■ fever ■ rash	**May be serious** Check with your doctor as soon as possible.
drowsiness ■ restlessness ■ tiredness ■ dizziness ■ constipation ■ diarrhea ■ headache ■ nausea or vomiting ■ sleeplessness ■ anxiety or agitation ■ depression ■ visual disturbances ■ urinary frequency or incontinence ■ dry mouth ■ breast swelling in men	If symptoms are disturbing or persist, let your doctor know.

STORAGE INSTRUCTIONS

This drug should be kept in a cool, dark place (not in a bathroom medicine cabinet). If your medicine is in a liquid form, make sure that it does not freeze.

STOPPING OR INTERRUPTING THERAPY

Take this drug exactly as directed by your doctor. Do not increase the dose or take it for longer than prescribed. If you miss a dose, take it as soon as possible. If it is almost time for your next dose, skip the missed dose and resume your regular schedule. Do not take two doses at the same time.

SPECIAL CONSIDERATIONS FOR THOSE OVER SIXTY-FIVE

None.

GALLSTONES

Gallstone disease is nothing new. Its symptoms and possible causes were discussed extensively in the medical literature of the last century. But many older people experience it for the first time because the incidence of the disease increases with advancing years. This condition is about two to four times more likely to develop in women than in men, is especially prevalent in obese individuals, and is most common in persons of both sexes over forty years of age. It is estimated that 30 percent of women and 15 percent of men over the age of seventy have gallstones.

Many people who have gallstone disease are not even aware they have this problem because they don't have any symptoms. Others do experience symptoms severe enough to require medical attention. The center of all this attention—the gallbladder—is a small, pear-shaped organ that is located in the upper right abdomen, tucked partway underneath the liver. Its purpose is to remove the excess water from bile, concentrate the bile, and then store it until it is needed for digestive work.

CAUSES

Researchers have found that the main culprit in gallstone disease is abnormal bile. There are three basic components of bile: cholesterol, bile acids, and phospholipids. In healthy people, these components are in proper balance, and the bile is in a freely moving, fluid state. But for rea-

sons not yet understood, this chemical balance is disturbed in some people. The ratio of cholesterol to bile acids increases, causing the bile to become supersaturated with cholesterol. This can lead to the formation of stones. (Although there are other types of gallstones, cholesterol stones are the most common.)

Incidentally, the development of these stones is not related to a high cholesterol level in the blood. Nor does it appear to be related to the amount of fat in the diet.

DIAGNOSIS

Depending on their number, size, and location, gallstones may cause either no problems at all, only mild discomfort, or the typical symptoms of a gallbladder attack—severe pain in the right upper or middle portion of the abdomen, sometimes accompanied by nausea, vomiting, and fever. Most often, this happens when one or more gallstones become lodged in the duct that carries bile to the duodenum. When this duct is blocked, the normal flow of bile is interrupted. As a result, the gallbladder may become severely inflamed or even infected.

If your doctor suspects that you might have gallstones, he or she will order some specific tests to confirm the diagnosis. A highly accurate test for this purpose, known as ultrasonography, involves transmitting high-pitched sound waves through the body over the area of the gallbladder.

A transducer, which is a sound-producing device, is placed over the skin and moved around from location to location. If you have a stone in the gallbladder or duct, an echo will be generated in that area. The echo is then transmitted through a computer onto a video screen, and a visual record is made from that image. Ultrasonography does not involve X rays.

TREATMENT

How your doctor manages your gallstone problem depends on various factors, including how severe your symptoms are, how long you have had gallbladder trouble, your overall health, and your age. The risks of surgically removing the gallbladder are higher in an older person, so more consideration might be given to a nonsurgical approach to the problem. If the gallstones have caused no symptoms, medical or surgical treatment may not be necessary.

Drugs Chenodiol (brand name Chenix) is currently the only drug on the market in the United States that is able to dissolve cholesterol gallstones in humans. For more detailed infor-mation on this drug, refer to the chart on pages 372–374.

Surgery Because of the current limitations of drug therapy and because people can function quite well without a gallbladder, gallstones are still most often treated by surgically removing the entire organ. This operation, called a cholecystectomy, is one of the safest and most frequently performed of all abdominal procedures. At the same time that the gallbladder is removed, any stones found in the bile duct are also extracted. Gallbladder surgery generally cures the gallstone problem but, like any form of major emergency surgery, there is a risk of complications, especially in older people.

OUTLOOK

Therapy with gallstone-dissolving drugs can, over time, eliminate the stones that are causing the difficulty; with long-term treatment, recurrence of the problem can be prevented. While this does not constitute a cure, it does mean relief from the severe pain and other symptoms of a gallbladder attack.

CONDITION: **GALLSTONES**

CATEGORY: **SOLVENTS**

GENERIC (CHEMICAL) NAME	BRAND (TRADE) NAME	DOSAGE FORMS AND STRENGTHS
Chenodiol	CHENIX	Tablets: 250 mg

DRUG PROFILE

Chenodiol is used to dissolve gallstones in patients in whom surgery is not necessary or should be avoided. This drug, also known as chenodeoxycholic acid, is one of the body's naturally occurring bile acids. By correcting the chemical imbalance in the gallbladder, it creates an environment that dissolves gallstones and prevents new ones from forming.

BEFORE USING THIS DRUG

Let your doctor know *IF*

You have ever had allergic reactions or other problems with ■ chenodiol.

You have ever had any of the following medical problems: ■ any other disease of the gallbladder or bile ducts ■ inflammatory bowel disease ■ liver disease ■ pancreas disease.

You are taking any of the following medicines: ■ antacids ■ estrogens (female hormones) ■ medicine for high cholesterol.

SPECIAL RESTRICTIONS WHILE TAKING THIS DRUG

FOOD AND DRUG INTERACTIONS

Foods and Beverages	Your doctor may prescribe a high-fiber diet to help stones dissolve faster and prevent new stones from forming. A weight-reduction diet may also be advised.

No special restrictions on other drugs, alcohol use, or smoking.

DAILY LIVING

Examinations or Tests	Your doctor will order regular blood tests and X rays or ultrasound tests to check whether chenodiol is dissolving the gallstones and the liver is functioning properly.
Other Precautions	If you have severe pain in your upper right side, or if you have fever, severe nausea and vomiting, yellowing of eyes or skin, or change in urine or stool color, contact your doctor immediately. These symptoms may reflect a worsening of your gallbladder condition.
Helpful Hints	Take this medicine with food or milk unless your doctor instructs you otherwise. This medicine often causes mild diarrhea; this will probably not last very long. If it bothers you, your doctor can reduce your dosage.

No special restrictions on driving, exertion and exercise, sun exposure, or exposure to excessive heat or cold.

POSSIBLE SIDE EFFECTS

Although this list of adverse effects may seem somewhat intimidating, keep in mind that some are quite rare. Of course, should these or any other problems arise while you are on medication, it is always a good idea to consult your doctor.

IF YOU DEVELOP	WHAT TO DO
severe diarrhea	**May be serious** Check with your doctor as soon as possible.

mild diarrhea ■ frequent urge for bowel movements ■ constipation ■ gas ■ loss of appetite ■ nausea or vomiting ■ stomach pain or cramps ■ heartburn

If symptoms are disturbing or persist, let your doctor know.

STORAGE INSTRUCTIONS

Store in a cool, dark place (not in a bathroom medicine cabinet).

STOPPING OR INTERRUPTING THERAPY

Chenodiol should be taken without interruption for the full length of time prescribed by your doctor, even once you begin to feel better. If stopped too soon, gallstones may not dissolve completely. If you miss a dose, take it as soon as possible. If it is almost time for your next dose, skip the missed dose and resume your regular schedule. Do not take two doses at the same time.

SPECIAL CONSIDERATIONS FOR THOSE OVER SIXTY-FIVE

None.

Chapter 4
Pain and Discomfort

PAIN

Pain is nature's distress signal, alerting us that something may be seriously awry and should be tended to. It's easy to forget, however, that pain is a symptom, not a disease. While it's important to relieve pain, it's even more important to discover what's causing it. As one grows older, one becomes more susceptible to certain conditions that cause pain. While medicine can sometimes help, relief is not always just a pill away.

THE MECHANISM OF PAIN

There are two types of pain—acute and chronic. Acute pain, which comes on suddenly and may last from a few hours to a few weeks, may be caused by such circumstances as an infection, accident, or surgery. Chronic pain, which may last for several months or persist throughout one's life, can be caused by a variety of conditions. In some cases, the underlying problem may defy detection.

Although there is a great deal still to be learned about the mechanism of pain, the basic way in which the "distress signal" is communicated to the brain is relatively clear. Apparently, a two-part process is involved. First, to trigger the body's protective reflexes, specialized nerve endings, known as pain receptors, pick up the sensation of injury and relay it via the spinal cord to the brain. Next, there is a more diffused and prolonged ache, perhaps a reminder of the damage that has been done. Chemicals are the actual communicators in the alarm system.

Tissue damage—caused by burning a finger, for example—releases tiny bursts of powerful substances that activate pain in nerve endings.

The alarm system is accompanied by another system—one that censors the messages of pain. When the body has been injured, the brain triggers the release of pain-killing chemicals known as endorphins. These natural pain-killers inhibit pain messages on their way up the spine.

THE PSYCHOLOGY OF PAIN

The way in which you experience pain is completely subjective. What is very painful to someone else may cause you only minor discomfort. Our experience of pain is modified by a number of factors. Some people have a higher or lower pain tolerance than others. For example, when stuck by a needle, some people will perceive the pain more strongly than others will—that is, they have a lower threshold.

Tolerance to pain depends, in part, on a general attitude toward pain; a high threshold may have been developed during childhood by such admonitions as "keep a stiff upper lip." Also, pain tolerance can be diminished by negative factors such as stress, fatigue, fear, anxiety, and depression.

Pain tolerance can be increased by positive factors, chief among which is distraction. Other positive factors that can modify pain include hypnosis and meditation. A study on the chemistry of pain indicates that men are less sensitive to pain than are women—and, interestingly, older people less sensitive than the young.

TREATMENT

Treatment for acute or chronic pain can range from relaxation techniques to acupuncture or biofeedback training to such drugs as aspirin, codeine, or stronger pain-killers. With chronic pain in particular, your doctor may design a regimen that incorporates both drug and nondrug therapies. By learning to minimize pain through distraction and relaxation, it is possible to keep doses of pain-killers at low levels, so side effects can be avoided or minimized.

Pain relief medicines fall into two categories—narcotics and others. *Nonnarcotic analgesics* are the most frequent drugs taken by older people, with aspirin the most popular choice. Aspirin is capable of reducing both fever and inflammation, as are other derivatives of salicylic acid (see chart on pages 379–383). You may prefer, however, using either acetaminophen or ibuprofen, which are also non-narcotic drugs available over the counter. Acetaminophen (see chart on pages 383–386) has little anti-inflammatory effect, but you may use it to reduce a fever or relieve pain if you find that aspirin upsets your stomach. Note, however, that, like many drugs, it tends to remain in an older person's system for a relatively long time, so any adverse reaction to the drug may be prolonged. Ibuprofen (see chart on pages 392–394), like aspirin, reduces pain, fever, and inflamma-

tion. Trial and error will help you determine which product works best for you.

Ibuprofen belongs to the group of pain-killers known as nonsteroidal anti-inflammatory agents. They are frequently used for arthritis, as well as other types of painful inflammatory conditions.

Keep in mind that no drug—including aspirin—is completely without potential side effects. Nevertheless, non-narcotics are generally safe if the instructions given on the package are followed.

Narcotic analgesics are available *only* with a doctor's prescription. These are potent drugs that should be used only in specific circumstances, such as to relieve acute pain after an injury or surgery or to ease the pain of the terminally ill (see pages 386–392). Narcotic analgesics include propoxyphene, codeine (and the similar drugs hydrocodone and oxycodone), meperidine, and hydromorphone. In older people, lower dosages are used. Common side effects of these drugs are drowsiness and constipation. In general, older people are more sensitive to the side effects of these medicines.

One hallmark of a narcotic is that the body builds up a tolerance to it, meaning that more drug is needed to produce the same effect. The danger of addiction after prolonged use is possible. Because of these hazards, narcotics generally should not be used to relieve persistent pain.

When all else fails, people who continue to suffer from chronic pain can seek help from a clinic specializing in pain disorders. At a multidisciplinary pain clinic, a team of specialists can prescribe or adjust medicines to achieve greater effectiveness without the dangers of abuse. Psychotherapy and behavioral modification may also be used. They may also offer such unconventional pain-reduction methods as acupuncture; nerve blocks, in which nerve paths are interrupted by injections; cryoanalgesia, the freezing of nerve fibers; and TENS (transcutaneous electrical nerve stimulation). Medicines may be prescribed or adjusted to achieve greater effectiveness without the danger of abuse. There are now estimated to be several hundred of these clinics around the country, some of which offer more comprehensive programs than others.

OUTLOOK

The search continues for a more complete understanding of the complexities of pain, as well as for potent pain-killers that don't have the drawbacks of narcotics. With all the innovative research being done in this area—and the increasing attention it is receiving from medical scientists—the next decade will likely produce more effective solutions to the challenges of pain management.

CONDITION: **PAIN**

CATEGORY: **ANALGESICS**

GENERIC (CHEMICAL) NAME	BRAND (TRADE) NAME	DOSAGE FORMS AND STRENGTHS

Aspirin and other salicylate
  drugs

Aspirin and other salicylate drugs are available over the counter under a variety of brand names, dosage forms, and strengths. Some of these preparations have a special coating to help protect the lining of the stomach against possible irritation. Because of the importance of salicylate drugs in the treatment of chronic pain, even though they are most often nonprescription drugs, they are included in this book for reader reference.

DRUG PROFILE

Aspirin and other drugs in the salicylate family are used to relieve pain, inflammation, and fever. Large doses are used to treat symptoms of arthritis and rheumatism such as swelling, stiffness, and joint pain. Aspirin and other salicylates are thought to control pain and swelling by blocking the production of naturally occurring triggers of pain and inflammation, called prostaglandins. These drugs also relieve fever by changing the way the body regulates its temperature.

Because aspirin also helps prevent the blood cells from clumping together, it is also sometimes prescribed to reduce the risk of recurrent ministrokes (transient ischemic attacks or TIAs) and stroke. The benefits of aspirin in ministrokes have to date been proven only in men—but not in women. Aspirin may also help prevent another heart attack in people who have survived a heart attack or who have the extremely severe type of chest pain known as unstable angina. Aspirin is also sometimes prescribed to prevent blood clots in people who are susceptible to this problem.

BEFORE USING THIS DRUG

Let your doctor know *IF*

You have ever had allergic reactions or other problems with ■ aspirin or any other salicylates ■ indomethacin ■ ibuprofen or any other nonsteroidal anti-inflammatory drugs ■ any other substance to which you are hypersensitive.

You have ever had any of the following medical problems: ■ hay fever ■ asthma ■ ulcers, gastritis, or any lesions of the digestive tract ■ liver disease ■ kidney disease ■ systemic lupus erythematosus ■ glucose-6-phosphate dehydrogenase (G-6-PD) deficiency ■ vitamin K deficiency ■ anemia ■ nasal polyps ■ pyruvate kinase deficiency ■ chronic hives ■ chronic stuffy nose ■ rheumatic fever ■ disease of the blood vessels ■ any bleeding disorder ■ recent oral surgery ■ diabetes ■ tinnitus (ringing in ears).

You are taking any of the following medicines: ■ acetaminophen ■ medicine for gout ■ medicine for arthritis ■ anticoagulants (blood thinners) ■ corticosteroids ■ antacids ■ any medicine containing magnesium ■ any medicine containing alcohol ■ beta-blockers ■ medicine for high blood pressure ■ diuretics ■ captopril (medicine for high blood pressure and congestive heart failure) ■ medicine for glaucoma ■ medicine for seizures ■ medicine for diabetes ■ methotrexate (medicine for severe psoriasis and cancer) ■ nitrates (medicine for chest pain) ■ medicine to make the urine more alkaline or more acidic ■ medicine for tuberculosis ■ medicine for nausea or vomiting.

■ *with a buffered aspirin or salicylate:* ■ tetracycline.

SPECIAL RESTRICTIONS WHILE TAKING THIS DRUG

FOOD AND DRUG INTERACTIONS

Other Drugs	Be especially careful about using other medicines that contain salicylates. Check the labels of all other drugs you are taking, including over-the-counter (OTC) products. If you use any laxative containing cellulose, take it at least two hours before or after your dose of a salicylate drug. If you are taking tetracycline, take it one hour before or after any dose of salicylate that contains a buffer.
Foods and Beverages	If you are on a low-salt diet, check with your doctor before taking buffered effervescent aspirin tablets or sodium salicylate because these preparations contain sodium.
Alcohol	It is a good idea to cut down on alcohol or avoid it while taking salicylates. Alcohol may add to the irritant effects of salicylates on your stomach.

Smoking	Smoking also creates excess stomach acid, which may worsen the stomach irritation caused by aspirin.

DAILY LIVING

Examinations or Tests	It is important for you to keep all appointments with your doctor so that your progress can be checked. If you are on long-term therapy with a salicylate drug, periodic blood or urine tests may be required.
Other Precautions	If you have diabetes, be aware that false urine-sugar tests may occur while you are taking a salicylate drug. Check with your doctor before increasing the dose of any diabetes medicine you may be taking.
	Tell any doctor or dentist you consult that you are taking a salicylate drug, especially if you will be undergoing any type of surgery.
	Let your doctor know if you notice a buzzing or ringing sound in your ears, since this may be a sign of aspirin overdose. If you should accidentally take an overdose of this drug, go to a hospital emergency room immediately.
	If you are taking aspirin or another salicylate for a fever that does not subside after three days, check with your doctor.
Helpful Hints	If this medicine upsets your stomach, taking it with a snack, after meals, or with milk or an antacid should help.
	The coated tablets should be swallowed whole without crushing, chewing, or breaking.
	The liquid may be mixed with fruit juice; drink a full glass of water afterwards.

No special restrictions on driving, exertion and exercise, sun exposure, or exposure to excessive heat or cold.

POSSIBLE SIDE EFFECTS

Although this list of adverse effects may seem somewhat intimidating, keep in mind that some are quite rare. Of course, should these or any other problems arise while you are on medication, it is always a good idea to consult your doctor.

IF YOU DEVELOP

seizures ■ confusion ■ severe or continuing headache ■ blood in urine or decreased urination ■ fast heartbeat ■ dizziness or light-headedness ■ severe drowsiness ■ personality changes ■ severe or continuing nausea or vomiting ■ difficulty in breathing or breathing changes ■ continuing stomach pain ■ fever ■ increased sweating ■ tearing eyes ■ fainting ■ rectal bleeding ■ shock (sweating, faintness, rapid pulse, nausea, panting, and pale, cold, moist skin) ■ bloody or black, tarry stools ■ vomiting, with blood or vomit that looks like coffee grounds ■ wheezing ■ rash, hives, or itching

WHAT TO DO

Urgent Get in touch with your doctor immediately.

---

stomach pain or tenderness ■ nausea or vomiting ■ ringing or buzzing in ears ■ tightness in chest ■ tiredness or weakness ■ bleeding or bruising ■ loss of taste for cigarettes

May be serious Check with your doctor as soon as possible.

---

heartburn ■ loss of appetite

With preparations that contain caffeine: sleeplessness or nervousness

With salicylamide only: drowsiness

If symptoms are disturbing or persist, let your doctor know.

STORAGE INSTRUCTIONS

Store in a cool, dark place (not in a bathroom medicine cabinet). If your medicine is in a liquid form, make sure that it does not freeze. If you notice a vinegarlike odor from a bottle of pills, this means that the drug is breaking down and should be discarded.

STOPPING OR INTERRUPTING THERAPY

If you are taking salicylate drugs for arthritis, you may have to take them for the rest of your life, since this medicine controls but does not cure arthritis. If you miss a dose, take it as soon as possible. If it is almost time for your next dose, skip the missed dose and resume your regular schedule. Do not take two doses at the same time.

SPECIAL CONSIDERATIONS FOR THOSE OVER SIXTY-FIVE

Those older people who have reduced kidney function tend not to eliminate the salicylates as readily as people with normal kidney function. In this case, a doctor may schedule regular checkups to make sure the person is receiving the proper dosage and that too much drug is not accumulating in the body.

CONDITION: **PAIN**

CATEGORY: **ANALGESICS**

GENERIC (CHEMICAL) NAME	BRAND (TRADE) NAME	DOSAGE FORMS AND STRENGTHS
Acetaminophen	Regular Strength ANACIN-3	Caplets: 500 mg Tablets: 325 mg
	Maximum Strength ANACIN-3	Capsules: 500 mg Tablets: 500 mg
	Aspirin-free ARTHRITIS PAIN FORMULA	Tablets: 500 mg
	Extra Strength DATRIL	Capsules: 500 mg Tablets: 500 mg

PANADOL	Capsules: 500 mg Tablets: 500 mg
Maximum Strength ST. JOSEPH Aspirin-Free	Tablets: 500 mg
Regular Strength TYLENOL	Caplets: 325 mg Tablets: 325 mg
Extra-Strength TYLENOL	Caplets: 500 mg Liquid: 500 mg per tbsp Tablets: 500 mg

DRUG PROFILE

Acetaminophen is used to relieve fever and pain. It is thought to work by blocking pain centers in the central nervous system and by resetting the body's thermostat to its normal temperature.

BEFORE USING THIS DRUG

Let your doctor know *IF*

You have ever had allergic reactions or other problems with ■ acetaminophen.

You have ever had any of the following medical problems: ■ anemia ■ asthma or other lung disease ■ kidney disease ■ liver disease.

You are taking any of the following medicines: ■ anticoagulants (blood thinners) ■ barbiturates ■ medicine for seizures ■ charcoal ■ antibiotics ■ sulfinpyrazone ■ medicine for Parkinson's disease ■ medicine for stomach cramps, ulcers, or irritable bowel syndrome ■ medicine for urinary tract spasms ■ medicine for asthma ■ atropine (eye medicine) ■ scopolamine (medicine for motion sickness).

SPECIAL RESTRICTIONS WHILE TAKING THIS DRUG

FOOD AND DRUG INTERACTIONS

Other Drugs	Be especially careful about using other medicines that contain acetaminophen. Check the labels of all other drugs you are taking, including over-the-counter (OTC) medicines.

Alcohol	Drinking large amounts of alcohol during long-term therapy with acetaminophen may lead to liver problems and should be avoided.

No special restrictions on foods and beverages or smoking.

DAILY LIVING

Examinations or Tests	It is important for you to keep all appointments with your doctor so that your progress can be checked.
Other Precautions	Take this medicine exactly as instructed on the package labeling. If you are taking acetaminophen for a fever that does not subside after three days, check with your doctor.

No special restrictions on driving, exertion and exercise, sun exposure, or exposure to excessive heat or cold.

POSSIBLE SIDE EFFECTS

Although this list of adverse effects may seem somewhat intimidating, keep in mind that some are quite rare. Of course, should these or any other problems arise while you are on medication, it is always a good idea to consult your doctor.

IF YOU DEVELOP

hoarseness ■ nausea or vomiting ■ stomach cramps or pain ■ excitement ■ delirium ■ severe dizziness or drowsiness ■ clammy skin ■ fast, shallow breathing ■ fast, weak, irregular pulse ■ yellowing of eyes or skin ■ diarrhea ■ loss of appetite ■ fever or sore throat ■ stomach swelling and tenderness ■ bloody or cloudy urine ■ decreased urination ■ pain or difficulty in urination

WHAT TO DO

Urgent Get in touch with your doctor immediately.

■ bleeding or bruising ■ rash, hives, or itching ■ tiredness or weakness	**May be serious** Check with your doctor as soon as possible.

STORAGE INSTRUCTIONS

Store in a cool, dark place (not in a bathroom medicine cabinet). If your medicine is in a liquid form, make sure that it does not freeze.

STOPPING OR INTERRUPTING THERAPY

Take this medicine exactly as directed on the package label unless otherwise instructed by your doctor.

SPECIAL CONSIDERATIONS FOR THOSE OVER SIXTY-FIVE

Exceeding recommended doses is dangerous because liver damage can occur more easily in this age group if too much acetaminophen is taken.

CONDITION: **PAIN**

CATEGORY: **ANALGESICS**

GENERIC (CHEMICAL) NAME	BRAND (TRADE) NAME	DOSAGE FORMS AND STRENGTHS
Codeine sulfate		Tablets: 15, 30, 60 mg
Codeine phosphate and acetaminophen	EMPRACET with Codeine	Tablets: 300 mg acetaminophen and 30 mg or 60 mg codeine phosphate
	PHENAPHEN with Codeine	Capsules: 325 mg acetaminophen and 15, 30, or 60 mg codeine phosphate
	PHENAPHEN-650 with Codeine	Tablets: 650 mg acetaminophen and

	TYLENOL with Codeine	30 mg codeine phosphate Capsules: 300 mg acetaminophen and 30 or 60 mg codeine phosphate Elixir: 120 mg acetaminophen and 12 mg codeine phosphate Tablets: 300 mg acetaminophen and 7.5, 15, 30, or 60 mg codeine phosphate
Codeine phosphate and aspirin	EMPIRIN with Codeine	Tablets: 325 mg aspirin and 15, 30, or 60 mg codeine phosphate
Hydrocodone bitartrate and acetaminophen	VICODIN	Tablets: 5 mg hydrocodone bitartrate and 500 mg acetaminophen
Hydromorphone hydrochloride	DILAUDID	Rectal suppositories: 3 mg Tablets: 1, 2, 3, 4 mg
Meperidine hydrochloride	DEMEROL	Syrup: 50 mg per tsp Tablets: 50, 100 mg
Meperidine hydrochloride and promethazine hydrochloride	MEPERGAN Fortis	Capsules: 50 mg meperidine hydrochloride and 25 mg promethazine hydrochloride
Methadone hydrochloride	DOLOPHINE Hydrochloride	Tablets: 5, 10 mg

Oxycodone hydrochloride and acetaminophen	PERCOCET	Tablets: 5 mg oxycodone hydrochloride and 325 mg acetaminophen
Oxycodone hydrochloride, oxycodone terephthalate, and acetaminophen	TYLOX	Capsules: 4.5 mg oxycodone hydrochloride, 0.38 mg oxycodone terephthalate, and 500 mg acetaminophen
Oxycodone hydrochloride, oxycodone terephthalate, and aspirin	PERCODAN	Tablets 4.5 mg oxycodone hydrochloride, 0.38 mg oxycodone terephthalate, and 325 mg aspirin
	PERCODAN-Demi	Tablets: 2.25 mg oxycodone hydrochloride, 0.19 mg oxycodone terephthalate, and 325 mg aspirin
Propoxyphene hydrochloride	DARVON	Capsules: 32, 65 mg
Propoxyphene hydrochloride and acetaminophen	WYGESIC	Tablets: 65 mg propoxyphene hydrochloride and 650 mg acetaminophen
Butalbital, aspirin, caffeine, and codeine phosphate	FIORINAL with Codeine	Capsules: 50 mg butalbital; 325 mg aspirin; 40 mg caffeine; and 7.5 mg (No. 1), 15 mg (No. 2), or 30 mg (No. 3) codeine phosphate
Propoxyphene hydrochloride, aspirin, and caffeine	DARVON COMPOUND	Capsules; 32 mg propoxyphene hydrochloride, 389 mg aspirin, and 32.4 mg

		caffeine; 65 mg propoxy-phene hydrochloride, 389 mg aspirin, and 32.4 mg caffeine
Propoxyphene napsylate	DARVON-N	Suspension: 50 mg per tsp Tablets: 100 mg
Propoxyphene napsylate and acetaminophen	DARVOCET-N	Tablets: 50 mg propoxyphene napsylate and 325 mg acetaminophen; 100 mg propoxyphene napsylate and 650 mg acetaminophen

DRUG PROFILE

This class of drugs is used to relieve pain. These medicines alter the perception of pain; although it is not known exactly how they work, they are thought to act on nerves located in the brain and spinal cord that transmit the sensation of pain.

BEFORE USING THIS DRUG

Let your doctor know *IF*

You have ever had allergic reactions or other problems with ■ any prescription pain-killers.

You have ever had any of the following medical problems: ■ head injury ■ seizures ■ asthma or other lung disease ■ enlarged prostate ■ urinary problems ■ glaucoma ■ kidney disease ■ liver disease ■ abnormal heart rhythms ■ stomach or intestinal disorders ■ underactive thyroid ■ Addison's disease ■ alcoholism ■ heart attack.

You are taking any of the following medicines: ■ other pain-killers ■ medicine for glaucoma ■ antihistamines ■ medicine for coughs, colds, or hay fever ■ medicine for seizures ■ barbiturates ■ muscle relaxants ■ tranquilizers ■ sleep medicines ■ medicine for depression (within the last two weeks) ■ cimetidine (medicine for ulcers) ■ anticoagulants (blood thinners) ■ amphetamines.

SPECIAL RESTRICTIONS WHILE TAKING THIS DRUG

FOOD AND DRUG INTERACTIONS

Other Drugs	These medicines increase the effect of drugs that affect the central nervous system, such as antihistamines; medicine for hay fever, allergies, or colds; sleep medicines; tranquilizers; other narcotics or prescription pain-killers; muscle relaxants, or medicines for seizures. Do not take any other drugs, including over-the-counter (OTC) drugs, before checking with your doctor.
Alcohol	These medicines increase the effect of alcohol, which is a central nervous system depressant. Avoid alcohol unless your doctor has approved its use.

No special restrictions on foods and beverages or smoking.

DAILY LIVING

Driving	These drugs may cause drowsiness, light-headedness, and dizziness and also affect mental alertness and physical coordination. Be careful when driving, operating household appliances, or doing any other tasks that require alertness until you know how this drug affects you.
Examinations or Tests	It is important for you to keep all appointments with your doctor so that your progress can be checked.
Other Precautions	Tell any doctor or dentist you consult that you are taking this medicine, especially if you will be undergoing any type of surgery.
	Take this medicine exactly as prescribed by your doctor; taking it more often or for a longer period of time than prescribed may make it habit forming.

If you accidentally take an overdose of this medicine, call your doctor or go to an emergency room immediately.

Helpful Hints	You may vomit or feel nauseated when you first start taking this medicine. If this happens, lie down until you feel better. You also may experience dizziness and light-headedness, especially when getting up from a reclining or sitting position. Getting up slowly may help prevent this problem.

If you have been storing the suppository form of this medicine in a warm place, it may be too soft to use. Put it in the refrigerator for half an hour or run cold water over the wrapped suppository before use. |

No special restrictions on exertion and exercise, sun exposure, or exposure to excessive heat or cold.

POSSIBLE SIDE EFFECTS

Although this list of adverse effects may seem somewhat intimidating, keep in mind that some are quite rare. Of course, should these or any other problems arise while you are on medication, it is always a good idea to consult your doctor.

IF YOU DEVELOP	WHAT TO DO
difficulty in breathing ■ severe dizziness or drowsiness ■ seizures ■ blurred vision or other visual disturbances ■ extreme restlessness or nervousness ■ severe weakness ■ irregular, slow, or fast heartbeat ■ shakiness, tremors, or other unusual body movements	**Urgent** Get in touch with your doctor immediately.
inability to concentrate ■ confusion ■ depression ■ "high" feeling or other mood changes ■ weakness ■ faintness ■ agitation or nervousness ■ sleeplessness ■ delirium ■ eye pain ■ rash, hives, or itching ■ dry mouth ■ hallucinations	**May be serious** Check with your doctor as soon as possible.

nausea or vomiting ■ constipation ■ dizziness or light-headedness, especially when getting up from a reclining or sitting position ■ drowsiness ■ flushing ■ sexual problems ■ difficulty in urination or decreased urination ■ increased sweating

With oxycodone only: headache

If symptoms are disturbing or persist, let your doctor know.

STORAGE INSTRUCTIONS

Store in a cool, dark place (not in a bathroom medicine cabinet). If your medicine is in a liquid form, make sure that it does not freeze. Suppositories should be stored in the refrigerator.

STOPPING OR INTERRUPTING THERAPY

If you have been taking this medicine regularly for several weeks, do not abruptly stop taking it; your doctor will advise you on how to decrease your dosage gradually.

SPECIAL CONSIDERATIONS FOR THOSE OVER SIXTY-FIVE

Older people may be more susceptible to such side effects of this medicine as difficulty in breathing, confusion or difficulty in thinking, agitation, drowsiness, weakness, nausea, difficulty in urination, and constipation.

CONDITION: **PAIN**

CATEGORY: **NONSTEROIDAL ANTI-INFLAMMATORY DRUGS**

GENERIC (CHEMICAL) NAME	BRAND (TRADE) NAME	DOSAGE FORMS AND STRENGTHS
Diflunisal	DOLOBID	Tablets: 250, 500 mg
Fenoprofen calcium	NALFON	Capsules: 200, 300 mg Tablets: 600 mg

Ibuprofen	ADVIL (OTC)	Tablets: 200 mg
	MOTRIN	Tablets: 300, 400, 600, 800 mg
	NUPRIN (OTC)	Tablets: 200 mg
	RUFEN	Tablets: 400, 600, 800 mg
Indomethacin	INDOCIN	Capsules: 25, 50 mg Rectal suppositories: 50 mg
	INDOCIN SR	Controlled-release capsules: 75 mg
Meclofenamate sodium	MECLOMEN	Capsules: meclofenamate sodium equivalent to 50 or 100 mg meclofenamic acid
Naproxen	ANAPROX	Tablets: 275 mg
	NAPROSYN	Tablets: 250, 375, 500 mg
Phenylbutazone	BUTAZOLIDIN	Capsules: 100 mg Tablets: 100 mg
Piroxicam	FELDENE	Capsules: 10, 20 mg
Sulindac	CLINORIL	Tablets: 150, 200 mg
Tolmetin sodium	TOLECTIN	Capsules: tolmetin sodium equivalent to 400 mg tolmetin Tablets: tolmetin sodium equivalent to 200 mg tolmetin

DRUG PROFILE

Nonsteroidal anti-inflammatory drugs, or NSAIDs, help relieve swelling, stiffness, joint pain, and inflammation in the long-term treatment of arthritis. These drugs are thought to act by blocking the production of naturally occurring pain and inflammation triggers called prostaglandins.

For complete information on these drugs, see pages 433–438.

Chapter 5
Disorders of the Muscles, Bones, and Joints

BACKACHE

Just about everyone has a backache at some time in life. For most people, back trouble is annoying but temporary and not disabling. For others, however, back pain is so chronic and intense that normal living is impossible.

CAUSES

The cause of a backache is not always clear, but an understanding of the structure of the back can suggest some possible reasons for discomfort. The bones of the back, or vertebrae, are like hollow spools with the spinal cord threaded through the holes. Nerves sprout off the spinal cord, emerging from smaller holes at the back of the vertebrae, to carry messages back and forth between the body parts and the cord. Between the vertebrae are little pads called discs, which are composed of a cushiony, elastic material inside a membrane.

Strong bands of tissue (ligaments) and the muscles of the back support this vertebral stack, holding it in a double curve that swoops gently outward at the mid-back area and arches inward at the neck and at the waistline.

Back problems can start in any part of the back and then expand to involve other structures. Discs don't really "slip"—the term is used in popular parlance—but they can bulge out of alignment, or their membranes can tear so that the material inside begins to ooze. In either case, nearby nerves can be squeezed, causing a painful "pinching." If the sciatic nerve, which extends from the lower back and runs down the leg to the foot, is the one that's being pinched, pain may be felt along the entire leg. This is sometimes called sciatica.

In other cases of back trouble, muscles of the back tighten in spasm as the body tries to realign the vertebrae surrounding the disc. Pain then occurs in the lower back, a condition that used to be referred to as "lumbago."

Back pain can also be associated with poor posture or excess weight, which causes the abdomen to sag forward, pulling on the muscles of the lower back. Or, muscles grown weak from lack of exercise can be strained if you lift a heavy parcel or simply turn or bend. Osteoporosis, arthritis, tumors, infections, and injuries can also lead to vertebral degeneration and pain in the back.

DIAGNOSIS AND TREATMENT

If you complain of back pain and your doctor suspects that you may have a spinal tumor, an infection, or an injury that requires specific kinds of therapy, he or she may order special tests, including X rays. Most backaches, however, can be relieved with aspirin or other anti-inflammatory drugs and/or pain-killers and muscle relaxants. These remedies are discussed in detail in the drug charts on pages 398–424. Heat on the tender area may also help.

Your doctor may also advise you to put a board under your mattress and to sleep on your back with a pillow under your knees or on your side with your knees drawn up. In these positions, the lumbar curve straightens, relieving pressure on the nerves in that part of your back.

If the pain is severe or has persisted for a long time, you might have to spend a couple of weeks in bed, lying on your back with your knees up, and not move except to use the bathroom. Or your doctor might have you wear a surgical corset, which has steel braces in it to support your back.

If none of these relatively mild measures provides you much relief, the next step might be traction. This means that you must lie in bed on your back while a system of weights and pulleys straightens your back. This can be done on a continuous basis in the hospital or on an outpatient basis for about a half hour a day. If that doesn't help, you and your doctor might want to consider an operation or a nonsurgical technique to remove all or part of an offending disc.

OUTLOOK

When your pain is gone, your doctor might suggest that you consult a physical therapist who can show you some back-strengthening exercises and can instruct you in back-sparing ways of standing, moving, lifting, and doing your daily tasks. If you modify some of the habits that contributed to your back pain, it's likely you'll be able to maintain a healthy back.

CONDITION: **MUSCLE INJURIES**

CATEGORY: **BENZODIAZEPINES**

GENERIC (CHEMICAL) NAME	BRAND (TRADE) NAME	DOSAGE FORMS AND STRENGTHS
Diazepam	VALIUM VALRELEASE	Tablets: 2, 5, 10 mg Controlled-release capsules: 15 mg

DRUG PROFILE

Benzodiazepines are used to treat a number of conditions, including anxiety, insomnia, muscle spasm, and seizures. Exactly how these drugs work is a matter of some debate. However, what they all seem to have in common is that they reduce nerve cell activity in those areas of the central nervous system (CNS) and peripheral nervous system (PNS) thought to be responsible for the experience of anxiety and muscular tension.

For complete information on this drug, see pages 478–483.

CONDITION: **MUSCLE INJURIES**

CATEGORY: **MUSCLE RELAXANTS**

GENERIC (CHEMICAL) NAME	BRAND (TRADE) NAME	DOSAGE FORMS AND STRENGTHS
Carisoprodol	SOMA	Tablets: 350 mg
Methocarbamol	ROBAXIN	Tablets: 500, 750 mg

DRUG PROFILE

Carisoprodol and methocarbamol are used to relieve muscle pain and discomfort from strains, sprains, and other muscle injuries. They work by relaxing the muscles. These medicines are used as part of a treatment program that may include rest, physical therapy, and other drugs.

BEFORE USING THIS DRUG

Let your doctor know *IF*

You have ever had allergic reactions or other problems with ■ carisoprodol ■ methocarbamol ■ carbromal ■ mebutamate ■ meprobamate ■ tybamate.

You have ever had any of the following medical problems: ■ kidney disease ■ liver disease.

■ *with carisoprodol only:* ■ drug abuse, including alcoholism ■ porphyria.

■ *with methocarbamol only:* ■ myasthenia gravis.

You are taking any of the following medicines ■ other muscle relaxants ■ barbiturates ■ medicine for depression (within the last two weeks) ■ medicine for seizures ■ antihistamines ■ medicine for hay fever, coughs, or colds ■ sleep medicines ■ narcotics or other prescription pain-killers ■ tranquilizers.

■ *with methocarbamol only:* ■ medicine for myasthenia gravis.

SPECIAL RESTRICTIONS WHILE TAKING THIS DRUG

FOOD AND DRUG INTERACTIONS

Other Drugs	Do not take any other drugs, including over-the-counter (OTC) drugs, before checking with your doctor. This medicine increases the effect of other drugs that depress the central nervous system, such as other muscle relaxants; antihistamines; medicine for hay fever, allergies, or colds; sleep medicines; tranquilizers; narcotics or other prescription pain-killers; and medicine for seizures.

Alcohol	This drug increases the effect of alcohol, a central nervous system depressant. Avoid alcohol unless your doctor has approved its use.

No special restrictions on foods and beverages or smoking.

DAILY LIVING

Driving	This drug may cause dizziness, light-headedness, or faintness. Be careful when driving, operating household appliances, or doing any other tasks that require alertness until you know how this drug affects you.
Exertion and Exercise	Discuss with your doctor which kinds of physical exercise are safe for you to undertake.
Examinations or Tests	It is important for you to keep all appointments with your doctor so that your progress can be checked.
Other Precautions	Tell any doctor or dentist you consult that you are taking either of these drugs, especially if you will be undergoing any type of surgery.
Helpful Hints	If you are taking methocarbamol, your urine may turn a black, brown, or green color. This is a harmless reaction and will subside once you have stopped taking this medicine.

If you find methocarbamol tablets difficult to swallow, try crushing them and mixing the powder with a little food or liquid. |

No special restrictions on sun exposure or exposure to excessive heat or cold.

POSSIBLE SIDE EFFECTS

Although this list of adverse effects may seem somewhat intimidating, keep in mind that some are quite rare. Of course, should these or any other problems arise while you are on medication, it is always a good idea to consult your doctor.

IF YOU DEVELOP	WHAT TO DO
inability to walk ■ extreme weakness ■ double vision or other visual disturbances ■ speech difficulties ■ confusion ■ difficulty in breathing ■ fever *With carisoprodol only:* "high" feeling	**Urgent** Get in touch with your doctor immediately.
fast heartbeat ■ fainting ■ smarting eyes ■ rash, hives, or itching ■ other skin problems ■ depression ■ excitement ■ anxiety ■ muscle weakness ■ bleeding or bruising ■ sore throat ■ swelling of face, lips, or tongue ■ yellowing of skin ■ bloody or black, tarry stools ■ tiredness or weakness *With carisoprodol only:* flushing *After you STOP taking carisoprodol:* stomach cramps ■ sleeplessness ■ chills ■ headache ■ nausea	**May be serious** Check with your doctor as soon as possible.
dizziness or light-headedness, especially when getting up from a reclining or sitting position ■ drowsiness ■ clumsiness ■ nausea or vomiting ■ more frequent bowel movements ■ hiccups ■ stomach cramps and pain ■ heartburn ■ constipation ■ diarrhea ■ stuffy nose ■ headache ■ tremors ■ restlessness ■ irritability ■ sleeplessness ■ loss of appetite	If symptoms are disturbing or persist, let your doctor know.

STORAGE INSTRUCTIONS

Store in a cool, dark place (not in a bathroom medicine cabinet).

STOPPING OR INTERRUPTING THERAPY

Do not suddenly stop taking this medicine; your doctor will advise you on how to decrease your dosage gradually. If you miss a dose of this medicine, take it as soon as possible. If it is not within an hour of the scheduled time for the missed dose, skip it and resume your regular schedule. Do not take two doses at the same time.

SPECIAL CONSIDERATIONS FOR THOSE OVER SIXTY-FIVE

Because liver function sometimes decreases with age, and both these drugs are metabolized by the liver, doctors may start people over sixty-five on a lower dosage.

CONDITION: **MUSCLE INJURIES**

CATEGORY: **MUSCLE RELAXANTS**

GENERIC (CHEMICAL) NAME	BRAND (TRADE) NAME	DOSAGE FORMS AND STRENGTHS
Cyclobenzaprine hydrochloride	FLEXERIL	Tablets: 10 mg

DRUG PROFILE

Cyclobenzaprine is used to relieve painful muscle spasms. It works by relaxing the muscles. Cyclobenzaprine is used as part of a treatment program that may include rest, physical therapy, and other drugs.

BEFORE USING THIS DRUG

Let your doctor know *IF*

You have ever had allergic reactions or other problems with ■ cyclobenzaprine.

You have ever had any of the following medical problems: ■ glaucoma ■ heart or blood vessel disease (especially recent heart attack, abnormal heart rhythms, or congestive heart failure) ■ overactive thyroid ■ difficulty in urination.

You are taking any of the following medicines: ■ other muscle relaxants ■ medicine for seizures ■ medicine for depression (within the last two weeks) ■ antihistamines ■ medicine for hay fever, coughs, or colds ■ appetite suppressants ■ barbiturates ■ sleep medicines ■ tranquilizers ■ medicine for narcolepsy ■ medicine for high blood pressure ■ medicine for asthma ■ thyroid hormones ■ anticoagulants (blood thinners) ■ narcotics or other prescription pain-killers.

SPECIAL RESTRICTIONS WHILE TAKING THIS DRUG

FOOD AND DRUG INTERACTIONS

Other Drugs	Do not take any other drugs, including over-the-counter (OTC) drugs, before checking with your doctor. This medicine increases the effect of other drugs that depress the central nervous system, such as other muscle relaxants; antihistamines; medicine for hay fever, allergies, or colds; sleep medicines; tranquilizers; narcotics or other prescription pain-killers; and medicine for seizures.
Alcohol	This drug increases the effects of alcohol, a central nervous system depressant. Avoid alcohol unless your doctor has approved its use.

No special restrictions on foods and beverages or smoking.

DAILY LIVING

Driving	This drug may cause dizziness, light-headedness, or faintness. Be careful when driving, operating household appliances, or doing any other tasks that require alertness until you know how this drug affects you.
Exertion and Exercise	Discuss with your doctor which kinds of physical exercise are safe for you to undertake.
Examinations or Tests	It is important for you to keep all appointments with your doctor so that your progress can be checked.

Other Precautions	Tell any doctor or dentist you consult that you are taking this drug, especially if you will be undergoing any type of surgery.
Helpful Hints	If your mouth or throat feels dry, chewing sugarless gum or sucking ice chips or sugarless hard candy will help.

No special restrictions on sun exposure or exposure to excessive heat or cold.

POSSIBLE SIDE EFFECTS

Although this list of adverse effects may seem somewhat intimidating, keep in mind that some are quite rare. Of course, should these or any other problems arise while you are on medication, it is always a good idea to consult your doctor.

IF YOU DEVELOP	**WHAT TO DO**
swelling of face, lips, or tongue ■ irregular or fast heartbeat ■ severe drowsiness ■ fainting ■ hallucinations ■ muscle stiffness	**Urgent** Get in touch with your doctor immediately.
clumsiness or unsteadiness ■ confusion ■ depression ■ difficulty in urination ■ urinary frequency ■ ringing or buzzing in ears ■ rash, hives, or itching ■ yellowing of eyes or skin ■ nervousness ■ agitation ■ anxiety ■ excitement ■ strange thoughts or dreams	**May be serious** Check with your doctor as soon as possible.
fatigue or weakness ■ dizziness or light-headedness ■ drowsiness ■ dry mouth ■ muscle twitching or weakness ■ increased thirst ■ increased sweating ■ numbness, tingling, or pain in hands or feet ■ tremors ■ sleeplessness ■ speech difficulties ■ headache ■ constipation ■ nausea ■ indigestion ■ bad taste in mouth or other taste changes ■ general feeling of unwell-	If symptoms are disturbing or persist, let your doctor know.

ness ■ loss of appetite ■ diarrhea ■ stomach pain
■ gas ■ blurred vision

After you STOP taking this medicine: nausea
■ headache ■ general feeling of unwellness

STORAGE INSTRUCTIONS

Store in a cool, dark place (not in a bathroom medicine cabinet).

STOPPING OR INTERRUPTING THERAPY

Do not suddenly stop taking this medicine; your doctor will advise you on how to gradually decrease your dosage. If you miss a dose of this medicine, take it as soon as possible. If it is not within an hour of the scheduled time for the missed dose, skip it and resume your regular schedule. Do not take two doses at the same time.

SPECIAL CONSIDERATIONS FOR THOSE OVER SIXTY-FIVE

Older people may be more prone to such side effects as dry mouth, difficulty in urination, and constipation.

CONDITION: **MUSCLE INJURIES**

CATEGORY: **MUSCLE RELAXANT–ANALGESIC COMBINATIONS**

GENERIC (CHEMICAL) NAME	BRAND (TRADE) NAME	DOSAGE FORMS AND STRENGTHS
Chlorzoxazone and acetaminophen	PARAFON FORTE	Tablets: 250 mg chlorzoxazone and 300 mg acetaminophen

DRUG PROFILE

The combination of chlorzoxazone and acetaminophen is used to relieve pain and discomfort from strains, sprains, and other muscle injuries. Chlorzoxazone relaxes the muscles, while acetaminophen alleviates pain. Chlorzoxazone-acetaminophen is used as part of a treatment program that may include rest, physical therapy, and other drugs.

BEFORE USING THIS DRUG

Let your doctor know *IF*

You have ever had allergic reactions or other problems with ■ acetaminophen ■ chlorzoxazone ■ tartrazine (FD&C Yellow Dye No. 5) ■ any other drug.

You have ever had any of the following medical problems: ■ eczema, hay fever, hives, or other allergic reactions ■ asthma or other lung disease ■ kidney disease ■ liver disease ■ heart disease ■ anemia.

You are taking any of the following medicines: ■ other muscle relaxants ■ antibiotics ■ charcoal ■ sleep medicines ■ tranquilizers ■ medicine for depression (within the last two weeks) ■ narcotics or other prescription pain-killers.

SPECIAL RESTRICTIONS WHILE TAKING THIS DRUG

FOOD AND DRUG INTERACTIONS

Other Drugs	Do not take any other drugs, including over-the-counter (OTC) drugs, before checking with your doctor. This medicine increases the effect of other drugs that depress the central nervous system, such as other muscle relaxants; antihistamines; medicines for hay fever, allergies, or colds; sleep medicines; tranquilizers; narcotics or other prescription pain-killers; and medicine for seizures. In addition, be especially careful about using other medicines that contain acetaminophen. Check the labels of all other drugs you are taking.
Alcohol	This drug increases the effect of alcohol, a central nervous system depressant. Avoid alcohol unless your doctor has approved its use.

No special restrictions on foods and beverages or smoking.

DAILY LIVING

Driving	This drug may cause dizziness, light-headedness, or faintness. Be careful when driving, operating house-

hold appliances, or doing any other tasks that require alertness until you know how this drug affects you.

Exertion and Exercise	Discuss with your doctor which kinds of physical exercise are safe for you to undertake.
Examinations or Tests	It is important for you to keep all appointments with your doctor so that your progress can be checked.
Other Precautions	If overdose of this medicine is suspected, call your doctor or go to a hospital emergency room immediately. Tell any doctor or dentist you consult that you are taking this drug, especially if you will be undergoing any type of surgery.
Helpful Hints	This drug may cause your urine to turn orange or reddish-purple. This effect will disappear once you stop taking this drug. Tablets may be crushed and mixed with soft foods, milk, or fruit juice.

No special restrictions on sun exposure or exposure to excessive heat or cold.

POSSIBLE SIDE EFFECTS

Although this list of adverse effects may seem somewhat intimidating, keep in mind that some are quite rare. Of course, should these or any other problems arise while you are on medication, it is always a good idea to consult your doctor.

IF YOU DEVELOP

swelling of lips, face, or tongue ■ shallow or fast breathing ■ increased sweating ■ muscle weakness ■ stomach cramps or pain ■ nausea or vom-

WHAT TO DO

Urgent Get in touch with your doctor immediately.

iting ■ diarrhea ■ loss of appetite ■ hoarseness ■ delirium ■ severe dizziness or drowsiness ■ clammy skin ■ fast, weak, or irregular pulse

bloody or black, tarry stools, ■ bloody or cloudy urine or other changes in urination ■ tiredness or weakness ■ skin redness, itching, rash, or hives	**May be serious** Check with your doctor as soon as possible.
drowsiness ■ dizziness or light-headedness ■ excitement ■ restlessness ■ anxiety ■ headache ■ constipation ■ upset stomach ■ general feeling of unwellness	If symptoms are disturbing or persist, let your doctor know.

STORAGE INSTRUCTIONS

Store in a cool, dark place (not in a bathroom medicine cabinet).

STOPPING OR INTERRUPTING THERAPY

Take this medicine exactly as instructed by your doctor. Do not take more of it or for a longer period of time than prescribed. If you miss a dose, take it as soon as possible. If it is almost time for your next dose, skip the missed dose and resume your regular schedule. Do not take two doses at the same time.

SPECIAL CONSIDERATIONS FOR THOSE OVER SIXTY-FIVE

None.

CONDITION: **MUSCLE INJURIES**

CATEGORY: **MUSCLE RELAXANT–ANALGESIC COMBINATIONS**

GENERIC (CHEMICAL) NAME	BRAND (TRADE) NAME	DOSAGE FORMS AND STRENGTHS
Orphenadrine citrate, aspirin, and caffeine	NORGESIC	Tablets: 25 mg orphenadrine citrate, 385 mg aspirin, and 30 mg caffeine

NORGESIC FORTE	Tablets: 50 mg orphenadrine citrate, 770 mg aspirin, and 60 mg caffeine

DRUG PROFILE

This combination of orphenadrine, aspirin, and caffeine is used to relieve pain and discomfort from strains, sprains, or other muscle injuries. Orphenadrine reduces muscle spasm, while aspirin controls pain and swelling by blocking the production of naturally occurring triggers of pain and inflammation, called prostaglandins. Caffeine strengthens the action of the aspirin. This medicine is used as part of a treatment program that may include rest, physical therapy, and additional drugs.

BEFORE USING THIS DRUG

Let your doctor know *IF*

You have ever had allergic reactions or other problems with ■ orphenadrine ■ caffeine ■ aspirin or any other salicylate drug ■ indomethacin ■ ibuprofen ■ mefenamic acid ■ phenylbutazone ■ sodium benzoate.

You have ever had any of the following medical problems: ■ hay fever ■ asthma ■ ulcers or gastritis ■ lesions of the digestive tract ■ liver disease ■ kidney disease ■ systemic lupus erythematosus ■ glucose-6-phosphate dehydrogenase (G-6-PD) deficiency ■ vitamin K deficiency ■ nasal polyps ■ pyruvate kinase deficiency ■ chronic hives ■ chronic stuffy nose ■ rheumatic fever ■ disease of the blood vessels ■ any bleeding disorder ■ recent oral surgery ■ diabetes ■ overactive thyroid ■ heart disease, including abnormal heart rhythms ■ high blood pressure ■ enlarged prostate ■ difficulty in urination ■ congestive heart failure ■ glaucoma.

You are taking any of the following medicines: ■ any other pain-killers ■ medicine for gout ■ medicine for arthritis ■ anticoagulants (blood thinners) ■ corticosteroids ■ antacids ■ any medicine containing magnesium ■ any medicine containing alcohol ■ beta-blockers ■ medicine for high blood pressure ■ thiazide diuretics (water pills) ■ captopril (medicine for congestive heart failure and high blood pressure) ■ medicine for glaucoma ■ medicine for seizures ■ medicine for diabetes ■ methotrexate (medicine for severe psoriasis or cancer) ■ nitrates (medicine for chest pain) ■ medicine to make the urine more alkaline or more acidic ■ medicine for tuberculosis ■ phenothiazines (medicine for nausea or severe anxiety) ■ acetaminophen ■ tranquilizers ■ digoxin, digitoxin, or digitalis (heart medicines) ■ antibiotics ■ medicine for Parkinson's disease ■ sleep medicines ■ quinidine or disopyramide (medicine for abnormal heart rhythms) ■ potassium-containing medicines or supplements ■ cimetidine (medicine for ulcers) ■ barbiturates ■ medicine for stomach cramps ■ medicine for hay fever, coughs, or colds ■ antihistamines ■ medicine for depression ■ nitrofurantoin (medicine for urinary tract infections).

SPECIAL RESTRICTIONS WHILE TAKING THIS DRUG

FOOD AND DRUG INTERACTIONS

Other Drugs	Do not take any other drugs, including over-the-counter (OTC) drugs, before checking with your doctor. This medicine increases the effect of other drugs that depress the central nervous system, such as other muscle relaxants; antihistamines; medicines for hay fever, allergies, or colds; sleep medicines; tranquilizers; narcotics or other prescription pain-killers; and medicine for seizures. In addition, be especially careful about using other medicines that contain salicylates. Check the labels of all other drugs you are taking, as well as such products as special shampoos, lotions, and creams, to see if they contain aspirin, salicylic acid, or other salicylate drugs.
Alcohol	This drug increases the effect of alcohol, a central nervous system depressant. Alcohol may also add to the irritant effects of aspirin on your stomach. Avoid alcohol unless your doctor has approved its use.

No special restrictions on foods and beverages or smoking.

DAILY LIVING

Driving	This drug may cause dizziness, light-headedness, or faintness. Be careful when driving, operating household appliances, or doing any other tasks that require alertness until you know how this drug affects you.

Exertion and Exercise	Discuss with your doctor which kinds of physical exercise are safe for you to undertake.
Examinations or Tests	It is important for you to keep all appointments with your doctor so that your progress can be checked.
Other Precautions	If you have diabetes, be aware that false urine-sugar tests may occur while you are taking an aspirin-containing drug. Check with your doctor before increasing the dose of any diabetes medicine you may be taking.
	Tell any doctor or dentist you consult that you are taking this drug, especially if you will be undergoing any type of surgery.
	Let your doctor know if you notice a buzzing or ringing sound in your ears, since this may be a sign of aspirin overdose.
	If you accidentally take an overdose of this drug, go to a hospital emergency room immediately.
Helpful Hints	To reduce risk of possible stomach upset, take this drug with meals, milk, snacks, or a full glass of water.
	If your mouth or throat feels dry, chewing sugarless gum or sucking ice chips or sugarless hard candy will help.

No special restrictions on sun exposure or exposure to excessive heat or cold.

POSSIBLE SIDE EFFECTS

Although this list of adverse effects may seem somewhat intimidating, keep in mind that some are quite rare. Of course, should these or any other problems arise while you are on medication, it is always a good idea to consult your doctor.

IF YOU DEVELOP	WHAT TO DO
seizures ■ confusion ■ severe or continuing headache ■ blood in urine or decreased urination ■ irregular or fast heartbeat ■ diarrhea ■ severe dizziness, light-headedness, or drowsiness ■ extreme excitement or nervousness ■ hallucinations ■ delirium ■ unusual talkativeness or incoherence ■ personality changes ■ tremors ■ severe or continuing nausea or vomiting ■ difficulty in breathing ■ rapid, deep breathing ■ continuing stomach pain ■ fever ■ increased sweating ■ increased thirst ■ blurred vision or other visual disturbances ■ uncontrollable flapping movements of the hands ■ tearing eyes ■ fainting	**Urgent** Get in touch with your doctor immediately.
stomach pain or tenderness ■ nausea or vomiting ■ bloody or black, tarry stools ■ vomiting, with blood or vomit that looks like coffee grounds ■ ringing or buzzing in ears ■ tightness in chest ■ wheezing ■ rash, hives, or itching ■ tiredness or weakness ■ bleeding or bruising ■ loss of taste for cigarettes ■ hoarseness ■ flushing ■ eye pain ■ hallucinations ■ excitement, nervousness, or restlessness ■ sleeplessness	**May be serious** Check with your doctor as soon as possible.
dry mouth ■ heartburn or indigestion ■ loss of appetite ■ anxiety ■ drowsiness, dizziness, or light-headedness ■ constipation ■ difficulty in urination ■ increased eye sensitivity to light ■ decreased sweating ■ loss of taste ■ bloating	If symptoms are disturbing or persist, let your doctor know.

STORAGE INSTRUCTIONS

Store in a cool, dark place (not in a bathroom medicine cabinet). If you notice a vinegarlike odor from the bottle, this means that the drug is breaking down and should be discarded.

STOPPING OR INTERRUPTING THERAPY

If you miss a dose of this medicine, take it as soon as possible. If it is not within an hour of the scheduled time for the missed dose, skip it and resume your regular schedule. Do not take two doses at the same time.

SPECIAL CONSIDERATIONS FOR THOSE OVER SIXTY-FIVE

Those older people who have reduced kidney function tend not to eliminate the salicylates as readily as people with normal kidney function. For this reason, doctors may check such people regularly to make sure they are receiving the proper dosage and that too much drug is not accumulating in the body.

CONDITION: **MUSCLE INJURIES**

CATEGORY: **MUSCLE RELAXANT–ANALGESIC COMBINATIONS**

GENERIC (CHEMICAL) NAME	BRAND (TRADE) NAME	DOSAGE FORMS AND STRENGTHS
Carisoprodol and aspirin	SOMA COMPOUND	Tablets: 200 mg carisoprodol and 325 mg aspirin
Methocarbamol and aspirin	ROBAXISAL	Tablets: 400 mg methocarbamol and 325 mg aspirin

DRUG PROFILE

These combination drugs are used to relieve pain and discomfort from strains, sprains, or other muscle injuries. Carisoprodol and methocarbamol relax the muscles, while aspirin controls pain by blocking the production of naturally occurring triggers of pain and inflammation, called prostaglandins. These medicines are used as part of a treatment program that may include rest, physical therapy, and other drugs.

BEFORE USING THIS DRUG

Let your doctor know *IF*

You have ever had allergic reactions or other problems with ■ carisoprodol ■ methocarbamol ■ carbromal ■ mebutamate ■ tybamate ■ aspirin or any other salicylate drug ■ indomethacin ■ ibuprofen ■ mefenamic acid ■ phenylbutazone ■ sodium benzoate ■ tartrazine (FD&C Yellow Dye No. 5).

You have ever had any of the following medical problems: ■ hay fever ■ asthma ■ ulcers or gastritis ■ lesions of the digestive tract ■ liver disease ■ kidney disease ■ systemic lupus erythematosus ■ glucose-6-phosphate dehydrogenase (G-6-PD) deficiency ■ vitamin K deficiency ■ pyruvate kinase deficiency ■ nasal polyps ■ chronic hives ■ chronic stuffy nose ■ rheumatic fever ■ disease of the blood vessels ■ any bleeding disorder ■ recent oral surgery ■ diabetes ■ hypoglycemia ■ hearing problems ■ anemia.

■ *with carisoprodol only:* ■ drug abuse, including alcoholism ■ porphyria.

■ *with methocarbamol only:* ■ myasthenia gravis.

If you are taking any of the following medicines: ■ other muscle relaxants ■ medicine for gout ■ medicine for arthritis ■ anticoagulants (blood thinners) ■ corticosteroids ■ antacids ■ any medicine containing magnesium ■ any medicine containing alcohol ■ beta-blockers ■ medicine for high blood pressure ■ diuretics ■ captopril (medicine for congestive heart failure) ■ medicine for glaucoma ■ medicine for seizures ■ medicine for diabetes ■ methotrexate (medicine for severe psoriasis and cancer) ■ nitrates (medicine for chest pain) ■ medicine to make the urine more alkaline or more acidic ■ medicine for tuberculosis ■ medicine for nausea or vomiting ■ acetaminophen ■ barbiturates ■ medicine for depression (within the last two weeks) ■ antihistamines ■ medicine for hay fever, coughs, or colds ■ sleep medicines ■ narcotics or other prescription painkillers ■ tranquilizers.

■ *with methocarbamol only:* ■ medicine for myasthenia gravis.

SPECIAL RESTRICTIONS WHILE TAKING THIS DRUG

FOOD AND DRUG INTERACTIONS

Other Drugs	Do not take any other drugs, including over-the-counter (OTC) drugs, before checking with your doctor. This medicine increases the effect of other drugs

that depress the central nervous system, such as other muscle relaxants; antihistamines; medicine for hay fever, allergies, and colds; sleep medicines; tranquilizers; narcotics or other prescription pain-killers; and medicine for seizures. In addition, be especially careful about using other medicines that contain salicylates. Check the labels of all other drugs you are taking, as well as such products as special shampoos, lotions, and creams, to see if they contain aspirin, salicylic acid, or other salicylate drugs.

Alcohol	This drug increases the effect of alcohol, a central nervous system depressant. Alcohol may also add to the irritant effects of aspirin on your stomach. Avoid alcohol unless your doctor has approved its use.

No special restrictions on foods and beverages or smoking.

DAILY LIVING

Driving	This drug may cause dizziness, light-headedness, or faintness. Be careful when driving, operating household appliances, or doing any other tasks that require alertness until you know how this drug affects you.
Exertion and Exercise	Discuss with your doctor which kinds of physical exercise are safe for you to undertake.
Examinations or Tests	It is important for you to keep all appointments with your doctor so that your progress can be checked.
Other Precautions	If you have diabetes, be aware that false urine-sugar tests may occur while you are taking an aspirin-containing drug. Check with your doctor before increasing the dose of any diabetes medicine you may be taking.

Tell any doctor or dentist you consult that you are taking either of these drugs, especially if you will be undergoing any type of surgery.

Let your doctor know if you notice a buzzing or ringing sound in your ears, as this may be a sign of aspirin overdose. If you accidentally take an overdose of either of these drugs, go to a hospital emergency room immediately.

Helpful Hints

If you are taking methocarbamol, your urine may turn a black, brown, or green color. This is a harmless reaction and will subside once you have stopped taking this medicine.

No special restrictions on sun exposure or exposure to excessive heat or cold.

POSSIBLE SIDE EFFECTS

Although this list of adverse effects may seem somewhat intimidating, keep in mind that some are quite rare. Of course, should these or any other problems arise while you are on medication, it is always a good idea to consult your doctor.

IF YOU DEVELOP

seizures ■ confusion ■ severe or continuing headache ■ blood in urine or decreased urination ■ fast heartbeat ■ diarrhea ■ severe dizziness, light-headedness, or drowsiness ■ extreme excitement or nervousness ■ hallucinations ■ talkativeness, incoherence, or speech difficulties ■ personality changes ■ tremors ■ severe or continuing nausea or vomiting ■ difficulty in breathing ■ rapid, deep breathing ■ continuing stomach pain ■ fever ■ increased sweating ■ increased thirst ■ uncontrollable flapping movements of the hands ■ tearing eyes ■ fainting ■ inability to walk ■ extreme weakness ■ blurred or double vision

With carisoprodol only: "high" feeling

WHAT TO DO

Urgent: Stop taking the drug and get in touch with your doctor immediately.

stomach pain or tenderness ■ nausea or vomiting ■ bloody or black, tarry stools ■ vomiting, with blood, or vomit that looks like coffee grounds ■ ringing or buzzing in ears ■ tightness in chest ■ wheezing ■ rash, hives, itching, or other skin problems ■ tiredness or weakness ■ bleeding or bruising ■ loss of taste for cigarettes ■ smarting eyes ■ depression ■ excitement ■ anxiety ■ muscle weakness ■ swelling of face, lips, or tongue ■ yellowing of eyes or skin

With carisoprodol only: flushing

After you STOP taking carisoprodol: stomach cramps ■ sleeplessness ■ chills ■ headache ■ nausea

May be serious Check with your doctor as soon as possible.

dizziness or light-headedness, especially when getting up from a reclining or sitting position ■ drowsiness ■ clumsiness ■ more frequent bowel movements ■ hiccups ■ headache ■ restlessness ■ irritability ■ sleeplessness ■ loss of appetite ■ heartburn or indigestion ■ diarrhea ■ constipation ■ stuffy nose ■ sore throat

If symptoms are disturbing or persist, let your doctor know.

STORAGE INSTRUCTIONS

Store in a cool, dark place (not in a bathroom medicine cabinet). If you notice a vinegarlike odor from the bottle, this means that the drug is breaking down and should be discarded.

STOPPING OR INTERRUPTING THERAPY

Do not suddenly stop taking this medicine; your doctor will advise you on how to gradually decrease your dosage. If you miss a dose of either of these medicines, take it as soon as possible. If it is not within an hour of the scheduled time for the missed dose, skip it and resume your regular schedule. Do not take two doses at the same time.

SPECIAL CONSIDERATIONS FOR THOSE OVER SIXTY-FIVE

Those older people who have decreased kidney or liver function tend not to eliminate the salicylates as readily as people with normal kidney or liver function. For this reason, doctors may check such people regularly to make sure they are receiving the proper dosage and that too much drug is not accumulating in the body.

CONDITION: **NIGHT CRAMPS**

CATEGORY: **MUSCLE RELAXANTS**

GENERIC (CHEMICAL) NAME	BRAND (TRADE) NAME	DOSAGE FORMS AND STRENGTHS
Quinine sulfate	QUINAMM	Tablets: 260 mg

DRUG PROFILE

Quinine is used to treat nighttime leg muscle cramps. This drug acts directly on the muscles to make them less excitable by nerve impulses.

BEFORE USING THIS DRUG

Let your doctor know *IF*

You have ever had allergic reactions or other problems with ■ quinine ■ quinidine.

You have ever had any of the following medical problems: ■ asthma ■ eye disease, including optic neuritis ■ glucose-6-phosphate dehydrogenase (G-6-PD) deficiency ■ blood disease ■ hearing problems (especially noises in the ear) ■ heart disease, including abnormal heart rhythms ■ blackwater fever.

You are taking any of the following medicines: ■ any medicine containing quinine (includes some cold products) ■ quinidine (medicine for abnormal heart rhythms) ■ digoxin, digitoxin, or digitalis (heart medicines) ■ medicine to make the urine less acidic ■ antacids containing aluminum ■ anticoagulants (blood thinners) ■ medicine for myasthenia gravis ■ tranquilizers.

SPECIAL RESTRICTIONS WHILE TAKING THIS DRUG

FOOD AND DRUG INTERACTIONS

Other Drugs	If you are taking any heart drugs (digoxin, digitoxin, or digitalis), consult your doctor, since the combination with quinine may result in dangerously high levels of these drugs.
	Avoid antacids that contain aluminum, since they may interfere with the body's absorption of quinine.

No special restrictions on foods and beverages, alcohol use, or smoking.

DAILY LIVING

Examinations or Tests	It is important for you to keep all appointments with your doctor so that your progress can be checked.
Other Precautions	Tell any doctor or dentist you consult that you are taking this drug, especially if you will be undergoing any type of surgery.
Helpful Hints	If this medicine upsets your stomach, taking it with milk, meals, or snacks should help.

No special restrictions on driving, exertion and exercise, sun exposure, or exposure to excessive heat or cold.

POSSIBLE SIDE EFFECTS

Although this list of adverse effects may seem somewhat intimidating, keep in mind that some are quite rare. Of course, should these or any other problems arise while you are on medication, it is always a good idea to consult your doctor.

IF YOU DEVELOP	WHAT TO DO
chest pain ■ irregular heartbeat ■ seizures ■ ringing or buzzing in the ears or other hearing disturbances ■ blurred vision or other visual disturbances ■ rash, hives, or itching ■ wheezing ■ shortness of breath ■ difficulty in breathing ■ fever ■ flushing ■ confusion ■ fainting	**Urgent** Get in touch with your doctor immediately.
dizziness ■ severe headache ■ swelling of face ■ increased sweating ■ feeling of dread ■ restlessness ■ increased eye sensitivity to light	**May be serious** Check with your doctor as soon as possible.
diarrhea ■ nausea or vomiting ■ stomach cramps or pain	If symptoms are disturbing or persist, let your doctor know.

STORAGE INSTRUCTIONS

Store in a cool, dark place (not in a bathroom medicine cabinet).

STOPPING OR INTERRUPTING THERAPY

If you miss a dose of this medicine, take it as soon as possible. If it is not within an hour of the scheduled time for the missed dose, skip it and resume your regular schedule. Do not take two doses at the same time.

SPECIAL CONSIDERATIONS FOR THOSE OVER SIXTY-FIVE

This drug is metabolized by the liver; since liver function sometimes decreases with age, doctors may start people over sixty-five on a lower dosage.

CONDITION: **MUSCLE CRAMPING AND STIFFENING**

CATEGORY: **MUSCLE RELAXANTS**

GENERIC (CHEMICAL) NAME	BRAND (TRADE) NAME	DOSAGE FORMS AND STRENGTHS
Baclofen	LIORESAL	Tablets: 10, 20 mg

DRUG PROFILE

Baclofen is used to relieve the spasm, cramping, and stiffening of muscles caused by multiple sclerosis or spinal cord injuries. This drug is thought to act on the spinal cord, blocking certain nerve impulses. Baclofen is used as part of a treatment program that may include rest, physical therapy, and other drugs.

BEFORE USING THIS DRUG

Let your doctor know *IF*

You have ever had allergic reactions or other problems with ■ baclofen.

You have ever had any of the following medical problems: ■ seizures ■ kidney disease ■ mental or emotional problems ■ stroke ■ stomach ulcer ■ diabetes.

You are taking any of the following medicines: ■ other muscle relaxants ■ medicine for seizures ■ antihistamines ■ medicine for hay fever, coughs, or colds ■ barbiturates ■ medicine for depression (within the last two weeks) ■ narcotics or other prescription pain-killers ■ tranquilizers ■ sleep medicines ■ medicine for diabetes.

SPECIAL RESTRICTIONS WHILE TAKING THIS DRUG

FOOD AND DRUG INTERACTIONS

Other Drugs	Do not take any other drugs, including over-the-counter (OTC) drugs, before checking with your doctor. This medicine increases the effect of other drugs

that depress the central nervous system, such as other muscle relaxants; antihistamines; medicine for hay fever, allergies, or colds; sleep medicines; tranquilizers; narcotics or other prescription pain-killers; and medicine for seizures.

Alcohol	This drug increases the effect of alcohol, a central nervous system depressant. Avoid alcohol unless your doctor has approved its use.

No special restrictions on foods and beverages or smoking.

DAILY LIVING

Driving	This drug may cause dizziness, light-headedness, or faintness. Be careful when driving, operating household appliances, or doing any other tasks that require alertness until you know how this drug affects you.
Exertion and Exercise	Discuss with your doctor which kinds of physical exercise are safe for you to undertake.
Examinations or Tests	It is important for you to keep all appointments with your doctor so that your progress can be checked.
Other Precautions	Tell any doctor or dentist you consult that you are taking this drug, especially if you will be undergoing any type of surgery.
	If you have diabetes, be aware that this medicine may affect blood-sugar levels. If you notice any change when testing sugar levels in your blood or urine, let your doctor know.

No special restrictions on sun exposure or exposure to excessive heat or cold.

POSSIBLE SIDE EFFECTS

Although this list of adverse effects may seem somewhat intimidating, keep in mind that some are quite rare. Of course, should these or any other problems arise while you are on medication, it is always a good idea to consult your doctor.

IF YOU DEVELOP	WHAT TO DO
seizures ■ difficulty in breathing ■ irregular heart-beat ■ blurred or double vision or other visual disturbances	**Urgent** Get in touch with your doctor immediately.
chest pain ■ bloody or dark urine ■ fainting ■ hallucinations ■ depression ■ anxiety ■ ringing or buzzing in ears ■ rash or itching ■ clumsiness ■ speech difficulties ■ tremors ■ rigid muscles ■ twitching ■ vomiting	**May be serious** Check with your doctor as soon as possible.
drowsiness, dizziness, or light-headedness ■ muscle weakness, pain, or stiffness ■ uncontrol-lable movements ■ nausea ■ confusion ■ weight gain ■ swelling of ankles ■ stomach pain ■ con-stipation ■ diarrhea ■ loss of appetite ■ numb-ness or tingling in hands or feet ■ slurred speech ■ male impotence ■ inability to ejaculate ■ excite-ment ■ "high" feeling ■ sleeplessness ■ stuffy nose ■ dry mouth ■ taste changes ■ positive test for occult blood in stool ■ pain or difficulty in urina-tion ■ urinary frequency ■ increased sweating	If symptoms are disturbing or persist, let your doctor know.

STORAGE INSTRUCTIONS

Store in a cool, dark place (not in a bathroom medicine cabinet).

STOPPING OR INTERRUPTING THERAPY

Do not suddenly stop taking this medicine; your doctor will advise you on how to decrease your dosage gradually. If you miss a dose of this medicine, take it as soon as possible. If it is not within an hour of the scheduled time for the missed dose, skip it and resume your regular schedule. Do not take two doses at the same time.

SPECIAL CONSIDERATIONS FOR THOSE OVER SIXTY-FIVE

Older people are more prone to such mental and emotional side effects as hallucinations, confusion, depression, anxiety, and excitement, as well as drowsiness.

MYASTHENIA GRAVIS

Myasthenia gravis, a disease marked by progressive muscle weakness, is most common among women in their twenties and thirties. In men, however, most cases of the disease occur after the age of forty.

CAUSES

Every voluntary movement, from scratching to swallowing to blinking your eyes, originates in the brain, which sends electrical signals along a complex network of nerve pathways leading to the muscles. In myasthenia gravis, the nerve-to-muscle transmission of these electrical impulses does not work properly because of a flaw in the muscles—specifically, in the structures known as receptors that are located on the muscle-cell surfaces. These receptors fail to take up a chemical messenger called acetylcholine (ACh), which is a vital link in the nerve-to-muscle pathway.

Myasthenia gravis is termed an autoimmune disease because the immune system produces antibodies that block off most of the ACh receptors. The result is mild to extreme muscle weakness. In many people with myasthenia gravis, the thymus gland appears to be involved. The thymus gland, which is located inside the chest, is part of the immune system. Seventy percent of people with myasthenia gravis have an enlarged thymus gland, and another 10 to 15 percent have tumors of the thymus gland.

DIAGNOSIS

Early symptoms of myasthenia gravis may be so subtle that they go unnoticed. In 50 percent of cases, double vision (which may be accompanied by drooping eyelids) first alerts the person that something is wrong. Within about a year, the symptoms generally progress to include weakness in the limbs, the other facial muscles, and, in the most severe cases, the muscles involved in swallowing and breathing. Another hallmark of the disease is a feeling of tiredness after only slight use of the affected muscles. Most of the time, the symptoms are least severe in the morning, after a long period of rest. As the day progresses, the weakness worsens. It also tends to become more pronounced with exercise and with emotional stress.

The course of myasthenia gravis varies widely; some people with the disease suffer a life-threatening near-paralysis of the respiratory muscles, while others have symptoms limited to the facial muscles. Early in the disease, about 25 percent of patients have spontaneous remissions, during which time symptoms improve markedly or disappear altogether. Such remissions, however, are never permanent in the absence of therapy.

If a pattern of symptoms leads the doctor to suspect that myasthenia gravis may be the problem, the diagnosis can be confirmed by injecting a small amount of a drug that temporarily increases the activity of ACh. In a person who has myasthenia gravis, the injection will cause the symptoms to improve greatly for a short time. Further tests—including electromyography, which charts a muscle's response to electrical stimulation, and blood tests for certain antibodies—may also be performed.

TREATMENT

The treatment used most often for myasthenia gravis is aimed at reducing the disease's symptoms and stopping its progression rather than halting the abnormal immune response itself. Many people with myasthenia gravis are on long-term therapy with anticholinesterase drugs; these work the same way as the drug used in diagnosing the condition. One of the most common of these drugs is pyridostigmine bromide (see drug chart on pages 427–429). These medicines work best for people who understand their disease and know what activities and times of day are associated with the worst symptoms. Such people can gauge the amount of medicine they'll need, much as a person who has diabetes can calculate the amount of insulin required in different circumstances.

Other drugs sometimes used to treat myasthenia gravis are corticosteroids (see drug chart on pages 439–443) and adrenocorticotropic hormone (ACTH).

These drugs suppress the immune system, thus reducing the level of circulating antibodies that block off ACh receptors. Another treatment that removes antibodies from the blood is plasma exchange, a process in which the plasma, which contains antibodies, is separated from other components of the blood.

Finally, thymectomy, or surgical removal of the thymus gland, is an option for many people with myasthenia gravis. After a thymectomy, medicine must be continued for some time—months to years, in some cases—but improvement eventually occurs in 85 percent of people who undergo the procedure. About one-third of those people experience total remission.

OUTLOOK

Myasthenia gravis varies greatly from person to person. Some individuals with the condition are severely disabled, while others are able to lead near-normal lives. The outlook for most people with myasthenia gravis has, however, improved greatly in the past several years as treatments effective against even its worst symptoms have been developed. Current research efforts, directed at understanding and correcting the immune disorder that underlies myasthenia gravis, hold promise for even better therapeutic approaches to this chronic disease.

CONDITION: **MYASTHENIA GRAVIS**

CATEGORY: **MUSCLE STIMULANTS**

GENERIC (CHEMICAL) NAME	BRAND (TRADE) NAME	DOSAGE FORMS AND STRENGTHS
Pyridostigmine bromide	MESTINON	Controlled-release tablets: 180 mg Syrup: 60 mg per tsp Tablets: 60 mg

DRUG PROFILE

Pyridostigmine is used to treat the muscular weakness and fatigue associated with myasthenia gravis. This drug acts both directly and through the nervous system to increase muscle tone.

BEFORE USING THIS DRUG

Let your doctor know *IF*

You have ever had allergic reactions or other problems with ■ pyridostigmine.

You have ever had any of the following medical problems: ■ asthma ■ intestinal or urinary tract blockage ■ seizures ■ slow heartbeat ■ blood vessel disease ■ spastic disorder ■ overactive thyroid ■ abnormal heart rhythms ■ stomach ulcers.

You are taking any of the following medicines: ■ corticosteroids ■ antibiotics ■ medicine for abnormal heart rhythms ■ quinine (medicine for malaria).

SPECIAL RESTRICTIONS WHILE TAKING THIS DRUG

FOOD AND DRUG INTERACTIONS

No special restrictions on other drugs, foods and beverages, alcohol use, or smoking.

DAILY LIVING

Driving	This drug may cause double vision or other visual disturbances. Be careful when driving, operating household appliances, or doing any other tasks that require alertness until you know how this drug affects you.
Examinations or Tests	It is important for you to keep all appointments with your doctor so that your progress can be checked.
Other Precautions	Tell any doctor or dentist you consult that you are taking this drug, especially if you will be undergoing any type of surgery.
	The controlled-release tablet should be swallowed whole, without crushing, breaking, or chewing.

No special restrictions on exertion and exercise, sun exposure, or exposure to excessive heat or cold.

POSSIBLE SIDE EFFECTS

Although this list of adverse effects may seem somewhat intimidating, keep in mind that some are quite rare. Of course, should these or any other problems arise while you are on medication, it is always a good idea to consult your doctor.

IF YOU DEVELOP	WHAT TO DO
seizures	**Urgent** Get in touch with your doctor immediately.
difficulty in breathing ■ slow or fast heartbeat ■ muscle cramps or pain ■ weakness ■ muscle weakness, especially in the neck ■ nausea or vomiting ■ diarrhea ■ stomach cramps ■ dilated pupils ■ increased salivation ■ increased sweating ■ fainting ■ dizziness ■ double vision or other visual disturbances ■ increased urination ■ diffi-	**May be serious** Check with your doctor as soon as possible.

culty in chewing or in swallowing ■ agitation
■ restlessness ■ tearing eyes ■ increased phlegm
production ■ clumsiness

STORAGE INSTRUCTIONS

Store in a cool, dark place (not in a bathroom medicine cabinet). If your medicine is in a liquid form, make sure that it does not freeze.

STOPPING OR INTERRUPTING THERAPY

If you miss a dose, take it as soon as possible. If it is almost time for your next dose, skip the missed dose (unless you are experiencing muscular weakness) and resume your regular schedule. Do not take two doses at the same time.

SPECIAL CONSIDERATIONS FOR THOSE OVER SIXTY-FIVE

None.

ARTHRITIS

Arthritis is a common ailment, affecting more than thirty-six million people in the United States. Yet it's not well understood by most people—even those who have it—partly because this single term actually refers to a host of different disorders.

Arthritis occurs when the delicate architecture of the joints—the meeting places of bones—is damaged. Just a few points can be affected or many; within a joint, the destruction of key components (such as the tough, shock-absorbing cartilage between bones) can be partial or total. The condition is marked by pain and sometimes by inflammation (swelling, redness, heat) in the joints. Arthritis sometimes causes disfigurement, ranging from gnarled fingers to a curved spine. Fortunately, though, new treatments reduce these crippling effects.

CAUSES

By far the most common form of the disease is osteoarthritis (OA). This condition affects an estimated sixteen million people in the United States, mainly older people. Older patients often assume that their symptoms are due to growing old; however, much OA results from a combination of the biological changes of aging, traumatic injuries to the body, and metabolic, immunologic, or inherited structural changes. Many doctors think that the major cause of osteoarthritis is the gradual wear and tear our joints experience over the years.

The main symptoms of OA are pain and stiffness in one or more joints. The joints most often affected include those of the fingers, the base of the thumb, the neck, the hips, the lower back, and the knees. The pain, which can range from dull aches to occasional sharp peaks, is often strongest first thing in the morning. Some people claim they can predict the weather by the severity of their pain. You may not want to plan a picnic by it, but arthritis pain sometimes is influenced by prevailing weather conditions.

Although the word *arthritis* literally means "joint inflammation," OA often occurs without significant inflammation. Swelling of the knee may occur, but there is no fever or other systemic symptom of inflammation.

The next most common type of arthritis is rheumatoid arthritis (RA), which affects about seven million people in the United States. This is the form of the disease most likely to be crippling. Although RA can strike at any age, it most often occurs in early to middle adulthood. However, it is not unusual for persons sixty to seventy years old to get it. About three-quarters of its victims are women. Researchers suspect that RA is an autoimmune disease, in which the body mistakenly perceives some of its own tissues as foreign and the immune system launches an attack against them. No one knows precisely what triggers this attack.

Unlike osteoarthritis, rheumatoid

arthritis can sometimes develop quite rapidly, and it *always* involves inflammation of the joints. In some cases, tissues other than joints become inflamed as well. Joints in the hands and feet are most commonly affected, but any and all joints can fall prey. The symptoms of the disease may subside for unpredictable lengths of time, only to flare up again.

Of the many other forms of arthritis, the most common in older people is gout. Gout usually strikes men over forty and involves acute pain in a single joint, usually the big toe. (See pages 450–451 for more on gout.) Another form, polymyalgia rheumatica, affects mostly people over sixty. Common symptoms are fever; weight loss; and pain in the neck, back, shoulders, upper arms, or thighs. An accompanying condition, known as giant-cell arteritis, may cause blindness.

DIAGNOSIS AND TREATMENT

If you have persistent pain, stiffness, or inflammation in any of your joints, see your doctor. A careful medical examination, along with various blood tests and possibly X rays, can help him or her determine whether you are suffering from arthritis and, if so, what form of the disease you have. Depending on the situation, your doctor may refer you to an arthritis specialist (rheumatologist).

Your treatment plan should be tailored to your particular case. One key to living with arthritis is to neither overwork nor underwork the affected joints; therefore, appropriate doses of moderate exercise and rest are likely to be part of your therapy program. A more formal physical therapy program may be part of your treatment plan. Electric blankets and other sources of heat may also be recommended to help ease your joint pain; at other times, your doctor may suggest you use cold compresses to relieve inflammation.

In some cases, joint-protection devices such as splints are useful both for relieving pain and preventing deformity. Your doctor will probably stress the importance of well-balanced meals and, if you are overweight, the need to cut calories. As a treatment of last resort, surgery, such as hip replacement, can provide great relief for some types of arthritis.

The cornerstone of arthritis treatment, however, is medicine. Most of the drugs prescribed for arthritis are both analgesic (pain-reducing) and anti-inflammatory (inflammation-reducing). Aspirin is often the initial drug of choice. The next to be tried, should there be gastric distress, is enteric-coated aspirin; the special coating prevents the medicine from being released or absorbed until it reaches the intestines. Steroids are another mainstay of arthritis therapy, but they should be given in low doses; these agents are particularly effective against polymyalgia rheumatica and giant-cell arteritis. Gold is sometimes prescribed, though its usefulness is limited by its toxicity. For detailed information on these drugs, see the charts on pages 433–449.

Even if you have a mild case of arthritis, don't try to diagnose and treat the problem yourself. Some people make the mistake of simply taking aspirin or a nonprescription-strength, nonsteroidal anti-inflammatory drug like ibuprofen on their own. But the dosages they're using may be too low for effectiveness or too high for safety, and the medicine they choose may not be the ideal one for their condition. A doctor's judgment is crucial in designing the treatment plan and in monitoring its effectiveness.

OUTLOOK

There is currently no cure for any form of arthritis. But the treatments and therapies available for making life livable with arthritis—even when severe—have grown in number and effectiveness in recent years. Meanwhile, our understanding of the various processes that can cause joint-tissue deterioration is steadily advancing. There's every reason to expect that modern medicine will continue to brighten the outlook for people who have an arthritic condition.

CONDITION: **ARTHRITIS**

CATEGORY: **SALICYLATE DRUGS**

GENERIC (CHEMICAL) NAME	BRAND (TRADE) NAME	DOSAGE FORMS AND STRENGTHS
Aspirin and other salicylate drugs		

Aspirin and other salicylate drugs are available over the counter under a variety of brand names, dosage forms, and strengths. Some of these preparations have a special coating to help protect the lining of the stomach against possible irritation. Because of the importance of salicylate drugs in the treatment of chronic pain, even though they are most often nonprescription drugs, they are included in this book for reader reference.

DRUG PROFILE

Aspirin and other drugs in the salicylate family are used to relieve pain, inflammation, and fever. Large doses are used to treat symptoms of arthritis and rheumatism such as swelling, stiffness, and joint pain. Aspirin and other salicylates are thought to control pain and swelling by blocking the production of naturally occurring triggers of pain and inflammation, called prostaglandins. These drugs relieve fever by changing the way the body regulates its temperature.

For complete information on these drugs, see pages 379–383.

CONDITION: **ARTHRITIS**

CATEGORY: **NONSTEROIDAL ANTI-INFLAMMATORY DRUGS**

GENERIC (CHEMICAL) NAME	BRAND (TRADE) NAME	DOSAGE FORMS AND STRENGTHS
Diflunisal	DOLOBID	Tablets: 250, 500 mg

Fenoprofen calcium	NALFON	Capsules: 200, 300 mg Tablets: 600 mg
Ibuprofen	ADVIL (OTC) MOTRIN NUPRIN (OTC) RUFEN	Tablets: 200 mg Tablets: 300, 400, 600, 800 mg Tablets: 200 mg Tablets: 400, 600, 800 mg

Indomethacin	INDOCIN
	
	INDOCIN SR
		Capsules: 25, 50 mg
		Rectal suppositories:
		  50 mg
		Controlled-release
		  capsules: 75 mg

Meclofenamate sodium	MECLOMEN	Capsules: meclofenamate
		  sodium equivalent to 50
		  or 100 mg meclofenamic
		  acid

Naproxen	ANAPROX NAPROSYN	Tablets: 275 mg Tablets: 250, 375, 500 mg
Phenylbutazone	BUTAZOLIDIN	Capsules: 100 mg Tablets: 100 mg
Piroxicam	FELDENE	Capsules: 10, 20 mg
Sulindac	CLINORIL	Tablets: 150, 200 mg

Tolmetin sodium	TOLECTIN	Capsules: tolmetin sodium
		  equivalent to 400 mg
		  tolmetin
		Tablets: tolmetin sodium
		  equivalent to 200 mg
		  tolmetin

DRUG PROFILE

Nonsteroidal anti-inflammatory drugs, or NSAIDs, help relieve swelling, stiffness, joint pain, and inflammation in the long-term treatment of arthritis. These drugs are thought to act by blocking the production of naturally occurring triggers of pain and inflammation, called prostaglandins.

BEFORE USING THIS DRUG

Let your doctor know *IF*

You have ever had allergic reactions or other problems with ■ the medicine prescribed for you or any other nonsteroidal anti-inflammatory agent ■ other medicines for arthritis or gout.

You have ever had any of the following medical problems: ■ asthma or bronchospasm ■ bleeding disorders ■ dizziness ■ heart disease ■ high blood pressure ■ congestive heart failure ■ kidney disease ■ liver disease ■ nasal polyps ■ water retention ■ stomach ulcer, intestinal bleeding, colitis, or other digestive disorders.

■ *with indomethacin and phenylbutazone only:* ■ seizures ■ mental illness ■ Parkinson's disease.

You are taking any of the following medicines:

■ *with diflunisal only:* ■ aspirin or aspirinlike medicine ■ anticoagulants (blood thinners) ■ medicine containing aluminum ■ benzodiazepines.

■ *with fenoprofen only:* ■ aspirin or aspirinlike medicine ■ anticoagulants (blood thinners) ■ barbiturates.

■ *with ibuprofen only:* ■ aspirin or aspirinlike medicine ■ anticoagulants (blood thinners) ■ bumentanide, ethacrynic acid, or furosemide (diuretics) ■ digoxin, digitoxin, or digitalis (heart medicines) ■ lithium ■ medicine for seizures.

■ *with indomethacin only:* ■ aspirin or aspirinlike medicine ■ anticoagulants (blood thinners) ■ beta-blockers ■ bumentanide, ethacrynic acid, furosemide, triamterene, or thiazide diuretics (water pills) ■ prazosin (medicine for high blood pressure) ■ captopril (medicine for high blood pressure and congestive heart failure) ■ cimetidine (medicine for ulcers) ■ digoxin, digitoxin, or digitalis (heart medicines) ■ lithium ■ probenecid (medicine for gout) ■ medicine for asthma ■ decongestants.

- *with meclofenamate only:* ■ aspirin or aspirinlike medicine ■ anticoagulants (blood thinners).

- *with naproxen only:* ■ aspirin or aspirinlike medicine ■ probenecid ■ anticoagulants (blood thinners).

- *with phenylbutazone only:* ■ aspirin or aspirinlike medicine ■ male hormones ■ anticoagulants (blood thinners) ■ barbiturates ■ digoxin, digitoxin, or digitalis (heart medicines) ■ medicine for seizures ■ medicine for diabetes.

- *with piroxicam and sulindac only:* ■ anticoagulants (blood thinners) ■ lithium.

- *with tolmetin only:* ■ anticoagulants (blood thinners).

SPECIAL RESTRICTIONS WHILE TAKING THIS DRUG

FOOD AND DRUG INTERACTIONS

Other Drugs	It is important to let your doctor know if you are taking any other drug, especially blood thinners or lithium, since their effects may be increased when taken with some NSAIDs. Also, be sure to tell your doctor if you have ever experienced asthma or an allergic reaction to aspirin or any other type of arthritis medicine.
Alcohol	Drinking alcohol while taking this drug may cause stomach upset. Avoid alcohol unless your doctor has approved its use.

No special restrictions on foods and beverages or smoking.

DAILY LIVING

Driving	This type of drug may cause drowsiness or loss of alertness. Be careful when driving, operating household appliances, or doing any other tasks that require alertness until you know how this drug affects you.

Examinations or Tests	It is important for you to keep all appointments with your doctor so that your progress can be checked.
Other Precautions	If you have diabetes, be aware that these medicines may cause fluctuations in blood-sugar levels. Your doctor may want to monitor your blood-sugar levels carefully during the first few weeks of use. Taking aspirin regularly with NSAIDs may cause stomach upset. If the drug you are taking upsets your stomach, ask your doctor if you can take it with an antacid.
Helpful Hints	NSAIDs reach the bloodstream more quickly if your stomach is empty. If the drug you are taking upsets your stomach, however, ask your doctor if you can take it with milk, meals, or snacks. If you have been storing the suppository form of this medicine in a warm place, it may be too soft to use. Put it in the refrigerator for half an hour or run cold water over the wrapped suppository before use.

No special restrictions on exertion and exercise, sun exposure, or exposure to excessive heat or cold.

POSSIBLE SIDE EFFECTS

Although this list of adverse effects may seem somewhat intimidating, keep in mind that some are quite rare. Of course, should these or any other problems arise while you are on medication, it is always a good idea to consult your doctor.

IF YOU DEVELOP

fever ■ rash, hives, or itching ■ difficulty in breathing ■ severe nausea or vomiting ■ vomiting, with blood ■ black, tarry stools ■ swelling of hands or feet ■ decreased urination

WHAT TO DO

Urgent Get in touch with your doctor immediately.

stomach pain ■ blurred vision or other visual disturbances ■ ringing or buzzing in ears or other hearing problems ■ yellowing of eyes or skin ■ any change in color of urine or stool ■ increased sweating ■ confusion ■ nervousness ■ agitation	**May be serious** Check with your doctor as soon as possible.
indigestion ■ heartburn ■ nausea or vomiting ■ diarrhea ■ constipation ■ loss of appetite ■ gas or bloating ■ drowsiness ■ sleeplessness ■ headache ■ dizziness, light-headedness, or faintness	If symptoms are disturbing or persist, let your doctor know.

STORAGE INSTRUCTIONS

Store in a cool, dark place (not in a bathroom medicine cabinet). Suppositories should be stored in the refrigerator.

STOPPING OR INTERRUPTING THERAPY

Because these medicines control but do not cure arthritis, you may have to take them for a long period of time. Your symptoms could take from one to four weeks to abate. Do not take more of this medicine or take it for a longer period of time than recommended by your doctor or the package labeling. If you are supposed to take your medicine once a day and you miss a dose, take it as soon as possible. If it is not within six hours of the scheduled time for the missed dose, skip it and resume your regular schedule. If you are supposed to take your medicine two or more times a day and you miss a dose, take it as soon as possible. If it is not within two hours of the scheduled time for the missed dose, skip it and resume your regular schedule.

SPECIAL CONSIDERATIONS FOR THOSE OVER SIXTY-FIVE

Because kidney function sometimes decreases with age, older people may be susceptible to urinary problems with these drugs. Indomethacin and meclofenamate should be used with great care by those over sixty, since side effects are more likely to occur.

CONDITION: **ARTHRITIS**

CATEGORY: **CORTICOSTEROIDS**

GENERIC (CHEMICAL) NAME	BRAND (TRADE) NAME	DOSAGE FORMS AND STRENGTHS
Betamethasone	CELESTONE	Syrup: 0.6 mg per tsp Tablets: 0.6 mg
Cortisone acetate		Tablets: 5, 10, 25 mg
Dexamethasone	DECADRON	Elixir: 0.5 mg per tsp Tablets: 0.25, 0.5, 0.75, 1.5, 4, 6 mg
Hydrocortisone Hydrocortisone cypionate	CORTEF CORTEF Oral Suspension	Tablets: 5, 10, 20 mg Suspension: hydrocortisone cypionate equivalent to 10 mg hydrocortisone per tsp
Methylprednisolone	MEDROL	Tablets: 2, 4, 8, 16, 24, 32 mg
Prednisone	DELTASONE	Tablets: 2.5, 5, 10, 20, 50 mg
Triamcinolone Triamcinolone diacetate	ARISTOCORT ARISTOCORT	Tablets: 1, 2, 4, 8 mg Syrup: 2 mg per tsp

DRUG PROFILE

Oral corticosteroids (also known as steroids) are used to treat a wide variety of inflammatory diseases, such as arthritis, and other rheumatic disorders, such as lupus. They are also used in conjunction with immunosuppressive agents to prevent reactions from kidney and heart transplants. Although these multifaceted drugs do not cure the underlying disease, they suppress the redness, swelling, and heat that signal inflammation.

BEFORE USING THIS DRUG

Let your doctor know *IF*

You have ever had allergic reactions or other problems with ■ any corticosteroids ■ corticotropin (ACTH).

You have ever had any of the following medical problems: ■ peptic ulcer or intestinal bleeding ■ diabetes ■ bone disease such as osteoporosis ■ slow healing of wounds ■ high blood pressure ■ mental illness ■ recent fungal infection ■ recent viral infection ■ herpes eye infection ■ colitis or diverticulitis ■ glaucoma ■ heart disease ■ disease of the blood vessels ■ kidney disease ■ liver disease ■ myasthenia gravis ■ congestive heart failure ■ tuberculosis ■ underactive thyroid ■ seizures ■ high cholesterol.

You are taking any of the following medicines: ■ other medicine for arthritis or other inflammatory conditions, including aspirin or aspirinlike medicine ■ antibiotics ■ digoxin, digitoxin, or digitalis (heart medicines) ■ medicine for abnormal heart rhythms ■ diuretics ■ medicine for high blood pressure ■ medicine for asthma ■ insulin or other medicine for diabetes ■ anticoagulants (blood thinners) ■ medicine for Parkinson's disease ■ barbiturates ■ medicine for seizures ■ female hormones (estrogens) ■ medicine for myasthenia gravis ■ antacids ■ muscle relaxants ■ medicine for high cholesterol ■ medicine for tuberculosis ■ potassium-containing medicines or supplements.

You have recently had a vaccination.

You are subjected to unusual stress in your daily life.

SPECIAL RESTRICTIONS WHILE TAKING THIS DRUG

FOOD AND DRUG INTERACTIONS

Other Drugs	These drugs interact with many other drugs; do not take any other drug, including over-the-counter (OTC) drugs, before checking with your doctor.
	These drugs may affect how your body absorbs medicine for diabetes, and your dosage may need to be adjusted.

Let your doctor know if you are planning to receive any kind of vaccine.

Foods and Beverages	Tell your doctor if you are on any kind of special diet. Your doctor may recommend a low-salt, high-potassium diet to counterbalance some of the side effects of this drug such as bloating.
	Long-term therapy with this drug makes you more prone to osteoporosis (thinning of the bones). Your doctor may recommend that you include more calcium in your diet or may prescribe a calcium supplement for you.
	You may also be advised to take vitamin A and/or C supplements while on this drug.
Alcohol	Drinking alcohol while taking this drug may cause stomach upset. Avoid alcohol unless your doctor has approved its use.

No special restrictions on smoking.

DAILY LIVING

Exertion and Exercise	Discuss with your doctor which kinds of physical exercises are safe for you to undertake.
Examinations or Tests	It is important for you to keep all appointments with your doctor so that your progress can be checked. Periodic blood, urine, and eye tests may be required.
Other Precautions	Tell any doctor or dentist you consult that you are presently taking or have taken any of these drugs in the past year, especially if you will be undergoing any type of surgery.

If you are undergoing some sort of unusual stress, or if you develop any signs of infection (fever, sore throat, muscle aches, pain in urination), call your doctor.

Helpful Hints

If this medicine upsets your stomach, taking it with milk, meals, or snacks should help. If you continue to experience distress, let your doctor know.

No special restrictions on sun exposure or exposure to excessive heat or cold.

POSSIBLE SIDE EFFECTS

Although this list of adverse effects may seem somewhat intimidating, keep in mind that some are quite rare. Of course, should these or any other problems arise while you are on medication, it is always a good idea to consult your doctor.

IF YOU DEVELOP

seizures ■ stomach pain ■ dizziness or faintness ■ fever ■ loss of appetite with weight loss ■ muscle or joint pain or weakness ■ nausea or vomiting ■ difficulty in breathing ■ tiredness ■ slow or fast heartbeat ■ palpitations ■ swelling of mouth or tongue ■ speech difficulties ■ pain in urination ■ urinary frequency

After you STOP taking this medicine: loss of appetite and/or weight loss ■ nausea or vomiting ■ drowsiness ■ headache ■ fever ■ joint or muscle pain ■ peeling of skin ■ dizziness ■ depression

WHAT TO DO

Urgent Get in touch with your doctor immediately.

back, hip, or rib pain ■ acne ■ increased sweating ■ hair growth ■ skin redness, rash, or hives ■ scaly skin or other skin changes ■ bruising ■ depression ■ nervousness or restlessness ■ anxiety ■ "high" feeling ■ other mood changes

May be serious Check with your doctor as soon as possible.

■ blood in stools ■ bloating ■ halos around lights or other visual disturbances ■ sore throat or hoarseness ■ wounds that take a long time to heal ■ swelling of hands, feet, or ankles ■ diarrhea ■ constipation ■ reactivation of an ulcer ■ any lung or throat infection ■ white patches in mouth or throat

indigestion ■ increase in appetite with weight gain ■ eruptions on mouth or lips ■ sleeplessness ■ headache ■ unusual roundness of the face	If symptoms are disturbing or persist, let your doctor know.

STORAGE INSTRUCTIONS

Store in a cool, dark place (not in a bathroom medicine cabinet). If your medicine is in a liquid form, make sure that it does not freeze.

STOPPING OR INTERRUPTING THERAPY

Take this medicine exactly as prescribed by your doctor. Do not suddenly stop taking this medicine; your doctor will advise you on how to gradually reduce your dosage. Ask your doctor what to do if you miss a dose. You may experience side effects from corticosteroids for up to a year after stopping therapy; let your doctor know if this should happen.

SPECIAL CONSIDERATIONS FOR THOSE OVER SIXTY-FIVE

Long-term use of corticosteroids may cause gradual bone loss; this can be serious in older people, particularly women, who are vulnerable to osteoporosis. This age group is particularly susceptible to adverse effects on the muscles and nerves as well.

CONDITION: **ARTHRITIS**

CATEGORY: **OTHER ANTIARTHRITIC AGENTS**

GENERIC (CHEMICAL) NAME	BRAND (TRADE) NAME	DOSAGE FORMS AND STRENGTHS
Auranofin	RIDAURA	Capsules: 3 mg

DRUG PROFILE

Auranofin is a gold compound used to treat rheumatoid arthritis. It is not known exactly how this drug works to relieve joint pain and inflammation. Because of its relatively serious potential side effects, auranofin is reserved for people who do not respond to therapy with nonsteroidal anti-inflammatory drugs and should be prescribed only by doctors who are familiar with its use.

BEFORE USING THIS DRUG

Let your doctor know *IF*

You have ever had allergic reactions or other problems with ■ auranofin or other gold compounds ■ gold or other metals.

You have ever had any of the following medical problems: ■ blood diseases, including bone marrow depression ■ kidney disease ■ systemic lupus erythematosus ■ skin disease, including rash, hives, or eczema ■ colitis ■ bleeding disease ■ any reaction to a drug that affected your blood, lungs, or digestive tract ■ irritable bowel disease ■ blood vessel disease.

You are taking any of the following medicines: ■ other arthritis medicine, especially penicillamine or phenylbutazone ■ medicine for cancer ■ medicine for malaria ■ phenytoin (medicine for seizures).

You have recently received radiation therapy.

SPECIAL RESTRICTIONS WHILE TAKING THIS DRUG

FOOD AND DRUG INTERACTIONS

No special restrictions on other drugs, foods and beverages, alcohol use, or smoking.

DAILY LIVING

Exertion and Exercise	Discuss with your doctor which kinds of physical exercise are safe for you to undertake.
Sun Exposure	If you experience skin problems with auranofin, prolonged exposure to sunlight will aggravate the prob-

lem. It is a good idea to apply a sunscreen to exposed skin surfaces before going outdoors.

Examinations or Tests	It is important for you to keep all appointments with your doctor so that your progress can be checked. Periodic blood and urine tests are usually required before and during therapy.

Other Precautions	Take this medicine exactly as instructed by your doctor; taking more than your prescribed dose may increase your chances of developing side effects.
	Let your doctor know if any side effect becomes bothersome. If you experience diarrhea, a dose change or even a break from taking this drug may be possible. Medicine for diarrhea or an oral iron preparation may be prescribed for you.

No special restrictions on driving or exposure to excessive heat or cold.

POSSIBLE SIDE EFFECTS

Although this list of adverse effects may seem somewhat intimidating, keep in mind that some are quite rare. Of course, should these or any other problems arise while you are on medication, it is always a good idea to consult your doctor.

IF YOU DEVELOP

red marks on skin ■ puffy face, hands, or feet ■ coughing, wheezing, or other difficulty in breathing

WHAT TO DO

Urgent Get in touch with your doctor immediately.

severe diarrhea or diarrhea lasting more than three days ■ rash, hives, or itching ■ sores or white spots in mouth or throat ■ bloody or cloudy urine ■ bleeding or bruising ■ vomiting, with blood or vomit that looks like coffee grounds ■ difficulty in swallowing ■ headache ■ dizziness ■ fever ■ irritation or soreness of tongue or gums ■ metal-

May be serious Check with your doctor as soon as possible.

lic taste ■ severe stomach pain ■ bloody or black, tarry stools ■ yellowing of eyes or skin ■ numbness, tingling, pain, or weakness in hands or feet ■ tiredness ■ sore throat

nausea or vomiting ■ stomach cramps or pain ■ increased bowel movements, loose stools, or diarrhea ■ indigestion ■ gas or bloating ■ loss of appetite ■ constipation ■ taste changes ■ hair loss ■ positive test for occult blood in stool	If symptoms are disturbing or persist, let your doctor know.

STORAGE INSTRUCTIONS

Store in a cool, dark place (not in a bathroom medicine cabinet).

STOPPING OR INTERRUPTING THERAPY

It may be three to six months before you see any improvement in your symptoms. If you are supposed to take your medicine once a day and miss a dose, take it as soon as possible. If you do not remember until the following day, skip the missed dose and resume your regular schedule. If you are supposed to take your medicine twice or more a day and miss a dose, take it as soon as possible. If it is almost time for your next dose, skip it and resume your regular schedule. Do not take two doses at the same time.

SPECIAL CONSIDERATIONS FOR THOSE OVER SIXTY-FIVE

None.

CONDITION: **ARTHRITIS**

CATEGORY: **OTHER ANTI-ARTHRITIC AGENTS**

GENERIC (CHEMICAL) NAME	BRAND (TRADE) NAME	DOSAGE FORMS AND STRENGTHS
Penicillamine	CUPRIMINE DEPEN	Capsules: 125, 250 mg Tablets: 250 mg

DRUG PROFILE

Penicillamine (a chemical relative of penicillin) is used in the treatment of several medical problems, including rheumatoid arthritis. With long-term use, this drug can reduce the swelling, stiffness, and joint pain of arthritis. How it works is not known, and penicillamine does not cure arthritis. Because of its relatively serious potential side effects, penicillamine is reserved for people who have not responded to other treatments.

BEFORE USING THIS DRUG

Let your doctor know *IF*

You have ever had allergic reactions or other problems with ■ penicillamine ■ penicillin ■ chrysotherapy (gold salts).

You have ever had any of the following medical problems: ■ kidney disease ■ stomach ulcer.

You are taking any of the following medicines: ■ oxyphenbutazone, phenylbutazone, or gold (other medicine for arthritis) ■ medicine for cancer ■ medicine or vitamins containing iron or magnesium ■ medicine for malaria ■ digoxin, digitoxin, or digitalis (heart medicines) ■ antacids containing aluminum ■ probenecid (medicine for gout) ■ medicine to prevent reactions after organ transplants ■ aspirin or aspirinlike medicine ■ corticosteroids.

SPECIAL RESTRICTIONS WHILE TAKING THIS DRUG

FOOD AND DRUG INTERACTIONS

Other Drugs	Do not take any other drugs, including over-the-counter (OTC) drugs, before checking with your doctor. If you require any drug or vitamin that contains iron, do not take it within two hours of your penicillamine dose, since iron can interfere with the action of penicillamine. If you are taking any other drug, do not take it within an hour of taking penicillamine.

No special restrictions on foods and beverages, alcohol use, or smoking.

DAILY LIVING

Examinations or Tests	It is important for you to keep all appointments with your doctor so that your progress can be checked. You will probably require blood and urine tests every two weeks during the first six months on penicillamine and monthly thereafter.
Helpful Hints	Penicillamine should be taken on an empty stomach —at least an hour before or more than two hours after eating—to speed its absorption into the body. If this drug upsets your stomach, however, taking it with milk, meals, or snacks should help.

No restrictions on driving, exertion and exercise, sun exposure, or exposure to excessive heat or cold.

POSSIBLE SIDE EFFECTS

Although this list of adverse effects may seem somewhat intimidating, keep in mind that some are quite rare. Of course, should these or any other problems arise while you are on medication, it is always a good idea to consult your doctor.

IF YOU DEVELOP

sore throat or fever ■ chills ■ bleeding ■ bruising, wounding, or dark spots on skin ■ spitting up blood ■ difficulty in breathing ■ wheezing ■ unexplained cough ■ difficulty in speech ■ difficulty in chewing or swallowing ■ yellowing of eyes or skin ■ sores or white spots in mouth or gums ■ any change in color of urine or stool

WHAT TO DO

Urgent Get in touch with your doctor immediately.

joint pain ■ rash, hives, or itching ■ wrinkling or any other skin problems ■ swelling of lymph glands ■ swelling of feet or lower legs ■ weight gain ■ tiredness or weakness ■ ringing in the ears ■ blurred vision or other visual disturbances ■ muscle weakness ■ tongue inflammation

May be serious Check with your doctor as soon as possible.

nausea or vomiting ■ stomach pain ■ loss of appetite ■ diarrhea ■ decreased sense of taste ■ upset stomach ■ hair loss ■ dry and scaly corners of the mouth ■ soreness of the vagina or vulva

If symptoms are disturbing or persist, let your doctor know.

STORAGE INSTRUCTIONS

Store in a cool, dark place (not in a bathroom medicine cabinet).

STOPPING OR INTERRUPTING THERAPY

Take this medicine exactly as prescribed, since it has been especially tailored to you and your particular symptoms. It may be two to three months before you notice improvement in your symptoms. If you are supposed to take this medicine once a day and miss a dose, take it as soon as possible. If you do not remember until the next day, skip the missed dose and resume your regular schedule. If you are supposed to take your medicine twice a day and miss a dose, take it as soon as possible. If it is almost time for your next dose, skip the missed dose and resume your regular schedule. If you are supposed to take penicillamine more than twice a day and miss a dose, take the missed dose within two hours of the scheduled time for that dose. If a longer time has passed, skip the missed dose and resume your regular schedule.

SPECIAL CONSIDERATIONS FOR THOSE OVER SIXTY-FIVE

Older people may be more prone to the side effects of this medicine, especially rashes and taste changes. Doctors may start people over sixty-five on a lower dosage and build it up gradually.

GOUT

Gout ranks high among human biology's great sources of exquisite agony. And much of the old folklore surrounding this disease is at least partly true. For example, gout has often been regarded as a disease of rotund gentlemen who ingest food and alcohol with abandon. Indeed, the disease almost exclusively strikes men over forty; obesity and alcohol can contribute to its risks, though they are *not* prerequisites. And the traditional caricatures of gout sufferers as having tender, swollen big toes do indeed show one of the main targets of the disease.

For nearly two million people in the United States, gout is no source of amusement. Rather, it is the cause of flare-ups of extreme pain and inflammation in the joints of large toes as well as other weight-bearing joints. Its sufferers' main consolation is that a variety of medicines can effectively relieve symptoms as well as treat the underlying problem.

CAUSES

At the root of gout is an excess of uric acid in the blood. Uric acid is produced naturally in the body and is also derived from foods containing substances called purines. Usually there is a proper balance between the production of uric acid and its disposal in the urine. Levels can rise because of overproduction, impaired excretion, or both.

Under certain conditions, excess uric acid in the blood will form tiny needle-shaped crystals, which typically settle in the joints of the legs and feet. This then triggers the body to dispatch white blood cells to attack the crystals, causing the swelling, redness, and extreme sensitivity in the affected joint. A doctor's clearest evidence of gout comes from a combination of white blood cells and uric acid crystals in a sample of fluid taken from the joint.

For a lucky few, the first flare-up of gout is also the last. Generally, though, gout attacks tend to recur and can increase in severity. Left uncorrected, high uric acid levels can collect in the kidneys, and may damage the kidneys' delicate blood-filtering apparatus and possibly form painful kidney stones. Over the years, untreated gout may lead to a condition called tophaceous gout, in which small clumps of uric acid crystals can trigger inflammation, pain, and tissue damage throughout the body—notably in the big toe, elbow, and inner ear.

TREATMENT

A number of treatments can relieve the pain of gout and the potential tissue damage caused by excess uric acid. Colchicine is one of the oldest medicines for quelling the inflammation and pain of an acute gout attack; also, small doses may be used to prevent acute gout attacks (see the chart on pages 452–454). As alternatives, a doctor may recommend one of the nonsteroidal anti-inflammatory drugs (NSAIDs) for use during attacks (see the charts on pages 433–438).

For long-term treatment of gout, several other medicines can help lower blood levels of uric acid in two ways—by helping the body get rid of uric acid through the urine and by inhibiting the production of uric acid in the first place (see the charts on pages 454–463).

Your doctor may advise you to avoid foods containing very high levels of purines—including organ meats such as liver, pancreas, or brain—and to use moderation in your eating habits. Losing weight, if you are obese, should also help. Other useful measures include controlling high blood pressure, high blood fat levels, and diabetes. Finally, alcohol helps block the excretion of uric acid, so you would be wise to cut back or abstain.

OUTLOOK

Managing gout and other uric acid-related disorders is a lifetime affair. If, after study, your doctor recommends drugs that help lower blood levels of uric acid, those agents should be taken indefinitely; uric acid levels can rise quickly when the drugs are discontinued. Because the compounds are quite expensive, the decision to institute therapy should be made with care. But the gains from sticking to antigout therapy, once begun, are great in preventing both the extreme pain of gout and the potential damage to various parts of the body.

CONDITION: **GOUT**

CATEGORY: **ANTIGOUT AGENTS (DRUGS FOR ACUTE ATTACKS)**

GENERIC (CHEMICAL) NAME	BRAND (TRADE) NAME	DOSAGE FORMS AND STRENGTHS
Colchicine		Granules: 0.5 mg Tablets: 0.432, 0.5, 0.6 mg

DRUG PROFILE

Colchicine is used to treat acute attacks of gouty arthritis and to prevent attacks from recurring. This drug works by reducing inflammation.

BEFORE USING THIS DRUG

Let your doctor know *IF*

You have ever had allergic reactions or other problems with ■ colchicine.

You have ever had any of the following medical problems: ■ heart disease ■ kidney disease ■ liver disease ■ blood disease ■ stomach ulcer or other digestive disorders.

You are taking any of the following medicines: ■ vitamin B_{12} .

SPECIAL RESTRICTIONS WHILE TAKING THIS DRUG

FOOD AND DRUG INTERACTIONS

Alcohol	Avoid alcohol while taking this drug; alcohol may increase the amount of uric acid in the blood, thus worsening your condition.

No special restrictions on other drugs, foods and beverages, or smoking.

DAILY LIVING

Examinations or Tests	It is important for you to keep all appointments with your doctor so that your progress can be checked. Periodic blood and urine tests may be required.
Helpful Hints	Be sure to drink plenty of fluids (at least ten to twelve full glasses of water a day) to prevent the formation of kidney stones.

No special restrictions on driving, exertion and exercise, sun exposure, or exposure to excessive heat or cold.

POSSIBLE SIDE EFFECTS

Although this list of adverse effects may seem somewhat intimidating, keep in mind that some are quite rare. Of course, should these or any other problems arise while you are on medication, it is always a good idea to consult your doctor.

IF YOU DEVELOP	WHAT TO DO
numbness, tingling, pain, or weakness in hands or feet ■ rash or other skin problems ■ fever ■ bleeding or bruising ■ sore throat ■ severe muscle weakness ■ blood in urine ■ decreased urination	**Urgent** Get in touch with your doctor immediately.
diarrhea ■ nausea or vomiting ■ stomach pain or discomfort	**May be serious** *Stop taking this medicine* and check with your doctor as soon as possible.
hair loss	If symptoms are disturbing or persist, let your doctor know.

STORAGE INSTRUCTIONS

Store in a cool, dark place (not in a bathroom medicine cabinet).

STOPPING OR INTERRUPTING THERAPY

If you are on long-term therapy with this drug and you miss a dose, take it as soon as possible. If it is almost time for your next dose, skip the missed dose and resume your regular schedule. Do not take two doses at the same time.

SPECIAL CONSIDERATIONS FOR THOSE OVER SIXTY-FIVE

Older people may be more prone to the side effects of colchicine.

CONDITION: **GOUT**

CATEGORY: **ANTIGOUT AGENTS (URIC ACID REDUCERS)**

GENERIC (CHEMICAL) NAME	BRAND (TRADE) NAME	DOSAGE FORMS AND STRENGTHS
Allopurinol	LOPURIN	Tablets: 100, 300 mg
	ZYLOPRIM	Tablets: 100, 300 mg

DRUG PROFILE

Allopurinol is used in such conditions as gout and kidney stones caused by an excess amount of uric acid in the body. This drug blocks xanthine oxidase, an enzyme necessary for the production of uric acid, and may be used in combination with other drugs. Although allopurinol can prevent gout attacks, it does not actually cure gout and cannot stop a gout attack in progress.

BEFORE USING THIS DRUG

Let your doctor know *IF*

You have ever had allergic reactions or other problems with ■ allopurinol ■ thiazide diuretics.

You have ever had any of the following medical problems: ■ kidney disease ■ hemochromatosis (excess iron in the blood).

You are taking any of the following medicines: ■ other medicine for gout or gouty arthritis ■ penicillin or any drug in the penicillin family, including amoxicillin, ampicillin, bacampicillin, and hetacillin ■ medicine for asthma ■ anticoagulants (blood thinners) ■ azothioprine, dacarbazine, mercaptopurine, or vidarabine (medicines for cancer) ■ chlorpropamide (medicine for diabetes) ■ medicine for high blood pressure ■ diuretics (water pills) ■ medicine to make the urine more acidic ■ pyrazinamide (medicine for tuberculosis) ■ co-trimoxazole (medicine for urinary tract infections) ■ medicine for seizures ■ captopril (medicine for congestive heart failure).

SPECIAL RESTRICTIONS WHILE TAKING THIS DRUG

FOOD AND DRUG INTERACTIONS

Alcohol	Avoid alcohol while taking this drug; alcohol may increase the amount of uric acid in the blood, thus worsening your condition.

No special restrictions on other drugs, foods and beverages, or smoking.

DAILY LIVING

Driving	This drug may cause drowsiness. Be careful when driving, operating household appliances, or doing any other tasks that require alertness until you know how this drug affects you.
Examinations or Tests	It is important for you to keep all appointments with your doctor so that your progress can be checked. Periodic blood and urine tests may be required.
Other Precautions	It may be several months before you notice the effects of this medicine, but continue to take it as instructed. Should you experience more frequent gout attacks during the first few months of treatment, your doctor may prescribe an additional medicine, such as colchicine.

Helpful Hints   If this drug upsets your stomach, taking it with milk, meals, or snacks should help. If you continue to experience distress, let your doctor know.

Be sure to drink plenty of fluids (at least ten to twelve full glasses) while taking this drug.

No special restrictions on exertion and exercise, sun exposure, or exposure to excessive heat or cold.

POSSIBLE SIDE EFFECTS

Although this list of adverse effects may seem somewhat intimidating, keep in mind that some are quite rare. Of course, should these or any other problems arise while you are on medication, it is always a good idea to consult your doctor.

IF YOU DEVELOP

rash, hives, or itching ■ chills ■ fever ■ muscle aches and pains ■ nausea or vomiting occurring shortly after rash ■ general feeling of unwellness ■ pain in urination ■ blood in urine ■ decreased urination ■ eye irritation ■ swelling of lips and mouth ■ red, thickened, or scaly skin ■ boils on nose ■ bleeding (including nosebleed) or bruising ■ yellowing of eyes or skin ■ loosening of fingernails ■ small red marks on skin

WHAT TO DO

Urgent Get in touch with your doctor immediately.

numbness, tingling, pain, or weakness in hands or feet ■ increase in gout attacks ■ loss of appetite ■ weight loss ■ swelling of hands or feet ■ hearing problems

May be serious Check with your doctor as soon as possible.

drowsiness ■ diarrhea ■ stomach pain ■ nausea or vomiting (without rash) ■ taste changes ■ upset stomach

If symptoms are disturbing or persist, let your doctor know.

STORAGE INSTRUCTIONS

Store in a cool, dark place (not in a bathroom medicine cabinet).

STOPPING OR INTERRUPTING THERAPY

Take this medicine exactly as instructed by your doctor. If you are supposed to take this medicine once a day and miss a dose, take it as soon as possible. If you do not remember until the next day, skip the missed dose and resume your regular schedule. Do not take two doses at the same time. If you are supposed to take this drug twice or more a day and miss a dose, take it as soon as possible. If it is almost time for your next dose and your dose is one 100 mg tablet, double the next dose; if your dose is two 100 mg tablets, take three tablets for your next dose. Then go back to your regular schedule.

SPECIAL CONSIDERATIONS FOR THOSE OVER SIXTY-FIVE

Those older people who have reduced kidney function tend not to eliminate this drug as readily as people with normal kidney function. Doctors may check such people regularly to make sure they are receiving the proper dosage and that too much drug is not accumulating in the body.

CONDITION: **GOUT**

CATEGORY: **ANTIGOUT AGENTS (URIC ACID REDUCERS)**

GENERIC (CHEMICAL) NAME	BRAND (TRADE) NAME	DOSAGE FORMS AND STRENGTHS
Probenecid	BENEMID	Tablets: 0.5 g

DRUG PROFILE

Probenecid increases the elimination of uric acid from the body through urination in people susceptible to chronic gout and gouty arthritis. Probenecid does not actually cure gout and cannot stop a gout attack in progress. Probenecid is also sometimes prescribed along with penicillin for the treatment of infections because it helps achieve extra ''mileage'' from a penicillin dose.

BEFORE USING THIS DRUG

Let your doctor know *IF*

You have ever had allergic reactions or other problems with ■ probenecid.

You have ever had any of the following medical problems: ■ blood disease ■ kidney disease, including kidney stones ■ stomach ulcer ■ glucose-6-phosphate dehydrogenase (G-6-PD) deficiency.

You are taking any of the following medicines: ■ other medicine for gout or gouty arthritis ■ any medicine for pain and inflammation ■ aspirin or aspirinlike medicine ■ methotrexate (medicine for severe psoriasis or cancer) ■ captopril (medicine for congestive heart failure) ■ clofibrate (medicine for high cholesterol) ■ medicine for diabetes ■ water pills (diuretics) ■ medicine for asthma ■ antibiotics ■ medicine for high blood pressure ■ pyrazinamide (medicine for tuberculosis) ■ vitamin B preparations ■ medicine for herpes infections.

SPECIAL RESTRICTIONS WHILE TAKING THIS DRUG

FOOD AND DRUG INTERACTIONS

Other Drugs	Do not take aspirin or aspirinlike medicines, since they reduce the effectiveness of probenecid. If you have pain or a fever, take acetaminophen instead.
	If you have diabetes and are taking an oral diabetes medicine, you may develop low blood sugar while on this drug. If this happens, stop taking the oral diabetes medicine and inform your doctor immediately.
	If you are taking cholestyramine (medicine for high cholesterol), take your dose of probenecid one hour before or four to six hours following your dose of cholestyramine.
Alcohol	Avoid alcohol while taking this drug; alcohol may increase the amount of uric acid in the blood, thus worsening your condition.

No special restrictions on smoking.

DAILY LIVING

Examinations or Tests	It is important for you to keep all appointments with your doctor so that your progress can be checked. Periodic blood and urine tests may be required.

Other Precautions	Tell any doctor or dentist you consult that you are taking this drug, especially if you will be undergoing any type of surgery or any kind of diagnostic tests.

It may be several weeks before you notice the effects of this medicine, but you should continue to take it as instructed. If you do experience gout attacks, your doctor will prescribe appropriate medicine to stop an attack in progress.

If you have diabetes, be aware that this drug may interfere with certain urine-sugar tests. Ask your doctor what kind of test is best to use while taking this medicine. |

Helpful Hints	Be sure to drink plenty of fluids (at least ten to twelve full glasses of water a day) while taking this drug to help prevent the formation of kidney stones.

If this drug upsets your stomach, taking it with milk, meals, or snacks should help. If you continue to experience distress, let your doctor know. |

No special restrictions on driving, exertion and exercise, sun exposure, or exposure to excessive heat or cold.

POSSIBLE SIDE EFFECTS

Although this list of adverse effects may seem somewhat intimidating, keep in mind that some are quite rare. Of course, should these or any other problems arise while you are on medication, it is always a good idea to consult your doctor.

IF YOU DEVELOP	WHAT TO DO
blood in urine ■ pain in urination ■ lower back pain ■ fever ■ extreme dizziness ■ tiredness ■ difficulty in breathing ■ sore throat ■ decreased urination ■ bleeding or bruising	**May be serious** Check with your doctor as soon as possible.
nausea or vomiting ■ loss of appetite ■ headache ■ urinary frequency ■ sore gums ■ flushing	If symptoms are disturbing or persist, let your doctor know.

STORAGE INSTRUCTIONS

Store in a cool, dark place (not in a bathroom medicine cabinet).

STOPPING OR INTERRUPTING THERAPY

Take this medicine exactly as instructed by your doctor. If you miss a dose, take it as soon as possible. If it is almost time for your next dose, skip the missed dose and resume your regular schedule. Do not take two doses at the same time.

SPECIAL CONSIDERATIONS FOR THOSE OVER SIXTY-FIVE

None.

CONDITION: **GOUT**

CATEGORY: **ANTIGOUT AGENTS (URIC ACID REDUCERS)**

GENERIC (CHEMICAL) NAME	BRAND (TRADE) NAME	DOSAGE FORMS AND STRENGTHS
Sulfinpyrazone	ANTURANE	Capsules: 200 mg Tablets: 100 mg

DRUG PROFILE

Sulfinpyrazone increases the elimination of uric acid from the body through urination in people susceptible to gouty arthritis. Sulfinpyrazone does not actually cure gouty arthritis and cannot stop an attack in progress.

BEFORE USING THIS DRUG

Let your doctor know *IF*

You have ever had allergic reactions or other problems with ■ sulfinpyrazone ■ oxyphenbutazone ■ phenylbutazone.

You have ever had any of the following medical problems: ■ blood disease ■ kidney disease, including kidney stones ■ stomach ulcer or other digestive disorders.

You are taking any of the following medicines: ■ other medicine for gout or gouty arthritis ■ any medicine for pain and inflammation ■ aspirin or aspirinlike medicine ■ medicine for cancer ■ medicine for high cholesterol ■ medicine for diabetes ■ water pills (diuretics) ■ medicine for asthma ■ antibiotics, especially sulfa drugs ■ medicine for high blood pressure ■ pyrazinamide (medicine for tuberculosis) ■ acetaminophen ■ niacin ■ verapamil (medicine for chest pain) ■ cholestyramine.

SPECIAL RESTRICTIONS WHILE TAKING THIS DRUG

FOOD AND DRUG INTERACTIONS

Other Drugs	Do not take aspirin or aspirinlike medicine, as they reduce the effectiveness of this drug. If you have pain or a fever, take acetaminophen instead.
	If you are taking cholestyramine for high cholesterol, take your dose of this drug at least one hour before or four to six hours after your dose of cholestyramine.
Alcohol	Avoid alcohol while taking this drug; alcohol may increase the amount of uric acid in the blood, thus worsening your condition.

No special restrictions on smoking.

DAILY LIVING

Examinations or Tests	It is important for you to keep all appointments with your doctor so that your progress can be checked. Periodic blood and urine tests may be required.
Other Precautions	It may be several weeks before you notice the effects of this medicine, but you should continue to take it as instructed. If you do experience gout attacks, your doctor will prescribe appropriate medicine to stop an attack in progress.
Helpful Hints	Take sulfinpyrazone with milk or meals to avoid stomach upset. Be sure to drink plenty of fluids (at least ten to twelve full glasses of water a day) to help prevent the formation of kidney stones.

No special restrictions on driving, exertion and exercise, sun exposure, or exposure to excessive heat or cold.

POSSIBLE SIDE EFFECTS

Although this list of adverse effects may seem somewhat intimidating, keep in mind that some are quite rare. Of course, should these or any other problems arise while you are on medication, it is always a good idea to consult your doctor.

IF YOU DEVELOP	WHAT TO DO
bleeding or bruising ■ clumsiness or unsteadiness ■ difficulty in breathing ■ seizures ■ diarrhea ■ severe or continuing nausea, vomiting, or stomach pain ■ sore throat ■ fever ■ tiredness or weakness	**Urgent** Get in touch with your doctor immediately.
rash ■ bloody or black, tarry stools ■ blood in urine ■ reactivation of stomach ulcer ■ dizziness ■ hearing problems ■ swelling of face, feet, or	**May be serious** Check with your doctor as soon as possible.

hands ■ yellowing of eyes or skin ■ lower back pain ■ pain or difficulty in urination

| nausea or vomiting ■ stomach pain ■ indigestion | If symptoms are disturbing or persist, let your doctor know. |

STORAGE INSTRUCTIONS

Store in a cool, dark place (not in a bathroom medicine cabinet).

STOPPING OR INTERRUPTING THERAPY

Take this medicine exactly as instructed by your doctor. If you miss a dose, take it as soon as possible. If it is almost time for your next dose, skip the missed dose and resume your regular schedule. Do not take two doses at the same time.

SPECIAL CONSIDERATIONS FOR THOSE OVER SIXTY-FIVE

None.

OSTEOPOROSIS

One out of every four women over the age of sixty is affected by osteoporosis, which has been called a silent epidemic. Bones weakened by osteoporosis cannot withstand normal strains and break easily, often during such routine activities as bending or lifting. There are 1.3 million osteoporosis-related fractures each year in people over forty-five. Although all bones are affected, fractures of the spine, wrist, and hip are most common.

CAUSES

What happens as we age to make us prone to osteoporosis? To understand this, let's first look at the relationship between calcium and bone. Your body has between two and four pounds of calcium. Most of it—98 percent—is found in your bones. Contrary to popular opinion, bone is *not* lifeless but a constantly changing, living tissue. Calcium is its most important component, giving bones their strength and solidity. Each day, new bone is added as old bone is broken down and removed from the body through a process called remodeling. The amount of bone present in the body is the result of a balance between the formation of new bone and the breakdown of old bone.

When we reach our mid-thirties, the balance tips a bit, and more bone is lost than gained. Some bone loss is a normal part of aging and affects both men and women, but osteoporosis involves a more extreme loss that results in dangerous weakening of the bones.

Women are far more likely to develop osteoporosis than men, however, for reasons that include inadequate amounts of calcium-rich foods during childbearing years, smaller frames, and a decrease in the level of estrogen that occurs after menopause. (Although the connection between estrogen and bone loss is not completely understood, researchers think that estrogen is needed to maintain the balance between deposit and loss of calcium in the bones.) Inactivity may also contribute to the development of osteoporosis in both sexes. Other, less important, reasons that affect both sexes are inadequate amounts of vitamin D in the diet, and inadequate exposure to sunlight. Sunlight helps the body manufacture vitamin D, which is necessary for calcium absorption.

Fair-skinned white women and Asian women are more likely to develop osteoporosis than are black women. Thin women with small frames are also likely candidates. In addition, women who have an early menopause and who smoke are more susceptible to this condition.

DIAGNOSIS

An early sign of osteoporosis is a gradual loss of height, which results from the compression of weakened bones of the spine. In its extreme form, this leads to the development of a curved spine. Often, the gradual loss of bone isn't recognized until a bone fractures. Your doctor may confirm the diagnosis of osteoporosis with X rays or with advanced techniques for measuring bone thickness and density.

TREATMENT

Because it is difficult, if not impossible, to replace lost bone, the goal of treatment is to stop further bone loss. A dietary approach may be one way to do this. Because your body cannot make calcium, you must supply it by eating calcium-rich foods. The current Recommended Dietary Allowance (RDA) for calcium is 1000 mg (milligrams). Most researchers believe that's less than what's needed, particularly for women past menopause, and probably for older men as well. They recommend increasing the amount to 1,500 mg a day. One cup of milk has about 300 mg, one ounce of cheese has about 200 mg, and eight sardines have about 350 mg of calcium.

Because many people don't eat enough calcium-rich food each day, doctors may recommend a calcium supplement to ensure an adequate daily supply. Keep in mind, however, that calcium supplements are not recommended for people who have ever had kidney stones and may not be advisable for people with a family history of this condition. If the calcium tablets are too large to swallow whole, you can crush them and mix them with something easy to swallow like applesauce or cottage cheese. Turn to the drug chart on pages 472–474 for more information on calcium supplements.

Recent research indicates that calcium supplementation is not, in itself, adequate for preventing bone loss during and after menopause. Estrogen replacement therapy has been found to be the most important preventive in postmenopausal women. The hormone estrogen is often prescribed for women in this category. Except in women who have undergone a hysterectomy, estrogen is given with intermittent doses of progesterone. Such hormonal treatment has been effective in limiting osteoporosis in some postmenopausal women. The drug chart on pages 467–472 will provide you with more information on estrogen.

The best regimen for preventing osteoporosis appears to be a combination of estrogen replacement therapy and calcium supplementation. The use of calcium supplements may permit a reduced dose of estrogen—and a lowered risk of unpleasant side effects connected with estrogen therapy, such as uterine bleeding and migraine headaches.

Make sure you get enough sunlight so that your body can manufacture vitamin D. If you can't get out into the sun for fifteen minutes to an hour a day or if you live in a climate where the sun doesn't shine every day, drink vitamin D–fortified milk, or ask your doctor about supplements. Do not decide on your own to take a vitamin D supplement as this can be dangerous.

Exercise regularly. Inactivity leads to bone loss, no matter what your age. Any weight-bearing exercise such as walking, dancing, or tennis is beneficial because it places stress on the skeleton, stimulating the formation of bone. Of course, it's wise to check with your doctor if you're contemplating embarking on a new exercise program.

OUTLOOK

Although we don't yet know how to reverse calcium loss from bones, we do know that further loss can be halted by weight-bearing exercise. For women, estrogen replacement is another possibility.

Combinations of substances (such as the hormone calcitonin) that show promise in reversing the bone loss of osteoporosis are currently under investigation. If they prove safe and effective, they may one day soon help to end this silent epidemic.

CONDITION: **OSTEOPOROSIS**

CATEGORY: **ESTROGENS**

GENERIC (CHEMICAL) NAME	BRAND (TRADE) NAME	DOSAGE FORMS AND STRENGTHS
Conjugated estrogens	PREMARIN	Tablets: 0.3, 0.625, 0.9, 1.25, 2.5 mg
Chlorotrianisene	TACE	Capsules: 12, 25, 72 mg
Diethylstilbestrol		Coated tablets: 0.1, 0.25, 0.5, 1, 5 mg Tablets: 1, 5 mg
Estradiol	ESTRACE ESTRADERM	Tablets: 1, 2 mg Skin patch: 0.05, 0.1 mg per 24 hours
Estropipate	OGEN	Tablets: 0.75, 1.5, 3, 6 mg
Ethinyl estradiol	ESTINYL	Tablets: 0.02, 0.05, 0.5 mg
Quinestrol	ESTROVIS	Tablets: 100 μg

DRUG PROFILE

Estrogens (female hormones) are used to help treat the bone loss that occurs in women after menopause or after surgical removal of the uterus and/or ovaries, when the body no longer produces natural estrogens. These drugs are also used in other medical conditions such as breast cancer or prostate cancer as well as for atrophic vaginitis (dryness of the vagina) and other symptoms of menopause. It is not known exactly how estrogens prevent bone loss, but they do help the bones absorb the calcium they need to stay healthy. Many studies have shown that estrogen deficiency contributes to bone loss after menopause. Estrogens are usually administered in low doses in a cycle: three weeks on therapy and one week off therapy. You may be given a low dose of progesterone along with estrogens, which will help counteract some of estrogen's side effects. Estrogens are used as part of a treatment program for osteoporosis that may include diet, calcium supplements, and exercise. Although estrogens can prevent further bone loss, they cannot rebuild bones or straighten bones that have already become thin.

BEFORE USING THIS DRUG

Let your doctor know *IF*

You have ever had allergic reactions or other problems with ■ estrogens.

■ *with Estinyl and Estrace only:* ■ tartrazine (FD&C Yellow Dye No. 5) ■ aspirin.

You have ever had any of the following medical problems: ■ asthma or other lung disease ■ circulation disorders or blood clots ■ breast lumps or breast cancer or a family history of breast cancer ■ any other kind of cancer ■ endometriosis ■ diabetes ■ epilepsy or other seizure disorders ■ gallbladder disease or gallstones ■ heart disease, including heart attacks ■ high blood pressure or a family history of high blood pressure ■ high blood calcium levels ■ jaundice ■ kidney disease ■ liver disease ■ depression ■ migraine headaches ■ stroke ■ high cholesterol or a family history of high cholesterol ■ high blood pressure or toxemia during pregnancy ■ weight gain or fluid retention in synchrony with menstrual cycle ■ abnormal bleeding from the vagina.

You are taking any of the following medicines: ■ corticosteroids or corticotropin (ACTH) ■ medicine for diabetes ■ medicine for seizures ■ barbiturates ■ rifampin (antibiotic) ■ antidepressants ■ vitamin C ■ anticoagulants (blood thinners) ■ aminocaproic acid (medicine for excessive bleeding) ■ chenodiol (medicine for gallstones) ■ dantrolene (muscle relaxant) ■ mineral oil ■ tamoxifen (medicine for cancer) ■ vitamin A ■ vitamin B_6 ■ thyroid hormones ■ meprobamate (sedative and muscle relaxant).

SPECIAL RESTRICTIONS WHILE TAKING THIS DRUG

FOOD AND DRUG INTERACTIONS

Foods and Beverages	Your doctor may prescribe a diet to help maintain healthy bones, which you should follow carefully. Such a diet is usually high in calcium; if it is difficult

for you to include enough calcium in your diet, your doctor may suggest that you take a calcium supplement.

Smoking	Smoking increases the chance of developing such serious side effects as blood clot, heart attack, and stroke with estrogen therapy. If you smoke, try to stop or at least cut down.

No special restrictions on other drugs or alcohol use.

DAILY LIVING

Exertion and Exercise	You should try to include some regular physical activity in your daily life to strengthen your bones. Discuss with your doctor which kinds of exercise are appropriate for you.
Sun Exposure	You may find that you sunburn more easily or that you develop brown, blotchy spots on your skin after exposure to the sun while taking estrogens. Try to minimize sun exposure. It is a good idea to apply a sunscreen to exposed skin surfaces before going outdoors.
Examinations or Tests	It is important for you to keep all appointments with your doctor so that your progress can be checked. You will need periodic gynecologic examinations, including Pap smears, breast examinations, and annual mammograms. Periodic blood pressure or blood and urine tests may be required while you are on estrogen therapy.
Other Precautions	Tell any doctor or dentist you consult that you are on estrogen therapy, especially if you will be undergoing any type of surgery or any kind of diagnostic testing.

If you wear contact lenses, you may find your eyes becoming sensitive to them during estrogen therapy. If this happens, discuss with your eye doctor whether it may be necessary for you to wear eyeglasses while you are on estrogen.

Estrogen therapy has been associated with a number of serious side effects. Long-term use of estrogens in women after menopause increases the possibility of developing endometrial cancer (cancer of the uterus [womb]). If you develop any abnormal bleeding from the vagina, let your doctor know. (If your uterus has been surgically removed [hysterectomy], there is no chance of you developing endometrial cancer.) Your doctor may be able to tailor your dosage schedule to minimize such a risk.

Studies of women taking oral contraceptives (which contain higher doses of estrogen and progesterone than are prescribed for women after menopause) have shown an increased risk of noncancerous live tumors, blood clots, heart attacks, and stroke. If you develop any warning sign of a blood clot (see ''Possible Side Effects''), call your doctor or go to an emergency room immediately.

Helpful Hints	*Tablets and capsules.* You may feel nauseated during the first few weeks of estrogen therapy. If this is a problem, try taking your daily dose during or directly after meals or with snacks.

Skin patch. Immediately after opening the package, apply the patch to a clean, dry, hairless area of skin. Avoid the breast area and waistline (wearing tight clothing may dislodge the patch). The skin at the site should not be open, irritated, or oily. If the patch becomes loose or falls off, reapply it or, if necessary, apply a new one. Apply patches to different areas of the body, allowing at least one week between applications to a particular site.

No special restrictions on driving or exposure to excessive heat or cold.

POSSIBLE SIDE EFFECTS

Although this list of adverse effects may seem somewhat intimidating, keep in mind that some are quite rare. Of course, should these or any other problems arise while you are on medication, it is always a good idea to consult your doctor.

IF YOU DEVELOP

Possible signs of a blood clot: pain or heavy feeling in chest; pains in groin or legs (especially the calf); weakness or numbness in arms or legs; severe and sudden headache, sometimes with vomiting; visual disturbances; difficulty in speech; sudden dizziness or faintness; unexplained cough or shortness of breath

WHAT TO DO

Urgent Get in touch with your doctor immediately.

---

pain, swelling, or tenderness in stomach or side ■ vaginal bleeding ■ vaginal discharge ■ vaginitis ■ breast lumps ■ discharge from nipples ■ depression ■ uncontrollable, jerky movements ■ yellowing of eyes or skin ■ bleeding ■ fever ■ joint pain ■ rash

May be serious Check with your doctor as soon as possible.

---

nausea or vomiting ■ increased or decreased appetite ■ weight gain or loss ■ swelling of arms or legs ■ tenderness and swelling of breasts ■ stomach cramps or bloating ■ diarrhea ■ headache, including migraine headaches ■ dizziness ■ change in sexual drive ■ hair growth or loss ■ intolerance to contact lenses or other eye problems ■ increased skin sensitivity to sunlight, including development of brown, blotchy spots

With patch only: redness and irritation at patch site ■ skin redness or other skin problems

If symptoms are disturbing or persist, let your doctor know.

STORAGE INSTRUCTIONS

Store in a cool, dark place (not in a bathroom medicine cabinet).

STOPPING OR INTERRUPTING THERAPY

If you miss a dose of the oral form of this medicine, take it as soon as possible. If you do not remember until the following day, skip the missed dose and resume your regular schedule. Do not take two doses at the same time.

SPECIAL CONSIDERATIONS FOR THOSE OVER SIXTY-FIVE

None.

CONDITION: **OSTEOPOROSIS**

CATEGORY: **CALCIUM SUPPLEMENTS**

GENERIC (CHEMICAL) NAME	BRAND (TRADE) NAME	DOSAGE FORMS AND STRENGTHS
Calcium carbonate	CALTRATE OS-CAL TUMS	Tablets: 600 mg Tablets: 250, 500 mg Chewable tablets: 500, 750 mg
Calcium phosphate	POSTURE	Tablets: 300, 600 mg
Dibasic calcium phosphate		Capsules: 500 mg

DRUG PROFILE

Calcium supplements are used along with estrogen as part of a treatment program to prevent the bone loss of osteoporosis for people who find it difficult to include sufficient calcium in their diets. Calcium is a major component of bone; a deficiency of this mineral can lead to the weakening of bones that is the hallmark of osteoporosis. Although calcium supplements are not prescription drugs, they are included in this book because of their importance in helping decrease bone loss in older women after menopause.

BEFORE USING THIS DRUG

Let your doctor know *IF*

You have ever had any of the following medical problems: ■ heart disease ■ kidney disease, including kidney stones ■ severe constipation ■ sarcoidosis ■ hyper-parathyroidism.

You are taking any of the following medicines: ■ aspirin, indomethacin, or other medicine for arthritis ■ sodium polystyrene sulfonate (medicine to lower the amount of potassium in the body) ■ tranquilizers ■ cimetidine or ranitidine (medicine for ulcers) ■ digoxin, digitoxin, or digitalis (heart medicines) ■ iron preparations ■ ketoconazole (medicine for fungal infections) ■ tetracyclines ■ levodopa (medicine for Parkinson's disease) ■ quinidine (medicine for abnormal heart rhythms) ■ beta-blockers ■ captopril (medicine for high blood pressure or congestive heart failure) ■ corticosteroids ■ medicine for seizures ■ verapamil (medicine for chest pain) ■ thiazide diuretics.

SPECIAL RESTRICTIONS WHILE TAKING THIS DRUG

FOOD AND DRUG INTERACTIONS

Other Drugs	Calcium preparations may interfere with the absorption of other drugs. If you are taking any other medicine by mouth, space your dose one to two hours before or after taking your calcium supplement.
Foods and Beverages	Avoid large amounts of foods that may interfere with the effectiveness of this medicine, such as spinach, rhubarb, bran, and whole-grain cereals.

No special restrictions on alcohol use or smoking.

DAILY LIVING

Examinations or Tests	It is important for you to keep all appointments with your doctor so that your progress can be checked.

No special restrictions on driving, exertion and exercise, sun exposure, or exposure to excessive heat or cold.

POSSIBLE SIDE EFFECTS

Although this list of adverse effects may seem somewhat intimidating, keep in mind that some are quite rare. Of course, should these or any other problems arise while you are on medication, it is always a good idea to consult your doctor.

IF YOU DEVELOP	WHAT TO DO
severe and continuing constipation ■ pain or difficulty in urination ■ tiredness ■ continuing headache ■ loss of appetite ■ anxiety ■ mood or mental changes ■ muscle pain or twitching	**May be serious** Check with your doctor as soon as possible.
mild constipation ■ gas or bloating ■ belching	If symptoms are disturbing or persist, let your doctor know.

STORAGE INSTRUCTIONS

Store in a cool, dark place (not in a bathroom medicine cabinet).

STOPPING OR INTERRUPTING THERAPY

If you miss a dose of this medicine, take it as soon as possible. If you do not remember until the following day, skip the missed dose and resume your regular schedule.

SPECIAL CONSIDERATIONS FOR THOSE OVER SIXTY-FIVE

Older people may be especially prone to constipation with calcium supplements.

Chapter 6
Sleep Disorders and Emotional Problems

INSOMNIA

As we get older, one of our most common complaints is poor sleep. Approximately one-half of people over sixty years of age report symptoms due to sleep disturbance. It takes longer to fall asleep, and we awaken more often during the night, are not as refreshed on arising in the morning, and are sleepy during the day. Studies done in sleep laboratories confirm these complaints. Older people spend more time in lighter sleep and have shorter periods of deeper sleep. While older people sleep less at night, they nap more during the day. Because insomnia is more common in this age group, older people use more sleeping pills.

CAUSES

For some, sleep becomes an elusive goal night after night. In fact, doctors estimate that one out of every five people who come to see them has some difficulty sleeping. Much of this difficulty is due to stress, such as that caused by family problems, job pressures, the loss of a job, or the death of a loved one. These stressful emotions are physically arousing; they make us more vigilant, less able to assume the relaxed state that permits sleep to begin and to progress normally. As a result, we sleep less, plagued with symptoms of insomnia at just those times when we may need more sleep.

Emotions aren't the only things that cause insomnia. It may be something that's more concrete, such as a bedroom that's too warm or too cold, too noisy, or too dry or an unfamiliar sleeping environment, such as a hospital. Lack of exercise can make it hard to get to sleep. Such medical disorders as peptic ulcer, asthma, angina, and insulin-dependent diabetes may produce insomnia. The pain of arthritis or other medical conditions may sometimes be so acute that it hinders sleep. In addition, some medicines, such as those for high blood pressure and Parkinson's disease or those that have a stimulating effect, can interfere with your normal sleeping pattern. If you are undergoing diuretic therapy, you may find your nights interrupted by visits to the bathroom. (This may also occur if you drink too much fluid too soon before retiring.)

DIAGNOSIS

The term *insomnia* covers several kinds of sleep problems, including these:

• Difficulty in falling asleep—lying in bed and tossing and turning, trying unsuccessfully to sleep.

• Broken sleep—repeatedly waking during the night.

• Early morning awakening—waking earlier than you want and being unable to go back to sleep before getting up for the day.

TREATMENT

• Have a medical checkup. Insomnia is a symptom that something is wrong—something physical or psychological or both.

• Start an exercise program. Regular, moderate exercise is helpful for those of us who lead basically sedentary lives. Late afternoon or early evening is the best time to exercise—never just before bedtime.

• Try a light snack of high-protein food right before bedtime. L-tryptophan, an amino acid found in small quantities in high-protein foods, such as turkey, beef, cheese, and milk, may help bring on sleep.

• Avoid coffee, tea, cola drinks, and cigarettes, especially in the evening. Lowering your caffeine (or nicotine) intake may be enough to "cure" your insomnia. Spicy foods or too much fluid in the evening may contribute to insomnia because of indigestion or having to get up to urinate.

• Take a warm (not hot) shower or bath just before getting into bed; warmth relaxes muscles.

• If your blankets cling together and your hair is full of static electricity, use a vaporizer or small room humidifier to add moisture to the air.

• Avoid excessive daytime napping if you have trouble sleeping at night.

• Some people cope with insomnia by using alcohol—but alcohol is not a good sedative. Even if you initially fall asleep easily, you're likely to wake up in the middle of the night unable to go back to sleep.

• If your insomnia is caused by a particularly stressful—but temporary—situation, your doctor may prescribe a sleep-inducing drug for a short period. See the drug charts on pages 478–491 for detailed information about these medicines. Drugs from the antihistamine family are sometimes prescribed for brief insomnia. Avoid alcohol completely if you're taking sleeping pills.

• Learn about normal changes in sleep throughout a person's life. Discuss your sleep pattern with your doctor to find out if you do have insomnia and to identify factors that contribute to it. Your doctor may be able to recommend relaxation techniques to help you fall asleep. Keeping regular bedtime and wake-up hours, making sure the bedroom is quiet and at a comfortable temperature, and avoiding activities such as reading or watching TV in bed (so that you learn to associate the bed/bedroom with only sleep) can help insomnia.

OUTLOOK

The key to solving a sleep problem is to find the cause. Physical problems as well as emotional concerns may cause sleeplessness, so the first step to a good night's sleep is a visit to your doctor. Steps you can take yourself to relieve insomnia include exercising regularly, taking a warm bath and/or eating a light snack before bed, and ensuring comfortable surroundings. Sleep-inducing drugs are a temporary solution for short-term problems and may help you get back into the pattern of sleeping through the night.

CONDITION: **INSOMNIA**

CATEGORY: **HYPNOTICS (BENZODIAZEPINES)**

GENERIC (CHEMICAL) NAME	BRAND (TRADE) NAME	DOSAGE FORMS AND STRENGTHS
Alprazolam	XANAX	Tablets: 0.25, 0.5, 1 mg
Chlorazepate dipotassium	TRANXENE TRANXENE-SD	Capsules: 3.75, 7.5, 15 mg Tablets: 3.75, 7.5, 15 mg Tablets: 11.25, 22.5 mg
Chlordiazepoxide hydrochloride	LIBRITABS LIBRIUM	Tablets: 5, 10, 25 mg Capsules: 5, 10, 25 mg
Clonazepam*	KLONOPIN	Tablets: 0.5, 1, 2 mg
Diazepam	VALIUM VALRELEASE	Tablets: 2, 5, 10 mg Controlled-release capsules: 15 mg
Flurazepam	DALMANE	Capsules: 15, 30 mg
Lorazepam	ATIVAN	Tablets: 0.5, 1, 2 mg
Oxazepam	SERAX	Capsules: 10, 15, 30 mg Tablets: 15 mg
Prazepam	CENTRAX	Capsules: 5, 10, 20 mg Tablets: 10 mg
Temazepam	RESTORIL	Capsules: 15, 30 mg

Triazolam	HALCION	Tablets: 0.125, 0.25, 0.5 mg

*Clonazepam is used only to treat seizures, and not to treat anxiety, insomnia, or muscle spasm. It is listed here because of its many similarities to the other benzodiazepines discussed in this chart.

DRUG PROFILE

Benzodiazepines are used to treat a number of conditions, including anxiety, insomnia, muscle spasm, and seizures. Exactly how these drugs work is a matter of some debate. However, what they all seem to have in common is that they reduce nerve cell activity in those areas of the central nervous system (CNS) and peripheral nervous system (PNS) thought to be responsible for the experience of anxiety and muscular tension. The benzodiazepines most often used as sleep-inducing drugs are flurazepam (Dalmane), temazepam (Restoril), triazolam (Halcion), and oxazepam (Serax). Low doses are usually prescribed for older people.

BEFORE USING THIS DRUG

Let your doctor know *IF*

You have ever had allergic reactions or other problems with ■ any benzodiazepines ■ tartrazine (FD&C Yellow Dye No. 5) (contained in Serax tablets) ■ aspirin.

You have ever had any of the following medical problems: ■ seizures ■ asthma or other lung disease ■ kidney disease ■ liver disease ■ depression or any other serious mental illness ■ myasthenia gravis ■ porphyria.

■ *with clonazepam only:* ■ glaucoma.

You are taking any of the following medicines: ■ other benzodiazepines ■ medicine for seizures ■ sleep medicines ■ tranquilizers ■ muscle relaxants ■ medicine for depression ■ narcotics or other prescription pain-killers ■ medicine for hay fever, coughs, or colds ■ antihistamines ■ medicine for ulcers ■ Antabuse (used in treatment of alcoholism) ■ antibiotics ■ levodopa (medicine for Parkinson's disease) ■ anticoagulants (blood thinners).

SPECIAL RESTRICTIONS WHILE TAKING THIS DRUG

FOOD AND DRUG INTERACTIONS

Other Drugs	Do not take any other drugs, including over-the-counter (OTC) drugs, before checking with your doctor. This drug increases the effect of other drugs that depress the central nervous system, such as antihistamines; medicine for hay fever, allergies, or colds; other sleep medicines; tranquilizers; narcotics or other prescription pain-killers; muscle relaxants; and medicine for seizures.
Foods and Beverages	Excessive consumption of caffeine (found in coffee, tea, cola drinks, cocoa, chocolate) may aggravate symptoms of anxiety and counteract the calming effects of benzodiazepines.
Alcohol	Avoid alcohol, another central nervous system depressant, while taking benzodiazepines; this combination can be dangerous.
Smoking	Cigarette smoking may reduce the effect of benzodiazepines. If you smoke, try to stop or at least cut down.

DAILY LIVING

Driving	This drug may cause drowsiness or loss of alertness. Be careful when driving, operating household appliances, or doing any other tasks that require alertness until you know how this drug affects you.
Examinations or Tests	It is important for you to keep all appointments with your doctor so that your progress can be checked. If you are on long-term therapy for prevention of seizures, periodic blood and urine tests may be required.

If you are taking this type of medicine for anxiety or insomnia, ask your doctor every few months if you need to keep taking it.

| Other Precautions | Taking this medicine more often or for a longer period of time than prescribed by your doctor may make it habit forming. If you suspect that this medicine is not working, do not increase the dose but check with your doctor.

Tell any doctor or dentist you consult that you are taking any of these drugs, especially if you will be undergoing any type of surgery. |

| Helpful Hints | Swallow the controlled-release capsules whole—do not break, crush, or chew them. |

No special restrictions on exertion and exercise, sun exposure, or exposure to excessive heat or cold.

POSSIBLE SIDE EFFECTS

Although this list of adverse effects may seem somewhat intimidating, keep in mind that some are quite rare. Of course, should these or any other problems arise while you are on medication, it is always a good idea to consult your doctor.

IF YOU DEVELOP

difficulty in speech ■ confusion ■ severe drowsiness or weakness ■ difficulty in walking ■ difficulty in breathing

With clonazepam only: loss of feeling on one side of the body

depression ■ hallucinations ■ sleeplessness ■ uncontrollable movements of the body, mouth, or cheek ■ excitement ■ agitation ■ nervousness

WHAT TO DO

Urgent Get in touch with your doctor immediately.

May be serious Check with your doctor as soon as possible.

■ irritability ■ talkativeness ■ restlessness ■ anxiety ■ nightmares ■ fainting ■ personality changes ■ tiredness or weakness ■ tremors ■ rage ■ burning or prickling feeling ■ irregular or fast heartbeat ■ flushing ■ increased sweating ■ shortness of breath ■ sores in mouth or throat ■ rash, hives, or itching ■ bleeding or bruising ■ sore throat or fever ■ yellowing of eyes or skin

With clonazepam only: abnormal eye movements ■ movement difficulties ■ glassy eyes ■ memory problems ■ hysteria ■ muscle pain or weakness ■ tightness in chest ■ runny nose ■ uncontrollable bowel movements ■ swelling of ankles or face ■ swollen lymph glands ■ changes in skin color

After you STOP taking this medicine: anxiety ■ sleeplessness ■ depression ■ clumsiness ■ tremors ■ loss of appetite ■ diarrhea ■ vomiting ■ stomach or muscle cramps ■ irritability ■ memory problems ■ personality changes ■ seizures ■ hallucinations ■ increased sweating

---

drowsiness ■ dizziness or light-headedness ■ ''high'' feeling ■ vivid dreams ■ clumsiness or poor balance ■ headache ■ blurred or double vision or other visual disturbances ■ stomach cramps or pain ■ constipation ■ diarrhea ■ nausea or vomiting ■ dry mouth ■ increased thirst ■ increased salivation ■ increased production of phlegm in lungs ■ difficulty in urination ■ urinary frequency ■ urinary retention ■ incontinence ■ hiccups ■ increase or decrease in appetite ■ weight gain or loss ■ swelling of tongue ■ bitter or metallic taste in mouth ■ increased or diminished sex drive ■ breast swelling in men ■ increased eye sensitivity to light

With clonazepam only: heartburn ■ excessive hair growth or loss

If symptoms are disturbing or persist, let your doctor know.

STORAGE INSTRUCTIONS

Store in a cool, dark place (not in a bathroom medicine cabinet).

STOPPING OR INTERRUPTING THERAPY

Take this medicine exactly as prescribed by your doctor. Do not suddenly discontinue taking this medicine, since uncomfortable and potentially serious withdrawal reactions may occur (see ''Possible Side Effects''). Your doctor will advise you how to reduce your dosage gradually and safely. If you miss a dose, take it as soon as possible. If it is not within an hour of the scheduled time of the missed dose, skip it and resume your regular schedule. Do not take two doses at the same time.

SPECIAL CONSIDERATIONS FOR THOSE OVER SIXTY-FIVE

Because older people may be especially prone to the side effects of benzodiazepines (particularly, drowsiness, difficulty in walking, confusion, agitation, and excitement), doctors may start people over sixty-five on a lower dosage.

CONDITION: **INSOMNIA**

CATEGORY: **HYPNOTICS (BARBITURATES)**

GENERIC (CHEMICAL) NAME	BRAND (TRADE) NAME	DOSAGE FORMS AND STRENGTHS
Butabarbital sodium	BUTICAPS BUTISOL Sodium	Capsules: 15, 30 mg Elixir: 30 mg per tsp Tablets: 15, 30, 50, 100 mg
Mephobarbital	MEBARAL	Tablets: 32, 50, 100 mg
Pentobarbital and Pentobarbital sodium	NEMBUTAL	Capsules: 50, 100 mg Elixir: 18.2 mg pentobarbital equivalent to 20 mg pentobarbital sodium per tsp Rectal suppositories: 30, 60, 120, 200 mg

Phenobarbital		Capsules: 16 mg
		Controlled-release
		  capsules: 65 mg
		Elixir: 15, 20 mg per tsp
		Tablets: 8, 16, 32, 65,
		  100 mg

Secobarbital sodium	SECONAL	Capsules: 50, 100 mg

DRUG PROFILE

Barbiturates are used to treat insomnia and to relieve anxiety or nervousness. Although it is not understood exactly how the barbiturates work, some experts believe that these drugs act on the part of the brain responsible for wakefulness. Barbiturates have a relatively high propensity for interactions with other drugs. Infrequently, they may cause agitation instead of relieving anxiety and nervousness. They are also associated with daytime drowsiness and morning "hangover." Doctors usually prefer not to prescribe these drugs for older people.

BEFORE USING THIS DRUG

Let your doctor know *IF*

You have ever had allergic reactions or other problems with ■ any barbiturates ■ tartrazine (FD&C Yellow Dye No. 5) (contained in Buticaps, Butisol, and Nembutal) ■ aspirin.

You have ever had any of the following medical problems: ■ asthma or other lung disease ■ kidney disease ■ liver disease ■ mental illness ■ porphyria ■ overactive thyroid ■ high or low blood pressure ■ drug abuse, including alcoholism.

You are taking any of the following medicines: ■ any medicine containing alcohol ■ antihistamines ■ medicine for hay fever, coughs, or colds ■ muscle relaxants ■ narcotics or other prescription pain-killers ■ medicine for seizures ■ medicine for depression ■ anticoagulants (blood thinners).

SPECIAL RESTRICTIONS WHILE TAKING THIS DRUG

FOOD AND DRUG INTERACTIONS

Other Drugs	Do not take any other drugs, including over-the-counter (OTC) drugs, before checking with your doctor. This drug increases the effect of other drugs that depress the central nervous system, such as antihistamines; medicine for hay fever, allergies, or colds; other sleep medicines; tranquilizers; narcotics or other prescription pain-killers; muscle relaxants; and medicine for seizures.
Alcohol	Avoid alcohol, another central nervous system depressant, while taking this drug; this combination can be very dangerous.
Smoking	Smoking may reduce the effectiveness of this drug. If you smoke, try to stop or at least cut down.

No special restrictions on foods and beverages.

DAILY LIVING

Driving	This drug may cause drowsiness or loss of alertness. Be careful when driving, operating household appliances, or doing any other tasks that require alertness until you know how this drug affects you.
Examinations or Tests	It is important for you to keep all appointments with your doctor so that your progress can be checked. Ask your doctor every couple of months if you need to keep taking this medicine.
Other Precautions	Taking this medicine more often or for a longer period of time than prescribed by your doctor may make it

habit forming. If you suspect that this medicine is not working, do not increase the dose, but check with your doctor.

Tell any doctor or dentist you consult that you are taking this drug, especially if you will be undergoing any type of surgery.

If you accidentally take an overdose, go to an emergency room immediately.

Helpful Hints

The controlled-release capsules should be swallowed whole—without chewing, breaking, or crushing.

If you have been storing the suppository form of this medicine in a warm place, it may be too soft to use. Put it in the refrigerator for half an hour or run cold water over the wrapped suppository before use.

No special restrictions on exertion or exercise, sun exposure, or exposure to excessive heat or cold.

POSSIBLE SIDE EFFECTS

Although this list of adverse effects may seem somewhat intimidating, keep in mind that some are quite rare. Of course, should these or any other problems arise while you are on medication, it is always a good idea to consult your doctor.

IF YOU DEVELOP

cold, clammy skin ■ slow or fast heartbeat ■ chest pain ■ confusion ■ slurred speech ■ wheezing or other difficulty in breathing ■ loss of balance ■ fever ■ severe headache ■ swelling of the tip of the penis ■ pain in urination

WHAT TO DO

Urgent Get in touch with your doctor immediately.

---

bleeding (including nosebleed or bleeding lip sores) or bruising ■ muscle or joint pain ■ any other unusual pain ■ scaly, red skin ■ yellowing of eyes or skin ■ rash or hives ■ mouth sores

May be serious Check with your doctor as soon as possible.

■ swelling of face or lips ■ red, itching, or swollen eyes ■ stuffy nose ■ depression ■ agitation ■ excitement ■ hallucinations ■ extreme tiredness

clumsiness ■ staggering ■ dizziness or light-headedness ■ drowsiness ■ "hangover" feeling ■ anxiety ■ nightmares ■ sleeplessness ■ irritability ■ constipation ■ diarrhea ■ nausea or vomiting

If symptoms are disturbing or persist, let your doctor know.

After you STOP taking this medicine: increased dreaming ■ nightmares ■ sleeplessness

STORAGE INSTRUCTIONS

Store in a cool, dark place (not in a bathroom medicine cabinet). If your medicine is in a liquid form, make sure that it does not freeze. Suppositories should be stored in the refrigerator.

STOPPING OR INTERRUPTING THERAPY

Do not suddenly discontinue taking this drug, since dangerous withdrawal reactions (for example, seizures) may occur. Your doctor will advise you on how to reduce your dosage gradually. Take this medicine exactly as prescribed by your doctor. If you miss a dose, take it as soon as possible. If it is almost time for your next dose, skip the missed dose and resume your regular schedule. Do not take two doses at the same time.

SPECIAL CONSIDERATIONS FOR THOSE OVER SIXTY-FIVE

Because older people may be especially prone to the side effects of barbiturates (particularly, excitement, depression, and confusion), doctors may start people over sixty-five on a lower dosage.

CONDITION: **INSOMNIA**

CATEGORY: **HYPNOTICS (NONBARBITURATES)**

GENERIC (CHEMICAL) NAME	BRAND (TRADE) NAME	DOSAGE FORMS AND STRENGTHS
Chloral hydrate	NOCTEC	Capsules: 250, 500 mg Syrup: 500 mg per tsp

DRUG PROFILE

Chloral hydrate is a sleep-inducing medicine. The way this drug works is not completely understood, but many experts believe that it acts on the part of the brain that controls sleeping and waking. Chloral hydrate, unlike some other sedatives, is usually not associated with worsening of insomnia after it is discontinued. It is inexpensive, has few side effects, and is considered to be the first-choice sleep medicine for older people when nondrug measures fail.

BEFORE USING THIS DRUG

Let your doctor know *IF*

You have ever had allergic reactions or other problems with ■ chloral hydrate.

You have ever had any of the following medical problems: ■ heart disease ■ liver disease ■ kidney disease ■ porphyria ■ ulcers ■ depression or other mental illness ■ drug abuse, including alcoholism.

You are taking any of the following medicines: ■ other sleep medicines ■ tranquilizers ■ any medicine containing alcohol ■ medicine for high blood pressure ■ antihistamines ■ medicine for hay fever, coughs, or colds ■ muscle relaxants ■ narcotics or other prescription pain-killers ■ medicine for Parkinson's disease ■ medicine for seizures ■ barbiturates ■ medicine for depression ■ anticoagulants (blood thinners).

SPECIAL RESTRICTIONS WHILE TAKING THIS DRUG

FOOD AND DRUG INTERACTIONS

Other Drugs	Do not take any other drugs, including over-the-counter (OTC) drugs, before checking with your doctor. This drug increases the effect of other drugs that depress the central nervous system, such as antihistamines; medicine for hay fever, allergies, or colds; other sleep medicines; tranquilizers; narcotics or other prescription pain-killers; muscle relaxants; and medicine for seizures.
Alcohol	Avoid alcohol, another central nervous system depressant, while taking chloral hydrate; this combination can be dangerous.
Smoking	Smoking may reduce the effectiveness of this drug. If you smoke, try to stop or at least cut down.

No special restrictions on foods and beverages.

DAILY LIVING

Driving	This drug will probably cause drowsiness or loss of alertness. Do not drive, operate household appliances, or do any other tasks that require alertness until you know how this drug affects you.
Examinations or Tests	Ask your doctor every few months if you need to keep taking this drug.
Other Precautions	Taking this medicine more often or for a longer period of time than prescribed by your doctor may make it habit forming. If you suspect that this medicine is not

working, do not increase the dose, but check with your doctor.

If you accidentally take an overdose, get in touch with your doctor immediately.

| Helpful Hints | If your medicine is in capsule form, swallow it whole without chewing, crushing, or breaking it. Taking the capsules with a full glass of water or other liquid lessens the chance of stomach upset.

Some people find the taste of the syrup unpleasant. To improve the taste and lessen the chance of upset stomach, mix your dose with water, juice, or other liquids. |

No special restrictions on exertion and exercise, sun exposure, or exposure to excessive heat or cold.

POSSIBLE SIDE EFFECTS

Although this list of adverse effects may seem somewhat intimidating, keep in mind that some are quite rare. Of course, should these or any other problems arise while you are on medication, it is always a good idea to consult your doctor.

IF YOU DEVELOP

confusion ■ loss of balance ■ paranoia (unreasonable suspiciousness) ■ irregular or slow heartbeat ■ difficulty in swallowing ■ severe drowsiness ■ continued nausea and vomiting ■ difficulty in breathing ■ severe weakness ■ low body temperature

WHAT TO DO

Urgent Get in touch with your doctor immediately.

---

rash or hives ■ blisters ■ purplish or brownish-red spots on skin ■ sleepwalking ■ hallucinations ■ extreme agitation or excitement

May be serious Check with your doctor as soon as possible.

nausea or vomiting ■ diarrhea ■ stomach pain ■ unpleasant taste in mouth ■ general feeling of unwellness ■ clumsiness ■ drowsiness ■ dizziness, or light-headedness ■ headache ■ "hangover" feeling ■ nightmares

If symptoms are disturbing or persist, let your doctor know.

STORAGE INSTRUCTIONS

Store in a cool, dark place (not in a bathroom medicine cabinet). If your medicine is in a liquid form, make sure that it does not freeze.

STOPPING OR INTERRUPTING THERAPY

Take this medicine exactly as prescribed by your doctor. If you have been using chloral hydrate for six months or longer, suddenly stopping the drug may result in serious withdrawal effects. Your doctor will advise you on how to reduce your dosage gradually. If you miss a dose, take it as soon as possible. If it is almost time for your next dose, skip the missed dose and resume your regular schedule. Do not take two doses at the same time.

SPECIAL CONSIDERATIONS FOR THOSE OVER SIXTY-FIVE

Because older people may be especially prone to the side effects of sleep medicines (particularly, drowsiness, confusion, agitation, and clumsiness), doctors may start people over sixty-five on a lower dosage.

ANXIETY

Virtually all of us have experienced the worry, uneasiness, and panic that characterize anxiety. Some people become so anxious that they think they're "going crazy" or "losing" their mind. Others fear that something awful is about to happen and experience exaggerated feelings of doom. These emotions are often associated with frightening physical symptoms as well; difficulty in breathing, pounding heart, dizziness, chest tightness, choking sensation, increased sweating, "jitters," insomnia, and nightmares are just some of them.

Some anxiety is normal, but when it becomes so extreme that it interferes with day-to-day living, it's time to get some help.

FORMS OF ANXIETY

Generalized anxiety disorder is a vague, persistent feeling that something is wrong. People suffering from generalized anxiety feel worried and on edge all the time. They find concentration and decision making difficult. They can't sleep well at night and feel fatigued during the day. The disorder is often accompanied by physical problems, such as chest pain and blurred vision, that have no apparent cause. In an effort to find relief, sufferers tend to go from doctor to doctor looking for a cure.

Panic attacks are sudden episodes of severe anxiety and fear that can be mistaken for heart attacks because of the accompanying physical symptoms.

Phobias are extreme anxieties that focus on a specific place, activity, or object.

Some people who experience severe panic attacks may limit normal activities such as shopping, going to the movies, driving, or visiting friends to avoid the frightening symptoms of such attacks when they're away from home. When their activities become so restricted that they won't leave home at all, they're said to be suffering from *agoraphobia*, a fear of public places.

CAUSES

Just as anxiety takes different forms, it has different causes. Physical problems such as heart conditions, endocrine disorders (such as an overactive or underactive thyroid), and neurologic and respiratory diseases can all cause feelings of anxiety. Other culprits include caffeine, alcohol withdrawal, certain vitamin deficiencies, and drug side effects. Anxiety may also be a prominent feature of depression.

Physical changes that occur as we get older may also provoke a good deal of anxiety. Some people become anxious because their hearing or sight becomes less sharp with age, others because of hair loss or prominent wrinkles. Not surprisingly, anxiety is also provoked by changes in lifestyle; financial strain; housing difficulties; failing health; and the loss of a spouse, family member, or close friend.

DIAGNOSIS

Because the condition can be caused by so many different physical and emotional factors, your doctor will do a complete physical examination and will also want to know exactly what prescription and over-the-counter drugs you're taking.

TREATMENT

If a medical problem is at the root of anxiety, treating the condition often relieves the anxious feelings.

If a specific situation caused the anxiety, just talking about the upsetting event may be enough to alleviate the symptoms.

If the anxiety isn't caused by physical problems or a specific event, your doctor may prescribe a medicine to relieve the anxiety, ease the physical symptoms it causes, and help you sleep at night. For detailed information on drugs commonly used to treat anxiety, see the charts on pages 494–505. As a rule, antianxiety agents should only be used when symptoms are intense and disruptive. Shorter-acting drugs (oxazepam, lorazepam, alprazolam) are preferred for older people and are usually only prescribed for several weeks. Your doctor may prescribe benzodiazepines for a longer period of time for disruptive chronic anxiety.

OUTLOOK

Some anxiety is part of living. However, if anxiety gets out of hand and becomes distressing, it can be relieved. Anxiety stemming from a physical illness often resolves itself once the illness is treated. Anxiety that is caused by a specific event can often be put into perspective by talking about it with a doctor or counselor. Anxiety for which no cause can be determined can now be eased by the use of one of several drugs.

CONDITION: **ANXIETY**

CATEGORY: **ANTIANXIETY AGENTS (BENZODIAZEPINES)**

GENERIC (CHEMICAL) NAME	BRAND (TRADE) NAME	DOSAGE FORMS AND STRENGTHS
Alprazolam	XANAX	Tablets: 0.25, 0.5, 1 mg
Chlorazepate dipotassium	TRANXENE	Capsules: 3.75, 7.5, 15 mg Tablets: 3.75, 7.5, 15 mg
	TRANXENE-SD	Tablets: 11.25, 22.5 mg
Chlordiazepoxide hydrochloride	LIBRITABS LIBRIUM	Tablets: 5, 10, 25 mg Capsules: 5, 10, 25 mg
Clonazepam*	KLONOPIN	Tablets: 0.5, 1, 2 mg
Diazepam	VALIUM VALRELEASE	Tablets: 2, 5, 10 mg Controlled-release capsules: 15 mg
Flurazepam	DALMANE	Capsules: 15, 30 mg
Lorazepam	ATIVAN	Tablets: 0.5, 1, 2 mg
Oxazepam	SERAX	Capsules: 10, 15, 30 mg Tablets: 15 mg
Prazepam	CENTRAX	Capsules: 5, 10, 20 mg Tablets: 10 mg
Temazepam	RESTORIL	Capsules: 15, 30 mg

Triazolam	HALCION	Tablets: 0.125, 0.25, 0.5 mg

*Clonazepam is used only to treat seizures, and not to treat anxiety, insomnia, or muscle spasms. It is listed here because of its many similarities to the other benzodiazepines discussed in this chart.

DRUG PROFILE

Benzodiazepines are used to treat a number of conditions, including anxiety, insomnia, muscle spasm, and seizures. Exactly how these drugs work is a matter of some debate. However, what they all seem to have in common is that they reduce nerve cell activity in those areas of the central nervous system (CNS) and peripheral nervous system (PNS) thought to be responsible for the experience of anxiety and muscular tension. The benzodiazepines most often used as antianxiety agents are alprazolam (Xanax), chlorazepate (Tranxene, Tranxene-SD), chlordiazepoxide (Libritabs, Librium), diazepam (Valium, Valrelease), lorazepam (Ativan), and prazepam (Centrax). Low doses are usually prescribed for older people.

For complete information on these drugs, see pages 478–483.

CONDITION: **ANXIETY**

CATEGORY: **ANTIANXIETY AGENTS (NONBENZODIAZEPINES)**

GENERIC (CHEMICAL) NAME	BRAND (TRADE) NAME	DOSAGE FORMS AND STRENGTHS
Meprobamate	EQUANIL	Capsules: 400 mg Coated tablets: 400 mg Tablets: 200, 400 mg
	MILTOWN	Tablets: 200, 400 mg
	MILTOWN 600	Tablets: 600 mg

DRUG PROFILE

Meprobamate is used to relieve short-term anxiety, including anxiety associated with such disorders as phobias and panic attacks. The way this drug works is not completely understood, though it is believed to act on the area of the brain that is the center of the emotions.

BEFORE USING THIS DRUG

Let your doctor know *IF*

You have ever had allergic reactions or other problems with ■ meprobamate ■ carbromal ■ carisoprodol ■ mebufamate ■ tybamate ■ tartrazine (FD&C Yellow Dye No. 5) (contained in Equanil tablets) ■ aspirin.

You have ever had any of the following medical problems: ■ seizures ■ kidney disease ■ liver disease ■ porphyria.

You are taking any of the following medicines: ■ other tranquilizers ■ sleep medicines ■ medicine for depression ■ narcotics or other prescription pain-killers ■ antihistamines ■ medicine for hay fever, coughs, or colds ■ medicine for seizures ■ medicine for Parkinson's disease ■ muscle relaxants ■ barbiturates.

SPECIAL RESTRICTIONS WHILE TAKING THIS DRUG

FOOD AND DRUG INTERACTIONS

Other Drugs	Do not take any other drugs, including over-the-counter (OTC) drugs, before checking with your doctor. This drug increases the effect of other drugs that depress the central nervous system, such as antihistamines; medicine for hay fever, allergies, or colds; sleep medicines; tranquilizers; narcotics or other prescription pain-killers; muscle relaxants; and medicine for seizures.
Alcohol	Avoid alcohol, another central nervous system depressant, while taking this drug; this combination can be dangerous.
Smoking	Smoking may reduce the effectiveness of this drug. If you smoke, try to stop or at least cut down.

No special restrictions on foods and beverages.

DAILY LIVING

Driving	Meprobamate may cause drowsiness or loss of alertness. Be careful when driving, operating household appliances, or doing any other tasks that require alertness until you know how this drug affects you.
Examinations or Tests	It is important for you to keep all appointments with your doctor so that your progress can be checked. Ask your doctor every several weeks if you need to keep taking this drug.
Other Precautions	Taking this medicine more often or for a longer period of time than prescribed by your doctor may make it habit forming. If you suspect that the drug is not working, do not increase the dose, but check with your doctor.
	Tell any doctor or dentist you consult that you are taking this drug, especially if you will be undergoing any type of surgery.
	If you accidentally take an overdose, go to an emergency room immediately.

No special restrictions on exertion and exercise, sun exposure, or exposure to excessive heat or cold.

POSSIBLE SIDE EFFECTS

Although this list of adverse effects may seem somewhat intimidating, keep in mind that some are quite rare. Of course, should these or any other problems arise while you are on medication, it is always a good idea to consult your doctor.

IF YOU DEVELOP

extreme drowsiness or weakness ■ difficulty in breathing ■ slurred speech ■ loss of balance

WHAT TO DO

Urgent Get in touch with your doctor immediately.

■ sore throat ■ fever ■ chills ■ bleeding or bruising ■ fainting ■ decreased urination ■ irregular, slow, or fast heartbeat

rash, hives, or itching ■ blisters ■ purplish or brownish-red spots on skin ■ agitation ■ excitement ■ tingling, burning, or prickling sensations ■ "high" feeling ■ swelling of feet or ankles ■ swollen glands ■ stomach pain	**May be serious** Get in touch with your doctor immediately.
clumsiness ■ headache ■ blurred vision or other visual disturbances ■ diarrhea ■ drowsiness ■ dizziness or light-headedness ■ nausea or vomiting ■ tiredness ■ loss of appetite	If symptoms are disturbing or persist, let your doctor know.

STORAGE INSTRUCTIONS

Store in a cool, dark place (not in a bathroom medicine cabinet).

STOPPING OR INTERRUPTING THERAPY

Take this medicine exactly as prescribed by your doctor. *Do not suddenly discontinue taking this medicine, since potentially serious withdrawal reactions may occur.* Your doctor will advise you how to reduce your dosage gradually. If you miss a dose, take it as soon as possible. If it is almost time for your next dose, skip the missed dose and resume your regular schedule. Do not take two doses at the same time.

SPECIAL CONSIDERATIONS FOR THOSE OVER SIXTY-FIVE

Because older people may be especially prone to the side effects of meprobamate, doctors may start people over sixty-five on a lower dosage.

CONDITION: **ANXIETY**

CATEGORY: **ANTIANXIETY AGENTS (ANTIHISTAMINES)**

GENERIC (CHEMICAL) NAME	BRAND (TRADE) NAME	DOSAGE FORMS AND STRENGTHS
Hydroxyzine hydrochloride	ATARAX	Syrup: 10 mg per tsp Tablets: 10, 25, 50 mg
	VISTARIL	Capsules: 25, 50, 100 mg Suspension: 25 mg per tsp

DRUG PROFILE

When you are exposed to a substance to which you are allergic, a chemical called *histamine* is released into the bloodstream and produces the itchy, watery eyes; runny nose; and rashes that are typical of an allergic reaction. Antihistamines work by blocking the action of histamine. They are used to treat allergies as well as to relieve the symptoms of a cold. Hydroxyzine is also used to treat anxiety. Exactly how it works to relieve anxiety is not completely understood.

For complete information on this drug, see pages 633–638.

CONDITION: **ANXIETY**

CATEGORY: **NEUROLEPTICS (PHENOTHIAZINES)**

GENERIC (CHEMICAL) NAME	BRAND (TRADE) NAME	DOSAGE FORMS AND STRENGTHS
Chlorpromazine hydrochloride	THORAZINE	Concentrate: 30, 100 mg per ml Controlled-release capsules: 30, 75, 150, 200, 300 mg

		Rectal suppositories: 25, 100 mg Syrup: 10 mg per tsp Tablets: 10, 25, 50, 100, 200 mg
Fluphenazine hydrochloride	PROLIXIN	Elixir: 2.5 mg per tsp Tablets: 1, 2.5, 5, 10 mg
Prochlorperazine	COMPAZINE	Controlled-release capsules: 10, 15, 30 mg Rectal suppositories: 2.5, 5, 25 mg Syrup: 5 mg per tsp Tablets: 5, 10, 25 mg
Thiethylperazine maleate*	TORECAN	Rectal suppositories: 10 mg Tablets: 10 mg
Thioridazine hydrochloride	MELLARIL	Concentrate: 30, 100 mg per ml Suspension: 25, 100 mg per tsp Tablets: 10, 15, 25, 50, 100, 150, 200 mg
Trifluoperazine hydrochloride	STELAZINE	Concentrate: 10 mg per ml Tablets: 1, 2, 5, 10 mg

*Triethylperazine is only used to relieve nausea and vomiting and not to treat emotional disorders. It is listed here because of its many similarities to the other phenothiazines discussed in this chart.

DRUG PROFILE

Phenothiazines are used to treat a variety of emotional disorders, including very severe anxiety, agitation, depression, and sleep disturbances. Some phenothiazines (prochlorperazine, thiethylperazine, and chlorpromazine) are also used to treat nausea and vomiting. These drugs are thought to work by inhibiting the action of dopamine, a chemical messenger, in the part of the brain that is the seat of the emotions as well as in the zone of the brain that controls nausea and vomiting.

BEFORE USING THIS DRUG

Let your doctor know *IF*

You have ever had allergic reactions or other problems with ■ any phenothiazines ■ tartrazine (FD&C Yellow Dye No. 5) ■ aspirin.

You have ever had any of the following medical problems: ■ seizures ■ anemia or other blood disease ■ asthma or other lung disease ■ respiratory tract infection, such as pneumonia ■ liver disease ■ kidney disease ■ heart or blood vessel disease ■ glaucoma ■ enlarged prostate ■ urinary problems ■ Parkinson's disease.

You are taking any of the following medicines: ■ medicine for seizures ■ antacids ■ appetite suppressants ■ medicine for high blood pressure ■ medicine for asthma ■ medicine for Parkinson's disease ■ medicine for depression ■ beta-blockers ■ antihistamines ■ medicine for hay fever, coughs, or colds ■ barbiturates ■ narcotics or other prescription pain-killers ■ sleep medicines ■ tranquilizers ■ cimetidine (medicine for ulcers) ■ Antabuse (used in the treatment of alcoholism) ■ medicine for nausea or vomiting ■ antibiotics ■ anticoagulants (blood thinners).

You are often exposed to extreme heat or cold or to organophosphate insecticides (e.g., if you work in a plant that manufactures this type of pesticide).

SPECIAL RESTRICTIONS WHILE TAKING THIS DRUG

FOOD AND DRUG INTERACTIONS

Other Drugs	Do not take any other drugs, including over-the-counter (OTC) drugs, before checking with your doctor. This drug increases the effects of other drugs that depress the central nervous system, such as antihistamines; medicine for hay fever, allergies, or colds; sleep medicines; other tranquilizers; narcotics or other prescription pain-killers; muscle relaxants; and medicine for seizures.

Alcohol	Avoid alcohol, another central nervous system depressant, while taking this drug; the combination can be dangerous.
Smoking	Smoking may reduce the effectiveness of this drug. If you smoke, try to stop or at least cut down.

No special restrictions on foods and beverages.

DAILY LIVING

Driving	These drugs may cause drowsiness or loss of alertness. Be careful when driving, operating household appliances, or doing any other tasks that require alertness until you know how this drug affects you.
Exertion and Exercise	This drug may cause you to sweat less than normally. Sweating is your body's natural way of cooling down, and not sweating enough can be dangerous. Use caution not to become overheated when you exercise or exert yourself.
Sun Exposure	Your skin may become more sensitive to sunlight and more likely to develop a sunburn while you are taking this drug. It is a good idea to avoid too much sun and to apply a sunscreen to exposed skin surfaces before going outdoors.
Excessive Heat	See ''Exertion and Exercise''; use caution during hot weather, since overexertion may result in heat stroke. Avoid extremely hot baths or saunas.
Excessive Cold	This drug may disturb your body's ability to regulate its temperature; use care during very cold weather and make sure all exposed parts are well covered. Also, do not swim in extremely cold water.

Examinations or Tests	It is important for you to keep all appointments with your doctor so that your progress can be checked.
Other Precautions	Tell any doctor or dentist you consult that you are taking this drug, especially if you will be undergoing any type of surgery or a spinal X ray.
Helpful Hints	Drink plenty of liquids, particularly water and fruit juices, while taking this drug.
	Taking this drug with food or a glass of water will lessen the chance of upset stomach.
	If you have been storing the suppository form of this medicine in a warm place, it may be too soft to use. Put it in the refrigerator for half an hour or run cold water over the wrapped suppository before use.
	If you are taking a controlled-release form, swallow the capsule or tablet whole without crushing, breaking, or chewing it.
	You may feel dizzy, light-headed, or faint when starting out on this type of drug. This should disappear in a few weeks or so. Getting up slowly from a reclining or sitting position should help.
	If your mouth or throat feels dry, chewing sugarless gum or sucking ice chips or sugarless hard candy will help.

POSSIBLE SIDE EFFECTS

Although this list of adverse effects may seem somewhat intimidating, keep in mind that some are quite rare. Of course, should these or any other problems arise while you are on medication, it is always a good idea to consult your doctor.

IF YOU DEVELOP

seizures ■ difficulty in breathing ■ increased sweating ■ incontinence ■ fainting ■ severe muscle stiffness ■ extreme tiredness or weakness ■ irregular or fast heartbeat ■ swelling in throat ■ yellowing of eyes or skin

WHAT TO DO

Urgent Get in touch with your doctor immediately.

cough, fever, or body aches ■ sore throat ■ blurred vision or other visual disturbances ■ dilated pupils, or other changes in pupil size ■ slurred speech ■ rigid facial expression ■ spasms of neck, back, feet, or other parts of the body ■ uncontrollable movements of the tongue, face, mouth, or jaw ■ shuffling walk ■ twisting of body ■ tremors ■ restlessness ■ agitation ■ jitters ■ inability to sit still ■ sleeplessness ■ swelling of hands or feet ■ urinary retention ■ rigidness ■ posture changes ■ difficulty in speech ■ difficulty in swallowing ■ drooling or excessive salivation ■ slow, monotonous speech ■ protrusion of tongue ■ slow movements or inability to move

May be serious Check with your doctor as soon as possible.

constipation ■ diarrhea ■ decreased sweating ■ drowsiness ■ dizziness, light-headedness, or fainting, especially when getting up from a reclining or sitting position ■ male sexual problems ■ increased skin sensitivity to sunlight ■ headache ■ anxiety ■ ''high'' feeling ■ depression ■ weakness ■ reddened skin, rash, or hives ■ loss of appetite ■ upset stomach ■ increased appetite ■ weight gain ■ breast pain or swelling in men and women ■ darkening or whitening of mouth membranes ■ loosened teeth ■ cracked lips and corners of mouth ■ tongue discoloration

If symptoms are disturbing or persist, let your doctor know.

STORAGE INSTRUCTIONS

Store in a cool, dark place (not in a bathroom medicine cabinet). If your medicine is in a liquid form, make sure that it does not freeze. Suppositories should be stored in the refrigerator.

STOPPING OR INTERRUPTING THERAPY

Take this medicine exactly as prescribed by your doctor; it may take several weeks before you see an effect. Do not suddenly discontinue taking this medicine, since this may result in withdrawal reactions (abnormal movements). Your doctor will advise you on how to reduce your dosage gradually. If you miss a dose, take it as soon as possible. If it is almost time for your next dose, skip the missed dose and resume your regular schedule. Do not take two doses at the same time.

SPECIAL CONSIDERATIONS FOR THOSE OVER SIXTY-FIVE

Because older people may be especially susceptible to the side effects of the phenothiazines, doctors may start people over sixty-five on a lower dosage.

DEPRESSION

All of us have depressed moods or feel "blue" about certain events or circumstances such as a serious illness, financial difficulties, the need to move from a familiar home to a new community, or the death of someone close. These are normal feelings that tend to ease with the passage of time. This kind of minor depression is sometimes called reactive depression because it's a reaction to a specific event. It usually doesn't require any medical treatment.

In some cases, the depression isn't relieved with time. In other instances, a depression occurs for no apparent reason and is severe enough to interfere with normal daily functioning. Such depressions are much more serious and may call for medical treatment.

Depression is the most common emotional disorder of older people. The first episode of depression most often occurs between ages fifty and sixty in women and fifty-five and sixty-five in men. Frequently, there is a history of depression in the family.

CAUSES

Depression may be caused by a chemical imbalance in the brain, according to current scientific thinking. Although emotional factors can trigger a depressive episode, diseases or drugs may also be responsible. Depression is known to accompany such illnesses as diabetes, thyroid disease, Parkinson's disease, influenza, hepatitis, and viral pneumonia. Certain cancers and rheumatoid arthritis can also depress mood. Unwanted side effects of some drugs—such as alcohol, sedatives, some antibiotics, some blood pressure medicines, antiarthritic drugs, and digitalis—may cause depressive symptoms.

DIAGNOSIS

Depression is a painful emotional experience. Typical symptoms of depression include weight loss, loss of appetite and energy, fatigue, and feelings of profound helplessness and hopelessness. Waking early in the morning (3:00 to 5:00 a.m.) and being unable to fall back to sleep, frequent or unexplained crying spells, and a loss of interest in people or pleasurable activities are other common signs. Depression may also wear the mask of a physical illness, such as a gastrointestinal problem, chest pain, or muscle or bone pain. In reality, depression is the underlying problem.

In another kind of depression, known as manic depression, there are extreme mood swings; periods of profound despair alternate with periods of intense animation and excitement.

Because depression may result from such a variety of conditions and can masquerade as many other problems, your doctor will do a thorough physical examination, including an electrocardiogram (ECG), blood pressure readings, and blood and urine tests. To further aid in the diagnosis, your doctor will inquire exactly which over-the-counter and prescription medicines you're taking. Your doctor will also conduct a diagnostic interview. This discussion of your problems and feelings will help differentiate true depression from grief, mourning, or dementia. True depression can be identified by the signs and symptoms described earlier.

TREATMENT

Fortunately, depression can be treated successfully with currently available techniques and medicines. If the depression is caused by drugs or by interactions of drugs, your doctor may discontinue a drug you don't really need or substitute one drug for another. Very often, this is all that's necessary to solve the problem. If the depression is related to a physical illness, treating the illness may lift the depression.

Your doctor may also prescribe an antidepressant that can help improve your mood. There are several kinds of antidepressant drugs, some of which are just recently available. All of them act on the areas of the brain that determine mood and probably affect substances in brain tissue that transmit nerve impulses. For a detailed description of these drugs, including their side effects, refer to the drug charts on pages 508–536.

In addition to prescribing medicine for your depression, your doctor may suggest that you talk over your feelings with a trained professional. Often, this will help you find ways to deal with the psychological factors that contribute to depression.

OUTLOOK

Depression can be a serious illness, but most people who suffer from this emotional disorder can be helped. In some cases, changing or foregoing certain medicines is enough. In others, treating a previously undetected medical condition will relieve the depression. In still others, an antidepressant medicine, perhaps combined with psychotherapy, is the suitable treatment approach.

The sense of hopelessness and helplessness that is an integral part of depression often prevents people from seeking help. But now that effective treatments are available, there is no longer any need to live with the pain of depression.

CONDITION: **DEPRESSION**

CATEGORY: **TRICYCLIC AND TETRACYCLIC ANTIDEPRESSANTS**

GENERIC (CHEMICAL) NAME	BRAND (TRADE) NAME	DOSAGE FORMS AND STRENGTHS
Amitriptyline hydrochloride	ELAVIL	Tablets: 10, 25, 50, 75, 100, 150 mg
	ENDEP	Tablets: 10, 25, 50, 75, 100, 150 mg
Amoxapine	ASENDIN	Tablets: 25, 50, 100, 150 mg
Desipramine hydrochloride	NORPRAMIN	Tablets: 10, 25, 50, 75, 100, 150 mg
	PERTOFRANE	Capsules: 25, 50 mg
Doxepin hydrochloride	ADAPIN	Capsules: 10, 25, 50, 75, 100 mg
	SINEQUAN	Capsules: 10, 25, 50, 75, 100, 150 mg Concentrate: 10 mg per ml
Imipramine hydrochloride	TOFRANIL	Tablets: 10, 25, 50 mg
Maprotiline hydrochloride	LUDIOMIL	Tablets: 25, 50, 75 mg
Nortriptyline hydrochloride	AVENTYL	Capsules: 10, 25 mg Solution: 10 mg per tsp
	PAMELOR	Capsules: 10, 25, 50, 75 mg Solution: 10 mg per tsp

Protriptyline hydrochloride VIVACTIL	Tablets: 5, 10 mg

Trimipramine maleate SURMONTIL	Capsules: 25, 50, 100 mg

DRUG PROFILE

The tricyclic and tetracyclic antidepressants are used to treat depressive illnesses and to relieve the anxiety and nervousness that may accompany these problems. According to one widely held theory, severe depression stems at least in part from having low levels of certain chemical messengers in the brain. These drugs may alleviate depression by increasing the amounts of chemical messengers available to the brain.

BEFORE USING THIS DRUG

Let your doctor know *IF*

You have ever had allergic reactions or other problems with ■ any tricyclic antidepressants ■ trazodone ■ tartrazine (FD&C Yellow Dye No. 5) (contained in Norpramin and Tofranil) ■ aspirin.

You have ever had any of the following medical problems: ■ other mental illness ■ heart disease, including heart attack, chest pain, and abnormal heart rhythms ■ alcoholism ■ asthma or other lung disease ■ seizures ■ difficulty in urination ■ enlarged prostate ■ glaucoma ■ kidney disease ■ liver disease ■ high or low blood pressure ■ overactive or underactive thyroid.

You are taking any of the following medicines: ■ other medicine for depression ■ antihistamines ■ medicine for hay fever, coughs, or colds ■ barbiturates ■ medicine for seizures ■ medicine for Parkinson's disease ■ narcotics or other prescription pain-killers ■ tranquilizers ■ sleep medicines ■ medicine for a thyroid condition ■ medicine for asthma ■ methylphenidate (medicine for narcolepsy) ■ anticoagulants (blood thinners) ■ male or female hormones ■ cimetidine (medicine for ulcers) ■ Antabuse (used in treatment of alcoholism) furazolidone (antibiotic) ■ muscle relaxants ■ medicine for high blood pressure ■ diltiazem, nifedipine, or verapamil (calcium blockers).

SPECIAL RESTRICTIONS WHILE TAKING THIS DRUG

FOOD AND DRUG INTERACTIONS

Other Drugs	Do not take any other drugs, including over-the-counter (OTC) drugs, before checking with your doctor. This drug increases the effects of other drugs that depress the central nervous system, such as antihistamines; medicine for hay fever, allergies, or colds; sleep medicines; tranquilizers; narcotics or other prescription pain-killers; muscle relaxants; and medicine for seizures.
Alcohol	Avoid alcohol, another central nervous system depressant, while taking this drug; this combination may cause drowsiness and reduce the effectiveness of this medicine.
Smoking	Smoking may reduce the effectiveness of this medicine. If you smoke, try to stop or at least cut down.

No special restrictions on foods and beverages.

DAILY LIVING

Driving	This drug may cause drowsiness or loss of alertness. Be careful—especially during the first two to four weeks of therapy—when driving, operating household appliances, or doing any other tasks that require alertness until you know how this drug affects you.
Exertion and Exercise	This drug may cause you to sweat less than normally. Sweating is your body's natural way of cooling down, and not sweating enough can be dangerous. Use caution not to become overheated when you exercise or exert yourself.

Sun Exposure	Your skin may become more sensitive to sunlight and more likely to develop a sunburn while you are taking this drug. It is a good idea to avoid too much sun and to apply a sunscreen to exposed skin surfaces before going outdoors.
Excessive Heat	See "Exertion and Exercise"; use caution during hot weather, since overexertion may result in heat stroke. Avoid extremely hot baths or saunas.
Examinations or Tests	It is important for you to keep all appointments with your doctor so that your progress can be checked. Periodic electrocardiograms and blood or urine tests may be required.
Other Precautions	Tell any doctor or dentist you consult that you are taking this drug, especially if you will be undergoing any type of surgery.
Helpful Hints	You may feel dizzy, light-headed, or faint when first starting out on this drug. This should disappear in a few weeks or so. Getting up slowly from a reclining or sitting position should help.
	If your mouth or throat feels dry, chewing sugarless gum or sucking ice chips or sugarless hard candy will help.
	If this medicine causes upset stomach, ask your doctor whether you can take it with food.

No special restrictions on excessive cold.

POSSIBLE SIDE EFFECTS

Although this list of adverse effects may seem somewhat intimidating, keep in mind that some are quite rare. Of course, should these or any other problems arise while you are on medication, it is always a good idea to consult your doctor.

IF YOU DEVELOP

collapse ■ seizures ■ hallucinations ■ agitation ■ difficulty in breathing ■ irregular, slow, or fast heartbeat

WHAT TO DO

Urgent Get in touch with your doctor immediately.

blurred vision ■ confusion ■ inability to concentrate ■ inability to sit still ■ personality changes ■ tremors ■ constipation ■ slurred speech ■ eye pain ■ fainting ■ nervousness ■ restlessness ■ excitement ■ flushing ■ chills ■ swollen glands ■ difficulty in urination ■ shuffling walk ■ sleeplessness ■ rigid facial expression ■ irritability ■ hair loss ■ sore throat or fever ■ swelling of face or tongue ■ nightmares ■ ringing in ears ■ numbness or tingling sensations ■ worsening of depression ■ "high" feeling ■ difficulty in swallowing ■ difficulty in speech ■ rash, hives, or itching ■ reddened skin or other skin changes

May be serious Check with your doctor as soon as possible.

drowsiness ■ dry mouth or throat ■ stuffy nose ■ headache ■ nausea or vomiting ■ tiredness or weakness ■ dizziness or light-headedness, especially when getting up from a reclining or sitting position ■ increased appetite ■ loss of appetite ■ weight gain ■ unpleasant taste in mouth ■ fatigue ■ diarrhea ■ increased sweating ■ increased skin sensitivity to sunlight ■ increased or diminished sex drive ■ male impotence ■ swelling of testicles ■ swelling of breasts in men and women ■ upset stomach ■ heartburn ■ stomach cramps ■ black tongue

After you STOP taking this medicine: restlessness ■ inability to sit still ■ anxiety ■ chills ■ runny nose ■ general feeling of unwellness ■ muscle ache ■ headache ■ dizziness ■ nausea or vomiting ■ worsening of depression

If symptoms are disturbing or persist, let your doctor know.

STORAGE INSTRUCTIONS

Store in a cool, dark place (not in a bathroom medicine cabinet). If your medicine is in a liquid form, make sure that it does not freeze.

STOPPING OR INTERRUPTING THERAPY

Take this medicine exactly as prescribed by your doctor; it may take several weeks before you see an effect. Do not suddenly discontinue taking this medicine. Your doctor will advise you on how to reduce your dosage gradually. For a week after you stop taking a tricyclic antidepressant, continue to follow the precautions listed in this chart, since some of the drug will still be in your body. If you miss a dose, take it as soon as possible. If it is almost time for your next dose, skip the missed dose and resume your regular schedule. Do not take two doses at the same time.

SPECIAL CONSIDERATIONS FOR THOSE OVER SIXTY-FIVE

Because older people may be more prone to side effects of tricyclic antidepressants (specifically—confusion, inability to concentrate, tremors, drowsiness, dry mouth, and difficulty in urination), doctors may start people over sixty-five on a lower dosage and build it up gradually over a period of weeks.

CONDITION: **DEPRESSION**

CATEGORY: **OTHER ANTIDEPRESSANTS**

GENERIC (CHEMICAL) NAME	BRAND (TRADE) NAME	DOSAGE FORMS AND STRENGTHS
Trazodone hydrochloride	DESYREL	Tablets: 50, 100, 150 mg

DRUG PROFILE

Trazodone is used to treat acute depression that occurs with or without anxiety. According to one widely held theory, severe depression stems at least in part from having low levels of certain chemical messengers in the brain. This drug may alleviate depression by increasing the amounts of chemical messengers available to the brain.

BEFORE USING THIS DRUG

Let your doctor know *IF*

You have ever had allergic reactions or other problems with ■ trazodone.

You have ever had any of the following medical problems: ■ heart disease, including heart attack or abnormal heart rhythms ■ kidney disease ■ liver disease ■ high or low blood pressure ■ alcoholism ■ anemia.

You are taking any of the following medicines: ■ other medicine for depression ■ medicine for high blood pressure ■ antihistamines ■ medicine for hay fever, coughs, or colds ■ barbiturates ■ medicine for seizures (especially phenytoin) ■ medicine for Parkinson's disease ■ narcotics or other prescription pain-killers ■ tranquilizers ■ sleep medicines ■ muscle relaxants ■ digoxin, digitoxin, or digitalis (heart medicine).

You are undergoing electroconvulsive shock therapy.

SPECIAL RESTRICTIONS WHILE TAKING THIS DRUG

FOOD AND DRUG INTERACTIONS

Other Drugs	Do not take any other drugs, including over-the-counter (OTC) drugs, before checking with your doctor. This drug increases the effects of other drugs that depress the central nervous system, such as antihistamines; medicine for hay fever, allergies, or colds; sleep medicines; tranquilizers; narcotics or other prescription pain-killers; muscle relaxants; and medicine for seizures.
Alcohol	Avoid alcohol, another central nervous system depressant, while taking this drug; the combination can be dangerous.
Smoking	Smoking may reduce the effectiveness of this medicine. If you smoke, try to stop or at least cut down.

No special restrictions on foods and beverages.

DAILY LIVING

Driving	This drug may cause drowsiness or blurred vision. Be careful when driving, operating household appliances, or doing any other tasks that require alertness until you know how this drug affects you.
Sun Exposure	Your skin may become more sensitive to sunlight and more likely to develop a sunburn while you are taking this drug. It is a good idea to avoid too much sun and to apply a sunscreen to exposed skin surfaces before going outdoors.
Excessive Heat	Use caution during hot weather since this drug may make you more sensitive to extremely hot temperatures. Avoid extremely hot baths or saunas.
Excessive Cold	You may be more sensitive to extreme cold while taking this drug.
Examinations or Tests	It is important for you to keep all appointments with your doctor so that your progress can be checked.
Other Precautions	Tell any doctor or dentist you consult that you are taking this drug, especially if you will be undergoing any type of surgery.
Helpful Hints	You may feel dizzy, light-headed, or faint while taking this drug. Getting up slowly from a reclining or sitting position should help.
	For maximum benefit, take this medicine shortly after eating a meal or snack. In addition to getting more of the medicine into your bloodstream, this will lessen the chance of dizziness or light-headedness.

If this medicine makes you feel drowsy, let your doctor know; you may be able to take most of your daily dose at bedtime.

If your mouth or throat feels dry, chewing sugarless gum or sucking ice chips or sugarless hard candy will help.

No special restrictions on exertion and exercise.

POSSIBLE SIDE EFFECTS

Although this list of adverse effects may seem somewhat intimidating, keep in mind that some are quite rare. Of course, should these or any other problems arise while you are on medication, it is always a good idea to consult your doctor.

IF YOU DEVELOP	WHAT TO DO
seizures ■ difficulty in breathing ■ prolonged or inappropriate penile erection ■ fainting ■ chest pain ■ irregular, slow, or fast heartbeat ■ sore throat or fever	**Urgent** Get in touch with your doctor immediately.
confusion ■ clumsiness ■ anger or hostility ■ agitation ■ excitement ■ restlessness ■ nervousness ■ inability to concentrate ■ memory problems ■ difficulty in speech ■ hallucinations ■ personality changes ■ "high" feeling ■ inability to sit still ■ muscle twitches ■ rash or hives ■ tingling or prickling sensations ■ blood in urine ■ difficulty in urination ■ urinary frequency	**May be serious** Check with your doctor as soon as possible.
blurred or double vision ■ dizziness or light-headedness, especially when getting up from a reclining or sitting position ■ drowsiness ■ dry mouth ■ headache ■ full or heavy feeling in head ■ nausea or vomiting ■ constipation ■ diarrhea ■ gas ■ muscle aches ■ tiredness ■ general feeling of unwellness ■ sleeplessness ■ unpleasant	If symptoms are disturbing or persist, let your doctor know.

taste in mouth ■ increased salivation ■ increased appetite ■ weight gain ■ acne ■ increased skin sensitivity to sunlight ■ swelling of skin ■ stuffy nose ■ increased sweating or clammy feeling ■ eye pain ■ ringing in ears ■ change in sexual drive ■ male impotence ■ problems with ejaculation in males

STORAGE INSTRUCTIONS

Store in a cool, dark place (not in a bathroom medicine cabinet).

STOPPING OR INTERRUPTING THERAPY

Take this medicine exactly as prescribed by your doctor; it may take several weeks before you see an effect. If you miss a dose, take it as soon as possible. If it is within four hours of your next dose, skip the missed dose and resume your regular schedule. Do not take two doses at the same time. Do not suddenly discontinue taking this medicine. Your doctor will advise you on how to reduce your dosage gradually.

SPECIAL CONSIDERATIONS FOR THOSE OVER SIXTY-FIVE

Because older people may be more prone to side effects of trazodone (especially drowsiness, dizziness, confusion, visual disturbances, dry mouth, and constipation), doctors may start people over sixty-five on a lower dosage.

CONDITION: **DEPRESSION**

CATEGORY: **MAO INHIBITORS**

GENERIC (CHEMICAL) NAME	BRAND (TRADE) NAME	DOSAGE FORMS AND STRENGTHS
Isocarboxazid	MARPLAN	Tablets: 10 mg
Phenelzine sulfate	NARDIL	Tablets: 15 mg
Tranylcypromine sulfate	PARNATE	Tablets: 10 mg

DRUG PROFILE

MAO (monoamine oxidase) activity increases after age forty-five. This enzyme is responsible for the breakdown of chemical messengers to the brain; reduced levels of these messengers may affect mood in older people. MAO inhibitors are used to treat severe depression. They block the action of monoamine oxidase, which, in turn, increases the levels of the messengers in the brain.

BEFORE USING THIS DRUG

Let your doctor know *IF*

You have ever had allergic reactions or other problems with ■ tranylcypromine, isocarboxazid, phenelzine sulfate, or any other MAO inhibitor drug ■ pargyline hydrochloride (medicine for high blood pressure).

You have ever had any of the following medical problems: ■ drug abuse, including alcohol and cocaine ■ heart disease, including angina (chest pain), coronary artery disease, and heart attack ■ diabetes ■ seizures ■ severe or frequent headaches ■ high blood pressure ■ kidney disease ■ liver disease ■ mental illness ■ overactive thyroid ■ Parkinson's disease ■ stroke ■ glaucoma ■ pheochromocytoma (adrenal gland tumor) ■ asthma or other lung disease ■ anemia ■ angioneurotic edema (accumulation of excess fluid under the skin, often associated with hives, redness, or purplish or brownish-red spots).

You are taking any of the following medicines: ■ other medicine for depression (within the past two weeks) ■ medicine for diabetes ■ medicine for high blood pressure ■ medicine for asthma ■ diuretics (water pills) ■ medicine for Parkinson's disease ■ medicine for seizures ■ barbiturates ■ muscle relaxants ■ antihistamines ■ medicine for hay fever, coughs, or colds ■ appetite suppressants ■ narcotics or other prescription pain-killers ■ sleep medicines ■ any medicine containing alcohol ■ any medicine containing caffeine ■ amphetamines ■ methylphenidate (medicine for narcolepsy) ■ Antabuse (used in treatment of alcoholism) ■ tranquilizers.

You are receiving electroconvulsive shock therapy.

SPECIAL RESTRICTIONS WHILE TAKING THIS DRUG

FOOD AND DRUG INTERACTIONS

Other Drugs	Do not take any other drugs, including over-the-counter (OTC) drugs, before checking with your doctor. OTC drugs that may interact adversely with this

drug include those used for colds, coughs, hay fever, and appetite suppression, as well as drugs containing caffeine.

Foods and Beverages	The combination of MAO inhibitors and food or beverages that contain caffeine or the chemicals tyramine or tryptophan can result in serious problems. Foods to avoid include cheese (Cheddar, Camembert, Stilton, or processed cheese), sour cream, yogurt, liver (especially chicken liver), pickled herring, canned figs, raisins, bananas, avocados, soy sauce, meat tenderizers, fava beans, cured meats (e.g., bologna, sausage, and salami), and yeast or meat extracts. Also, avoid large quantities of cocoa, coffee, tea, and cola beverages. Ask your doctor to provide you with a full list of foods to avoid; also, let your doctor know if you are on any special kind of diet. Continue to avoid the above foods and beverages for two weeks after stopping therapy with an MAO inhibitor.
Alcohol	Avoid alcohol while taking this drug; the combination can cause serious reactions. Beer and Chianti wine are especially dangerous.

No special restrictions on smoking.

DAILY LIVING

Driving	MAO inhibitors may cause drowsiness or loss of alertness. Be careful when driving, operating household appliances, or doing any other tasks that require alertness until you know how this drug affects you.

Examinations or Tests	It is important for you to keep all appointments with your doctor so that your progress can be checked. Periodic blood and urine tests may be required.
Other Precautions	Tell any doctor or dentist you consult that you are taking this drug, especially if you will be undergoing any type of surgery or radiologic diagnostic test.
Helpful Hints	You may feel dizzy, light-headed, or faint while taking this drug. Getting up slowly from a reclining or sitting position should help. If you become extremely dizzy, lie down until you feel better. If you continue to experience these symptoms, let your doctor know.

No special restrictions on exertion and exercise, sun exposure, or exposure to excessive heat or cold.

POSSIBLE SIDE EFFECTS

Although this list of adverse effects may seem somewhat intimidating, keep in mind that some are quite rare. Of course, should these or any other problems arise while you are on medication, it is always a good idea to consult your doctor.

IF YOU DEVELOP

severe headache ■ stiff or sore neck ■ chest pain ■ irregular, slow, or fast heartbeat ■ nausea or vomiting ■ excessive sweating with clammy skin ■ chills or fever ■ increased eye sensitivity to light ■ confusion ■ incoherence ■ difficulty in breathing ■ seizures ■ personality changes ■ hallucinations ■ jaw spasms or difficulty in opening mouth ■ body spasms

WHAT TO DO

Urgent Get in touch with your doctor immediately.

severe dizziness, light-headedness, or fainting ■ dilated pupils ■ swelling of feet or legs ■ agitation ■ nervousness ■ clumsiness ■ rash ■ purplish or brownish-red spots ■ aggravation of glaucoma ■ aching joints ■ diarrhea ■ pounding heartbeat ■ yellowing of eyes or skin

May be serious Check with your doctor as soon as possible.

After you STOP taking this medicine: restlessness
■ anxiety ■ confusion ■ hallucinations ■ depression ■ weakness ■ diarrhea ■ headache

blurred vision or other visual disturbances ■ constipation ■ difficulty in urination ■ numbness, tingling, or pain in hands or feet ■ tremors ■ dizziness or light-headedness, especially when getting
up from a reclining or sitting position ■ headache
■ drowsiness ■ dry mouth ■ weight gain ■ tiredness ■ restlessness ■ sleeplessness ■ male
impotence ■ loss of appetite ■ flushing ■ urinary
frequency ■ weakness ■ increased appetite
■ stomach pain

If symptoms are disturbing
or persist, let your doctor
know.

STORAGE INSTRUCTIONS

Store in a cool, dark place (not in a bathroom medicine cabinet).

STOPPING OR INTERRUPTING THERAPY

Take this medicine exactly as prescribed by your doctor. Do not suddenly discontinue taking this medicine. Your doctor will advise you on how to reduce your dosage gradually. If you miss a dose, take it as soon as possible. If it is within two
hours of your next dose, skip the missed dose and resume your regular schedule.
Do not take two doses at the same time. For two weeks after stopping this drug,
continue to follow the precautions listed in this chart, since some of the drug will
still be in your body.

SPECIAL CONSIDERATIONS FOR THOSE OVER SIXTY-FIVE

None.

CONDITION: **DEPRESSION**

CATEGORY: **ANTIDEPRESSANTS (COMBINATIONS)**

GENERIC (CHEMICAL) NAME	BRAND (TRADE) NAME	DOSAGE FORMS AND STRENGTHS
Perphenazine and amitriptyline hydrochloride	ETRAFON	Tablets: 2 mg perphenazine and 10 mg amitriptyline; 2 mg perphenazine and 25 mg amitriptyline; 4 mg perphenazine and 10 mg amitriptyline; 4 mg perphenazine and 25 mg amitriptyline
	TRIAVIL	Tablets: 2 mg perphenazine and 10 mg amitriptyline; 2 mg perphenazine and 25 mg amitriptyline; 4 mg perphenazine and 10 mg amitriptyline; 4 mg perphenazine and 25 mg amitriptyline; 4 mg perphenazine and 50 mg amitriptyline

DRUG PROFILE

This drug—a combination of a phenothiazine (perphenazine) and a tricyclic antidepressant (amitriptyline)—is used to treat depressive illnesses and to relieve the anxiety and nervousness that may accompany them. Phenothiazines are thought to work by inhibiting the action of dopamine, a chemical messenger, in the part of the brain that is the seat of the emotions. According to one widely held theory, severe depression stems at least in part from having low levels of certain chemical messengers in the brain. Tricyclic antidepressants may alleviate depression by increasing the amounts of chemical messengers available to the brain.

BEFORE TAKING THIS DRUG

Let your doctor know *IF*

You have ever had allergic reactions or other problems with ■ any phenothiazines ■ any tricyclic antidepressants.

You have ever had any of the following medical problems: ■ other mental illness ■ seizures ■ anemia or other blood disease ■ asthma or other lung disease ■ respiratory tract infection, such as pneumonia ■ liver disease ■ kidney disease ■ heart or blood vessel disease, including heart attack, chest pain, and abnormal heart rhythms ■ glaucoma ■ enlarged prostate ■ urinary problems ■ alcoholism ■ high or low blood pressure ■ overactive thyroid.

You are taking any of the following medicines: ■ other medicine for depression ■ medicine for seizures ■ antacids ■ appetite suppressants ■ medicine for high blood pressure ■ medicine for asthma ■ medicine for Parkinson's disease ■ beta-blockers ■ antihistamines ■ medicine for hay fever, coughs, or colds ■ barbiturates ■ narcotics or other prescription pain-killers ■ sleep medicines ■ tranquilizers ■ vitamin C ■ cimetidine (medicine for ulcers) ■ Antabuse (used in treatment of alcoholism) ■ medicine for nausea or vomiting ■ antibiotics ■ medicine for a thyroid condition ■ methylphenidate (medicine for narcolepsy) ■ anticoagulants (blood thinners) ■ male or female hormones.

You are often exposed to extreme heat or cold or to organophosphate insecticides (e.g., if you work in a plant that manufactures this type of pesticide).

SPECIAL RESTRICTIONS WHILE TAKING THIS DRUG

FOOD AND DRUG INTERACTIONS

Other Drugs	Do not take any other drugs, including over-the-counter (OTC) drugs, before checking with your doctor. This drug increases the effect of other drugs that depress the central nervous system, such as antihistamines; medicine for hay fever, allergies, or colds; sleep medicines; other tranquilizers; narcotics or other prescription pain-killers; muscle relaxants; and medicine for seizures.
Alcohol	Avoid alcohol, another central nervous system depressant, while taking this drug; the combination can be dangerous.

Smoking	Smoking may reduce the effectiveness of this drug. If you smoke, try to stop or at least cut down.

No special restrictions on foods and beverages.

DAILY LIVING

Driving	This drug may cause drowsiness or loss of alertness. Be careful when driving, operating household appliances, or doing any other tasks that require alertness until you know how this drug affects you.
Exertion and Exercise	This drug may cause you to sweat less than normally. Sweating is your body's natural way of cooling down, and not sweating enough can be dangerous. Use caution not to become overheated when you exercise or exert yourself.
Sun Exposure	Your skin may become more sensitive to sunlight and more likely to develop a sunburn while you are taking this drug. It is a good idea to avoid too much sun and to apply a sunscreen to exposed skin surfaces before going outdoors.
Excessive Heat	See "Exertion and Exercise"; use caution during hot weather, since overexertion may result in heat stroke. Avoid extremely hot baths or saunas.
Excessive Cold	This drug may disturb your body's ability to regulate its temperature; use care during very cold weather and make sure all exposed parts are well covered. Also, do not swim in extremely cold water.
Examinations or Tests	It is important for you to keep all appointments with your doctor so that your progress can be checked. A

blood test and an electrocardiogram may be necessary before you start therapy on this drug.

Other Precautions	Tell any doctor or dentist you consult that you are taking this drug, especially if you will be undergoing any type of surgery or a spinal X ray.

Helpful Hints	You may feel dizzy, light-headed, or faint when first starting out on this drug. This should disappear in a few weeks or so. Getting up slowly from a reclining or sitting position should help.

If your mouth or throat feels dry, chewing sugarless gum or sucking ice chips or sugarless hard candy will help.

If this medicine causes upset stomach, ask your doctor whether you can take it with food.

POSSIBLE SIDE EFFECT

Although this list of adverse effects may seem somewhat intimidating, keep in mind that some are quite rare. Of course, should these or any other problems arise while you are on medication, it is always a good idea to consult your doctor.

IF YOU DEVELOP

collapse ■ seizures ■ hallucinations ■ agitation ■ difficulty in breathing ■ irregular, slow, or fast heartbeat ■ incontinence ■ fainting ■ severe muscular stiffness ■ extreme tiredness or weakness ■ swelling in throat ■ sore throat or fever

WHAT TO DO

Urgent Get in touch with your doctor immediately.

blurred vision or other visual disturbances ■ confusion ■ inability to concentrate ■ inability to sit still ■ jitters ■ personality changes ■ tremors ■ slurred speech ■ eye pain ■ weakness ■ nervousness ■ restlessness ■ excitement ■ flushing ■ chills ■ swollen glands ■ difficulty in urination ■ shuffling walk ■ sleeplessness ■ rigid facial

May be serious Check with your doctor as soon as possible.

expression ■ irritability ■ hair loss ■ flulike symptoms ■ swelling of face or tongue ■ nightmares ■ ringing in ears ■ numbness or tingling sensations ■ worsening of depression ■ ''high'' feeling ■ difficulty in swallowing ■ difficulty in speech ■ twisting of torso ■ rash, hives, or itching ■ reddened skin or other skin changes ■ spasms of the neck, back, feet, or other parts of the body ■ uncontrollable movements of the tongue, face, mouth, or jaw ■ protrusion of tongue ■ swelling of hands or feet ■ posture changes ■ drooling or excessive salivation ■ yellowing of eyes or skin ■ slow, monotonous speech ■ difficulty in movement or slow movements

drowsiness ■ dry mouth ■ sore throat ■ stuffy nose ■ headache ■ nausea or vomiting ■ dizziness or light-headedness, especially when getting up from a reclining or sitting position ■ increased appetite ■ weight gain ■ unpleasant taste in mouth ■ diarrhea ■ constipation ■ loss of appetite ■ increased sweating ■ increased skin sensitivity to sunlight ■ change in sex drive ■ male impotence ■ swelling of testicles ■ swelling of breasts in men and women ■ upset stomach ■ heartburn ■ stomach cramps ■ black tongue or other tongue discoloration ■ anxiety ■ darkening or whitening of mouth membranes ■ loosened teeth ■ cracked lips and corners of mouth

After you STOP taking this medicine: restlessness ■ inability to sit still ■ anxiety ■ chills ■ runny nose ■ general feeling of unwellness ■ muscle ache ■ headache ■ dizziness ■ nausea or vomiting

If symptoms are disturbing or persist, let your doctor know.

STORAGE INSTRUCTIONS

Store in a cool, dark place (not in a bathroom medicine cabinet).

STOPPING OR INTERRUPTING THERAPY

Take this medicine exactly as prescribed by your doctor; it may take several weeks before you see an effect. If you miss a dose, take it as soon as possible. If it is almost time for your next dose, skip the missed dose and resume your regular schedule. Do not take two doses at the same time. Do not suddenly discontinue taking this medicine. Your doctor will advise you on how to reduce your dosage gradually. For a week after you stop, continue to follow the precautions listed in this chart, since some of the drug will still be in your body.

SPECIAL CONSIDERATIONS FOR THOSE OVER SIXTY-FIVE

Because older people may be especially susceptible to the side effects of this drug, doctors may start people over sixty-five on a lower dosage.

CONDITION: **DEPRESSION**

CATEGORY: **ANTIDEPRESSANTS (COMBINATIONS)**

GENERIC (CHEMICAL) NAME	BRAND (TRADE) NAME	DOSAGE FORMS AND STRENGTHS
Chlordiazepoxide and amitriptyline hydrochloride	LIMBITROL	Tablets: 5 mg chlordiazepoxide and 12.5 mg amitriptyline; 10 mg chlordiazepoxide and 25 mg amitriptyline

DRUG PROFILE

This drug—a combination of a benzodiazepine (chlordiazepoxide) and a tricyclic antidepressant (amitriptyline)—is used to treat depressive illnesses and to relieve the anxiety and nervousness that may accompany these illnesses. According to one widely held theory, severe depression stems at least in part from having low levels of certain chemical messengers in the brain. Tricyclic antidepressants may alleviate depression by increasing the amounts of chemical messengers available to the brain.

BEFORE USING THIS DRUG

Let your doctor know *IF*

You have ever had allergic reactions or other problems with ■ any benzodiazepines ■ any tricyclic antidepressants ■ trazodone.

You have ever had any of the following medical problems: ■ other mental illness ■ alcoholism ■ asthma or other lung disease ■ seizures ■ difficulty in urination ■ enlarged prostate ■ glaucoma ■ heart disease, including heart attack, chest pain, and abnormal heart rhythms ■ kidney disease ■ liver disease ■ high or low blood pressure ■ overactive thyroid ■ myasthenia gravis ■ porphyria.

You are taking any of the following medicines: ■ other medicine for depression ■ any benzodiazepines ■ antihistamines ■ medicine for hay fever, coughs, or colds ■ barbiturates ■ medicine for seizures ■ medicine for Parkinson's disease ■ narcotics or other prescription pain-killers ■ tranquilizers ■ sleep medicines ■ medicine for a thyroid condition ■ medicine for asthma ■ methylphenidate (medicine for narcolepsy) ■ anticoagulants (blood thinners) ■ male or female hormones ■ cimetidine (medicine for ulcers) ■ Antabuse (used in treatment of alcoholism) ■ medicine for arthritis ■ antacids ■ medicine for high blood pressure ■ digoxin, digitoxin, or digitalis (heart medicines) ■ antibiotics ■ medicine for tuberculosis ■ muscle relaxants ■ timolol, naldolol, propranolol, metoprolol, acebutolol, atenolol, pindolol, or labetolol (beta-blockers).

You are receiving electroconvulsive shock therapy.

SPECIAL RESTRICTIONS WHILE TAKING THIS DRUG

FOOD AND DRUG INTERACTIONS

Other Drugs	Do not take any other drugs, including over-the-counter (OTC) drugs, before checking with your doctor. This drug increases the effect of other drugs that depress the central nervous system, such as antihistamines; medicine for hay fever, allergies, or colds; sleep medicines; tranquilizers; narcotics or other prescription pain-killers; muscle relaxants; and medicine for seizures.
Alcohol	Avoid alcohol, another central nervous system depressant, while taking this drug; the combination can be dangerous.
Smoking	Smoking may reduce the effectiveness of this drug. If you smoke, try to stop or at least cut down.

No special restrictions on foods and beverages.

DAILY LIVING

Driving	This drug may cause drowsiness or loss of alertness. Be careful when driving, operating household appliances, or doing any other tasks that require alertness until you know how this drug affects you.
Exertion and Exercise	This drug may cause you to sweat less than normally. Sweating is your body's natural way of cooling down, and not sweating enough can be dangerous. Use caution not to become overheated when you exercise or exert yourself.
Sun Exposure	Your skin may become more sensitive to sunlight and more likely to develop a sunburn while you are taking this drug. It is a good idea to avoid too much sun and to apply a sunscreen to exposed skin surfaces before going outdoors.
Excessive Heat	See "Exertion and Exercise"; use caution during hot weather, since overexertion may result in heat stroke. Avoid extremely hot baths or saunas.
Examinations or Tests	It is important for you to keep all appointments with your doctor so that your progress can be checked. Periodic electrocardiograms and blood or urine tests may be required.
Other Precautions	Do not take more of this medicine or take it for a longer period of time than prescribed. If you suspect that this drug is not working, do not increase the dosage, but check with your doctor.

Tell any doctor or dentist you consult that you are taking this drug, especially if you will be undergoing any type of surgery.

Helpful Hints

You may feed dizzy, light-headed, or faint when first starting out on this drug. This should disappear in a few weeks or so. Getting up slowly from a reclining or sitting position should help.

If your mouth or throat feels dry, chewing sugarless gum or sucking ice chips or sugarless hard candy will help.

If this medicine causes upset stomach, ask your doctor whether you can take it with food.

No special restrictions on exposure to excessive cold.

POSSIBLE SIDE EFFECTS

Although this list of adverse effects may seem somewhat intimidating, keep in mind that some are quite rare. Of course, should these or any other problems arise while you are on medication, it is always a good idea to consult your doctor.

IF YOU DEVELOP

confusion ■ severe drowsiness or weakness ■ staggering ■ difficulty in breathing ■ collapse ■ seizures ■ hallucinations ■ sore throat or fever ■ yellowing of eyes or skin

WHAT TO DO

Urgent Get in touch with your doctor immediately.

depression ■ sleeplessness ■ uncontrollable movements of the body, mouth, or cheek ■ excitement ■ nervousness ■ irritability ■ talkativeness ■ restlessness ■ inability to sit still ■ inability to concentrate ■ anxiety ■ nightmares ■ fainting ■ personality changes ■ tremors ■ rage ■ burning or prickling sensation ■ irregular or fast heartbeat ■ flushing ■ increased sweating ■ shortness of breath ■ tiredness or weakness ■ sores in mouth or throat ■ rash, hives, or itching ■ bleeding or bruising ■ eye pain

May be serious Check with your doctor as soon as possible.

After you STOP taking this medicine: anxiety
■ sleeplessness ■ depression ■ loss of appetite
■ increased sweating ■ diarrhea ■ nausea or
vomiting ■ irritability ■ memory problems ■ clumsiness ■ tremors ■ stomach or muscle cramps
■ personality changes ■ seizures ■ hallucinations
■ restlessness ■ chills ■ runny nose ■ general
feeling of unwellness ■ muscle ache ■ headache
■ dizziness ■ hair loss ■ ringing in ears ■ numbness or tingling sensations ■ worsening of depression ■ twisting of torso

---

drowsiness ■ dizziness or light-headedness, especially when getting up from a reclining or sitting
position ■ "high" feeling ■ vivid dreams ■ clumsiness or poor balance ■ headache ■ blurred or
double vision or other visual disturbances ■ stomach cramps or pain ■ constipation ■ diarrhea
■ nausea or vomiting ■ upset stomach ■ dry
mouth or throat ■ increased thirst ■ increased
salivation ■ increased phlegm production in lungs
■ difficulty in urination ■ urinary frequency or
other urinary problems ■ hiccups ■ increase or
decrease in appetite ■ weight gain or loss ■ swelling of face or tongue ■ bitter or metallic taste in
mouth ■ change in sex drive ■ male impotence
■ swelling of breasts in men and women
■ increased skin sensitivity to sunlight ■ stuffy
nose ■ swelling of testicles ■ black tongue
■ heartburn

If symptoms are disturbing
or persist, let your doctor
know.

STORAGE INSTRUCTIONS

Store in a cool, dark place (not in a bathroom medicine cabinet).

STOPPING OR INTERRUPTING THERAPY

Take this medicine exactly as prescribed by your doctor; it may take several weeks
before you see an effect. Do not suddenly discontinue taking this medicine. Your
doctor will advise you on how to reduce your dosage gradually. If you miss a dose,
take it as soon as possible. If it is almost time for your next dose, skip the missed
dose and resume your regular schedule. Do not take two doses at the same time.
For a week after you stop taking this medicine, continue to follow the precautions
listed in this chart, since some of the drug will still be in your body.

SPECIAL CONSIDERATIONS FOR THOSE OVER SIXTY-FIVE

Because older people may be more prone to side effects of this drug, doctors may start people over sixty-five on a lower dosage.

CONDITION: **MANIC DEPRESSION**

CATEGORY: **ANTIDEPRESSANT AND ANTIMANIC DRUGS**

GENERIC (CHEMICAL) NAME	BRAND (TRADE) NAME	DOSAGE FORMS AND STRENGTHS
Lithium carbonate	ESKALITH	Capsules: 300 mg Tablets: 300 mg
	ESKALITH CR	Controlled-release tablets: 450 mg
	LITHOBID	Controlled-release tablets: 300 mg
	LITHONATE	Capsules: 300 mg
	LITHOTABS	Tablets: 300 mg
Lithium citrate	CIBALITH-S	Syrup: 8 milliequivalents (equivalent to 300 mg lithium carbonate) per tsp

DRUG PROFILE

Lithium is used to treat manic-depressive illness—severe mood swings between an excited, "high," or irritable state and a state of extreme depression. It is not known exactly how this drug produces its therapeutic effect.

BEFORE USING THIS DRUG

Let your doctor know *IF*

You have ever had allergic reactions or other problems with ■ lithium.

You have ever had any of the following medical problems: ■ diabetes ■ difficulty in urination ■ seizures ■ heart disease, including abnormal heart rhythms ■ kidney disease ■ thyroid disease ■ Parkinson's disease ■ recent infection ■ high blood pressure.

You are taking any of the following medicines: ■ other medicine for depression ■ medicine for asthma ■ medicine for arthritis ■ diuretics ■ appetite suppressants ■ medicine for thyroid disease ■ baking soda ■ antacids ■ antibiotics ■ tranquilizers ■ medicine for mental illness ■ medicine for diabetes ■ medicine for seizures ■ muscle relaxants ■ narcotics or other prescription pain-killers ■ medicine to make the urine less acidic ■ verapamil (calcium blocker) ■ any medicine containing caffeine ■ salt pills.

You are undergoing electroconvulsive shock therapy.

SPECIAL RESTRICTIONS WHILE TAKING THIS DRUG

FOOD AND DRUG INTERACTIONS

Other Drugs	Do not take any other drugs, including over-the-counter (OTC) drugs, before checking with your doctor.
Foods and Beverages	It is important for you to drink plenty of liquids (two and a half to three quarts a day) while you are taking this medicine. If you become ill and develop fever, vomiting, or diarrhea, be sure to drink more liquids to supplement the fluids you are losing. Let your doctor know if you are on any type of special diet.

No special restrictions on alchohol use or smoking.

DAILY LIVING

Driving	This drug may cause drowsiness or loss of alertness. Be careful when driving, operating household appliances, or doing any other tasks that require alertness until you know how this drug affects you.

Exertion and Exercise	The loss of fluids and salt from your body can cause a dangerous buildup of lithium in your body. Use caution while exercising or exerting yourself, and drink fluids to replace those lost by sweating.
Excessive Heat	See above; use caution during hot weather, and drink fluids to replace those lost by sweating. Avoid extremely hot baths or saunas.
Examinations or Tests	It is important for you to keep all appointments with your doctor so that your progress can be checked. Blood and urine tests are required during lithium therapy in order to check the level of lithium in the blood and to evaluate its effects on various organs, especially the thyroid gland and kidneys.
Other Precautions	Tell any doctor or dentist you consult that you are taking this drug, especially if you will be undergoing any type of surgery. If you become ill and develop fever, excessive sweating, diarrhea, or vomiting, let your doctor know immediately. The loss of fluid can result in a dangerous buildup of lithium in your body.
Helpful Hints	If you are taking the controlled-release capsules, swallow them whole without breaking, crushing, or chewing. If your mouth or throat feels dry, chewing sugarless gum or sucking ice chips or sugarless hard candy will help.

No special restrictions on sun exposure or exposure to excessive cold.

POSSIBLE SIDE EFFECTS

Although this list of adverse effects may seem somewhat intimidating, keep in mind that some are quite rare. Of course, should these or any other problems arise while you are on medication, it is always a good idea to consult your doctor.

IF YOU DEVELOP	WHAT TO DO
diarrhea ■ drowsiness ■ muscle weakness ■ vomiting ■ tremors ■ clumsiness ■ confusion ■ seizures ■ delirium ■ blackouts ■ difficulty in moving ■ severe dizziness ■ incontinence ■ fainting ■ severe muscle twitching ■ jerky or writhing movements ■ irregular or fast heartbeat	**Urgent** Get in touch with your doctor immediately.
difficulty in breathing ■ tiredness ■ weight gain ■ swelling of neck, wrist, feet, or lower legs ■ hair loss ■ headache ■ memory problems ■ inability to concentrate ■ dulled senses ■ rigidity ■ difficulty in speech ■ confusion ■ restlessness ■ blurred vision	**May be serious** Check with your doctor as soon as possible.
increased thirst ■ nausea ■ stomach pain ■ bloating ■ mild tremors or muscle twitching ■ rash or dry skin ■ numbness in skin ■ skin ulcers ■ inflammation of the hair follicles ■ acne ■ thinning of hair or change in hair texture ■ stomach discomfort ■ increased urination ■ unpleasant taste in mouth ■ dry mouth ■ weight loss	If symptoms are disturbing or persist, let your doctor know.

STORAGE INSTRUCTIONS

Store in a cool, dark place (not in a bathroom medicine cabinet). If your medicine is in a liquid form, make sure that it does not freeze.

STOPPING OR INTERRUPTING THERAPY

Take this medicine exactly as prescribed by your doctor; it may take several weeks before you see an effect. if you miss a dose, take it as soon as possible. If it is within two hours (with the regular-acting form) or six hours (with the controlled-release form) of your next dose, skip the missed dose and resume your regular schedule. Do not take two doses at the same time.

SPECIAL CONSIDERATIONS FOR THOSE OVER SIXTY-FIVE

Because older people may be especially susceptible to the side effects of lithium, doctors may start people over sixty-five on a lower dosage.

Chapter 7
Diet, Nutrition, and Health Maintenance

NUTRITIONAL DEFICIENCIES

For one reason or another, many older people tend to eat less. Some diet to control their weight, and others have reduced appetites. But maintaining proper intake of nutrients, particularly vitamins and minerals, is of crucial importance to overall health.

This can be a particular challenge for people with a chronic illness, such as heart disease, diabetes, hypertension, or cancer. These conditions can increase the body's need for certain vitamins and minerals. Surgery, stress, digestive problems such as constipation, and alcohol abuse are other factors that make it especially important to consume ample amounts of these nutrients.

Taking vitamin or mineral supplements is not always the right answer (unless directed by your doctor) because megadoses of vitamins and minerals can cause problems of their own. Sometimes they also interfere with the effectiveness of prescription drugs. The question of what, if any, supplements to take should be handled by a doctor as part of your overall health care. (Many vitamin supplements are available without a prescription and are not included in this book. Those supplements that do require a prescription are discussed in the drug charts on pages 540–556.) What you should do, on your own, is maintain a balanced diet as much as possible, including meats, poultry, fish, fresh vegetables and fruit, whole grains, and dairy products.

SOURCES AND RECOMMENDED DOSES OF CRITICAL NUTRIENTS

Advertisements would have us believe that all older people are deficient in iron ("iron-poor blood" is the slogan). The reality is quite different. Because the body stores iron as we get older, an older person has a higher amount of iron stored in the body than does a young person. Studies have shown that the iron content in the diet of most older people is adequate. Foods that are good sources of iron are red meats, liver, soybeans, and fortified bread.

Calcium is the nutrient in which older people, especially women, are most likely to be deficient. As we age, our bodies absorb calcium less efficiently. A lack of calcium has been linked to osteoporosis—the gradual loss of bone tissue—which weakens the bones and makes them more vulnerable to fracture (see also pages 464–466). In some people the problem is a low calcium intake, but in others the problem is poor absorption of calcium. Everyone, regardless of age, should consume at least 800 milligrams (mg) of calcium a day. Women who have passed menopause should get 1,500 mg of calcium a day. Foods that are rich in calcium include milk (whole or skim), yogurt, cheese, greens, and sardines and canned salmon with the bones. Alternatively, your doctor may recommend that you take a calcium supplement, such as calcium carbonate or calcium gluconate.

Vitamin D is another nutrient crucial for healthy bones. Proper amounts of this vitamin can prevent or even reverse osteomalacia, a weakening of the bones that can lead to bone fractures. A quart of fortified milk a day, plus fifteen minutes of sunshine twice a week, will probably give you all the vitamin D you need (400–600 International Units [IU] per day). In addition to milk, fish oils and deep-sea fish are good sources of vitamin D. (If you suspect that you may not be getting enough vitamin D, discuss this with your doctor.) However, because vitamin D is stored in the body, too much of a good thing may be toxic. Steer clear of high-dose vitamin D supplements—some contain as much as 50,000 IU and should not be taken.

Zinc is important for maintaining the body's immune system and its ability to heal wounds. Red meat, liver, fish, and dark poultry are all good sources of this mineral. Supplements are usually not necessary, but people who have chronic illnesses or serious infections might benefit from supplements as prescribed by a doctor. High doses of zinc can cause diarrhea and nausea.

Consuming adequate amounts of vitamin A in foods may help to prevent some forms of cancer, but there is no evidence that large doses of this vitamin can reverse visual or skin problems, as many people believe. Too much vitamin A can actually do damage. For example, 50,000 IU or more per day can cause bone disease, liver disease, hair loss, drowsiness, and itching. The recommended daily intake is 5,000 IU. Carrots, sweet potatoes, spinach, and liver are good sources of this vitamin.

Beware of any "miracle products" promoted to prevent aging. In general, it's a good idea to check with your doctor before taking anything to supplement your normal diet.

OUTLOOK

As we age, our nutritional requirements change, and a diet that once supplied us with plentiful nutrients may no longer be adequate for our needs. Some minor menu modifications are usually enough to make up the difference, though the use of vitamin and mineral supplements is sometimes helpful. The most important thing to remember is that eating well is important to living well, and that as we grow older, we can learn to do both better.

CONDITION: **NUTRITIONAL DEFICIENCIES**

CATEGORY: **VITAMINS**

GENERIC (CHEMICAL) NAME	BRAND (TRADE) NAME	DOSAGE FORMS AND STRENGTHS
Vitamins A, B_1, B_2, B_6, B_{12}, niacin, pantothenic acid, biotin, folic acid, iron, chromium, magnesium, manganese, copper, zinc	BERROCA PLUS	Tablets
Vitamins A, B_1, B_2, B_6, B_{12}, niacinamide, pantothenic acid, folic acid, zinc, magnesium, manganese	VICON FORTE	Capsules

This type of drug is available both by prescription and over the counter under a variety of brand names and dosage forms.

DRUG PROFILE

Multivitamins are used as nutritional supplements in people with inadequate diets. They are also used in people recovering from surgery or in those with medical conditions (such as severe illness or injury or overactive thyroid) for which nutritional requirements are increased. Those with conditions in which the body is unable to absorb enough essential nutrients or excretes excessive nutrients, those who abuse alcohol, and those whose chronic use of certain medicines results in specific nutrient deficiencies may also need multivitamins.

BEFORE USING THIS DRUG

Let your doctor know *IF*

You have ever had any of the following medical problems: ■ severe vitamin deficiency ■ anemia ■ Parkinson's disease ■ any other chronic disease.

You are taking any of the following medicines: ■ levodopa (medicine for Parkinson's disease) ■ diuretics (water pills) ■ laxatives ■ medicine for seizures ■ medicine for high cholesterol ■ isoniazid (medicine for tuberculosis).

SPECIAL RESTRICTIONS WHILE TAKING THIS DRUG

FOOD AND DRUG INTERACTIONS

Other Drugs	Many drugs affect vitamin requirements. Let your doctor know about any other drugs you are taking, including over-the-counter (OTC) drugs.
Foods and Beverages	Before prescribing a vitamin supplement, your doctor will probably evaluate your diet and make specific recommendations, which you should follow carefully.
Alcohol	Excessive alcohol intake may cause depletion of vitamins. It may also prevent the body from absorbing a vitamin supplement.
Smoking	Smokers have lower levels of vitamin C in their blood. But a small supplement (40 mg/day—the amount contained in a glass of orange juice) should be sufficient to meet this extra need. However, taking vitamins does not protect against the other harmful effects of smoking.

DAILY LIVING

No special restrictions on driving, exertion and exercise, sun exposure, or exposure to excessive heat or cold.

POSSIBLE SIDE EFFECTS

Although this list of adverse effects may seem somewhat intimidating, keep in mind that some are quite rare. Of course, should these or any other problems arise while you are on medication, it is always a good idea to consult your doctor.

IF YOU DEVELOP

flushing (from large doses of niacin) ■ headache ■ confusion ■ weakness ■ rash or hives ■ heart disturbances ■ increased thirst ■ increased urination ■ indigestion ■ kidney stones

WHAT TO DO

Urgent Get in touch with your doctor immediately.

---

nausea, vomiting, or other digestive disorders

May be serious Check with your doctor as soon as possible.

STORAGE INSTRUCTIONS

Store in a cool, dark place (not in a bathroom medicine cabinet).

STOPPING OR INTERRUPTING THERAPY

Try to remember to take this supplement every day. If you should miss a day, skip the missed dose and resume your regular schedule.

SPECIAL CONSIDERATIONS FOR THOSE OVER SIXTY-FIVE

Vitamin toxicity is more apt to occur in older people (see "Possible Side Effects" for symptoms).

CONDITION: **NUTRITIONAL DEFICIENCIES**

CATEGORY: **VITAMINS**

GENERIC (CHEMICAL) NAME	BRAND (TRADE) NAME	DOSAGE FORMS AND STRENGTHS
Vitamins B_1, B_2, B_6, B_{12}, C, niacin, pantothenic acid, folic acid		

This type of drug is available both by prescription and over the counter under a variety of brand names and dosage forms.

DRUG PROFILE

Vitamin B complex and vitamin B complex with C are used as nutritional supplements in people with inadequate diets. They are also used in people recovering from surgery or in those with medical conditions (such as severe illness or injury or overactive thyroid) for which nutritional requirements are increased. Those with conditions in which the body is unable to absorb enough essential nutrients or excretes excessive nutrients, those who abuse alcohol, and those whose use of certain medicines results in specific nutrient deficiencies may also need multivitamins.

BEFORE USING THIS DRUG

Let your doctor know *IF*

You have ever had allergic reactions or other problems with ■ vitamin C.

You have ever had any of the following medical problems: ■ anemia ■ any serious or chronic medical condition.

You are taking any of the following medicines: ■ medicine for seizures ■ sulfasalazine (medicine for inflammatory bowel disease) ■ aspirin ■ isoniazid (medicine for tuberculosis) ■ penicillamine (medicine for arthritis) ■ aluminum hydroxide (antacid) ■ cimetidine or ranitidine (medicine for ulcers).

SPECIAL RESTRICTIONS WHILE TAKING THIS DRUG

FOOD AND DRUG INTERACTIONS

Other Drugs	Many drugs affect vitamin requirements. Let your doctor know about any other drugs you are taking, including over-the-counter (OTC) drugs.
Foods and Beverages	Before prescribing a vitamin supplement, your doctor will probably evaluate your diet and make specific recommendations, which you should follow carefully.
Alcohol	Excessive alcohol intake may cause depletion of vitamins. It may also prevent the body from absorbing a vitamin supplement.

Smoking	Smokers have lower levels of vitamin C in their blood, but a small supplement (40 mg/day—the amount contained in a glass of orange juice) should be sufficient to meet this extra need. However, taking vitamins does not protect against the other harmful effects of smoking.

DAILY LIVING

No special restrictions on driving, exertion and exercise, sun exposure, or exposure to excessive heat or cold.

POSSIBLE SIDE EFFECTS

Although this list of adverse effects may seem somewhat intimidating, keep in mind that some are quite rare. Of course, should these or any other problems arise while you are on medication, it is always a good idea to consult your doctor.

IF YOU DEVELOP	WHAT TO DO
skin redness ■ rash or itching ■ difficulty in breathing	**Urgent** Get in touch with your doctor immediately.
nausea or vomiting ■ flushing ■ diarrhea ■ kidney stones	**May be serious** Check with your doctor as soon as possible.

STORAGE INSTRUCTIONS

Store in a cool, dark place (not in a bathroom medicine cabinet).

STOPPING OR INTERRUPTING THERAPY

Try to remember to take this supplement every day. If you should miss a day, skip the missed dose and resume your regular schedule.

SPECIAL CONSIDERATIONS FOR THOSE OVER SIXTY-FIVE

None.

CONDITION: **NUTRITIONAL DEFICIENCIES**

CATEGORY: **VITAMINS**

GENERIC (CHEMICAL) NAME	BRAND (TRADE) NAME	DOSAGE FORMS AND STRENGTHS

Vitamin B_{12} (cobalamin)

This drug is available both by prescription and over the counter under a variety of brand names and dosage forms.

DRUG PROFILE

Vitamin B_{12} (cobalamine) is involved in the production of red blood cells and is important in maintaining healthy nerves. This nutritional supplement is used to treat people with severe deficiency, those with certain metabolic disorders, and those with conditions in which the body is unable to absorb this vitamin from food.

BEFORE USING THIS DRUG

Let your doctor know *IF*

You have ever had any of the following medical problems: ■ heart disease ■ Leber's disease (atrophy of the optic nerve) ■ pernicious anemia ■ stomach or intestinal problems.

You are taking any of the following medicines: ■ folic acid ■ vitamin C ■ aspirin or aspirinlike medicine ■ medicine for seizures ■ prednisone (corticosteroid) ■ neomycin, chloramphenicol, or aminoglycosides (antibiotics) ■ cholestyramine (medicine for high cholesterol).

You are undergoing cobalt irradiation of the small intestine.

SPECIAL RESTRICTIONS WHILE TAKING THIS DRUG

FOOD AND DRUG INTERACTIONS

No special restrictions on other drugs, foods and beverages, alcohol use, or smoking.

DAILY LIVING

Examinations or Tests	Some experts believe that your body's requirement for potassium may increase while you are on B_{12} therapy. It is important for you to keep all doctor or laboratory appointments so that your doctor can check on this.
Other Precautions	Vitamin B_{12} is often taken by people who do not need it. If you are anemic, it is important that the cause of anemia be determined before B_{12} therapy is started.

No special restrictions on driving, exertion and exercise, sun exposure, or exposure to excessive heat or cold.

POSSIBLE SIDE EFFECTS

It is unlikely that any side effects will occur with this supplement.

STORAGE INSTRUCTIONS

Store in a cool, dark place (not in a bathroom medicine cabinet).

STOPPING OR INTERRUPTING THERAPY

If you should miss a dose, skip the missed dose and resume your regular schedule.

SPECIAL CONSIDERATIONS FOR THOSE OVER SIXTY-FIVE

None.

CONDITION: **NUTRITIONAL DEFICIENCIES**

CATEGORY: **VITAMINS**

GENERIC (CHEMICAL) NAME	BRAND (TRADE) NAME	DOSAGE FORMS AND STRENGTHS
Niacin	NICOBID	Controlled-release capsules: 125, 250, 500 mg

This drug is available both by prescription and over the counter under a variety of brand names and dosage forms.

DRUG PROFILE

Niacin helps the body break down food so that it can be used for energy. This type of supplement is used to prevent or treat niacin deficiency, or pellagra. Niacin is also used to lower blood levels of fats and cholesterol.

BEFORE USING THIS DRUG

Let your doctor know *IF*

You have ever had allergic reactions or other problems with ■ niacin or niacinamide.

You have ever had any of the following medical problems: ■ diabetes ■ ulcer ■ gout ■ liver disease.

You are taking any of the following medicines: ■ isoniazid (medicine for tuberculosis) ■ medicine for cancer.

SPECIAL RESTRICTIONS WHILE TAKING THIS DRUG

FOOD AND DRUG INTERACTIONS

Foods and Beverages	Before prescribing vitamin supplements, your doctor will probably evaluate your diet and make specific recommendations, which you should follow carefully.

Alcohol	Alcohol abuse commonly causes niacin deficiency.

No special restrictions on other drugs or smoking.

DAILY LIVING

Precautions	If you have diabetes, be aware that this medicine may affect blood-sugar levels. If you notice any change when testing sugar levels in your blood or urine, let your doctor know.
Helpful Hints	Swallow the capsule whole—without chewing, crushing, or breaking. If the capsule is too large for you, try swallowing it with a spoonful of jelly.
	If this medicine upsets your stomach, taking it with milk, meals, or snacks should help.

No special restrictions on driving, exertion and exercise, sun exposure, or exposure to excessive heat or cold.

POSSIBLE SIDE EFFECTS

Although this list of adverse effects may seem somewhat intimidating, keep in mind that some are quite rare. Of course, should these or any other problems arise while you are on medication, it is always a good idea to consult your doctor.

IF YOU DEVELOP	**WHAT TO DO**
flushing (especially of the face and neck) or feeling of warmth ■ dizziness or fainting ■ fast heartbeat ■ itching ■ "burning" sensation, stinging, or tingling of skin ■ dry skin or skin color changes ■ bloating or gas ■ headache ■ nausea or vomiting ■ heartburn ■ diarrhea ■ hunger pangs or other stomach pain ■ worsening of stomach ulcer	If symptoms are disturbing or persist, let your doctor know.

■ yellowing of eyes or skin ■ worsening of diabetes ■ visual disturbances ■ nervousness
■ vasovagal attacks (paleness, nausea, increased sweating, slow heartbeat, faintness) ■ gout

---

STORAGE INSTRUCTIONS

Store in a cool, dark place (not in a bathroom medicine cabinet).

STOPPING OR INTERRUPTING THERAPY

If you should miss a dose, skip the missed dose and resume your regular schedule.

SPECIAL CONSIDERATIONS FOR THOSE OVER SIXTY-FIVE

None.

CONDITION: **NUTRITIONAL DEFICIENCIES**

CATEGORY: **VITAMINS**

GENERIC (CHEMICAL) NAME	BRAND (TRADE) NAME	DOSAGE FORMS AND STRENGTHS
Folic acid		

This drug is available both by prescription and over the counter under a variety of brand names and dosage forms.

DRUG PROFILE

Folic acid helps produce red blood cells. This supplement is used to treat certain types of anemia that may be the result of disease, alcoholism, drug therapy, or kidney dialysis.

BEFORE USING THIS DRUG

Let your doctor know *IF*

You have ever had any of the following medical problems: ■ seizures ■ malnutrition

■ long illness or serious injury ■ anemia (hemolytic or pernicious) ■ alcoholism ■ chronic diarrhea ■ intestinal disease ■ liver disease.

You are taking any of the following medicines: ■ tetracycline ■ chloramphenicol ■ aspirin ■ antacids ■ anti-inflammatory drugs ■ diuretics (water pills) ■ sulfasalazine (medicine for inflammatory bowel disease) ■ phenytoin (medicine for seizures).

SPECIAL RESTRICTIONS WHILE TAKING THIS DRUG

FOOD AND DRUG INTERACTIONS

Foods and Beverages	Before prescribing vitamin supplements, your doctor will probably evaluate your diet and make specific recommendations, which you should follow carefully.
Alcohol	Alcohol abuse is a leading cause of folic acid deficiency.
Smoking	Some scientists believe that folic acid may have anticancer properties; however, taking vitamins does not protect against the harmful effects of smoking.

No special restrictions on other drugs.

DAILY LIVING

No special restrictions on driving, exertion and exercise, sun exposure, or exposure to excessive heat or cold.

POSSIBLE SIDE EFFECTS

It is unlikely that any side effects will occur with this supplement.

STORAGE INSTRUCTIONS

Store in a cool, dark place (not in a bathroom medicine cabinet).

STOPPING OR INTERRUPTING THERAPY

Try to remember to take this supplement every day. If you should miss a day, skip the missed dose and resume your regular schedule.

SPECIAL CONSIDERATIONS FOR THOSE OVER SIXTY-FIVE

None.

CONDITION: **NUTRITIONAL DEFICIENCIES**

CATEGORY: **VITAMINS**

GENERIC (CHEMICAL) NAME	BRAND (TRADE) NAME	DOSAGE FORMS AND STRENGTHS
Vitamin D (calcitrol)	ROCALTROL	Capsules: 0.25, 0.5 μg

DRUG PROFILE

Calcitrol is a synthetic form of vitamin D and is used when the body does not absorb enough of this vitamin. This may occur in people with medical conditions like rickets, osteomalacia, and osteoporosis; those undergoing kidney dialysis; those taking certain drugs; or in homebound people who do not get enough sunlight. Vitamin D regulates the metabolism of calcium and phosphorus, which are primary components of bone.

BEFORE USING THIS DRUG

Let your doctor know *IF*

You have ever had any of the following medical problems: ■ milk intolerance ■ kidney disease, including kidney stones ■ heart disease ■ sarcoidosis ■ disease of the parathyroid gland ■ bone disease ■ liver disease ■ intestinal problems.

You are taking any of the following medicines: ■ thiazide diuretics (water pills) ■ cholestyramine or colestipol (medicine for high cholesterol) ■ corticosteroids ■ antacids containing magnesium ■ diltiazem, nifedipine, or verapamil (calcium blockers) ■ laxatives ■ antibiotics ■ sucralfate (medicine for ulcers) ■ medicine for seizures.

SPECIAL RESTRICTIONS WHILE TAKING THIS DRUG

FOOD AND DRUG INTERACTIONS

Foods and Beverages	Before prescribing vitamin supplements, your doctor will probably evaluate your diet and make specific recommendations, which you should follow carefully.
	It is important to drink plenty of fluids while you are taking this supplement.
Alcohol	Alcohol will not cause vitamin D deficiency unless you have a malabsorption condition or advanced liver disease.
Smoking	Smoking increases the risk of osteoporosis. You should not smoke, particularly if you are being treated for bone disease.

No special restrictions on other drugs.

DAILY LIVING

Examinations or Tests	It is important for you to keep all doctor and laboratory appointments so that your progress can be checked. Depending on what you are being treated for, periodic blood and urine tests may be required to determine your body levels of vitamin D, calcium, and phosphorus.
Other Precautions	Take this supplement exactly as instructed. Vitamin D toxicity develops very rapidly if excess doses are taken.

No special restrictions on driving, exertion and exercise, sun exposure, or exposure to excessive heat or cold.

POSSIBLE SIDE EFFECTS

Although this list of adverse effects may seem somewhat intimidating, keep in mind that some are quite rare. Of course, should these or any other problems arise while you are on medication, it is always a good idea to consult your doctor.

IF YOU DEVELOP	WHAT TO DO
severe stomach pain ■ seizures ■ irregular heartbeat	**Urgent** Get in touch with your doctor immediately.
weakness ■ headache ■ dizziness ■ drowsiness ■ constipation ■ ringing in ears ■ nausea or vomiting ■ dry mouth ■ metallic taste ■ clumsiness ■ mood or mental changes ■ muscle or bone pain ■ increased urination or need to urinate at night ■ increased thirst ■ loss of appetite or weight loss ■ eye irritation ■ stomach cramps or pain ■ fever ■ decreased sex drive ■ rash or itching	**May be serious** Check with your doctor as soon as possible.

STORAGE INSTRUCTIONS

Store in cool, dark place (not in a bathroom medicine cabinet).

STOPPING OR INTERRUPTING THERAPY

Try to remember to take this supplement every day. If you should miss a day, skip the missed dose and resume your regular schedule.

SPECIAL CONSIDERATIONS FOR THOSE OVER SIXTY-FIVE

Older people are particularly prone to developing vitamin D toxicity (see "Possible Side Effects" for symptoms).

CONDITION: **NUTRITIONAL DEFICIENCIES**

CATEGORY: **VITAMINS**

GENERIC (CHEMICAL) NAME	BRAND (TRADE) NAME	DOSAGE FORMS AND STRENGTHS
Vitamin K_4 (menadiol sodium diphosphate)	SYNKAYVITE	Tablets: 5 mg
Vitamin K_1 (phytonadione)	MEPHYTON	Tablets: 5 mg

DRUG PROFILE

Vitamin K promotes certain substances in the body that help blood clot. Your doctor will prescribe vitamin K if your body is having trouble absorbing it from your regular diet because of a medical condition or because you are taking certain drugs (antibiotics, quinidine, quinine, or aspirin). Vitamin K is also used to treat certain types of bleeding disorders.

BEFORE USING THIS DRUG

Let your doctor know *IF*

You have ever had any of the following medical conditions: ■ liver disease ■ cystic fibrosis ■ prolonged diarrhea ■ intestinal problems.

You are taking any of the following medicines: ■ anticoagulants (blood thinners) ■ mineral oil or other laxatives ■ aspirin or aspirinlike medicine ■ antibiotics ■ medicine for high cholesterol ■ vitamin E.

SPECIAL RESTRICTIONS WHILE TAKING THIS DRUG

FOOD AND DRUG INTERACTIONS

Other Drugs	Many drugs affect the absorption of vitamin K. Let your doctor know about all other drugs you are taking, including over-the-counter (OTC) drugs.

No special restrictions on foods and beverages, alcohol use, or smoking.

DAILY LIVING

Examinations or Tests	It is important for you to keep all appointments with your doctor so that your progress can be checked. Periodic blood tests are usually required.
Other Precautions	Tell any doctor or dentist you consult that you are taking vitamin K, especially if you will be undergoing any type of surgery.

No special restrictions on driving, exertion and exercise, sun exposure, or exposure to excessive heat or cold.

POSSIBLE SIDE EFFECTS

Although this list of adverse effects may seem somewhat intimidating, keep in mind that some are quite rare. Of course, should these or any other problems arise while you are on medication, it is always a good idea to consult your doctor.

IF YOU DEVELOP

abnormal bleeding ■ abnormal clotting

WHAT TO DO

Urgent Get in touch with your doctor immediately.

STORAGE INSTRUCTIONS

Store in a cool, dark place (not in a bathroom medicine cabinet).

STOPPING OR INTERRUPTING THERAPY

If you are taking vitamin K for bleeding disorders, keep your doctor informed about any change from your usual dosage schedule.

SPECIAL CONSIDERATIONS FOR THOSE OVER SIXTY-FIVE

Older people are particularly prone to developing vitamin K toxicity (see ''Possible Side Effects'' for symptoms).

CONDITION: **NUTRITIONAL DEFICIENCIES**

CATEGORY: **POTASSIUM SUPPLEMENTS**

GENERIC (CHEMICAL) NAME	BRAND (TRADE) NAME	DOSAGE FORMS AND STRENGTHS
Potassium chloride	K-LOR	Powder: 1.125, 1.5 g per packet
	KLOTRIX	Controlled-release tablets: 750 mg
	K-LYTE	Powder: 1.86 g per measured scoop
	K-TAB	Controlled-release tablets: 750 mg
	MICRO-K	Controlled-release capsules: 600, 750 mg
	SLOW-K	Controlled-release tablets: 600 mg

DRUG PROFILE

Potassium supplements are used to prevent and treat the lack of potassium, a vital element in the body, when this lack cannot be made up by diet. Hypokalemia (lack of potassium) occurs in various medical conditions or with the administration of potassium-depleting drugs such as some diuretics (see pages 28–33).

BEFORE USING THIS DRUG

Let your doctor know *IF*

You have ever had allergic reactions or other problems with ■ any form of potassium.

You have ever had any of the following medical problems: ■ heart disease ■ muscle problems or congenital muscle disease ■ kidney disease ■ urinary problems ■ intestinal blockage or motility (movement) problems ■ diabetes.

You are taking any of the following medicines: ■ any potassium-containing medicines or supplements ■ appetite suppressants ■ decongestants ■ aminophylline, oxtriphylline, or theophylline (medicine for asthma) ■ laxatives ■ baking soda ■ flecainide or mexilitine (medicine for abnormal heart rhythms) ■ medicine for diabetes ■ diuretics (water pills) ■ digoxin, digitoxin, or digitalis (heart medicines).

SPECIAL RESTRICTIONS WHILE TAKING THIS DRUG

FOOD AND DRUG INTERACTIONS

Other Drugs	Many drugs interact with potassium supplements. Let your doctor know about all other drugs you are taking, including over-the-counter (OTC) drugs.
Foods and Beverages	Too much potassium can be harmful. Let your doctor know if you use salt substitutes or if you drink low-salt milk, as these substances contain potassium.
Alcohol	It is all right to drink alcohol in small amounts while taking this supplement.

No special restrictions on smoking.

DAILY LIVING

Exertion and Exercise	Some potassium-deficient people may experience cramps or weakness after exercise due to additional potassium lost through sweating.
Sun Exposure/ Excessive Heat	Some potassium-deficient people may experience cramps, weakness, irregular heartbeat, and other signs of dehydration due to additional potassium lost through sweating.

Examinations or Tests

It is important for you to keep all appointments with your doctor so that your progress can be checked. Periodic blood and urine tests may be required.

Helpful Hints

If you are taking a soluble granule or powder, dissolve the medicine in at least four ounces of cold water or juice. Wait until the mixture has stopped fizzing before drinking.

Controlled-release tablets or capsules should be swallowed whole without crushing or chewing. If you have trouble swallowing tablets or capsules, let your doctor know.

To prevent nausea, vomiting, upset stomach, or diarrhea, take this medicine directly after meals.

No special restrictions on driving or exposure to excessive cold.

POSSIBLE SIDE EFFECTS

Although this list of adverse effects may seem somewhat intimidating, keep in mind that some are quite rare. Of course, should these or any other problems arise while you are on medication, it is always a good idea to consult your doctor.

IF YOU DEVELOP	WHAT TO DO
numbness or tingling in hands or feet ■ tiredness or weakness ■ confusion ■ irregular heartbeat ■ heaviness of limbs ■ cold, grayish skin ■ dizziness ■ difficulty in breathing ■ vomiting ■ diarrhea	**Urgent** Get in touch with your doctor immediately.
nausea or stomach discomfort	If symptoms are disturbing or persist, let your doctor know.

STORAGE INSTRUCTIONS

Store in a cool, dark place (not in a bathroom medicine cabinet).

STOPPING OR INTERRUPTING THERAPY

If you miss a dose, take it as soon as possible. If it is not within two hours of the missed dose, skip it and resume your regular schedule.

SPECIAL CONSIDERATIONS FOR THOSE OVER SIXTY-FIVE

The side effects of dehydration (signalled by irregular heartbeat or weakness), nausea, and vomiting are particularly serious in older people.

SMOKING

Until fairly recently, smoking was considered a bad habit—but one that anyone could control with a little willpower. Recent evidence has shown, however, that cigarette smoking is a stubborn form of drug addiction; the smoker has a true physical dependence on nicotine, the active ingredient in tobacco. In fact, nicotine is probably one of the most addictive drugs used in our society.

Nicotine is a stimulant, leading to an increase in heart rate and blood pressure and the narrowing of blood vessels. In addition, the nicotine in tobacco smoke reaches the brain within ten seconds of inhaling it. If the amount of nicotine contained in a single cigarette were injected directly into the bloodstream rather than being absorbed through the lungs, it would paralyze the centers in the brain controlling breathing and cause death.

Nicotine is not the only culprit in cigarette smoke. *Tar*—the short name for the condensed solid particles in smoke—contains several thousand chemicals that have been implicated in a number of diseases. Among the chemicals are hydrocarbons, phenols, and ketones; the corrosive gases hydrogen cyanide and nitrogen oxide; and carbon monoxide. The presence of carbon monoxide interferes with oxygen delivery to the brain, heart, and other tissues.

WHY YOU SHOULD QUIT

We are all familiar with the link between cigarette smoking and lung cancer. The risk of lung cancer is ten times greater for a smoker than for a nonsmoker. But smoking has also been identified as a major cause, or at least a contributing factor, in many other forms of cancer. In total, three out of every ten cancer deaths can be attributed to the use of tobacco. Cigarette smoking also takes its toll in terms of heart disease, as well as such lung diseases as emphysema and chronic bronchitis.

These are compelling arguments not to start smoking—but what about stopping? Hasn't the damage been done after years of inhaling all the dangerous components of cigarette smoke? Isn't it too late?

A growing body of evidence shows that even people in their sixties and seventies who have smoked since adolescence can benefit substantially from giving it up. For example, if a man who has smoked a half pack to one pack of cigarettes a day all his life quits smoking at age sixty-five, he will add two years to his life expectancy. If he has smoked more than two packs a day, the gain will be four years. (This information is based on a study of more than one million people who were studied over a twenty-year period.) A more recent study of more than two thousand five hundred people between the ages of sixty-five and seventy-four showed that stopping smoking substantially decreases the death rate from coronary heart disease. In a study of more than forty thousand British doctors (the majority of them middle-aged or older), it was found that the lung cancer rate was cut in half in the group that stopped smoking within two and a half years after the cessation of smoking. Clearly, even older people can achieve substantial health benefits—and increased odds of living longer—from stopping smoking.

BUT HOW DO I STOP?

It's hard to stop smoking. Some smokers seem to be able to do so without much trouble, but most people go through a period of withdrawal that includes agitation, nausea, headache, and other physical symptoms. Drowsiness and the persistent inability to concentrate are other common complaints. These symptoms usually abate within ten days to two weeks, but sometimes they last longer than that.

If you really decide to stop and feel that you need something more than willpower, your doctor may prescribe nicotine polacrilex (Nicorette), a nicotine chewing gum. (See the chart on pages 563–566.) Each piece of gum delivers about the same amount of nicotine as a cigarette. Nicorette relieves the craving for nicotine and relieves the withdrawal symptoms that so often cause people to start smoking again.

Using Nicorette is most helpful when it's combined with a program to eliminate the psychological dependency on cigarette smoking. This involves, for example, learning other ways to relax, cope with stress, and handle boredom. Once this is achieved, the next goal is to withdraw from all sources of nicotine—including Nicorette. Research has shown that a comprehensive treatment program, including the use of nicotine gum and group counseling is more successful than reliance on the gum alone.

Questions have been raised about the safety of Nicorette in older people who may suffer from a chronic lung problem or cerebrovascular or cardiovascular disease. Currently, it is up to the doctor to weigh the risks of short-term (three to six months) exposure to the low levels of nicotine contained in the gum against the risks of continued smoking—long-term exposure to nicotine, carbon monoxide, and carcinogens.

A number of other treatments can help people stop smoking. These include such behavior-modification techniques as rapid smoking. This consists of having the person inhale his or her own cigarette smoke every six seconds until he or she no longer wants to take another puff; as part of this approach, the doctor or therapist teaches alternative coping skills to replace smoking. Recent studies have shown that rapid smoking therapy poses no particular danger for older people, including those who have heart and lung ailments. In fact, it produces no greater physiologic changes than does smoking at a regular rate.

Smokenders, which involves behavior modification in a group format similar to that of Alcoholics Anonymous, is a ten-week program that is believed to have a success rate of about 25 percent (though whether this is permanent abstinence is unknown). The American Cancer Society (ACS) also offers a program, known as Fresh Start, to help people stop smoking. It is a four-session, group program that is led by former smokers who understand well the difficulties of quitting. Videotapes and audiotapes of the ACS program, which uses behavioral and other techniques, are also available. They can be purchased at commercial outlets. (For more information on Fresh Start, call your local ACS office.) Other approaches to quitting smoking include acupuncture and hypnosis, as well as self-help manuals for those who prefer doing it on their own.

OUTLOOK

Smoking is the number one preventable cause of premature death and disability in this country—and an addiction that's hard to break. But more than thirty million Americans have quit; you can too. It may be difficult, but it's not impossible. The benefits, a healthy and longer life, make it worthwhile.

CONDITION: **SMOKING**

CATEGORY: **SMOKING DETERRENTS**

GENERIC (CHEMICAL) NAME	BRAND (TRADE) NAME	DOSAGE FORMS AND STRENGTHS
Nicotine polacrilex	NICORETTE	Chewing gum: nicotine polacrilex equivalent to 2 mg nicotine per piece of gum

DRUG PROFILE

This drug, which comes in the form of chewing gum, is used as part of a medically supervised behavior-modification program to stop smoking for people who have a strong physical dependence on nicotine. The drug is absorbed through the lining of the cheek into the bloodstream and helps reduce nicotine withdrawal symptoms.

BEFORE USING THIS DRUG

Let your doctor know *IF*

You have ever had allergic reactions or other problems with ■ nicotine.

You have ever had any of the following medical problems: ■ angina (chest pain) ■ heart attack ■ abnormal heart rhythms ■ disease of the blood vessels ■ high blood pressure ■ temperomandibular (jaw muscle) joint disease (TMJ) ■ dental problems ■ inflammation of the vocal cords ■ stomach ulcer ■ heartburn ■ diabetes ■ overactive thyroid ■ pheochromocytoma (adrenal gland tumor) ■ gout.

You are taking any of the following medicines: ■ aminophylline, oxtriphylline, or theophylline (medicine for asthma) ■ medicine containing caffeine ■ decongestants ■ medicine for migraine or vascular headaches ■ pentazocine or propoxyphene (prescription pain-killers) ■ beta-blockers ■ medicine for high blood pressure ■ nitrates (medicine for angina) ■ sulfinpyrazone (medicine for gout) ■ ergoloid mesylate (vasodilator) ■ imipramine (medicine for depression) ■ furosemide (diuretic).

You wear dentures.

SPECIAL RESTRICTIONS WHILE TAKING THIS DRUG

FOOD AND DRUG INTERACTIONS

Other Drugs	Stopping smoking may change the body's response to drugs. Let your doctor know about all other drugs you are taking, including over-the-counter (OTC) drugs.
Smoking	You must stop smoking completely when you start using this drug. In addition, you may not use any other form of tobacco, such as chewing tobacco.

No special restrictions on foods and beverages or alcohol use.

DAILY LIVING

Precautions	Read the accompanying pamphlet carefully; your doctor may want you to chew one piece of the gum in the office to make sure you have mastered the technique.
	To use: When you feel the urge to smoke, chew one piece of gum slowly until you can taste it or until you feel a tingling sensation in your mouth. Resume chewing when the taste or sensation disappears. Adverse effects from this drug usually subside after the first few days of use.
	Your doctor will probably warn you that you may experience withdrawal symptoms after stopping this drug, such as craving for tobacco, irritability, anxiety, restlessness, impatience, depression, inability to concentrate, hostility, headache, drowsiness, and upset stomach.
	Overdose may occur if too many pieces are chewed in rapid succession or if the gum is chewed too fast. If overdose occurs (see ''Possible Side Effects'' for

symptoms) or if a child should accidentally chew the gum, call your doctor or a poison control center immediately.

If dental problems or damage to your dental work occurs, stop use of this drug and check with your doctor or dentist.

| Helpful Hints | If your mouth feels dry or irritated, sucking hard sugarless candy in between pieces of gum will help. |

No special restrictions on driving, exertion and exercise, sun exposure, or exposure to excessive heat or cold.

POSSIBLE SIDE EFFECTS

Although this list of adverse effects may seem somewhat intimidating, keep in mind that some are quite rare. Of course, should these or any other problems arise while you are on medication, it is always a good idea to consult your doctor.

IF YOU DEVELOP	WHAT TO DO
signs of overdose: cold sweat; hearing problems; visual disturbances; confusion; extreme weakness; fainting; dizziness; difficulty in breathing; seizures; weak, irregular pulse; diarrhea	**Urgent** Get in touch with your doctor immediately.
light-headedness or dizziness ■ nausea or vomiting ■ upset stomach ■ loss of appetite ■ heartburn ■ mouth or throat irritation ■ sleeplessness ■ irritability ■ headache ■ ringing in ears ■ palpitations ■ gas ■ belching ■ laxative effect ■ constipation ■ flushing ■ aching jaw muscles ■ hiccups ■ increased salivation ■ hoarseness ■ dry mouth ■ cough ■ sneezing	If symptoms are disturbing or persist, let your doctor know.

STORAGE INSTRUCTIONS

Store in a cool, dark place (not in a bathroom medicine cabinet).

STOPPING OR INTERRUPTING THERAPY

Use this drug exactly as instructed by your doctor and the pamphlet that accompanies the chewing gum. Your doctor will probably direct you to cut down on the gum gradually to avoid withdrawal symptoms.

SPECIAL CONSIDERATIONS FOR THOSE OVER SIXTY-FIVE

Older people may be especially sensitive to the adverse effects of this drug.

Chapter 8
Hormonal Disorders

DIABETES MELLITUS

From the sugar in your tea to last night's spaghetti, all sugars and starchy foods eventually break down in your body, in part to glucose, a form of carbohydrate. Carbohydrate supplies a major amount of the body's fuel; it travels through the blood and readily enters cells to give them the energy they need. When diabetes mellitus ("sugar diabetes") complicates the picture, glucose has trouble entering the cells that need it, causing an energy crisis. In addition, glucose builds up to high levels in the blood, where it can cause further trouble.

CAUSES

Two types of illnesses account for the vast majority of cases of diabetes. In insulin-dependent (Type I) diabetes, a person loses the ability to make the hormone insulin. Insulin is the key that unlocks the cells and permits glucose to enter. Without insulin, body cells literally starve for glucose, even as this sugar rises to higher and higher levels in the blood. A person with Type I diabetes must take daily insulin injections to survive.

Non-insulin-dependent (Type II) diabetes is most common in older people. In Type II diabetes, the body produces less than the required amount of insulin, and the cells show resistance to insulin's action.

Type I diabetes most often develops in childhood or adolescence, which is why it used to be called juvenile-onset diabetes. Type II diabetes generally occurs in people over forty. Most Type II diabetics are overweight. If you've recently developed diabetes, chances are it is Type II diabetes—this is the form of diabetes we will focus on here.

Many people, doctors included, mistakenly think of Type II diabetes as a mild form of the disease. However, Type II diabetes can cause some serious complications. In the short run (especially during times of illness or stress), high blood-sugar levels can lead to diabetic coma, which can be fatal if not treated quickly in a hospital. And, over the years, Type II diabetes, like Type I diabetes, can lead to conditions as varied as infection, nerve impairment, kidney disease, cataract formation, and changes in the retina of the eye that impair vision. It can also contribute (along with other factors, such as high blood pressure, high blood fat levels, and smoking) to heart disease, stroke, and gangrene of the feet and legs.

Fortunately, proper control and care of diabetes can practically eliminate problems like diabetic coma. And most authorities believe that working to keep blood-sugar levels close to normal can help prevent many long-term complications as well.

DIAGNOSIS

Extreme thirst, urinary frequency, and unusual hunger are the three "classic" symptoms of diabetes—if you have these symptoms, diabetes will be the first thing to come to a doctor's mind. However, the classic symptoms do not always occur in people with non-insulin-dependent diabetes. Sometimes more subtle signs—such as constant fatigue, blurred vision, or cuts that take unusually long to heal—are the only outward indications of the disease. Or there may be no symptoms at all, with the first sign of trouble being an unusually high glucose level in a routine blood or urine test.

In any event, once diabetes is suspected, your doctor may use one or more blood tests to confirm the diagnosis. Your doctor may want to perform a fasting blood-sugar test, in which a blood sample will be taken in the morning, before you've eaten anything.

In addition, your doctor may order an oral glucose tolerance test, in which you swallow a measured dose of glucose and your blood sugar is sampled several times over the following hours. This test creates a graph showing how your body handles, or tolerates, glucose. It can help distinguish between a diagnosis of diabetes and one of impaired glucose tolerance, which is a milder condition.

TREATMENT

If you are diagnosed as having Type II diabetes, the first course of action is to try to control blood sugar through diet and exercise alone. Dietary needs vary, so you'll need to work out a diet plan individually with your doctor or dietitian. Appropriate diet will successfully control diabetes in about one-half of older diabetics.

Lifestyle Changes In general, a healthy diet for a person with diabetes includes a variety of food groups, derives most of its calories from whole-grain starchy foods, and is low in fats (especially saturated fats and cholesterol). Sugary foods, of course, need to be restricted. In addition, four out of five people with Type II diabetes need to lose weight, so there's a good chance your diet will be designed to cut calories. Losing weight improves your body's ability to use its own insulin effectively to lower blood sugar.

Exercise is also essential in treating Type II diabetes. Aerobic exercise, the kind that gets your heart and lungs pumping, lowers blood sugar by burning glucose, and it can contribute to needed weight loss. Moreover, regular aerobic exercise, like weight loss, conditions your body cells to be more receptive to insulin and therefore to take glucose in from the blood with less of a struggle.

Medicine—The Next Step If diet and exercise don't succeed in keeping your blood sugar at desired levels, medicine is the next option. Insulin is one choice, and some doctors consider it the first choice. However, most doctors prefer to try an oral diabetes medicine first (see the chart on pages 571–575). At least 80 percent of older diabetics requiring medicine are controlled with oral medicine. Oral diabetes medicines are *not* substitutes for diet and exercise; to be most effective, they should be an addition to a treatment plan that already includes diet and exercise.

Insulin—There If You Need It If an oral diabetes medicine fails to lower blood sugar adequately, you can count on daily injections of insulin to do the job. About 30 percent of older diabetics require insulin sometime in the course of their disease. If you do need to take insulin injections, you will need to eat your meals regularly and always carry some form of sugary food with you to treat low blood sugar (hypoglycemia) if it occurs. Signs of hypoglycemia include sweating, fainting, feeling very hot, weakness, tremors, unsteadiness, hunger, blurred vision, slurred speech, headache, tingling in feet or hands, seizures, nervousness, shakiness, and a general feeling of unwellness.

Keeping an Eye on Things In addition to following your diet and exercise routine and taking medicine if necessary, your doctor may also want you to test your urine or blood for glucose regularly. Urine tests are less accurate than self-performed blood tests, but they can be useful as a general indication that blood sugar is rising too high.

OUTLOOK

The list of tools for helping people with diabetes normalize their blood-sugar levels has grown tremendously in the last decade. By making the best use of these tools, doctors hope to prevent the long-term complications of the disease. Meanwhile, techniques for treating those complications if they occur have also improved; the most dramatic has been the perfection of laser treatments to prevent vision loss from diabetes-related eye disease.

Through such techniques as manipulating the immune system and transplanting insulin-making cells, researchers are looking at ways of preventing or curing insulin-dependent diabetes. And continuing research into how cells use insulin may lead to improved oral medicines for Type II diabetes.

CONDITION: **DIABETES MELLITUS**

CATEGORY: **ORAL ANTIDIABETIC AGENTS (SULFONYLUREAS)**

GENERIC (CHEMICAL) NAME	BRAND (TRADE) NAME	DOSAGE FORMS AND STRENGTHS
Acetohexamide	DYMELOR	Tablets: 250, 500 mg
Chlorpropamide	DIABINESE	Tablets: 100, 250 mg
Glipizide	GLUCOTROL	Tablets: 5, 10 mg
Glyburide	DIAβETA MICRONASE	Tablets: 1.25, 2.5, 5 mg Tablets: 1.25, 2.5, 5 mg
Tolazamide	RONASE TOLINASE	Tablets: 100, 250, 500 mg Tablets: 100, 250, 500 mg
Tolbutamide	ORINASE	Tablets: 250, 500 mg

DRUG PROFILE

These drugs, known collectively as sulfonylureas, are used to lower blood-glucose (sugar) levels in people with non-insulin-dependent diabetes (also called maturity-onset, or Type II diabetes) that is not controlled by diet alone. These agents are thought to work by stimulating the pancreas to produce insulin, a hormone that helps the body break down glucose for energy.

A 1970 study reported that tolbutamide increases the risk of death from heart disease. You should discuss the benefits and risks of sulfonylurea treatment with your doctor.

BEFORE USING THIS DRUG

Let your doctor know *IF*

You have ever had allergic reactions or other problems with ■ any sulfonylureas

■ sulfonamides (sulfa drugs) ■ thiazide diuretics (water pills).

You have ever had any of the following medical problems: ■ porphyria ■ under-active pituitary gland ■ Addison's disease (underactive adrenal glands) ■ thyroid disease ■ kidney disease ■ liver disease ■ heart disease ■ recent severe infection.

You are taking any of the following medicines: ■ any other medicine for diabetes, including insulin or other sulfonylureas ■ anticoagulants (blood thinners) ■ medicine for asthma ■ medicine for seizures ■ aspirin or aspirinlike medicine ■ nonsteroidal anti-inflammatory agents ■ medicine for gout ■ diuretics, especially thiazide diuretics ■ sulfonamides (sulfa drugs) ■ medicine for depression ■ timolol, nadolol, propranolol, metoprolol, atenolol, pindolol, acebutolol, or labetolol (beta-blockers) ■ cimetidine or ranitidine (medicine for ulcers) ■ diltiazem, nifedipine, or verapamil (calcium blockers) ■ estrogens ■ thyroid hormones ■ corticosteroids ■ tranquilizers ■ medicine for nausea or vomiting ■ androgens (male sex hormones) ■ nicotinic acid ■ isoniazid (medicine for tuberculosis) ■ antibiotics ■ clofibrate (medicine for high cholesterol) ■ medicine for high blood pressure ■ digoxin, digitoxin, or digitalis (heart medicines) ■ appetite suppressants ■ barbiturates ■ any medicine containing alcohol ■ medicine to make the urine more or less acidic.

SPECIAL RESTRICTIONS WHILE TAKING THIS DRUG

FOOD AND DRUG INTERACTIONS

Other Drugs	It is a good idea to check with your doctor before taking any other medicines. Many drugs affect the way these drugs work. Let your doctor know about any other drugs you are taking, including over-the-counter (OTC) drugs.
Foods and Beverages	It is important to follow your doctor's diet recommendations. Do not skip meals. You may be advised to go on a weight-reduction diet.
Alcohol	Drinking alcohol while taking this drug may cause you to become hypoglycemic (to have low blood sugar). Some of these drugs, when combined with alcohol,

may make you very sick. Avoid alcohol unless your doctor has approved its use.

No special restrictions on smoking.

DAILY LIVING

Exertion and Exercise	Appropriate exercise is an important part of the management of diabetes. Ask your doctor about an exercise program for you. Keep in mind that severe or prolonged exercise can sometimes result in hypoglycemia, so be careful not to overexert yourself.
Sun Exposure	Your skin may become more sensitive to sunlight and more likely to develop a sunburn while you are taking this drug. It is a good idea to avoid too much sun and to apply a sunscreen to exposed skin surfaces before going outdoors.
Examinations or Tests	It is very important for you to keep all appointments with your doctor so that your progress and reactions to therapy can be checked. Your doctor may instruct you to perform tests at home for sugar in blood or urine. If you are being switched from insulin to a sulfonylurea, you may be asked to perform a urine ketone test as well.
Other Precautions	Tell any doctor or dentist you consult that you are taking any of these drugs, especially if you will be undergoing any type of surgery. If you become sick with a fever, let your doctor know; your body is under added stress when fighting off an infection, and you may need insulin to maintain blood sugar at normal levels. Also, let your doctor know if you are unable to eat because of severe nausea or vomiting.

You should keep something sweet with you (a piece of candy, for example) to eat immediately if you become hypoglycemic. Also, you should check your blood-sugar levels if you experience symptoms of hypoglycemia.

If you experience upset stomach with a sulfonylurea, let your doctor know; it may be possible to reduce your dosage.

No special restrictions on driving or exposure to excessive heat or cold.

POSSIBLE SIDE EFFECTS

Although this list of adverse effects may seem somewhat intimidating, keep in mind that some are quite rare. Not all of these effects have been reported with all sulfonylureas. Of course, should these or any other problems arise while you are on medication, it is always a good idea to consult your doctor.

IF YOU DEVELOP

signs of hypoglycemia: increased sweating; fainting; feeling very hot; weakness; tremors; unsteadiness; hunger; blurred vision; slurred speech; headache; tingling in feet or hands; seizures; nervousness; shakiness; pale, moist skin; pounding heart; rapid breathing; and a general feeling of unwellness

WHAT TO DO

Urgent Get in touch with your doctor immediately.

---

rash, hives, itching, skin redness, or other skin problems ■ bleeding or bruising ■ sore throat or fever ■ yellowing of eyes or skin ■ pale stools ■ dark urine ■ severe diarrhea ■ confusion ■ nausea or vomiting ■ loss of appetite ■ depression ■ dizziness

May be serious Check with your doctor as soon as possible.

---

full feeling ■ heartburn ■ diarrhea ■ headache ■ increased skin sensitivity to sunlight ■ upset stomach ■ stomach cramps ■ constipation ■ weakness or tiredness ■ tingling or prickling feeling ■ drowsiness ■ gas ■ taste changes

If symptoms are disturbing or persist, let your doctor know.

STORAGE INSTRUCTIONS

Store in a cool, dark place (not in a bathroom medicine cabinet).

STOPPING OR INTERRUPTING THERAPY

If you miss a dose of this medicine, take it as soon as possible. If it is almost time for your next dose, skip the missed dose and resume your regular schedule. Do not take two doses at the same time.

SPECIAL CONSIDERATIONS FOR THOSE OVER SIXTY-FIVE

Older people are more prone to developing hypoglycemia with these drugs. Doctors may want to start people over sixty-five on a lower dosage and check their progress often.

THYROID DISEASE

Just as a conductor sets a proper tempo for a musical performance, your thyroid gland helps set the tempo for daily life. When the thyroid works properly, your many bodily processes, such as your heartbeat, digestion, and metabolism, all function at their optimum speeds. But when thyroid problems develop, it can seem as if the body's conductor has gone out of control, causing the body's tempo to speed up or slow down abnormally.

Problems with the thyroid—a butterfly-shaped gland perched around the windpipe in the neck—become somewhat more common in older persons. They also tend to be more common in women. Fortunately, though, the treatments for most thyroid conditions are very effective.

CAUSES

Your thyroid influences metabolic rate by means of several hormones it secretes into the bloodstream. The two main ones are T-4 (thyroxine) and T-3 (triiodothyronine). The gland varies its secretion of thyroid hormones in response to a number of chemical messages. In particular, another gland, the pituitary, strongly influences thyroid activity by secreting or withholding a substance called thyroid-stimulating hormone (TSH). This elaborate system of chemical checks and balances helps ensure that the body gets only as much thyroid hormone as it needs.

Thyroid disease can result if this series of controls goes awry. Some thyroid diseases are caused when the body's immune system mistakenly attacks the gland. Others may develop as a side effect of other diseases. Often, the cause of thyroid disease cannot be found.

Regardless of the cause, however, the result is generally either an overactive or an underactive gland. If you have an overactive thyroid (*hyperthyroidism*), your thyroid gland is usually enlarged (goiter) and you may experience such symptoms as fast heartbeat, increased sweating, high blood pressure, agitation, difficulty in sleeping, diarrhea, and bulging eyes. You may also find that you lose weight no matter how much you eat. However, about 40 percent of older people with hyperthyroidism do not experience an enlarged thyroid gland, nervousness, increased sweating, fast heartbeat, or bulging eyes. Instead, older patients may show such symptoms as abnormal heart rhythm, congestive heart failure, muscle wasting, poor appetite, and fatigue.

Symptoms of an underactive thyroid (*hypothyroidism*) are much the opposite. You may experience constant fatigue, a slow pulse, a feeling of coldness, constipation, coarse hair and puffy skin, slowness of movement, and mental dullness. People with an underactive thyroid often have high levels of lipids (fats) in the blood and can be at greater risk of developing atherosclerosis.

An enlarged thyroid gland, or goiter, can occur in a variety of thyroid conditions, both hyperthyroid and hypothyroid. Sometimes a goiter can develop even though there is no change in thyroid activity at all. Unless a goiter grows very large, it is seldom harmful in itself, though the condition that gave rise to it may need treatment. Iodine deficiency, once a major cause of goiters, is now rare in the United States.

Another possible thyroid problem is the growth of nodules, or lumps, on the gland. "Hot" thyroid nodules actively produce thyroid hormone and can contribute to hyperthyroidism; "cold" nodules produce no thyroid hormone. Thyroid nodules deserve special attention because they can sometimes become cancerous.

DIAGNOSIS

Symptoms can be useful in detecting thyroid trouble, but they can also be deceiving. In particular, many of the signs of hypothyroidism can look a great deal like the normal signs of aging. Fortunately, doctors have a wide range of tests at their disposal to help them diagnose thyroid problems.

Measurements of T-4 and T-3 in the blood are often the most direct evidence of an over- or underactive thyroid. In addition, the doctor will probably measure TSH. In hypothyroidism, TSH levels are high.

TREATMENT

In older persons, thyroid problems are most likely to involve an underactive gland. Treatment generally consists of replacing the missing thyroid hormones with oral thyroid supple-ments. Most doctors prescribe a drug called levothyroxine sodium, which is a synthetic form of T-4. Thyroid hormone derived from animal glands is also still available and just as effective.

Oral thyroid hormone is generally taken once a day in the morning. Your doctor will probably start you on a low dose and increase it gradually over a period of several weeks. To work properly, it must be taken consistently over a long period of time. It should start improving some symptoms, such as fatigue, in a matter of weeks. Other symptoms will take longer to correct. To learn more about this type of treatment, check the drug chart on pages 579–582.

If you have an overactive thyroid, there are a number of treatments your doctor may initiate. Two medicines, propylthiouracil and methimazole, work directly on the thyroid gland to inhibit the secretion of thyroid hormone. Depending on the specific condition you have, it may be necessary for you to take these oral drugs for many years, or your doctor may tell you to discontinue their use once your thyroid activity is back to normal.

A more direct treatment approach is to partially destroy an overactive thyroid gland by using radioactive iodine. This highly effective treatment usually has to be done only once. About half the time, it turns an overactive thyroid into an underactive one—still a plus, since hypothyroidism is much easier to control (using thyroid hormone tablets) than is hyperthyroidism.

Several medicines are commonly used in hyperthyroid states. Beta-blockers can be very effective in controlling a number of the consequences of hyperthyroidism, such as high blood pressure and rapid heart rate. Less frequently, oral iodide can be used to quickly return thyroid levels to normal by blocking the release of thyroid hormone from the gland.

Finally, surgical removal of part or all of a diseased thyroid gland is sometimes necessary, especially in the case of thyroid cancer or a dangerously enlarged goiter. If the entire thyroid must be taken out, the shortage of thyroid hormone can, again, easily be corrected with thyroid hormone tablets.

OUTLOOK

The number and range of thyroid tests continue to increase, making it easier for specialists to diagnose or rule out thyroid disease in the face of confusing symptoms. Meanwhile, doctors are becoming more adept at using such tools as medicine or radiation to make appropriate changes in thyroid functioning. As the trend toward more precise monitoring and control of thyroid activity continues, we can expect it to become easier and easier for doctors to keep the body running at a satisfying tempo. And it will be easier for people who have a thyroid condition to achieve a satisfying tempo in their daily lives.

CONDITION: **HYPOTHYROIDISM**

CATEGORY: **THYROID HORMONES**

GENERIC (CHEMICAL) NAME	BRAND (TRADE) NAME	DOSAGE FORMS AND STRENGTHS
Levothyroxine sodium	LEVOTHROID	Tablets: 25, 50, 75, 100, 125, 150, 175, 200, 300 μg
	SYNTHROID	Tablets: 25, 50, 75, 100, 125, 150, 200, 300 μg
Liothyronine sodium	CYTOMEL	Tablets: 5, 25, 50 μg
Liotrix	EUTHROID	Tablets: 30, 60, 120, 180 mg
Thyroglobulin	PROLOID	Tablets: 32, 65, 100, 130, 200 mg
Thyroid, desiccated	ARMOUR Thyroid	Tablets: 15, 30, 60, 90, 120, 180, 240, 300 mg

DRUG PROFILE

Replacement thyroid hormones are prescribed when the thyroid gland does not produce enough natural thyroid hormone. This condition is called hypothyroidism, and it may occur spontaneously or as the result of thyroid surgery. Depending on the exact preparation used, your symptoms of thyroid deficiency should gradually disappear.

BEFORE USING THIS DRUG

Let your doctor know *IF*

You have ever had allergic reactions or other problems with ■ any thyroid medicines ■ pork products ■ corn ■ milk products (contained in levothyroxine) ■ tartrazine (FD&C Yellow Dye No. 5) (contained in Synthroid and some strengths of Euthroid).

You have ever had any of the following medical problems: ■ overactive thyroid ■ diabetes ■ heart disease, including heart attack and angina (chest pain) ■ high blood pressure ■ kidney disease ■ underactive adrenal gland or pituitary gland.

You are taking any of the following medicines: ■ anticoagulants (blood thinners) ■ timolol, nadolol, propranolol, metoprolol, atenolol, pindolol, acebutolol, or labetalol (beta-blockers) ■ medicine for depression ■ digoxin, digitoxin, or digitalis (heart medicines) ■ medicine for asthma containing adrenaline, ephedrine, or isoproterenol ■ cholestyramine (medicine for high cholesterol) ■ medicine for diabetes ■ estrogens (female hormones) ■ androgens (male hormones) ■ corticosteroids ■ aspirin or aspirinlike medicine ■ phenylbutazone (medicine for arthritis) ■ tranquilizers ■ sleep medicines ■ narcotics or other prescription painkillers.

SPECIAL RESTRICTIONS WHILE TAKING THIS DRUG

FOOD AND DRUG INTERACTIONS

No special restrictions on other drugs, foods and beverages, alcohol use, or smoking.

DAILY LIVING

Exertion and Exercise	In some kinds of heart disease, thyroid medicine may cause chest pain or shortness of breath when you exert yourself. If you have ever had any kind of heart disease, let your doctor know, and discuss what type of exercise and how much of it is safe for you.
Examinations or Tests	It is important for you to keep all appointments for laboratory or blood tests, since these tests will help your doctor adjust your dosage.

Other Precautions   Tell any doctor or dentist you consult that you are taking this medicine, especially if you will be undergoing any type of surgery.

If you have diabetes, the dosage of your diabetes medicine may need to be adjusted while you are on thyroid hormone therapy. Your doctor may give you special instructions on testing your blood or urine for sugar.

No special restrictions on driving, sun exposure, or exposure to excessive heat or cold.

POSSIBLE SIDE EFFECTS

Although this list of adverse effects may seem somewhat intimidating, keep in mind that some are quite rare. Of course, should these or any other problems arise while you are on medication, it is always a good idea to consult your doctor.

IF YOU DEVELOP

chest pain ■ irregular or fast heartbeat ■ shortness of breath ■ rash or hives ■ increased sweating ■ nervousness ■ sensitivity to heat

WHAT TO DO

Urgent Get in touch with your doctor immediately.

---

increase in appetite ■ diarrhea ■ nausea or vomiting ■ tremors ■ headache ■ sleeplessness ■ fever ■ stomach cramps ■ weight loss

May be serious Check with your doctor as soon as possible.

STORAGE INSTRUCTIONS

Store in a cool, dark place (not in a bathroom medicine cabinet).

STOPPING OR INTERRUPTING THERAPY

If you have had thyroid surgery, you may need to take this medicine for the rest of your life. Do not stop taking this medicine without first checking with your doctor. If you miss a dose, take it as soon as possible. If it is almost time for your next dose, skip the missed dose and resume your regular schedule. Do not take two doses at the same time.

SPECIAL CONSIDERATIONS FOR THOSE OVER SIXTY-FIVE

Older people are often more sensitive to the effects of thyroid medicines. Doctors may start people over sixty-five on a low dosage and gradually increase the amount until it reaches a level that is effective. Older patients require a lower total dosage.

Chapter 9
Disorders of the
Respiratory System

RESPIRATORY INFECTIONS

THE COMMON COLD

It's been said that if you don't treat a cold, it'll last seven days, and that if you do take care of it, you'll be well in a week.

Colds are caused by viruses—lots of them. Doctors have identified more than one hundred sixty different types of viruses, which explains why you can catch so many colds in a lifetime. The immunity you develop to one type of cold virus doesn't help protect you against the other one hundred fifty-nine.

Cold viruses are spread through the air, from sneezing and coughing—we've known that for years. But what's now being shown is that cold viruses are often spread through hand-to-hand contact. For example, if you handle a phone or a glass that has been used by somebody with a cold, your chances of catching a cold rise sharply.

Colds often start slowly with that little tickle in the back of the throat. Within a few hours, your eyes begin to water, and you start sneezing and feeling congested. Within a day or two, you may develop a dry, hacking cough.

Treatment The diagnosis of a cold is not difficult. Doctors look at the season and the symptoms and prescribe accordingly. Although there's no cure for the cold, a variety of medicines can help you feel better while you're recovering.

Antihistamines, which are fre- quently used to relieve allergy symptoms, can help cold sufferers feel better by drying up the excess amounts of mucus that a cold produces. Decongestants shrink swollen blood vessels in the nose and the sinuses, thus clearing the passages to make breathing easier. Antihistamines and decongestants are also found in combination form. All three types of products are available over the counter, with somewhat stronger formulations available by prescription (see the drug charts on pages 589–591).

Analgesics, or pain-killers, such as aspirin or acetaminophen, can help you feel better during a cold by relieving fever, headache, and muscular pain. To help you cough up mucus or to quiet the cough so that you can get a good night's sleep, a cough suppressant may be prescribed (see the drug charts on pages 610–623).

Some over-the-counter pills for colds combine all these ingredients, serving as a kind of shotgun approach to cold symptoms.

Outlook Since time immemorial, people with colds have been told to stay warm, take it easy, and drink plenty of fluids. Fruit juices and hot drinks like tea and soups thin the mucus, making breathing easier. Studies have shown that chicken soup, which was called *Bubbiemycetin* by the *New England Journal of Medicine*, actually does make people feel better. The therapeutic benefit of chicken soup has been attributed to a combination of the steam, the liquid, the protein content, and maybe a little love.

Simple colds are self-limiting, and people usually feel better within a few days. However, a cold can sometimes develop into a more serious problem, such as acute sinusitis or acute bronchitis.

ACUTE SINUSITIS

The sinuses are nothing but trouble. No one knows their exact function, and we only notice them when they become infected.

Technically, the sinuses are hollow spaces in the bones of the face. There are four pairs of sinuses around the nose and eyes, all of which connect to the nasal passages by a narrow duct. Both the duct and the sinus cavities are lined with cilia, tiny little hairlike filaments that sweep mucus, as well as particles of dirt and bacteria, out of the nose and down the throat, finally to be destroyed in the stomach.

Trouble starts when a cold virus seemingly paralyzes the cilia. Mucus and bacteria accumulate in the sinuses, causing infection. As the cold runs its course, the trapped mucus causes pressure and facial pain, as well as headache, especially when a person bends over. Coming in the middle of a bad cold, such symptoms are a good sign of acute sinus infection. However, since they also signal an allergy, or even a dental infection, it may be necessary for the doctor to confirm the diagnosis by taking X rays of the face from different angles. Normally, the sinus bones appear hollow and empty on an X ray, but if there's an infection, an accumulation of mucus and fluid will make the sinuses seem filled and solid.

Treatment If your symptoms and X rays all point to acute sinusitis, antibiotics and decongestants are called for. Antibiotics, such as tetracycline and penicillin (see the drug charts on pages 591–595 and 599–603), given for ten days to two weeks, are necessary to knock out the bacterial infection. Your doctor may recommend that you take a decongestant to help drain the nasal passages (see section on colds). He or she may also suggest that you take an over-the-counter analgesic such as aspirin (see the drug chart on pages 628–629), acetaminophen, or ibuprofen (see the drug chart on pages 629–630) to relieve sinus headache.

Outlook Most of the symptoms of even a bad sinus infection can be cleared up within a week. If acute sinusitis is not taken care of, you can develop chronic sinusitis that reappears over months or even years.

ACUTE BRONCHITIS

While most colds clear up within a week, some can develop into bronchitis—an inflammation of the bronchi, or air tubes, in the lungs. The hallmarks of bronchitis are an exhausting cough and fever. Usually, the cough produces thick, yellowish mucus, but many people can have a dry, hacking cough. Bronchitis can also follow a bout of influenza. Your doctor will usually rely on your description of your symptoms and a physical exam to make the diagnosis of bronchitis, though he or she may order a chest X ray to rule out pneumonia.

Treatment Although the cough of bronchitis is annoying and exhausting, doctors are reluctant to give medicine simply to still the cough reflex. The cough is an automatic reflex that helps the body clear airways of secretions and obstructions. Generally, coughs are divided into two types—productive coughs that bring up mucus and nonproductive, or dry, coughs.

Productive coughs should not be discouraged, inasmuch as bringing up mucus helps clear infection. Dry coughs should actually be made more productive to help rid the body of bacteria-laden phlegm. Expectorant drugs are sometimes prescribed to do just this—loosen mucus, though there is no evidence that these drugs actually work. If a cough is keeping you awake at night, your doctor may prescribe a cough suppressant (see the drug charts on pages 610–623). These products often contain codeine, which acts by blocking the nerve signals in the brain that trigger the cough reflex.

Outlook With proper medicine, acute bronchitis due to influenza or a bad cold should clear up within ten days to two weeks. However, if you suffer from chronic bronchitis and are a smoker, you may take longer to recover from the acute infection.

INFLUENZA

Each winter, along with snow, New Year's Eve, and football, comes the flu. The influenza season starts in late November and continues until March. During these months, up to 60 percent of people develop cough, high fever, and body ache, the classic trio of flu symptoms.

Influenza is not hard to diagnose. The symptoms, the season, and a physical exam will usually give the doctor the information he or she needs.

Prevention In most cases, flu means about a week of discomfort and time lost from work and other activities. But if you're over sixty-five, especially if you have a chronic health problem such as chronic lung disease, asthma, heart disease, or diabetes, the flu can develop into a serious form of pneumonia. Individuals with sarcoidosis or those who have recently undergone an organ transplant or are being treated for cancer by drug therapy are at risk as well.

Thus, with influenza, the best offense is a good defense. Medical authorities, such as the American College of Physicians, the Centers for Disease Control, and the American Geriatric Society, strongly recommend an annual flu vaccination (see the drug chart on pages 625–627) to protect against the current flu virus.

Unlike vaccinations for such other common viral diseases as measles or chickenpox, where a single shot confers long-lasting protection, flu shots must be given each year. The flu virus changes slightly from year to year, so the immunity you have against one type may not protect you against another.

The best time for the shot is in the early fall to allow the body to build up enough immunity in time for the flu season. The shots are safe and up to 80 percent protective in older people. Even in those cases where flu does develop, it is usually far milder than if you hadn't been immunized at all.

Treatment If the flu does strike, bed rest, aspirin or acetaminophen (see the drug charts on pages 628–629), fluids and the appropriate cough medicine (see the drug charts on pages 610–623) will relieve symptoms until the disease runs its course. Unless bronchitis or pneumonia develops, there is usually no need for antibiotics.

In addition to these time-honored flu remedies, there is a drug that relieves symptoms and speeds recovery from some strains of influenza. Called amantadine, this medicine works by interfering with the replication and growth of the flu virus (see the drug chart on page 628). To be effective, amantadine must be given twenty-four to forty-eight hours after the onset of flu symptoms. The added benefit of amantadine is that it lessens the spread of disease to friends and family.

Short-lived side effects of amantadine are usually limited to insomnia and light-headedness. This drug also can be given to prevent influenza during an epidemic, but must be taken for four to six weeks to confer protection. Frequently, it is given to people with chronic illnesses as well as to older residents of nursing homes and hospitals to boost vaccination immunity.

Outlook The acute stages of influenza usually last a week to ten days. It may take another week to feel fully well and energetic. If the flu symptoms persist, or actually worsen after a week, it's a good idea to check with your doctor.

PNEUMOCOCCAL PNEUMONIA

While a variety of bacteria can cause pneumonia, most cases are due to a tiny organism called the pneumococcus. Each year, more than half a million people develop pneumococcal pneumonia, and nearly half of them are over the age of sixty.

Prevention Fortunately, there is a safe and effective vaccine that can protect adults against pneumococcal pneumonia (see the drug chart on pages 623–625). Only one shot of the vaccine is needed to confer permanent immunity.

Treatment If pneumococcal pneumonia does occur, its hallmark is severe chest pain in combination with fever; a dry, hacking cough; headache; and body ache. If a person who has had influenza or a cold develops these symptoms, a doctor might well suspect pneumonia and do further tests to confirm the diagnosis. He or she may look for the pneumococcus bacteria in the sputum that the person coughs up and do a chest X ray as well.

People with pneumococcal pneumonia are usually hospitalized and treated with antibiotics to reduce infection and with strong analgesics to relieve the chest pain. In addition, doctors can prescribe oxygen to help breathing and intravenous fluids to guard against dehydration.

VIRAL PNEUMONIA

Viral pneumonia is less serious than pneumococcal pneumonia but is still an important health problem during the winter months. It often begins with coldlike symptoms of sore throat, sneezing, and nasal congestion but soon develops into chest pains and a bad cough. By listening to the chest with a stethoscope the doctor can hear the characteristic rumbles called *rales* that are typical of pneumonia.

Treatment Bed rest, fluids, and a cough suppressant (see the drug charts on pages 610–623) are usually all that's required for recovery. Some doctors prescribe antibiotics (see the drug charts on pages 591–610) to prevent secondary infections such as bronchitis or bacterial pneumonia.

CONDITION: **RESPIRATORY INFECTIONS**

CATEGORY: **ANTIHISTAMINES AND ANTIHISTAMINE-DECONGESTANT COMBINATIONS**

GENERIC (CHEMICAL) NAME	BRAND (TRADE) NAME	DOSAGE FORMS AND STRENGTHS
Azatadine maleate	OPTIMINE	Tablets: 1 mg
Clemastine fumarate	TAVIST	Syrup: 0.67 mg per tsp Tablets: 1.34, 2.68 mg
Dexchlorpheniramine maleate	POLARAMINE	Controlled-release tablets: 4, 6 mg Syrup: 2 mg per tsp Tablets: 2 mg
Diphenhydramine hydrochloride	BENADRYL	Capsules: 25, 50 mg Elixir: 12.5 mg per tsp
Hydroxyzine	ATARAX VISTARIL	Syrup: 10 mg per tsp Tablets: 10, 25, 50, 100 mg Capsules: 25, 50, 100 mg Suspension: 25 mg per tsp
Promethazine hydrochloride	PHENERGAN	Rectal suppositories: 12.5, 25, 50 mg Syrup: 6.25, 25 mg per tsp Tablets: 12.5, 25, 50 mg
Tripelennamine hydrochloride	PBZ	Elixir: tripelennamine citrate equivalent to 25 mg tripelennamine hydrochloride per tsp Tablets: 25, 50 mg

	PBZ-SR	Controlled-release tablets: 100 mg
Phenylpropanolamine hydrochloride and chlorpheniramine maleate	DEHIST	Controlled-release capsules: 75 mg phenylpropanolamine hydrochloride and 8 mg chlorpheniramine maleate

Many brands of antihistamines and antihistamine-decongestant combinations are sold over the counter as well.

DRUG PROFILE

When you are exposed to a substance to which you are allergic, a chemical called histamine is released into the bloodstream and produces the itchy, watery eyes; runny nose; and rashes that are typical of an allergic reaction. Antihistamines work by blocking the action of histamine. They are used to treat allergies as well as to relieve the symptoms of a cold. Antihistamines are sometimes combined in the same preparation with a decongestant, such as phenylpropanolamine. Phenyl-propanolamine is thought to work by constricting blood vessels in the respiratory tract, shrinking the swollen membranes so that you are less congested and can breathe more easily. Hydroxyzine is also used to treat anxiety. Exactly how it works to relieve anxiety is not completely understood.

For complete information on these drugs, see pages 633–638.

CONDITION: **RESPIRATORY INFECTIONS**

CATEGORY: **ANTIHISTAMINES**

GENERIC (CHEMICAL) NAME	BRAND (TRADE) NAME	DOSAGE FORMS AND STRENGTHS
Terfenadine	SELDANE	Tablets: 60 mg

DRUG PROFILE

When you are exposed to a substance to which you are allergic, a chemical called histamine is released into the bloodstream and produces the itchy, watery eyes; runny nose; and rashes that are typical of an allergic reaction. Terfenadine, an antihistamine, blocks the action of histamine and is used to treat the symptoms of allergies, especially such seasonal allergies as hay fever.

For complete information on this drug, see pages 638–641.

CONDITION: **RESPIRATORY INFECTIONS**

CATEGORY: **ANTIBIOTICS (TETRACYCLINES)**

GENERIC (CHEMICAL) NAME	BRAND (TRADE) NAME	DOSAGE FORMS AND STRENGTHS
Demeclocycline hydrochloride	DECLOMYCIN	Capsules: 150 mg Tablets: 150, 300 mg
Doxycycline	VIBRAMYCIN	Capsules: 50, 100 mg Suspension: 25 mg per tsp Syrup: 50 mg per tsp
	VIBRATABS VIVOX	Tablets: 100 mg Capsules: 50, 100 mg Tablets: 100 mg
Methacycline hydrochloride	RONDOMYCIN	Capsules: 150, 300 mg
Minocycline	MINOCIN	Capsules: 50,100 mg Suspension: 50 mg per tsp Tablets: 50, 100 mg
Oxytetracycline	TERRAMYCIN	Capsules: 250 mg

Tetracycline hydrochloride	ACHROMYCIN V	Capsules: 250, 500 mg Suspension: 125 mg per tsp
	PANMYCIN	Capsules: 250 mg
	ROBITET	Capsules: 250, 500 mg
	SUMYCIN	Capsules: 250, 500 mg Syrup: 125 mg per tsp Tablets: 250, 500 mg

This type of drug is available under other brand names as well.

DRUG PROFILE

Tetracyclines are antibiotics that are used to treat a wide variety of bacterial infections, including skin eruptions and bronchitis and pneumonia. These antibiotics suppress the growth of the bacteria by interfering with their manufacture of protein.

BEFORE USING THIS DRUG

Let your doctor know *IF*

You have ever had any allergic reactions or other problems with ■ any tetracyclines.

You have ever had any of the following medical problems: ■ liver disease ■ kidney disease ■ diabetes ■ systemic lupus erythematosus ■ pancreas disease ■ myasthenia gravis ■ asthma, allergies, or hay fever.

You are taking any of the following medicines: ■ antacids ■ calcium supplements ■ iron supplements ■ any medicine containing magnesium, aluminum, or zinc ■ baking soda ■ penicillin ■ anticoagulants (blood thinners) ■ medicine for diarrhea ■ medicine to make the urine less acidic ■ methotrexate (medicine for cancer and severe psoriasis).

SPECIAL RESTRICTIONS WHILE TAKING THIS DRUG

FOOD AND DRUG INTERACTIONS

Other Drugs	Antacids containing calcium or magnesium; calcium, zinc, and iron supplements; and antidiarrheal preparations interfere with the absorption of this drug.

Allow one to three hours between the time you take tetracycline and the time you take any of these substances.

Foods and Beverages	Some food (especially certain dairy products) interferes with the absorption of this drug. To avoid this interaction, it is best to take this drug on an empty stomach, at least one hour before or two hours after meals. This does not apply to doxycycline or minocycline.

No special restrictions on alcohol use or smoking.

DAILY LIVING

Driving	Minocycline may cause dizziness and drowsiness. If you are taking minocycline, be careful when driving, operating household appliances, or doing any other tasks that require alertness until you know how this drug affects you.
Sun Exposure	You are more likely to get a sunburn while taking this medicine. Therefore, it is a good idea to avoid too much sun while you are taking this medicine. If you feel a tingling or burning sensation on your hands, feet, or nose or any other unusual reaction after being exposed to the sun, let your doctor know right away.
Examinations or Tests	It is important for you to keep all appointments with your doctor, even if you feel well, so that your progress can be checked. If you are on long-term tetracycline therapy, periodic blood and urine tests are usually required.
Other Precautions	Tell any doctor or dentist you consult that you are taking this drug, especially if you will be undergoing any type of surgery.

This drug causes tooth staining if given to children younger than fourteen.

Helpful Hints

This drug should be taken with a full glass of water.

If this drug upsets your stomach, ask your doctor if it may be taken with food.

No special restrictions on exposure to excessive heat or cold.

POSSIBLE SIDE EFFECTS

Although this list of adverse effects may seem somewhat intimidating, keep in mind that some are quite rare. Of course, should these or any other problems arise while you are on medication, it is always a good idea to consult your doctor.

IF YOU DEVELOP

fever ■ severe diarrhea ■ difficulty in breathing ■ headache ■ joint pain ■ loose or discolored nails ■ worsening of any skin cuts ■ tingling and burning of hands, feet, or nose (after sun exposure) ■ tongue inflammation or discoloration ■ sore throat ■ hoarseness

With democycline only: increased urination ■ extreme thirst ■ extreme fatigue or weakness

WHAT TO DO

May be serious Check with your doctor as soon as possible.

---

cramps ■ diarrhea ■ bulky, loose stools ■ loss of appetite ■ gas ■ indigestion ■ difficulty in swallowing ■ rash, hives, or itching ■ nausea or vomiting ■ change in skin color ■ skin flushing ■ vaginal discharge ■ itching or swelling in the rectal or genital area ■ increased skin sensitivity to sunlight

With minocycline only: light-headedness or dizziness ■ drowsiness ■ tiredness ■ clumsiness

If symptoms are disturbing or persist, let your doctor know.

STORAGE INSTRUCTIONS

Store in a cool, dark place (not in a bathroom medicine cabinet). If your medicine is in a liquid form, make sure that it does not freeze. If the color, appearance, or taste of the medicine changes, or if the expiration date has passed, discard it immediately. If you are uncertain whether your medicine is all right, consult your pharmacist or doctor.

STOPPING OR INTERRUPTING THERAPY

Tetracyclines should be taken without interruption for the full length of time prescribed by your doctor even if you begin to feel better. This will ensure that the infection clears up completely and that your symptoms don't return. If after several days of therapy, your symptoms either do not improve or worsen, contact your doctor. If you miss a dose, take it as soon as possible. If it is almost time for your next dose, space the next two doses half the time apart they would usually be (for instance, if you were taking two doses a day twelve hours apart, space the missed dose and the next dose five to six hours apart).

SPECIAL CONSIDERATIONS FOR THOSE OVER SIXTY-FIVE

None.

CONDITION: **RESPIRATORY INFECTIONS**

CATEGORY: **ANTIBIOTICS (ERYTHROMYCINS)**

GENERIC (CHEMICAL) NAME	BRAND (TRADE) NAME	DOSAGE FORMS AND STRENGTHS
Erythromycin	E-MYCIN ERYC ERY-TAB	Tablets: 250, 333 mg Capsules: 125, 250 mg Tablets: 250, 333, 500 mg
Erythromycin estolate	ILOSONE	Capsules: 125, 250 mg Chewable tablets: 125, 250 mg Drops: 100 mg per ml Suspension: 125, 250 mg per tsp Tablets: 500 mg

Erythromycin ethylsuccinate	E.E.S.	Chewable tablets: 200 mg Drops: 100 mg per 2.5 ml Suspension: 200, 400 mg per tsp Suspension granules: 200 mg per tsp Tablets: 400 mg
	E-MYCIN E	Suspension: 200, 400 mg per tsp
	WYAMYCIN E	Suspension: 200, 400 mg per tsp
Erythromycin stearate	ERYTHROCIN Stearate WYAMYCIN S	Tablets: 250, 500 mg Tablets: 250, 500 mg

This type of drug is available under other brand names as well.

DRUG PROFILE

Erythromcycins are antibiotics that are used to treat a variety of bacterial infections, including such respiratory tract infections as bronchitis and pneumonia. These drugs suppress the growth of the bacteria and keep them from multiplying by blocking the bacteria's ability to manufacture protein.

BEFORE USING THIS DRUG

Let your doctor know *IF*

You have ever had allergic reactions or other problems with ■ any erythromycins.

You have ever had the following medical problem: ■ liver disease.

You are taking any of the following medicines: ■ other antibiotics ■ theophylline (medicine for asthma) ■ carbamazepine (medicine for seizures) ■ anticoagulants (blood thinners) ■ corticosteroids ■ digoxin, digitoxin, or digitalis (heart medicines).

SPECIAL RESTRICTIONS WHILE TAKING THIS DRUG

FOOD AND DRUG INTERACTIONS

No special restrictions on other drugs, foods and beverages, alcohol use, or smoking.

DAILY LIVING

Examinations or Tests	It is important for you to keep all appointments with your doctor, even if you feel well, so that your progress can be checked.
Other Precautions	While you are taking this drug, you may develop fungal infections of the mouth, anus, or vagina. Let your doctor know if you develop itching, burning, soreness, or general irritation in the anal or vaginal area; a white vaginal discharge; or a white coating on the inside of your mouth.
Helpful Hints	This drug is best taken with a full glass of water on an empty stomach unless otherwise directed by your doctor.
	Chewable tablets should be chewed or crushed before swallowing; do not swallow them whole. Capsules or coated tablets should be swallowed whole.

No special restrictions on driving, exertion and exercise, sun exposure, or exposure to excessive heat or cold.

POSSIBLE SIDE EFFECTS

Although this list of adverse effects may seem somewhat intimidating, keep in mind that some are quite rare. Of course, should these or any other problems arise while you are on medication, it is always a good idea to consult your doctor.

IF YOU DEVELOP	WHAT TO DO
severe stomach pain or cramps ■ dark urine ■ pale stools ■ extreme tiredness or weakness ■ yellowing of eyes or skin ■ vomiting, with blood ■ bloody stools	**Urgent** Get in touch with your doctor immediately.
hearing loss	**May be serious** Check with your doctor as soon as possible.
diarrhea ■ nausea or vomiting ■ upset stomach ■ heartburn ■ loss of appetite ■ sore mouth or tongue ■ rash, hives, or itching ■ itching in the vaginal or anal area	If symptoms are disturbing or persist, let your doctor know.

STORAGE INSTRUCTIONS

Store in a cool, dark place (not in a bathroom medicine cabinet). If your medicine is in a liquid form, make sure that it does not freeze.

STOPPING OR INTERRUPTING THERAPY

Erythromycins should be taken without interruption for the full length of time prescribed by your doctor, even if you begin to feel better. This will ensure that the infection clears up completely and that your symptoms do not return. If you miss a dose, take it as soon as possible and resume your regular schedule. If it is almost time for your next dose, double that next dose.

SPECIAL CONSIDERATIONS FOR THOSE OVER SIXTY-FIVE

None.

CONDITION:　**RESPIRATORY INFECTIONS**

CATEGORY:　**ANTIBIOTICS (PENICILLINS)**

GENERIC (CHEMICAL) NAME	BRAND (TRADE) NAME	DOSAGE FORMS AND STRENGTHS
Amoxicillin	AMOXIL	Capsules: 250, 500 mg Chewable tablets: 125, 250 mg Suspension: 125, 250 mg per tsp
	LAROTID	Capsules: 250, 500 mg Suspension: 125, 250 mg per tsp
	POLYMOX	Capsules: 250, 500 mg Suspension: 125, 250 mg per tsp
	TRIMOX	Capsules: 250, 500 mg Suspension: 125, 250 mg per tsp
Ampicillin	AMCILL	Capsules: 250, 500 mg Suspension: 125, 250 mg per tsp
	OMNIPEN	Capsules: 250, 500 mg Suspension: 125, 250 mg per tsp
	POLYCILLIN	Capsules: 250, 500 mg Suspension: 125, 250, 500 mg per tsp
	SK-AMPICILLIN	Capsules: 250, 500 mg Suspension: 125, 250 mg per tsp
	TOTACILLIN	Capsules: 250, 500 mg Suspension: 125, 250 mg per tsp

Bacampicillin hydrochloride	SPECTROBID	Suspension: 125 mg per tsp Tablets: 400 mg
Carbenicillin indanyl sodium	GEOCILLIN	Tablets: 382 mg
Cloxacillin sodium	TEGOPEN	Capsules: 250, 500 mg Solution: 125 mg per tsp
Cyclacillin	CYCLAPEN-W	Suspension: 125, 250 mg per tsp Tablets: 250, 500 mg
Nafcillin sodium	UNIPEN	Capsules: 250 mg Solution: 250 mg per tsp Tablets: 500 mg
Oxacillin sodium	PROSTAPHLIN	Capsules: 250, 500 mg Solution: 250 mg per tsp
Penicillin G potassium	PENTIDS	Tablets: 200,000, 400,000 units
Penicillin V potassium	LEDERCILLIN VK	Solution: 125, 250 mg per tsp Tablets: 250, 500 mg
	PEN•VEE•K	Solution: 125, 250 mg per tsp Tablets: 250, 500 mg
	V-CILLIN K	Solution: 125, 250 mg per tsp Tablets: 125, 250, 500 mg

This type of drug is available under other brand names as well.

DRUG PROFILE

Penicillins are antibiotics that are used to treat a wide variety of bacterial infections, including infections of the ear, nose, and throat and such respiratory tract infections as bronchitis and pneumonia. Penicillins suppress the growth of bacteria by interfering with the bacteria's ability to form new protective cell walls.

BEFORE USING THIS DRUG

Let your doctor know *IF*

You have ever had allergic reactions or other problems with ■ any penicillins ■ procaine (an anesthetic or heart drug) ■ cephalosporins or griseofulvin (antibiotics) ■ penicillamine (medicine for arthritis) ■ tartrazine (FD&C Yellow Dye No. 5) ■ aspirin ■ any other medicine.

You have ever had any of the following medical problems: ■ any allergy ■ bleeding problems ■ kidney disease ■ liver disease ■ stomach or intestinal problems.

You are taking any of the following medicines: ■ any other medicine for infection (antibiotics) ■ medicine for gout ■ medicine for arthritis ■ medicine for seizures ■ anticoagulants (blood thinners) ■ Antabuse (used in treatment of alcoholism) ■ aspirin or aspirinlike medicine ■ triamterene, spironolactone, or amiloride (potassium-sparing diuretics) ■ medicine for high cholesterol ■ medicine for diarrhea.

SPECIAL RESTRICTIONS WHILE TAKING THIS DRUG

FOOD AND DRUG INTERACTIONS

Other Drugs	If you need to take medicine for diarrhea, check with your doctor. Penicillin, when taken with medicine for diarrhea, may make the diarrhea more severe. If you are taking the drug colestipol for high cholesterol, take your dose of penicillin at least one hour before or four hours after your dose of colestipol.
Foods and Beverages	If you are taking penicillin G, do not drink any acidic juices (e.g., orange, grapefruit, tomato) for at least an hour before and after you take your medicine. Such juices may reduce the effect of this type of penicillin.

No special restrictions on alcohol use or smoking.

DAILY LIVING

Examinations or Tests	It is important for you to keep all appointments with your doctor, even if you feel well, so that your progress can be checked. If you are on long-term penicillin therapy, periodic blood and urine tests may be required.
Other Precautions	Tell any doctor or dentist you consult that you are taking this drug, especially if you will be undergoing any type of surgery.

People with diabetes may find that this drug causes false results in urine-sugar tests. Check with your doctor to see if you need another kind of diabetes medicine or if you should use a different kind of test.

While you are taking this drug, you may develop fungal infections of the mouth, anus, or vagina. Let your doctor know if you develop itching, burning, soreness, or general irritation in the anal or vaginal area; a white vaginal discharge; or a white coating on the inside of your mouth. |
| Helpful Hints | This drug is best taken with a full glass of water on an empty stomach unless otherwise directed by your doctor.

Chewable tablets should be chewed or crushed before swallowing; do not swallow them whole. |

No special restrictions on driving, exertion and exercise, sun exposure, or exposure to excessive heat or cold.

POSSIBLE SIDE EFFECTS

Although this list of adverse effects may seem somewhat intimidating, keep in mind that some are quite rare. Of course, should these or any other problems arise while you are on medication, it is always a good idea to consult your doctor.

IF YOU DEVELOP	WHAT TO DO
difficulty in breathing ■ fever or chills ■ severe dizziness or fainting ■ tightness in throat ■ severe stomach cramps ■ severe diarrhea ■ rash or hives ■ purplish or brownish-red spots on skin ■ extreme tiredness or weakness ■ seizures ■ bleeding or bruising ■ extreme thirst ■ blood in urine or other urine changes ■ difficulty in urination ■ swelling of face or ankles ■ yellowing of eyes or skin ■ pale stools ■ bluish tinge to the skin ■ severe nausea and vomiting ■ excessive sweating	**Urgent** Get in touch with your doctor immediately.
itching ■ general feeling of unwellness ■ bone or muscle pain ■ swollen lymph glands ■ rapid weight loss	**May be serious** Check with your doctor as soon as possible.
mild diarrhea or loose stools ■ gas ■ nausea or vomiting ■ upset stomach ■ sore mouth ■ sore tongue or black, hairy tongue ■ stomach cramps ■ headache ■ dizziness	If symptoms are disturbing or persist, let your doctor know.

STORAGE INSTRUCTIONS

Store in a cool, dark place (not in a bathroom medicine cabinet). If your medicine is in a liquid form, make sure that it does not freeze.

STOPPING OR INTERRUPTING THERAPY

Penicillins should be taken without interruption for the full length of time prescribed by your doctor, even if you begin to feel better. This will ensure that the infection clears up completely and that your symptoms do not return. If you miss a dose, take it as soon as possible and resume your regular schedule. If it is almost time for your next dose, double that next dose.

SPECIAL CONSIDERATIONS FOR THOSE OVER SIXTY-FIVE

Older people may be more prone to developing diarrhea while taking amoxicillin, ampicillin, bacampicillin, and cyclacillin.

CONDITION: **RESPIRATORY INFECTIONS**

CATEGORY: **ANTIBIOTICS (CEPHALOSPORINS)**

GENERIC (CHEMICAL) NAME	BRAND (TRADE) NAME	DOSAGE FORMS AND STRENGTHS
Cefaclor	CECLOR	Capsules: 250, 500 mg Suspension: 125, 250 mg per tsp
Cefadroxil	DURICEF	Capsules: 500 mg Suspension: 125, 250, 500 mg per tsp Tablets: 1 g
	ULTRACEF	Capsules: 500 mg Suspension: 125, 250 mg per tsp Tablets: 1 g
Cephalexin	KEFLEX	Capsules: 250, 500 mg Suspension: 125, 250 mg per tsp Tablets: 1 g
Cephradine	ANSPOR	Capsules: 250, 500 mg Suspension: 125, 250 mg per tsp
	VELOSEF	Capsules: 250, 500 mg Suspension: 125, 250 mg per tsp

This type of drug is available under other brand names as well.

DRUG PROFILE

Cephalosporins are antibiotics that are used to treat a wide variety of bacterial infections, including such upper respiratory tract infections as bronchitis and pneumonia. These drugs work by interfering with the bacteria's ability to multiply and to form new protective cell walls.

BEFORE USING THIS DRUG

Let your doctor know *IF*

You have ever had any allergic reactions or other problems with ■ any cephalosporins ■ any penicillins ■ any other antibiotics ■ penicillamine (medicine for arthritis) ■ any other medicine.

You have ever had any of the following medical problems: ■ stomach or intestinal problems, especially colitis ■ kidney disease ■ liver disease ■ bleeding disorders.

You are taking any of the following medicines: ■ medicine for diarrhea ■ probenicid (medicine for gout) ■ any medicine containing alcohol ■ anticoagulants (blood thinners) ■ any other antibiotics.

SPECIAL RESTRICTIONS WHILE TAKING THIS DRUG

FOOD AND DRUG INTERACTIONS

Other Drugs	If you need to take medicine for diarrhea, check with your doctor. Cephalosporins, when taken with medicine for diarrhea, may make the diarrhea more severe.
Alcohol	Avoid alcohol while on cephalosporin therapy. The combination of alcohol and a cephalosporin may cause flushing, headache, shortness of breath, nausea, vomiting, dizziness, fainting, chest pain, and irregular or fast heartbeat.

No special restrictions on foods and beverages or smoking.

DAILY LIVING

Examinations or Tests	It is important for you to keep all appointments with your doctor, even if you feel well, so that your progress can be checked.
Other Precautions	People with diabetes may find that this drug causes false results in urine-sugar tests. Check with your doctor to see if you need another kind of diabetes medicine or if you should use a different kind of test. While you are taking this drug, you may develop fungal infections of the mouth, anus, or vagina. Let your doctor know if you develop itching, burning, soreness, or general irritation in the anal or vaginal area; a white vaginal discharge; or a white coating on the inside of your mouth.
Helpful Hints	If this medicine causes upset stomach, taking it with milk, meals, or snacks should help.

No special restrictions on driving, exertion and exercise, sun exposure, or exposure to excessive heat or cold.

POSSIBLE SIDE EFFECTS

Although this list of adverse effects may seem somewhat intimidating, keep in mind that some are quite rare. Of course, should these or any other problems arise while you are on medication, it is always a good idea to consult your doctor.

IF YOU DEVELOP

severe stomach cramps ■ severe diarrhea ■ fever or chills ■ extreme weakness or fatigue ■ excessive thirst ■ swelling in any part of the body

WHAT TO DO

Urgent Get in touch with your doctor immediately.

joint pain ■ rapid weight loss ■ difficulty in urination or defecation	**May be serious** Check with your doctor as soon as possible.
mild diarrhea ■ upset stomach ■ nausea or vomiting ■ stomach pain ■ sore mouth or tongue ■ heartburn ■ skin redness, rash, hives, itching, or other skin problems	If symptoms are disturbing or persist, let your doctor know.

STORAGE INSTRUCTIONS

Store in a cool, dark place (not in a bathroom medicine cabinet). If your medicine is in a liquid form, make sure that it does not freeze.

STOPPING OR INTERRUPTING THERAPY

Cephalosporins should be taken without interruption for the full length of time prescribed by your doctor, even if you begin to feel better. This will ensure that the infection clears up completely and that your symptoms don't return. If you miss a dose, take it as soon as possible and resume your regular schedule. If it is almost time for your next dose, double that next dose.

SPECIAL CONSIDERATIONS FOR THOSE OVER SIXTY-FIVE

Because this drug is metabolized by the kidneys, and kidney function commonly decreases with age, doctors may start people over sixty-five on a lower dosage.

CONDITION: **RESPIRATORY INFECTIONS**

CATEGORY: **OTHER ANTIBIOTICS**

GENERIC (CHEMICAL) NAME	BRAND (TRADE) NAME	DOSAGE FORMS AND STRENGTHS
Clindamycin hydrochloride	CLEOCIN HCl	Capsules: 75, 150 mg

DRUG PROFILE

Clindamycin is used to treat bacterial infections, including such infections of the respiratory tract as strep throat and pneumonia. This drug suppresses the growth of bacteria and keeps them from multiplying by blocking the bacteria's ability to manufacture cell protein.

BEFORE USING THIS DRUG

Let your doctor know *IF*

You have ever had allergic reactions or other problems with ■ clindamycin ■ lincomycin ■ tartrazine (FD&C Yellow Dye No. 5) ■ aspirin.

You have ever had any of the following medical problems: ■ kidney disease ■ liver disease ■ stomach or intestinal problems ■ myasthenia gravis.

You are taking any of the following medicines: ■ other antibiotics ■ medicine for diarrhea ■ narcotics or other prescription pain-killers.

SPECIAL RESTRICTIONS WHILE TAKING THIS DRUG

FOOD AND DRUG INTERACTIONS

Other Drugs	If you need to take medicine for diarrhea, check with your doctor. Clindamycin, when taken with medicine for diarrhea, may make the diarrhea more severe.

No special restrictions on foods and beverages, alcohol use, or smoking.

DAILY LIVING

Examinations or Tests	It is important for you to keep all appointments with your doctor, even if you feel well, so that your progress can be checked. If you are on long-term therapy or if you have liver or kidney disease, periodic blood and urine tests may be required.

Other Precautions	Tell any doctor or dentist you consult that you are taking this drug, especially if you will be undergoing any type of surgery.
	While you are taking this drug, you may develop fungal infections of the mouth, anus, or vagina. Let your doctor know if you develop itching, burning, soreness, or general irritation in the anal or vaginal area; a white vaginal discharge; or a white coating on the inside of your mouth.
Helpful Hints	Take this medicine with a full glass of water to avoid irritating the esophagus.

No special restrictions on driving, exertion and exercise, or exposure to excessive heat or cold.

POSSIBLE SIDE EFFECTS

Although this list of adverse effects may seem somewhat intimidating, keep in mind that some are quite rare. Of course, should these or any other problems arise while you are on medication, it is always a good idea to consult your doctor.

IF YOU DEVELOP	WHAT TO DO
stomach pain or cramps ■ severe diarrhea ■ severe nausea and vomiting ■ fever ■ extreme thirst ■ extreme weakness	**Urgent** Get in touch with your doctor immediately.
rapid weight loss ■ joint pain ■ difficulty in urination or defecation ■ loss of appetite	**May be serious** Check with your doctor as soon as possible.
diarrhea ■ gas or bloating ■ rash or itching ■ itching in genital or anal area	If symptoms are disturbing or persist, let your doctor know.

STORAGE INSTRUCTIONS

Store in a cool, dark place (not in a bathroom medicine cabinet).

STOPPING OR INTERRUPTING THERAPY

Clindamycin should be taken without interruption for the full length of time prescribed by your doctor, even if you begin to feel better. This will ensure that the infection clears up completely and that your symptoms do not return. If you miss a dose, take it as soon as possible and resume your regular schedule. If it is almost time to take your next dose, double that next dose.

SPECIAL CONSIDERATIONS FOR THOSE OVER SIXTY-FIVE

Older people who are very ill can be particularly susceptible to such side effects of clindamycin as diarrhea.

CONDITION: **COUGH**

CATEGORY: **COUGH SUPPRESSANTS**

GENERIC (CHEMICAL) NAME	BRAND (TRADE) NAME	DOSAGE FORMS AND STRENGTHS
Benzonatate	TESSALON	Capsules: 100 mg

DRUG PROFILE

Benzonatate is used to treat the dry cough associated with acute infections including the common cold, bronchitis, and pneumonia, as well as such chronic conditions as emphysema, bronchial asthma, and tuberculosis. This drug works by inhibiting the cough reflex, both in the brain center that stimulates coughing and in the nerves of the respiratory tract.

BEFORE USING THIS DRUG

Let your doctor know *IF*

You have ever had allergic reactions or other problems with ■ benzonatate.

You are taking any of the following medicines: ■ any local anesthetics.

SPECIAL RESTRICTIONS WHILE TAKING THIS DRUG

FOOD AND DRUG INTERACTIONS

No special restrictions on other drugs, foods and beverages, alcohol use, or smoking.

DAILY LIVING

Examinations or Tests	It is important for you to keep all appointments with your doctor so that your progress can be checked.
Helpful Hints	Swallow the capsules whole. They contain an anesthetic that could make your mouth temporarily numb if you chew or crush them.

No special restrictions on driving, exertion and exercise, sun exposure, or exposure to excessive heat or cold.

POSSIBLE SIDE EFFECTS

Although this list of adverse effects may seem somewhat intimidating, keep in mind that some are quite rare. Of course, should these or any other problems arise while you are on medication, it is always a good idea to consult your doctor.

IF YOU DEVELOP	WHAT TO DO
convulsions ■ restlessness ■ tremors	**Urgent** Get in touch with your doctor immediately.
numbness in chest	**May be serious** Check with your doctor as soon as possible.
headache ■ drowsiness ■ dizziness ■ rash or itching ■ stuffy nose ■ constipation ■ upset stomach ■ nausea ■ eye irritation ■ chills	If symptoms are disturbing or persist, let your doctor know.

STORAGE INSTRUCTIONS

Store in a cool, dark place (not in a bathroom medicine cabinet).

STOPPING OR INTERRUPTING THERAPY

Benzonatate should be taken without interruption for the full length of time prescribed by your doctor. If you miss a dose, take it as soon as possible. If it is almost time for your next dose, skip the missed dose and resume your regular schedule. Do not take two doses at the same time.

SPECIAL CONSIDERATIONS FOR THOSE OVER SIXTY-FIVE

None.

CONDITION: **COUGH**

CATEGORY: **COUGH SUPPRESSANTS**

GENERIC (CHEMICAL) NAME	BRAND (TRADE) NAME	DOSAGE FORMS AND STRENGTHS
Hydrocodone bitartrate and homatropine methylbromide	HYCODAN	Syrup: 5 mg hydrocodone bitartrate and 1.5 mg homatropine methylbromide per tsp Tablets: 5 mg hydrocodone bitartrate and 1.5 mg homatropine methylbromide

DRUG PROFILE

This combination drug is used to treat coughs. Hydrocodone inhibits the cough reflex in the brain center that stimulates coughing, dries the membranes of the respiratory tract, and thins out the mucus in the respiratory tract so that it can be coughed up more easily. Homatropine also has a drying effect on the respiratory tract.

BEFORE USING THIS DRUG

Let your doctor know *IF*

You have ever had allergic reactions or other problems with ■ hydrocodone ■ homatropine ■ atropine ■ belladonna.

You have ever had any of the following medical problems: ■ head injury ■ seizures ■ asthma or other lung disease ■ enlarged prostate ■ urinary problems ■ glaucoma ■ kidney disease ■ liver disease ■ abnormal heart rhythms ■ alcoholism ■ colitis or other intestinal problems ■ underactive thyroid ■ gallbladder disease.

You are taking any of the following medicines: ■ medicine for glaucoma ■ antihistamines ■ medicine for seizures ■ barbiturates ■ muscle relaxants ■ tranquilizers ■ sleep medicines ■ medicine for depression ■ narcotics or other prescription pain-killers ■ cimetidine (medicine for ulcers).

SPECIAL RESTRICTIONS WHILE TAKING THIS DRUG

FOOD AND DRUG INTERACTIONS

Other Drugs	Do not take any other drugs, including over-the-counter (OTC) drugs, before checking with your doctor. This medicine increases the effect of drugs that depress the central nervous system, such as antihistamines; medicine for hay fever, allergies, or colds; sleep medicines; tranquilizers; narcotics or other prescription pain-killers; muscle relaxants; and medicine for seizures.
Alcohol	This drug increases the effect of alcohol, a central nervous system depressant. Avoid alcohol unless your doctor has approved its use.

No special restrictions on foods and beverages or smoking.

DAILY LIVING

Driving	This drug may cause drowsiness, light-headedness, or dizziness, as well as loss of alertness and coordination. Be careful when driving, operating household appliances, or doing any other tasks that require alertness until you know how this drug affects you.
Examinations or Tests	It is important for you to keep all appointments with your doctor so that your progress can be checked.
Other Precautions	Tell any doctor or dentist you consult that you are taking this drug, especially if you will be undergoing any type of surgery.
	Taking this medicine more often or for a longer period of time than prescribed by your doctor may make it habit forming. If you accidentally take an overdose of this medicine, call your doctor or go to an emergency room immediately.
Helpful Hints	You may vomit or feel nauseated when you first start taking this drug. If this happens, lie down until you feel better. You also may experience dizziness or light-headedness, especially when getting up from a reclining or sitting position. Getting up slowly may help prevent this.

No special restrictions on exertion and exercise, sun exposure, or exposure to excessive heat or cold.

POSSIBLE SIDE EFFECTS

Although this list of adverse effects may seem somewhat intimidating, keep in mind that some are quite rare. Of course, should these or any other problems arise while you are on medication, it is always a good idea to consult your doctor.

IF YOU DEVELOP

difficulty in breathing ■ severe dizziness ■ severe drowsiness ■ blurred vision or other visual disturbances ■ agitation ■ delirium ■ extreme restlessness or nervousness ■ slow heartbeat ■ severe weakness ■ seizures ■ confusion ■ hallucinations ■ swelling of face

WHAT TO DO

Urgent Get in touch with your doctor immediately.

---

eye pain ■ rash, hives, or itching ■ depression ■ sleeplessness ■ faintness ■ ringing in the ears ■ fast heartbeat ■ shallow breathing ■ stomach pain

May be serious Check with your doctor as soon as possible.

---

dizziness or light-headedness, especially when getting up from a reclining or sitting position ■ constipation ■ drowsiness ■ nausea or vomiting ■ flushing or warm feeling ■ sexual problems ■ difficulty in urination or decreased urination ■ increased sweating ■ dry mouth

If symptoms are disturbing or perist, let your doctor know.

STORAGE INSTRUCTIONS

Store in a cool, dark place (not in a bathroom medicine cabinet). If your medicine is in a liquid form, make sure that it does not freeze.

STOPPING OR INTERRUPTING THERAPY

If you have been taking this medicine for three weeks or more, do not abruptly stop taking it; you must cut down on your dosage gradually in order to avoid the side effects that occur when this drug is abruptly stopped. Your doctor will advise you on how to reduce your dosage gradually. If you miss a dose, take it as soon as possible. If it is almost time for your next dose, skip the missed dose and resume your regular schedule. Do not take two doses at the same time.

SPECIAL CONSIDERATIONS FOR THOSE OVER SIXTY-FIVE

Older people may be more susceptible to such side effects of this medicine as breathing problems, confusion, agitation, or drowsiness.

CONDITION: **COUGH**

CATEGORY: **COUGH SUPPRESSANTS**

GENERIC (CHEMICAL) NAME	BRAND (TRADE) NAME	DOSAGE FORMS AND STRENGTHS
Hydrocodone and phenyltoloxamine	TUSSIONEX	Capsules: 5 mg hydrocodone and 10 mg phenyltoloxamine Suspension: 5 mg hydrocodone and 10 mg phenyltoloxamine per tsp Tablets: 5 mg hydrocodone and 10 mg phenyltoloxamine

DRUG PROFILE

This combination drug is used to treat the cough associated with acute infections, including the common cold, bronchitis, and pneumonia, as well as such chronic conditions as emphysema, bronchial asthma, and tuberculosis. Hydrocodone inhibits the cough reflex in the brain center that stimulates coughing, while phenyltoloxamine, an antihistamine, dries out the mucous secretions in the lungs and provides a mild sedative effect.

BEFORE USING THIS DRUG

Let your doctor know *IF*

You have ever had any allergic reactions or other problems with ■ hydrocodone ■ any antihistamines.

You have ever had any of the following medical problems: ■ head injury ■ seizures ■ asthma or other lung disease ■ enlarged prostate ■ urinary problems ■ glaucoma ■ kidney disease ■ liver disease ■ abnormal heart rhythms ■ high blood pressure ■ overactive thyroid ■ alcoholism ■ colitis or other intestinal problems ■ gallbladder disease.

You are taking any of the following medicines: ■ medicine for glaucoma ■ antihista-mines ■ medicine for hay fever, allergies, or colds ■ medicine for seizures ■ barbiturates ■ muscle relaxants ■ tranquilizers ■ sleep medicines ■ medicine for depression ■ narcotics or other prescription pain-killers ■ cimetidine (medi-cine for ulcers) ■ appetite suppressants ■ medicine for cancer ■ medicine for abnormal heart rhythms ■ medicine for high blood pressure.

SPECIAL RESTRICTIONS WHILE TAKING THIS DRUG

FOOD AND DRUG INTERACTIONS

Other Drugs	Do not take any other drugs, including over-the-counter (OTC) drugs, before checking with your doctor. This medicine increases the effect of drugs that depress the central nervous system, such as antihis-tamines; medicine for hay fever, allergies, or colds; sleep medicines; tranquilizers; narcotics or other pre-scription pain-killers; muscle relaxants; and medi-cines for seizures.
Alcohol	This drug increases the effect of alcohol, a central nervous system depressant. Avoid alcohol unless your doctor has approved its use.

No special restrictions on foods and beverages or smoking.

DAILY LIVING

Driving	This drug may cause drowsiness, light-headedness, or dizziness, as well as loss of alertness and coordi-nation. Be careful when driving, operating household appliances, or doing any other tasks that require alertness until you know how this drug affects you.
Examinations or Tests	It is important for you to keep all appointments with your doctor so that your progress can be checked.

Other Precautions	Tell any doctor or dentist you consult that you are taking this medicine, especially if you will be undergoing any type of surgery.
	Taking this medicine more often or for a longer period of time than prescribed by your doctor may make it habit forming. If you accidentally take an overdose of this medicine, call your doctor or go to an emergency room immediately.

Helpful Hints	You may vomit or feel nauseated when you first start taking this medicine. If this happens, lie down until you feel better. You may also experience dizziness or light-headedness, especially when getting up from a reclining or sitting position. Getting up slowly will help prevent this.

No special restrictions on exertion and exercise, sun exposure, or exposure to excessive heat or cold.

POSSIBLE SIDE EFFECTS

Although this list of adverse effects may seem somewhat intimidating, keep in mind that some are quite rare. Of course, should these or any other problems arise while you are on medication, it is always a good idea to consult your doctor.

IF YOU DEVELOP

difficulty in breathing ■ severe dizziness ■ severe drowsiness ■ blurred vision or other visual disturbances ■ extreme restlessness or nervousness ■ delirium ■ slow heartbeat ■ severe weakness ■ seizures ■ clammy skin ■ unsteadiness or clumsiness ■ hallucinations ■ dilated pupils ■ confusion ■ difficulty in speech ■ difficulty in swallowing ■ irritability ■ tremors ■ tightness in chest

WHAT TO DO

Urgent Get in touch with your doctor immediately.

facial itching ■ rash, hives, or itching ■ depression ■ sleeplessness ■ faintness ■ irregular or fast heartbeat ■ sore throat or fever ■ bleeding or bruising ■ tiredness

May be serious Check with your doctor as soon as possible.

dizziness or light-headedness, especially when getting up from a reclining or sitting position ■ constipation ■ drowsiness ■ nausea or vomiting ■ flushing or warm feeling ■ male impotence ■ difficulty in urination ■ decreased urination ■ increased sweating ■ thickened phlegm ■ dry or stuffy nose ■ increased skin sensitivity to sunlight ■ nightmares ■ loss of appetite ■ upset stomach ■ diarrhea ■ chills ■ ringing in the ears or other hearing problems

If symptoms are disturbing or persist, let your doctor know.

STORAGE INSTRUCTIONS

Store in a cool, dark place (not in a bathroom medicine cabinet). If your medicine is in a liquid form, make sure that it does not freeze.

STOPPING OR INTERRUPTING THERAPY

If you have been taking this medicine for three weeks or more, do not abruptly stop taking it; you must cut down on your dosage gradually in order to avoid the side effects that occur when this drug is abruptly stopped. Your doctor will advise you on how to reduce your dosage gradually. If you miss a dose, take it as soon as possible. If it is almost time for your next dose, skip the missed dose and resume your regular schedule. Do not take two doses at the same time.

SPECIAL CONSIDERATIONS FOR THOSE OVER SIXTY-FIVE

Because older people are more sensitive to the effects of this drug, as well as less able to metabolize it, doctors may start people over sixty-five on a lower dosage.

CONDITION: **COUGH**

CATEGORY: **COUGH SUPPRESSANTS**

GENERIC (CHEMICAL) NAME	BRAND (TRADE) NAME	DOSAGE FORMS AND STRENGTHS
Codeine		Tablets: 15, 30, 60 mg
Codeine with terpin hydrate	SK-TERPIN HYDRATE AND CODEINE	Elixir: 85 mg terpin hydrate and 10 mg codeine per tsp

DRUG PROFILE

Codeine is prescribed to relieve a cough associated with colds, influenza, or hay fever. It suppresses coughing by acting directly on the cough center of the brain. Terpin hydrate is an expectorant, which means that it loosens and helps you get rid of mucus in your airways.

BEFORE USING THIS DRUG

Let your doctor know *IF*

You have ever had allergic reactions or other problems with ■ codeine ■ terpin hydrate ■ any prescription pain-killers.

You have ever had any of the following medical problems: ■ head injury ■ brain disease ■ stomach or intestinal problems ■ seizures ■ asthma or other lung disease ■ enlarged prostate ■ urinary problems ■ heart disease ■ kidney disease ■ liver disease ■ underactive thyroid.

You are taking any of the following medicines: ■ antibiotics ■ anticoagulants (blood thinners) ■ barbiturates ■ antihistamines ■ medicine for hay fever, coughs, or colds ■ diuretics or other high blood pressure medicine ■ medicine for abnormal heart rhythms ■ medicine for depression ■ bromocriptine or other medicine for Parkinson's disease ■ medicine for diarrhea, stomach spasms, or cramps ■ metoclopramide (medicine for nausea and vomiting) ■ muscle relaxants ■ naltrexone (medicine for opiate abuse) ■ narcotics or other prescription pain-killers ■ medicine for seizures ■ sleep medicines ■ tranquilizers.

SPECIAL RESTRICTIONS WHILE TAKING THIS DRUG

FOOD AND DRUG INTERACTIONS

Other Drugs	Do not take any other drugs, including over-the-counter (OTC) drugs, before checking with your doctor. This drug increases the effect of drugs that depress the central nervous system, such as antihistamines; medicine for hay fever, allergies, or colds; sleep medicines; tranquilizers; narcotics or other prescription pain-killers; muscle relaxants; and medicine for seizures.
Alcohol	This drug increases the effect of alcohol, a central nervous system depressant. Avoid alcohol while taking this drug.

No special restrictions on foods and beverages or smoking.

DAILY LIVING

Driving	This drug may cause drowsiness, light-headedness, or dizziness as well as loss of alertness and coordination. Be careful when driving, operating household appliances, or doing any other tasks that require alertness until you know how this drug affects you.
Examinations or Tests	It is important for you to keep all appointments with your doctor so that your progress can be checked.
Other Precautions	Tell any doctor or dentist you consult that you are taking this drug, especially if you will be undergoing any type of surgery.

Taking this medicine more often or for a longer period of time than prescribed by your doctor may make it |

habit forming. If you have been taking this medicine for a few weeks and you think that it is no longer working as well as it did before, do not increase your dose, but check with your doctor.

If you continue to have a cough for more than seven days or you have a high fever, rash, headache, or sore throat with your cough, let your doctor know.

Helpful Hints

You may vomit or feel nauseated when you first start taking this medicine. If this happens, lie down until you feel better. You may also experience dizziness or light-headedness, especially when getting up from a reclining or sitting position. Getting up slowly will help prevent this.

To help loosen mucus in the lungs, drink a glass of water with each dose of this medicine.

No special restrictions on exertion and exercise, sun exposure, or exposure to excessive heat or cold.

POSSIBLE SIDE EFFECTS

Although this list of adverse effects may seem somewhat intimidating, keep in mind that some are quite rare. Of course, should these or any other problems arise while you are on medication, it is always a good idea to consult your doctor.

IF YOU DEVELOP

seizures ■ severe dizziness ■ severe drowsiness ■ difficulty in breathing ■ severe weakness ■ extreme restlessness or nervousness ■ low blood pressure ■ slow heart rate ■ cold, clammy skin ■ severe confusion

WHAT TO DO

Urgent Get in touch with your doctor immediately.

confusion ■ hallucinations ■ depression ■ "high" feeling or other mood change ■ irregular or fast heartbeat ■ rash, hives, or itching ■ swelling of

May be serious Get in touch with your doctor as soon as possible.

face ■ ringing or buzzing in ears ■ shortness of breath ■ jerky movements, twitching, or tremors

dizziness or light-headedness, especially when getting up from a reclining or sitting position ■ drowsiness ■ constipation ■ nausea or vomiting

If symptoms are disturbing or persist, let your doctor know.

STORAGE INSTRUCTIONS

Store in a cool, dark place (not in a bathroom medicine cabinet). If your medicine is in a liquid form, make sure that it does not freeze.

STOPPING OR INTERRUPTING THERAPY

If you have been taking this medicine for several weeks or more, do not abruptly stop taking it; you must cut down on your dosage gradually in order to avoid the side effects that occur when this drug is abruptly stopped. Your doctor will advise you on how to reduce your dosage gradually. If you are taking this medicine according to a regular schedule and you miss a dose, take it as soon as possible. If it is almost time for your next dose, skip the missed dose and resume your regular schedule. Do not take two doses at the same time.

SPECIAL CONSIDERATIONS FOR THOSE OVER SIXTY-FIVE

Older people may be more susceptible to such side effects of this medicine as breathing problems.

CONDITION: **PNEUMOCOCCAL PNEUMONIA**

CATEGORY: **VACCINES**

GENERIC (CHEMICAL) NAME	BRAND (TRADE) NAME	DOSAGE FORMS AND STRENGTHS
Pneumococcal vaccine	PNEUMOVAX 23 PNU-IMUNE 23	Injection: 25 μg Injection: 25 μg

DRUG PROFILE

This vaccine is given to prevent pneumococcal pneumonia. It is often recommended for people over the age of sixty-five and for people who have chronic illnesses or are undergoing cancer chemotherapy. Other people who may face a higher risk of pneumonia include those who live in closed groups in which infection can easily spread (such as nursing homes) or in communities experiencing a pneumonia epidemic. The vaccine consists of extract from the pneumonia bacteria, which, when injected, causes the body to form antibodies against pneumonia.

BEFORE USING THIS DRUG

Let your doctor know *IF*

You have ever had any of the following medical problems: ■ Hodgkin's disease (cancer of the lymph nodes) ■ heart disease ■ lung disease ■ infection of the respiratory tract, including pneumonia ■ recent fever ■ any recent infection.

You are taking any of the following medicines: ■ medicine for cancer.

You have recently been given a flu vaccine.

You have ever been given a vaccine for pneumonia.

SPECIAL RESTRICTIONS WHILE TAKING THIS DRUG

FOOD AND DRUG INTERACTIONS

No special restrictions on other drugs, foods and beverages, alcohol use, or smoking.

DAILY LIVING

Examinations or Tests	If you have a serious heart or lung condition, your doctor may want to check you regularly after you receive this vaccine.
Other Precautions	You may experience redness, soreness, swelling, or formation of a hard spot at the site of injection. This should disappear in a few days.

No special restrictions on driving, exertion and exercise, sun exposure, or exposure to excessive heat or cold.

POSSIBLE SIDE EFFECTS

Although this list of adverse effects may seem somewhat intimidating, keep in mind that some are quite rare. Of course, should these or any other problems arise while you are on medication, it is always a good idea to consult your doctor.

IF YOU DEVELOP	WHAT TO DO
wheezing or difficulty in breathing ■ faintness ■ skin eruptions ■ fast heartbeat	**Urgent** Get in touch with your doctor immediately.
fever ■ redness, soreness, swelling, or formation of a hard spot at the injection site ■ weakness ■ muscle or joint pain ■ headache ■ increased eye sensitivity to light ■ chills ■ nausea ■ rash	If symptoms are disturbing or persist, let your doctor know.

SPECIAL CONSIDERATIONS FOR THOSE OVER SIXTY-FIVE

None.

CONDITION: **INFLUENZA**

CATEGORY: **VACCINES**

GENERIC (CHEMICAL) NAME	BRAND (TRADE) NAME	DOSAGE FORMS AND STRENGTHS
Influenza virus vaccine	INFLUENZA VIRUS VACCINE, TRIVALENT	Injection: 15 μg
	FLUOGEN	Injection: 15 μg
	FLUOGEN-A	Injection: 15 μg
	FLUZONE	Injection: 15 μg
	FLUZONE-A	Injection: 15 μg

DRUG PROFILE

This vaccine is given to prevent influenza, or flu. It is often recommended for people over the age of sixty-five, for heavy smokers, and for people with such medical problems as certain types of heart conditions, lung disease, or kidney disease. It is also often recommended for people who live in closed groups in which infection can easily spread (such as people in nursing homes), or for those who come into contact with many unvaccinated people (such as those in a public health or service job).

BEFORE USING THIS DRUG

Let your doctor know *IF*

You have ever had allergic reactions or other problems with ■ chicken or chicken eggs.

You have ever had any of the following medical problems: ■ Guillain-Barré syndrome ■ any nerve disorder ■ heart disease ■ lung disease ■ infection of the respiratory tract ■ blood vessel disease ■ cancer ■ recent fever ■ any recent infection.

You are taking any of the following medicines: ■ anticoagulants (blood thinners) ■ theophylline (medicine for asthma) ■ medicine for cancer ■ corticosteroids ■ medicine for seizures.

You have recently been given any other vaccine.

SPECIAL RESTRICTIONS WHILE TAKING THIS DRUG

FOOD AND DRUG INTERACTIONS

No special restrictions on other drugs, foods and beverages, alcohol use, or smoking.

DAILY LIVING

Examinations or Tests	If you have a serious heart or lung condition, your doctor may want to check you regularly after you receive this vaccine.

Other Precautions

You may experience soreness, redness, or formation of a hard spot at the site of injection. This should disappear in a few days.

No special restrictions on driving, exertion and exercise, sun exposure, or exposure to excessive heat or cold.

POSSIBLE SIDE EFFECTS

Although this list of adverse effects may seem somewhat intimidating, keep in mind that some are quite rare. Of course, should these or any other problems arise while you are on medication, it is always a good idea to consult your doctor.

IF YOU DEVELOP	WHAT TO DO
difficulty in breathing ■ rash or hives	**Urgent** Get in touch with your doctor immediately.
fever ■ redness, soreness, swelling, or formation of a hard spot at the injection site ■ general feeling of unwellness ■ headache ■ muscle or joint pain	If symptoms are disturbing or persist, let your doctor know.

SPECIAL CONSIDERATIONS FOR THOSE OVER SIXTY-FIVE

None.

CONDITION: **INFLUENZA**

CATEGORY: **ANTIVIRAL AGENTS**

GENERIC (CHEMICAL) NAME	BRAND (TRADE) NAME	DOSAGE FORMS AND STRENGTHS
Amantadine hydrochloride	SYMMETREL	Capsules: 100 mg Syrup: 50 mg per tsp

DRUG PROFILE

Amantadine is used to treat Parkinson's disease and other movement disorders. Many experts think that the rigidity, shaking, and walking disturbances associated with these conditions result from a deficiency of a chemical called dopamine in the brain. Amantadine makes more dopamine available to the brain, thereby helping restore the chemical balance that regulates the nervous system. This drug is sometimes used along with levodopa or other antiparkinson medicine. Amantadine is also used to treat influenza. It works by interfering with the ability of the influenza virus to multiply.

For complete information on this drug, see pages 252–255.

CONDITION: **RESPIRATORY INFECTIONS**

CATEGORY: **ANALGESICS**

GENERIC (CHEMICAL) NAME	BRAND (TRADE) NAME	DOSAGE FORMS AND STRENGTHS
Aspirin and other salicylate drugs		

Aspirin and other salicylate drugs are available over the counter under a variety of brand names, dosage forms, and strengths. Some of these preparations have a special coating to help protect the lining of the stomach against possible irritation. Because of the importance of salicylate drugs in the treatment of chronic pain, even though they are most often nonprescription drugs, they are included in this book for reader reference.

For complete information on this drug, see pages 379-383.

DRUG PROFILE

Aspirin and other drugs in the salicylate family are used to relieve pain, inflammation, and fever. Large doses are used to treat symptoms of arthritis and rheumatism such as swelling, stiffness, and joint pain. Aspirin and other salicylates are thought to control pain and swelling by blocking the production of naturally occurring triggers of pain and inflammation, called prostaglandins. These drugs also relieve fever by changing the way the body regulates its temperature.

CONDITION: **RESPIRATORY INFECTIONS**

CATEGORY: **ANALGESICS**

GENERIC (CHEMICAL) NAME	BRAND (TRADE) NAME	DOSAGE FORMS AND STRENGTHS
Acetaminophen	Regular Strength ANACIN-3	Caplets: 500 mg Tablets: 325 mg
	Maximum Strength ANACIN-3	Capsules: 500 mg Tablets: 500 mg
	Aspirin-free ARTHRITIS PAIN FORMULA	Tablets: 500 mg
	Extra Strength DATRIL	Capsules: 500 mg Tablets: 500 mg
	PANADOL	Capsules: 500 mg Tablets: 500 mg
	Maximum Strength ST. JOSEPH Aspirin-Free	Tablets: 500 mg

Regular Strength TYLENOL	Caplets: 325 mg Tablets: 325 mg
Extra-Strength TYLENOL	Caplets: 500 mg Liquid: 500 mg per tbsp Tablets: 500 mg

DRUG PROFILE

Acetaminophen is used to relieve fever and pain. It is thought to work by blocking pain centers in the central nervous system and by resetting the body's thermostat to its normal temperature.

For complete information on this drug, see pages 383–386.

CONDITION: **RESPIRATORY INFECTIONS**

CATEGORY: **ANALGESICS**

GENERIC (CHEMICAL) NAME	BRAND (TRADE) NAME	DOSAGE FORMS AND STRENGTHS
Ibuprofen	ADVIL (OTC) MOTRIN	Tablets: 200 mg Tablets: 300, 400, 600, 800 mg
	NUPRIN (OTC) RUFEN	Tablets: 200 mg Tablets: 400, 600, 800 mg

DRUG PROFILE

Nonsteroidal anti-inflammatory drugs, or NSAIDs, help relieve swelling, stiffness, joint pain, and inflammation in the long-term treatment of arthritis. These drugs are thought to act by blocking the production of naturally occurring pain and inflammation triggers called prostaglandins.

For complete information on this drug, see pages 433–438.

ALLERGIC RHINITIS

If you think you've got a cold that just won't quit—complete with drippy nose, teary eyes, and nonstop sneezing, you might actually be suffering from a condition known as allergic rhinitis. This means that an abnormal sensitivity reaction, an allergy, has caused the mucous membranes lining your nose to become inflamed. The symptoms are very much like those of a cold, but colds generally run their course in a week or so, while allergic symptoms hang on for several weeks or even months. Another difference is that the sore throat, fever, and muscle aches that often accompany a cold are not part of an allergy attack.

The tendency to have allergies is genetic, passed from parent to child. An allergy generally appears for the first time during adolescence, but it can begin earlier or later, striking people of any age. While more than fifteen million Americans have allergies of one kind or another, about six million have allergic rhinitis, meaning that the reaction is confined to the nose.

CAUSES

An allergic reaction occurs when the body mistakes a harmless substance like pollen or animal dander for an invader, or antigen, and mounts a defense against it. The body defends itself by producing antibodies, which are designed to neutralize the antigen. The antigen and antibody lock together in combat. In response to the binding of the antigen and antibody, a chemical called histamine is released, which causes the swelling and itching.

The substance that most often sets off an episode of allergic rhinitis is pollen, from trees or grass in the spring and from ragweed in the late summer or early fall. Ragweed allergy is sometimes referred to as hay fever. The tiny mites that float in house dust, the microscopic flakes of dry skin shed into the air by household pets, or the mold spores spewed into the atmosphere by air-conditioning systems are a few of the other substances that can also set off allergy attacks. A person who is sensitive to one substance can subsequently become sensitive to others.

TREATMENT

Preventing an allergy attack by avoiding the allergen is the best strategy. If you're allergic to animal fur, for example, it's not hard to figure out how to stay away from it (though if you're an animal lover, you might not want to). People allergic to pollens should stay indoors as much as possible, with windows closed and air-conditioners running, during their allergy seasons. Their rooms should be cleaned regularly; bedrooms, especially, should be free of knickknacks, books, and other dust collectors. (This also applies to people who are allergic to house dust.) Down comforters are not for people allergic to feathers, nor is a cashmere sweater ideal for the individual whose nose tickles at the mere mention of wool.

But you can't completely avoid your allergens, so if your allergic reaction is troublesome enough, you will probably need some medicine to relieve your symptoms. The kinds of drugs generally used for allergy include antihistamines and decongestants. Another group of potent drugs, the corticosteroids, block the allergic response and reduce inflammation. Further information on all these medicines can be found in the drug charts on pages 641–642. A relatively new prescription drug used to treat chronic allergies is cromolyn sodium (brand names, Intal and Nasalcrom).

OUTLOOK

Medical therapy generally provides relief to sufferers of allergic rhinitis. But in some cases, no medicines seem to do the job, or their side effects prove worse than the dripping and sneezing of an allergic attack. Your doctor may then refer you to an allergist, who can do skin tests to determine the precise sources of your symptoms and, if your condition is severe enough, administer a series of allergy shots to desensitize your system.

CONDITION: **ALLERGIC RHINITIS**

CATEGORY: **ANTIHISTAMINES AND ANTIHISTAMINE-DECONGESTANT COMBINATIONS**

GENERIC (CHEMICAL) NAME	BRAND (TRADE) NAME	DOSAGE FORMS AND STRENGTHS
Azatadine maleate	OPTIMINE	Tablets: 1 mg
Clemastine fumarate	TAVIST	Syrup: 0.67 mg per tsp Tablets: 1.34, 2.68 mg
Dexchlorpheniramine maleate	POLARAMINE	Controlled-release tablets: 4, 6 mg Syrup: 2 mg per tsp Tablets: 2 mg
Diphenhydramine hydrochloride	BENADRYL	Capsules: 25, 50 mg Elixir: 12.5 mg per tsp
Hydroxyzine	ATARAX VISTARIL	Syrup: 10 mg per tsp Tablets: 10, 25, 50, 100 mg Capsules: 25, 50, 100 mg Suspension: 25 mg per tsp
Promethazine hydrochloride	PHENERGAN	Rectal suppositories: 12.5, 25, 50 mg Syrup: 6.25, 25 mg per tsp Tablets: 12.5, 25, 50 mg

Tripelennamine hydrochloride	PBZ	Elixir: tripelennamine citrate equivalent to 25 mg tripelennamine hydrochloride per tsp Tablets: 25, 50 mg
	PBZ-SR	Controlled-release tablets: 100 mg
Phenylpropanolamine hydrochloride and chlorpheniramine maleate	DEHIST	Controlled-release capsules: 75 mg phenylpropanolamine hydrochloride and 8 mg chlorpheniramine maleate

Many brands of antihistamines and antihistamine-decongestant combinations are sold over the counter as well.

DRUG PROFILE

When you are exposed to a substance to which you are allergic, a chemical called histamine is released into the bloodstream and produces the itchy, watery eyes; runny nose; and rashes that are typical of an allergic reaction. Antihistamines work by blocking the action of histamine. They are used to treat allergies as well as to relieve the symptoms of a cold. Antihistamines are sometimes combined in the same preparation with a decongestant, such as phenylpropanolamine. Phenylpropanolamine is thought to work by constricting blood vessels in the respiratory tract, shrinking the swollen membranes so that you are less congested and can breathe more easily. Hydroxyzine is also used to treat anxiety. Exactly how it works to relieve anxiety is not completely understood.

BEFORE USING THIS DRUG

Let your doctor know *IF*

You have ever had allergic reactions or other problems with ■ any antihistamines or decongestants ■ amphetamines ■ medicine for asthma.

You have ever had any of the following medical problems: ■ asthma or other lung disease ■ enlarged prostate ■ urinary problems or difficulty in urination ■ glaucoma ■ epilepsy or other seizure disorders ■ high blood pressure ■ overactive thyroid.

■ *with medicine containing a decongestant only:* ■ diabetes ■ ulcers.

You are taking any of the following medicines: ■ any other antihistamines ■ medicine for Parkinson's disease ■ medicine for seizures ■ aspirin or aspirinlike medicine ■ medicine for arthritis ■ medicine for cancer ■ antibiotics ■ digoxin, digitoxin, or digitalis (heart medicines) ■ medicine for abnormal heart rhythms ■ barbiturates ■ muscle relaxants ■ medicine for hay fever, coughs, or colds ■ narcotic or other prescription pain-killers ■ sleep medicines ■ tranquilizers ■ medicine for depression ■ medicine for high blood pressure ■ appetite suppressants ■ medicine for asthma.

SPECIAL RESTRICTIONS WHILE TAKING THIS DRUG

FOOD AND DRUG INTERACTIONS

Other Drugs	Do not take any other drugs, including over-the-counter (OTC) drugs, before checking with your doctor. This medicine increases the effect of drugs that depress the central nervous system, such as other antihistamines; medicine for hay fever, allergies, or colds; sleep medicines; tranquilizers; narcotics or other prescription pain-killers; muscle relaxants; and medicine for seizures. Antihistamines may mask ringing in the ears caused by aspirin. Let your doctor know if you are taking aspirin or aspirinlike medicine.
Alcohol	Antihistamines increase the effect of alcohol, a central nervous system depressant. Avoid alcohol unless your doctor has approved its use.

No special restrictions on foods and beverages or smoking.

DAILY LIVING

Driving	This drug may cause dizziness, drowsiness, weakness, or blurred vision. Be careful when driving, operating household appliances, or doing any other tasks that require alertness until you know how this drug affects you.
Other Precautions	Tell any doctor or dentist you consult that you are taking this drug, especially if you will be undergoing any type of surgery.
	If you are going to be tested for allergies, tell the doctor in charge that you are taking this drug, since it affects the results of allergy tests.
Helpful Hints	If this drug upsets your stomach, taking it with food, milk, or water should help.
	If your mouth or throat feels dry, chewing sugarless gum or sucking ice chips or sugarless hard candy will help.
	This drug may sometimes cause insomnia, which can be avoided by taking your last dose several hours before bedtime; check with your doctor about the best dosing schedule for you.
	If you have been storing the suppository form of this medicine, it may be too soft to use. Put it in the refrigerator for half an hour or run cold water over the wrapped suppository before use.

No special restrictions on exertion and exercise, sun exposure, or exposure to excessive heat or cold.

POSSIBLE SIDE EFFECTS

Although this list of adverse effects may seem somewhat intimidating, keep in mind that some are quite rare. Of course, should these or any other problems arise while you are on medication, it is always a good idea to consult your doctor.

IF YOU DEVELOP	WHAT TO DO
seizures ■ unsteadiness or clumsiness ■ severe drowsiness ■ fainting ■ flushing ■ hallucinations ■ difficulty in breathing ■ dilated pupils ■ sleeplessness ■ confusion ■ difficulty in speech ■ difficulty in swallowing ■ nervousness or restlessness ■ irritability ■ excitement or other mood changes ■ muscle weakness ■ tremors ■ tightness of chest ■ irregular or fast heartbeat	**Urgent** Get in touch with your doctor immediately.
sore throat or fever ■ bleeding or bruising ■ tiredness	**May be serious** Check with your doctor as soon as possible.
drowsiness ■ dizziness ■ thickening phlegm ■ blurred or double vision or other visual disturbances ■ pain or difficulty in urination ■ urinary frequency ■ dry mouth or throat ■ dry or stuffy nose ■ increased skin sensitivity to sunlight ■ nightmares ■ rash ■ loss of appetite ■ upset stomach ■ constipation ■ diarrhea ■ nausea or vomiting ■ male impotence ■ chills ■ increased sweating ■ ringing in the ears or other hearing problems	If symptoms are disturbing or persist, let your doctor know.

With phenylpropanolamine only: headache

STORAGE INSTRUCTIONS

Store in a cool, dark place (not in a bathroom medicine cabinet). If your medicine is in a liquid form, make sure that it does not freeze. Suppositories should be stored in the refrigerator.

STOPPING OR INTERRUPTING THERAPY

This drug should be taken without interruption for the full length of time prescribed by your doctor. If you miss a dose, take it as soon as possible. If it is almost time for your next dose, skip the missed dose and resume your regular schedule. Do not take two doses at the same time.

SPECIAL CONSIDERATIONS FOR THOSE OVER SIXTY-FIVE

Older people taking this drug may be more prone to develop confusion, difficulty in urination, dizziness, drowsiness, fainting, visual disturbances, fever, or dry mouth. Nightmares, restlessness, and irritability are also more apt to occur in those over sixty-five.

CONDITION: **ALLERGIC RHINITIS**

CATEGORY: **ANTIHISTAMINES**

GENERIC (CHEMICAL) NAME	BRAND (TRADE) NAME	DOSAGE FORMS AND STRENGTHS
Terfenadine	SELDANE	Tablets: 60 mg

DRUG PROFILE

When you are exposed to a substance to which you are allergic, a chemical called histamine is released into the bloodstream and produces the itchy, watery eyes; runny nose; and rashes that are typical of an allergic reaction. Terfenadine, an antihistamine, blocks the action of histamine and is used to treat the symptoms of allergies, especially such seasonal allergies as hay fever.

BEFORE USING THIS DRUG

Let your doctor know *IF*

You have ever had allergic reactions or other problems with ■ any antihistamines.

You have ever had any of the following medical problems: ■ asthma or other lung disease ■ enlarged prostate ■ glaucoma ■ urinary problems or difficulty in urination.

You are taking any of the following medicines: ■ any other antihistamines ■ antibiotics ■ medicine for Parkinson's disease ■ medicine for stomach spasms or cramps ■ medicine for arthritis ■ aspirin or aspirinlike medicine ■ medicine for cancer ■ medicine for high blood pressure ■ medicine for abnormal heart rhythms ■ tranquilizers ■ medicine for depression ■ medicine for seizures ■ narcotics or other prescription pain-killers ■ sleep medicines ■ medicine for hay fever, coughs, or colds ■ metyrosine (medicine for adrenal gland tumor) ■ muscle relaxants ■ paromomycin (medicine for amebic infection).

SPECIAL RESTRICTIONS WHILE TAKING THIS DRUG

FOOD AND DRUG INTERACTIONS

Other Drugs	Do not take any other drugs, including over-the-counter (OTC) drugs, before checking with your doctor. This medicine may increase the effect of drugs that depress the central nervous system, such as other antihistamines; medicine for hay fever, allergies, or colds; sleep medicines; tranquilizers, narcotics or other prescription pain-killers; muscle relaxants; and medicine for seizures. However, such problems occur to a lesser extent with this antihistamine than with other antihistamines.
	Antihistamines may mask ringing in the ears caused by aspirin. Let your doctor know if you are taking aspirin or apirinlike medicine.
Alcohol	This drug increases the effect of alcohol, a central nervous system depressant. Avoid alcohol unless your doctor has approved its use.

No special restrictions on foods and beverages or smoking.

DAILY LIVING

Driving	Although this drug rarely causes drowsiness, antihistamines may cause dizziness, drowsiness, weakness,

or blurred vision in some individuals. Be careful when driving, operating household appliances, or doing any other tasks that require alertness until you know how this drug affects you.

Other Precautions	Tell any doctor or dentist you consult that you are taking this medicine, especially if you will be undergoing any type of surgery.
	If you are going to be tested for allergies, tell the doctor in charge that you are taking this drug, since it affects the results of allergy tests.
Helpful Hints	If this drug upsets your stomach, taking it with food, milk, or water should help.

No special restrictions on exertion and exercise, sun exposure, or exposure to excessive heat or cold.

POSSIBLE SIDE EFFECTS

Although this list of adverse effects may seem somewhat intimidating, keep in mind that some are quite rare. Of course, should these or any other problems arise while you are on medication, it is always a good idea to consult your doctor.

IF YOU DEVELOP	WHAT TO DO
seizures ■ unsteadiness or clumsiness ■ severe drowsiness ■ fainting ■ flushing ■ hallucinations ■ confusion ■ difficulty in breathing ■ sleeplessness	**Urgent** Get in touch with your doctor immediately.
sore throat or fever ■ bleeding or bruising ■ tiredness ■ excitement ■ nervousness or restlessness ■ irritability	**May be serious** Check with your doctor as soon as possible.

blurred vision or other visual disturbances ■ pain or difficulty in urination ■ dizziness ■ dry mouth or throat ■ dry or stuffy nose ■ increased skin sensitivity to sunlight ■ loss of appetite ■ nightmares ■ ringing in the ears or other hearing problems ■ fast heartbeat ■ rash ■ upset stomach or stomach pain ■ nausea or vomiting ■ increased sweating ■ drowsiness ■ thickening phlegm

If symptoms are disturbing or persist, let your doctor know.

STORAGE INSTRUCTIONS

Store in a cool, dark place (not in a bathroom medicine cabinet).

STOPPING OR INTERRUPTING THERAPY

This drug should be taken without interruption for the full length of time prescribed by your doctor. If you miss a dose, take it as soon as possible. If it is almost time for your next dose, skip the missed dose, and resume your regular schedule. Do not take two doses at the same time.

SPECIAL CONSIDERATIONS FOR THOSE OVER SIXTY-FIVE

This drug has not long been in widespread use, and the full extent of its effects in older people are not yet known.

CONDITION:　**ALLERGIC RHINITIS**

CATEGORY:　**CORTICOSTEROIDS**

GENERIC (CHEMICAL) NAME	BRAND (TRADE) NAME	DOSAGE FORMS AND STRENGTHS
Beclomethasone dipropionate	BECLOVENT	Inhaler: 42 μg per inhalation
	VANCERIL Inhaler	Inhaler: 42 μg per inhalation

DRUG PROFILE

Inhaled corticosteroids such as beclomethasone are used as long-term therapy to prevent asthma attacks. They work by shrinking the swollen membranes of the respiratory tract, allowing the lungs to take in more air and making the flow of air easier. Inhaled steroids are sometimes used along with inhaled bronchodilators such as albuterol or terbutaline (see the charts on pages 653–656).

For complete information on this drug, see pages 657–661.

ASTHMA

If you have asthma, you're probably all too familiar with its symptoms—the coughing, the struggle for breath, the wheezing and whistling as air rushes through tightened passages in your lungs. But you may be less aware of what causes these sometimes disabling symptoms to occur.

In asthma, a chronic condition that can occur for the first time even after the age of fifty, the muscles of the bronchioles—the tubes that carry air back and forth from the lungs—tighten. This causes the bronchioles to narrow, go into spasm, and fill with mucus. The coughing and rattling sounds in the chest that accompany asthma result from the accumulation of mucus. Because of the narrowing of the bronchial passages, some of the air that has delivered its oxygen content and that should be exhaled is stuck in the lungs, and fresh air cannot be properly inhaled. Asthmatic breathing is hard physical work.

CAUSES

The tendency for muscles in the airways to go into spasm is hereditary and is sometimes related to allergies to pollen, dust, pet dander, mold spores, or particular foods, such as eggs or milk. In other people, the airways may be supersensitive to cold air, smoke (including cigarette smoke), smog, lint, chalk dust, or chemical fumes. Sometimes, a respiratory infection can bring on an asthma attack. Physical exercise is another common trigger of asthmatic symptoms.

The role of emotional pressure in causing asthma is debatable, though many experts believe that the existing illness is worsened by any form of stress. One thing is certain: The breathing problems caused by an attack of asthma and the ongoing frustration of being an asthmatic can lead to a lot of anxiety and emotional strain.

DIAGNOSIS

To determine whether your asthmatic symptoms can be caused by such diseases as chronic bronchitis, emphysema, or heart failure, your doctor may perform tests to rule out these problems. An important guide to an accurate assessment of your condition is your history of symptoms, especially if the attacks are worse during allergy seasons. Because of the genetic component to asthma, your doctor will also inquire whether anyone in your family is or has been allergic or asthmatic.

To confirm the diagnosis, your doctor may also perform blood tests and measurements of your ability to exhale air. One of the characteristics of asthma is that the airway obstruction is eased by a class of medicines called bronchodilators, which open the bronchial tubes. The doctor may therefore use this kind of medicine as a diagnostic tool before deciding whether it's an appropriate treatment for your condition.

TREATMENT

Although the large array of drugs available for asthma may seem confusing, there are actually only a few basic types. None can cure the asthma, but they may relieve its symptoms. In deciding what kind of medicine you should take and the proper dosage, your doctor will consider a number of factors, including the frequency and severity of your asthma attacks.

The most widely used preparations for treating asthma are bronchodilators. They relax the muscles that have tightened around the bronchioles and reduce the swelling of the mucous membranes. These drugs are available in tablet, liquid, and aerosol form. More information on bronchodilators can be found in the drug charts on pages 649–656.

If bronchodilators don't stop your attacks, your doctor may prescribe a corticosteroid (described in the drug charts on pages 657–661). These medicines must be used under close medical supervision, since they can produce severe side effects. Some people need these drugs only occasionally, while others require long-term steroid therapy.

Antihistamines may be prescribed as well because they help dry up the accumulated mucus in the lungs. Other available measures are aimed at stopping asthma attacks before they begin. For example, if your particular allergy is identified through skin tests or other diagnostic procedures, you may be given allergy injections to decrease your sensitivity—and the severity of your asthmatic condition. If you smoke, you should do everything possible to stop and also stay away from people who smoke.

Your bedroom should be scrupulously cleaned on a regular basis with a damp mop (avoid using a vacuum cleaner because it can send dust particles back into the air). If possible, have someone else do the cleaning, and don't enter the room until at least an hour after the cleaning has been finished. Avoid sleeping with a feather pillow, and get rid of such dust collectors as thick rugs, heavy drapes, and knickknacks. You may even have to find a new home for your dog or cat.

If cold air triggers your attacks, keep your mouth and nose covered with a scarf when you go outdoors in cold weather. If a particular food seems to contribute to your asthmatic symptoms, exclude it from your diet.

OUTLOOK

Most of the time, asthma can be managed by control of the environment, preventive medicine, and medicines that relieve the attacks. Sometimes, however, an attack of asthma can be so severe that you require hospitalization, where respiratory help is available and medicine can be given in the most effective manner.

It's important to remember that, while asthma is not a psychosomatic disease, it can produce emotional problems involving the affected individual as well as other family members. Emotional support is an important part of the overall treatment plan, making it easier for everyone involved to live with asthma.

BRONCHITIS

You may not consider a cough anything to worry about, but if you're told that it's a result of bronchitis, you should take it seriously.

Bronchitis is an inflammation of the bronchial tubes, the passages that bring air into the lungs. When the tubes are inflamed, either because of an infection or persistent irritation, they produce a heavy secretion of mucus. The coughing that is characteristic of bronchitis is the body's attempt to clear the mucus. If not properly treated, this condition can cause further health complications, especially in older people.

CAUSES

Bronchitis is characterized as either acute or chronic. An acute attack is generally caused by a virus but may be caused by bacteria. Typically, a head cold becomes a chest cold, or a case of the flu lingers and starts to affect your bronchial tubes. A bronchial cough may be accompanied by fever, aches and pains, and difficulty in breathing. Usually this type of bronchitis lasts about ten days. But it can lead to a more serious disorder—one that extends deeper into the lungs—if not treated promptly.

Chronic bronchitis keeps you coughing up mucus almost every day for months at a time, year after year, especially during cold weather. Its most common cause is cigarette smoking, which irritates the bronchial lining. Air pollution and the development of respiratory illnesses in childhood may predispose you to developing chronic bronchitis as an adult. In some cases, a series of attacks of acute bronchitis or chronic allergic asthma leads to chronic bronchitis. A rare condition known as alpha$_1$-antitrypsin deficiency may result in chronic bronchitis.

Periodically, the bronchitis may get so bad that you are breathless, have even more frequent coughing spells, and bring up pus along with the mucus. The danger of chronic bronchitis is that it can make you vulnerable to pneumonia.

TREATMENT

It's especially important for older people to seek medical help whenever they have breathing difficulty or coughing spells. Before making the diagnosis of bronchitis, your doctor will perform tests that rule out heart disease, lung infections, cancer, and other disorders that may produce the symptoms typical of bronchitis. A chest X ray certainly will be part of your exam. Your doctor may ask you to breathe into a tube as a way of measuring how seriously your airways are obstructed; if your breathing is severely impaired, you may need to have oxygen at home. Specially designed exercises may also be recommended to improve your ability to breathe.

The treatment of acute bronchitis generally includes staying indoors if the weather is cold, avoiding fatigue, and drinking plenty of fluids. If you're a smoker, you'll be told to give it up, at least while you're ill, because airways cannot heal if they're constantly irritated. Expectorant drugs are sometimes prescribed to loosen mucus, though there is no evidence that these drugs actually work. Antibiotics are not routinely prescribed, as acute bronchitis is generally caused by a virus. However, some doctors prescribe them to older people to eliminate the risk of serious bacterial infection resulting from lowered resistance. See the drug charts on pages 661-667 for further information.

If you have chronic bronchitis, you'll be told to stop smoking altogether, even when you feel fine. This will help prevent further damage to your bronchial airways. A vaporizer may come in handy (for acute as well as chronic sufferers) because the steam can help relieve the chest congestion. And you're almost certain to be given a prescription for an antibiotic, especially if your airways are severely obstructed. You may also be put on a bronchodilator, a drug class covered in the charts on pages 649–656. If you don't feel somewhat better within three or four days of starting medicine, a corticosteroid may be added to your drug therapy. (See the drug charts on pages 657–661.) This is usually given in cases in which the person is sick enough to be hospitalized.

OUTLOOK

Bronchitis should not be dismissed as "just an annoying cough" that will go away. It can do serious damage if left untreated. But effective treatment *is* available. If you let your doctor know about any breathing trouble or coughing spells you experience, you'll be less likely to cough the winter away.

EMPHYSEMA

Emphysema is a long-term illness in which breathing becomes increasingly difficult over the years. Known also as chronic obstructive pulmonary disease (COPD), it most often strikes men and women between the ages of fifty and the late seventies.

Normally, the oxygen in the air we breathe passes through the walls of air sacs in the lungs, called alveoli, and into the small blood vessels of the lungs. At the same time, carbon dioxide passes out of the blood vessels, into the air sacs, and then up through the bronchial tubes so that it can be exhaled. But in emphysema, the lungs' small airways are damaged, and the walls of the alveoli rupture. Therefore, less oxygen and carbon dioxide can move back and forth. In fact, some of the carbon dioxide gets stuck in the lungs, preventing the inhalation of fresh air.

CAUSES

Emphysema is a disease that would hardly exist if people didn't smoke cigarettes. Generally, years and years of smoking lead to the rupture of the alveoli, and continued smoking only worsens this life-threatening condition. Sometimes, other factors come into play. For example, genetic factors, exposure to industrial chemicals over a long period of time, other diseases of the lungs, and the physical stress of certain occupations may all contribute to the development of emphysema.

DIAGNOSIS

The main symptom of emphysema is difficulty in breathing, which may become so severe that you feel as if you're suffocating. You may have to puff in order to move enough air in and out of your lungs. All this straining will cause muscles in your chest to over-expand, giving your chest a barrel shape. Your neck and shoulder muscles may also become over-developed because of the effort it takes to breathe. Even with all that extra effort, you may not get enough air, and your skin may take on a blue tone because of oxygen deprivation.

Chronic bronchitis usually precedes emphysema, and you may have the persistent wet cough of that disease, as well. For some people, the cough is more severe than the breathing difficulty. During a respiratory infection, the symptoms of emphysema often become worse, and wheezing and shortness of breath occur.

To determine the cause of your breathing difficulties, your doctor will take a medical history and perform a physical examination, paying special attention to your chest sounds. As part of the exam, you'll probably be asked to blow into a device that provides a measurement of your ability to exhale. Blood tests, sputum analysis, and a chest X ray will also aid the doctor in arriving at a correct diagnosis.

TREATMENT

Therapy is aimed at easing your breathing and slowing the rate at which damage occurs. Your doctor is likely to prescribe a bronchodilator, which relieves the tightening of the bronchial tubes and loosens mucus. (See the drug charts on pages 649–656.) Your treatment may also include use of a portable oxygen tank to help prevent oxygen deprivation.

First and foremost, people with emphysema should stop smoking. They should also avoid areas of air pollution. Respiratory infections can worsen your problems, so stay away from people with such contagious diseases as influenza. If you have been exposed, your doctor might prescribe antibiotics for you to take as a preventive measure.

Being unable to breathe can cause a great deal of emotional stress, and emotional stress can increase difficulty in breathing. Many people with emphysema become depressed and angry; they may also feel frustrated that there is currently no cure for their illness. Such medicines as tranquilizers and antidepressants are often prescribed to help relieve those feelings and to enhance the effectiveness of treatment.

OUTLOOK

Emphysema is an irreversible condition that can lead to such other problems as pulmonary hypertension and heart failure. (Be sure to tell your doctor if your ankles begin to swell or your breathing problems suddenly become much worse—these are possible signals of complications.) Keep in mind, however, that there have been significant advances in the treatment of emphysema and that continuing research will undoubtedly lead to even more effective therapeutic approaches. Meanwhile, follow your current treatment plan, and don't hesitate to seek help if you feel emotionally overwhelmed by the effects of your illness.

CONDITION: **ASTHMA, BRONCHITIS, AND EMPHYSEMA**

CATEGORY: **BRONCHODILATORS (THEOPHYLLINE AND RELATED DRUGS)**

GENERIC (CHEMICAL) NAME	BRAND (TRADE) NAME	DOSAGE FORMS AND STRENGTHS
Theophylline	Available under a number of brand names and dosage forms and strengths.*	
Oxtriphylline	CHOLEDYL CHOLEDYL SA	Elixir: 100 mg per tsp Tablets: 100, 200 mg Controlled-release tablets: 400, 600 mg
Oxtriphylline and guaifenesin	BRONDECON	Elixir: 100 mg oxtriphylline and 50 mg guaifenesin per tsp Tablets: 200 mg oxtriphylline and 100 mg guaifenesin

*Common brand names for theophylline include BRONKODYL, CONSTANT-T, DURAPHYL, ELIXICON, ELIXOPHYLLIN, QUIBRON, RESPBID, SLO-BID, SLO-PHYLLIN, SOMOPHYLLIN-T, THEO-24, THEO-DUR, THEOBID, THEOLAIR, THEOPHYL, and UNIPHYL.

DRUG PROFILE

Theophylline and its relative, oxtriphylline, are used to treat the wheezing, cough, and breathing problems associated with bronchial asthma, chronic bronchitis, and emphysema. They work by relaxing the muscles of the respiratory tract, allowing the lungs to take in more air and making the flow of air easier. These drugs also increase the supply of blood to the lungs. Guaifenesin is an expectorant—it thins and loosens the mucus in the lungs so that it can be coughed up more easily.

BEFORE USING THIS DRUG

Let your doctor know *IF*

You have ever had allergic reactions or other problems with ▪ theophylline ▪ oxtriphylline ▪ caffeine ▪ theobromine.

   ▪ *with Brondecon only:* ▪ guaifenesin.

You have ever had any of the following medical problems: ▪ other respiratory infections, including influenza ▪ heart disease or any disease of the blood vessels ▪ stomach problems ▪ liver disease ▪ kidney disease ▪ overactive thyroid ▪ diabetes ▪ glaucoma ▪ high blood pressure ▪ abnormal heart rhythms ▪ diarrhea.

You are taking any of the following medicines: ▪ other medicine for respiratory problems ▪ medicine for gout ▪ antibiotics ▪ medicine for seizures ▪ medicine for tuberculosis ▪ barbiturates ▪ appetite suppressants ▪ beta-blockers ▪ calcium blockers ▪ lithium (medicine for depression) ▪ medicine for diarrhea ▪ influenza vaccine ▪ cimetidine or ranitidine (medicine for ulcers) ▪ diuretics ▪ tranquilizers ▪ muscle relaxants ▪ drugs for thyroid disease ▪ sleep medicines ▪ baking soda.

SPECIAL RESTRICTIONS WHILE TAKING THIS DRUG

FOOD AND DRUG INTERACTIONS

Other Drugs	Because many other drugs interact with this drug, check with your doctor before taking any other medicine, including over-the-counter (OTC) drugs. Also, tell your doctor if you are planning to be vaccinated for influenza.
Foods and Beverages	Limit your intake of foods and beverages that contain caffeine, such as cocoa, chocolate, coffee, tea, and colas. These may add to the stimulant effects of this drug. Also, cut down on charcoal-broiled foods because they decrease the effectiveness of this drug.
Smoking	Tell your doctor if you smoke or have given up smoking within the last two years. Your dosage may need to be adjusted accordingly.

No special restrictions on alcohol use.

DAILY LIVING

Examinations or Tests

It is important for you to keep all appointments with your doctor so that your progress can be checked. Periodic blood tests are usually required to keep track of how much of this drug is in your body.

Other Precautions

Taking this medicine more often or for a longer period of time than prescribed by your doctor may make you more prone to developing side effects.

If you develop diarrhea, fever, or flu symptoms (cough, fever, or body aches), contact your doctor. Your dosage may need to be adjusted. Do not switch brands or dosage forms without consulting your doctor.

Tell any doctor or dentist you consult that you are taking this medicine, especially if you will be undergoing any type of surgery.

Helpful Hints

Make sure you take this drug in regularly spaced doses exactly as instructed by your doctor, in order to maintain a constant level of medicine in your blood.

For maximum benefit, take the tablets and liquid form of this medicine with a glass of water on an empty stomach (half an hour before or two hours after meals).

If this drug causes upset stomach, taking it with an antacid should help.

Both the regular and controlled-release tablets should be swallowed whole, without chewing or crushing.

No special restrictions on driving, exertion and exercise, sun exposure, or exposure to excessive heat or cold.

POSSIBLE SIDE EFFECTS

Although this list of adverse effects may seem somewhat intimidating, keep in mind that some are quite rare. Of course, should these or any other problems arise while you are on medication, it is always a good idea to consult your doctor.

IF YOU DEVELOP	WHAT TO DO
behavior changes ■ frequent vomiting ■ fever ■ ringing in ears ■ irregular heartbeat ■ muscle twitching ■ vomiting, with blood or vomit that looks like coffee grounds ■ excessive sweating ■ seizures ■ rapid, shallow breathing ■ bloody or black, tarry stools ■ tremors ■ confusion	**Urgent** Get in touch with your doctor immediately.
dizziness ■ headache ■ urinary frequency ■ stomach pain or cramps ■ sleeplessness ■ fast heartbeat ■ flushing ■ rash or hives	**May be serious** Check with your doctor as soon as possible.
diarrhea ■ nausea or vomiting ■ loss of appetite ■ nervousness or restlessness ■ irritability	If symptoms are disturbing or persist, let your doctor know.

STORAGE INSTRUCTIONS

Store in a cool, dark place (not in a bathroom medicine cabinet). If your medicine is in a liquid form, make sure that it does not freeze.

STOPPING OR INTERRUPTING THERAPY

Take this medicine exactly as prescribed by your doctor. If you miss a dose, take it as soon as possible. If it is almost time for your next dose, skip the missed dose and resume your regular schedule. Do not take two doses at the same time.

SPECIAL CONSIDERATIONS FOR THOSE OVER SIXTY-FIVE

Older people, especially men, may be more prone to side effects. Doctors may want to monitor them especially closely and check their blood levels of this drug to make sure they are receiving the correct dosage. This drug can cause urinary frequency, particularly in women, and this may be an important problem for those over sixty-five.

CONDITION: **ASTHMA, BRONCHITIS, AND EMPHYSEMA**

CATEGORY: **BRONCHODILATORS (BETA-AGONISTS)**

GENERIC (CHEMICAL) NAME	BRAND (TRADE) NAME	DOSAGE FORMS AND STRENGTHS
Albuterol	PROVENTIL Inhaler	Inhaler: 90 μg per inhalation
	VENTOLIN Inhaler	Inhaler: 90 μg per inhalation
Albuterol sulfate	PROVENTIL	Syrup: 2 mg per tsp Tablets: 2, 4 mg
	VENTOLIN	Syrup: 2 mg per tsp Tablets: 2, 4 mg
Isoetharine hydrochloride	BRONKOMETER BRONKOSOL	Inhalation aerosol: 0.61% Inhalation solution: 0.25%, 1%
Metaproterenol sulfate	ALUPENT	Inhalation solution: 0.6%, 5% Metered-dose inhaler: 0.65 mg per inhalation Syrup: 10 mg per tsp Tablets: 10, 20 mg
	METAPREL	Inhalation solution: 5% Metered-dose inhaler: 0.65 mg per inhalation Syrup: 10 mg per tsp Tablets: 10, 20 mg

Terbutaline sulfate	BRETHAIRE	Inhaler: 200 μg per inhalation
	BRETHINE	Tablets: 2.5, 5 mg
	BRICANYL	Tablets: 2.5, 5 mg

DRUG PROFILE

Beta-agonists are used to treat the bronchial spasm and wheezing associated with asthma, bronchitis, and emphysema. These drugs work by relaxing the muscles of the respiratory tract, allowing the lungs to take in more air and making the flow of air easier. The inhalant form of albuterol is also used to prevent bronchial spasm triggered by exercise.

BEFORE USING THIS DRUG

Let your doctor know *IF*

You have ever had allergic reactions or other problems with ■ albuterol ■ isoetharine ■ metaproterenol ■ terbutaline ■ medicines with a stimulant effect (amphetamines, ephedrine, isoproterenol, and phenylpropanolamine).

You have ever had any of the following medical problems: ■ diabetes ■ heart disease, including abnormal heart rhythms ■ high blood pressure ■ overactive thyroid ■ enlarged prostate ■ seizures.

You are taking any of the following medicines: ■ medicine for asthma ■ beta-blockers ■ tricyclic antidepressants ■ appetite suppressants ■ medicine for Parkinson's disease ■ medicine for high blood pressure ■ nitrates (medicine for chest pain) ■ any medicine containing caffeine ■ antihistamines ■ medicine for hay fever or other allergies (including nose drops or nose sprays) ■ thyroid hormones ■ digoxin, digitoxin, or digitalis (heart medicines).

SPECIAL RESTRICTIONS WHILE TAKING THIS DRUG

FOOD AND DRUG INTERACTIONS

| Other Drugs | Do not take any other drugs, including over-the-counter (OTC) drugs, before checking with your doctor. Drugs that may add to the stimulant effects of this drug include appetite suppressants, medicine con- |

taining caffeine, decongestants, and some medicines for allergies or colds.

If you are also using an inhalant corticosteroid, allow fifteen minutes between the use of the corticosteroid and this drug.

Smoking	Smoking aggravates any kind of lung disease. If you smoke, try to stop or at least cut down.

No special restrictions on foods and beverages or alcohol use.

DAILY LIVING

Examinations or Tests	It is important for you to keep all appointments with your doctor so that your progress can be checked.
Other Precautions	Taking this medicine more often or for a longer period of time than prescribed by your doctor may make you more prone to developing side effects. If this medicine fails to relieve your symptoms or if your condition worsens, call your doctor immediately.
Helpful Hints	If your mouth or throat feels dry, rinse your mouth with water after each dose.

No special restrictions on driving, exertion and exercise, sun exposure, or exposure to excessive heat or cold.

POSSIBLE SIDE EFFECTS

Although this list of adverse effects may seem somewhat intimidating, keep in mind that some are quite rare. Of course, should these or any other problems arise while you are on medication, it is always a good idea to consult your doctor.

IF YOU DEVELOP	WHAT TO DO
chest pain or tight feeling in chest ■ pounding heartbeat ■ rapid, shallow breathing ■ wheezing	**Urgent** Get in touch with your doctor immediately.
severe dizziness ■ muscle cramps ■ irregular or fast heartbeat ■ excitement ■ irritability ■ tremors ■ increased sweating ■ dilated pupils ■ weakness ■ nosebleed ■ severe headache	**May be serious** Check with your doctor as soon as possible.
nervousness or restlessness ■ headache ■ nausea or vomiting ■ unusual taste in mouth ■ heartburn ■ dry mouth or throat ■ cough ■ sleeplessness ■ increased appetite ■ dizziness or light-headedness	If symptoms are disturbing or persist, let your doctor know.

STORAGE INSTRUCTIONS

Store in a cool, dark place (not in a bathroom medicine cabinet). Do not allow the inhalant to freeze.

STOPPING OR INTERRUPTING THERAPY

Take this medicine exactly as prescribed by your doctor. If you miss a dose, take it as soon as possible. If it is almost time for your next dose, skip the missed dose and resume your regular schedule. Do not take two doses at the same time.

SPECIAL CONSIDERATIONS FOR THOSE OVER SIXTY-FIVE

Older people may be more prone to the side effects of this drug. Doctors will probably start people over sixty-five on a lower than normal dosage and check them regularly. This drug can cause urinary frequency, particularly in women, and this may be an important problem for those over sixty-five.

CONDITION: **ASTHMA, BRONCHITIS, AND EMPHYSEMA**

CATEGORY: **CORTICOSTEROIDS**

GENERIC (CHEMICAL) NAME	BRAND (TRADE) NAME	DOSAGE FORMS AND STRENGTHS
Beclomethasone dipropionate	BECLOVENT	Inhaler: 42 μg per inhalation
	VANCERIL Inhaler	Inhaler: 42 μg per inhalation

DRUG PROFILE

Inhaled corticosteroids such as beclomethasone are used as long-term therapy to prevent asthma attacks. They work by shrinking the swollen membranes of the respiratory tract, allowing the lungs to take in more air and making the flow of air easier. Inhaled steroids are sometimes used along with inhaled bronchodilators such as albuterol or terbutaline (see the charts on pages 653–656).

BEFORE USING THIS DRUG

Let your doctor know *IF*

You have ever had allergic reactions or other problems with ■ any corticosteroids ■ aerosol sprays.

You have ever had any of the following medical problems: ■ colitis or diverticulitis ■ diabetes ■ bone disease, such as osteoporosis ■ recent fungal infection ■ glaucoma ■ heart disease ■ disease of the blood vessels ■ herpes eye infection ■ any viral infection, such as chickenpox ■ high blood pressure ■ kidney disease ■ liver disease ■ myasthenia gravis ■ stomach ulcer ■ stomach cramps ■ tuberculosis ■ underactive thyroid ■ mental illness ■ seizures ■ recent infection of the mouth, throat, or lungs ■ high cholesterol.

You are taking any of the following medicines: ■ any other medicine for asthma ■ antibiotics ■ digoxin, digitoxin, or digitalis (heart medicines) ■ medicine for abnormal heart rhythms ■ diuretics ■ medicine for high blood pressure ■ medicine for inflammation, such as medicine for arthritis (including aspirin or aspirin-like medicine) ■ insulin or other medicine for diabetes ■ anticoagulants (blood thinners) ■ medicine for Parkinson's disease ■ phenobarbital ■ medicine for seizures ■ estrogens (female hormones) ■ thiazides or furosemide (potassium-depleting diuretics) ■ medicine for myasthenia gravis.

You have recently had a vaccination.

SPECIAL RESTRICTIONS WHILE TAKING THIS DRUG

FOOD AND DRUG INTERACTIONS

Other Drugs	Corticosteroids interact with many other drugs. Do not take any other drugs, including over-the-counter (OTC) drugs, before checking with your doctor.
	If you are using a bronchodilator inhaler, allow at least fifteen minutes between the use of the bronchodilator and the beclomethasone inhaler.
	Corticosteroids may affect how your body absorbs medicine for diabetes, and your dosage may need to be adjusted.
	Tell your doctor if you are planning to receive any kind of vaccine.
Foods and Beverages	As this drug may deplete your body of calcium and potassium, your doctor may recommend a diet rich in these minerals. You may also be advised to go on a low-salt diet.
Smoking	Smoking aggravates any kind of lung disease. If you smoke, try to stop or at least cut down.

No special restrictions on alcohol use.

DAILY LIVING

Examinations or Tests	It is important for you to keep all appointments with your doctor so that your progress can be checked. If you are on long-term therapy with this drug, your doctor may want to perform periodic blood and urine tests.
Other Precautions	Tell any doctor or dentist you consult that you are taking this medicine, especially if you will be undergoing any type of surgery.

Taking this medicine more often or for a longer period of time than prescribed by your doctor may make you more prone to developing side effects. If this medicine fails to relieve your symptoms or if your condition worsens, call your doctor immediately.

You should also inform your doctor if you are undergoing some sort of unusual stress or if you develop a respiratory infection.

You may become more prone to fungal infections of the mouth and throat while using a corticosteroid inhaler. Let your doctor know if you develop signs of such an infection (white patches in the mouth or throat). You may also have a sore throat and hoarseness. Gargling with salt water or a special mouthwash prescribed by your doctor after each use and cleaning the inhaler daily should help prevent these effects.

No special restrictions on driving, exertion and exercise, sun exposure, or exposure to excessive heat or cold.

POSSIBLE SIDE EFFECTS

Although this list of adverse effects may seem somewhat intimidating, keep in mind that some are quite rare. Of course, should these or any other problems arise while you are on medication, it is always a good idea to consult your doctor.

IF YOU DEVELOP	WHAT TO DO
stomach pain ■ dizziness or faintness ■ fever ■ muscle or joint pain or weakness ■ nausea or vomiting ■ difficulty in breathing ■ tiredness ■ weight loss ■ slow or fast heartbeat ■ palpitations ■ swelling of mouth or tongue ■ difficulty in speech ■ seizures ■ loss of appetite ■ pain in urination ■ urinary frequency *After you STOP taking this medicine:* loss of appetite or weight loss ■ nausea or vomiting ■ drowsiness ■ headache ■ fever ■ joint or muscle pain ■ skin problems ■ dizziness ■ depression	**Urgent** Get in touch with your doctor immediately.
back, hip, or rib pain ■ acne ■ increased sweating ■ hair growth ■ rash, hives, or other skin changes ■ bruising ■ depression or other mood changes ■ nervousness or restlessness ■ bloody stools ■ bloating ■ halos around lights or other visual disturbances ■ wounds that take a long time to heal ■ swelling of hands, feet, or ankles ■ diarrhea ■ constipation ■ reactivation of an ulcer ■ any lung or throat infection ■ white patches in mouth or throat ■ skin redness ■ hoarseness or sore throat ■ dry mouth ■ swelling of face ■ "high feeling"	**May be serious** Check with your doctor as soon as possible.
indigestion ■ bloating ■ increased appetite ■ weight gain ■ eruptions on mouth or lips ■ sleeplessness	If symptoms are disturbing or persist, let your doctor know.

STORAGE INSTRUCTIONS

Store in a cool, dark place (not in a bathroom medicine cabinet). Do not let your medicine freeze.

STOPPING OR INTERRUPTING THERAPY

Take this medicine exactly as prescribed by your doctor. Inhaled corticosteroids need to be used at regular intervals to be effective; it may be one to four weeks before you notice improvement of your symptoms. If you miss a dose, take it as soon as possible. If it is almost time for your next dose, skip the missed dose and resume your regular schedule. Do not take two doses at the same time.

SPECIAL CONSIDERATIONS FOR THOSE OVER SIXTY-FIVE

Long-term use of corticosteroids may cause gradual bone loss; this can be serious in older people—particularly women, who are vulnerable to osteoporosis.

CONDITION: **BRONCHITIS**

CATEGORY: **ANTIBIOTICS (TETRACYCLINES)**

GENERIC (CHEMICAL) NAME	BRAND (TRADE) NAME	DOSAGE FORMS AND STRENGTHS
Demeclocycline hydrochloride	DECLOMYCIN	Capsules: 150 mg Tablets: 150, 300 mg
Doxycycline	VIBRAMYCIN	Capsules: 50, 100 mg Suspension: 25 mg per tsp Syrup: 50 mg per tsp
	VIBRATABS	Tablets: 100 mg
	VIVOX	Capsules: 50, 100 mg Tablets: 100 mg
Methacycline hydrochloride	RONDOMYCIN	Capsules: 150, 300 mg
Minocycline	MINOCIN	Capsules: 50,100 mg Suspension: 50 mg per tsp Tablets: 50, 100 mg
Oxytetracycline	TERRAMYCIN	Capsules: 250 mg

Tetracycline hydrochloride	ACHROMYCIN V	Capsules: 250, 500 mg Suspension: 125 mg per tsp
	PANMYCIN	Capsules: 250 mg
	ROBITET	Capsules: 250, 500 mg
	SUMYCIN	Capsules: 250, 500 mg Syrup: 125 mg per tsp Tablets: 250, 500 mg

This type of drug is available under other brand names as well.

DRUG PROFILE

Tetracyclines are antibiotics that are used to treat a wide variety of bacterial infections, including skin eruptions and bronchitis and pneumonia. These antibiotics suppress the growth of the bacteria by interfering with their manufacture of protein.

For complete information on these drugs, see pages 591–595.

CONDITION: **BRONCHITIS**

CATEGORY: **ANTIBIOTICS (ERYTHROMYCINS)**

GENERIC (CHEMICAL) NAME	BRAND (TRADE) NAME	DOSAGE FORMS AND STRENGTHS
Erythromycin	E-MYCIN ERYC ERY-TAB	Tablets: 250, 333 mg Capsules: 125, 250 mg Tablets: 250, 333, 500 mg
Erythromycin estolate	ILOSONE	Capsules: 125, 250 mg Chewable tablets: 125, 250 mg Drops: 100 mg per ml Suspension: 125, 250 mg per tsp Tablets: 500 mg

Erythromycin ethylsuccinate	E.E.S.	Chewable tablets: 200 mg Drops: 100 mg per 2.5 ml Suspension: 200, 400 mg per tsp Suspension granules: 200 mg per tsp Tablets: 400 mg
	E-MYCIN E	Suspension: 200, 400 mg per tsp
	WYAMYCIN E	Suspension: 200, 400 mg per tsp
Erythromycin stearate	ERYTHROCIN Stearate WYAMYCIN S	Tablets: 250, 500 mg Tablets: 250, 500 mg

This type of drug is available under other brand names as well.

DRUG PROFILE

Erythromcycins are antibiotics that are used to treat a variety of bacterial infections, including such respiratory tract infections as bronchitis and pneumonia. These drugs suppress the growth of the bacteria and keep them from multiplying by blocking the bacteria's ability to manufacture protein.

For complete information on these drugs, see pages 595–598.

CONDITION: **BRONCHITIS**

CATEGORY: **ANTIBIOTICS (PENICILLINS)**

GENERIC (CHEMICAL) NAME	BRAND (TRADE) NAME	DOSAGE FORMS AND STRENGTHS
Amoxicillin	AMOXIL	Capsules: 250, 500 mg Chewable tablets: 125, 250 mg Suspension: 125, 250 mg per tsp
	LAROTID	Capsules: 250, 500 mg Suspension: 125, 250 mg per tsp
	POLYMOX	Capsules: 250, 500 mg Suspension: 125, 250 mg per tsp
	TRIMOX	Capsules: 250, 500 mg Suspension: 125, 250 mg per tsp
Ampicillin	AMCILL	Capsules: 250, 500 mg Suspension: 125, 250 mg per tsp
	OMNIPEN	Capsules: 250, 500 mg Suspension: 125, 250 mg per tsp
	POLYCILLIN	Capsules: 250, 500 mg Suspension: 125, 250, 500 mg per tsp
	SK-AMPICILLIN	Capsules: 250, 500 mg Suspension: 125, 250 mg per tsp
	TOTACILLIN	Capsules: 250, 500 mg Suspension: 125, 250 mg per tsp

Bacampicillin hydrochloride	SPECTROBID	Suspension: 125 mg per tsp Tablets: 400 mg
Carbenicillin indanyl sodium	GEOCILLIN	Tablets: 382 mg
Cloxacillin sodium	TEGOPEN	Capsules: 250, 500 mg Solution: 125 mg per tsp
Cyclacillin	CYCLAPEN-W	Suspension: 125, 250 mg per tsp Tablets: 250, 500 mg
Nafcillin sodium	UNIPEN	Capsules: 250 mg Solution: 250 mg per tsp Tablets: 500 mg
Oxacillin sodium	PROSTAPHLIN	Capsules: 250, 500 mg Solution: 250 mg per tsp
Penicillin G potassium	PENTIDS	Tablets: 200,000, 400,000 units
Penicillin V potassium	LEDERCILLIN VK	Solution: 125, 250 mg per tsp Tablets: 250, 500 mg
	PEN•VEE•K	Solution: 125, 250 mg per tsp Tablets: 250, 500 mg
	V-CILLIN K	Solution: 125, 250 mg per tsp Tablets: 125, 250, 500 mg

This type of drug is available under other brand names as well.

DRUG PROFILE

Penicillins are antibiotics that are used to treat a wide variety of bacterial infections, including infections of the ear, nose, and throat and such respiratory tract infections as bronchitis and pneumonia. Penicillins suppress the growth of bacteria by interfering with the bacteria's ability to form new protective cell walls.

For complete information on these drugs, see pages 599–603.

CONDITION: **BRONCHITIS**

CATEGORY: **ANTIBIOTICS (CEPHALOSPORINS)**

GENERIC (CHEMICAL) NAME	BRAND (TRADE) NAME	DOSAGE FORMS AND STRENGTHS
Cefaclor	CECLOR	Capsules: 250, 500 mg Suspension: 125, 250 mg per tsp
Cefadroxil	DURICEF	Capsules: 500 mg Suspension: 125, 250, 500 mg per tsp Tablets: 1 g
	ULTRACEF	Capsules: 500 mg Suspension: 125, 250 mg per tsp Tablets: 1 g
Cephalexin	KEFLEX	Capsules: 250, 500 mg Suspension: 125, 250 mg per tsp Tablets: 1 g
Cephradine	ANSPOR	Capsules: 250, 500 mg Suspension: 125, 250 mg per tsp

VELOSEF

Capsules: 250, 500 mg
Suspension: 125, 250 mg
per tsp

This type of drug is available under other brand names as well.

DRUG PROFILE

Cephalosporins are antibiotics that are used to treat a wide variety of bacterial infections, including such upper respiratory tract infections as bronchitis and pneumonia. These drugs work by interfering with the bacteria's ability to multiply and to form new protective cell walls.

For complete information on these drugs, see pages 604–607.

TUBERCULOSIS

We tend to think of tuberculosis (TB) as a disease of the past—until it strikes us or someone we know. Its incidence is declining, but every year thousands of Americans are diagnosed as having an active case of TB. The most likely candidates for the white plague, as it has been called, are people forty-five and older. To understand why requires a brief review of the origins of this disorder.

TB is an infection that usually lodges in the lungs, though it can also affect other organs. Its cause is invasion of the body by a bacillus, a rod-shaped type of bacteria. In many cases, the body's own immune system fights back successfully, walling off the bacteria and keeping them inactive for years or even decades.

In the first half of this century, TB was a major public health hazard, affecting people of all ages. In many people, however, the disease has remained dormant. But with aging, their immune systems might have been weakened by other diseases, by immunosuppressive medicines, or just by getting older; the bacteria are thus able to break free and multiply, causing widespread damage in the lungs. Such a scenario is common to most people now being diagnosed as victims of TB—they are older people who were probably infected long ago.

DIAGNOSIS

The classic symptoms of TB are fatigue, fever, night sweats, weight loss, chronic wet cough, and blood in the mucus that is coughed up. But in older people, the symptoms are often more subtle—a slight cough, a little fever, and a general feeling of unwellness. Sometimes this decline in health is wrongly attributed to emotional depression or to the natural aging process. This kind of decline is *not* a normal part of the aging process but a signal that medical help is needed.

During your visit to the doctor, you will be asked to provide a detailed medical history. At that time, if you think you were ever infected with TB, or even just exposed to it, you should make a point of explaining the circumstances to your doctor.

If your doctor suspects that TB is the reason for your discomfort, you will probably be injected with a substance that causes a skin reaction if you have, or have ever had, a TB infection. This procedure, known as a tuberculin skin test, may have to be done twice in order to get an accurate result.

If you test positive, a chest X ray will be taken to check for the presence of TB-caused abnormalities in your lungs. These are signs of an active case of TB. A sputum sample may also be collected for analysis. If your doctor has reason to believe that the bacillus has invaded other body systems, you may be hospitalized for more comprehensive testing.

TREATMENT

Modern medicine has produced a real revolution in the treatment of TB.

The sanitariums where TB patients used to stay isolated while they rested, breathed fresh air, and hoped to get well no longer exist. Instead, people with TB take a combination of anti-TB drugs that can stop the infectious stage of the disease in two to four weeks. (See the drug charts on pages 670–676 for more information on these medicines.) Bed rest is not generally necessary, and even during the initial period of drug therapy, hospitalization and isolation are not always required.

The most effective drug can, however, have some very serious side effects, especially if the person is alcoholic, has vision problems, or suffers from kidney or liver disease. In those cases, substitute medicines are prescribed. Whatever drugs are prescribed, the doctor may insist on monthly office visits, with sputum and urine analyses and periodic chest X rays, to be sure the drugs are working without damaging vulnerable organs.

Your doctor may also want to test members of your family and other people you have been close to for possible TB infection. If they test positive, they will be instructed to take the anti-TB medicine also, as a preventive measure.

OUTLOOK

If your system is able to handle the most effective anti-TB drugs, and if you take them conscientiously as your doctor orders, you can expect to return to at least some of your normal activities within a month. In as little as nine months, your TB may be completely cured. But if you have drug-resistant bacteria or have to use second-choice medicines because you react adversely to the faster-acting drugs, your treatment period could stretch to twice that long.

You may have to return for checkups on a regular basis for six months to a year after you've stopped taking medicines. If, during that time, there are no signs of reactivation of TB, you may consider yourself not only cured but also out of danger of recurrence.

CONDITION: **TUBERCULOSIS**

CATEGORY: **ANTITUBERCULOSIS DRUGS**

GENERIC (CHEMICAL) NAME	BRAND (TRADE) NAME	DOSAGE FORMS AND STRENGTHS
Isoniazid	DOW-ISONIAZID	Tablets: 300 mg
	INH	Tablets: 300 mg
	NYDRAZID	Tablets: 100 mg

DRUG PROFILE

Isoniazid is used to treat tuberculosis or prevent it from developing in people who have a positive tuberculin skin test. This drug arrests the growth of the tuberculosis bacteria.

BEFORE USING THIS DRUG

Let your doctor know *IF*

You have ever had allergic reactions or other problems with ■ isoniazid or any other medicine for tuberculosis ■ niacin (vitamin B_6) when taken with isoniazid.

You have ever had any of the following medical problems: ■ alcoholism ■ kidney disease ■ liver disease ■ diabetes ■ seizures.

You are taking any of the following medicines: ■ other medicine for tuberculosis ■ antacids ■ anticoagulants (blood thinners) ■ medicine for seizures ■ antibiotics ■ niacin (vitamin B_6) ■ sleep medicines ■ tranquilizers ■ corticosteroids ■ Antabuse (used in treating alcoholism) ■ theophylline (medicine for asthma) ■ aspirin.

SPECIAL RESTRICTIONS WHILE TAKING THIS DRUG

FOOD AND DRUG INTERACTIONS

Other Drugs	Allow at least one hour between taking isoniazid and any antacid containing aluminum.

Alcohol	Avoid alcohol while taking this medicine. Alcohol decreases the effect of this drug, and liver problems may develop as a result of this combination.
Smoking	Smoking aggravates any kind of lung disease. If you smoke, try to stop or at least cut down.

No special restrictions on foods and beverages.

DAILY LIVING

Examinations or Tests	It is important for you to keep all appointments with your doctor so that your progress can be checked. Periodic eye examinations may be required.
Other Precautions	Tell any doctor or dentist you consult that you are taking this drug, especially if you will be undergoing any type of surgery.
	If you have diabetes, be aware that this drug may affect the results of urine-sugar tests. Do not change the dose of your diabetes medicine, but check with your doctor.
	Your doctor will probably recommend that you take vitamin B_6 along with your daily dose of this drug; vitamin B_6 helps reduce the side effects of this drug.
Helpful Hints	If this medicine upsets your stomach, taking it with food should help. Or instead, you may take an antacid, but allow at least one hour between the antacid and your dose of this drug.

No special restrictions on driving, exertion and exercise, sun exposure, or exposure to excessive heat or cold.

POSSIBLE SIDE EFFECTS

Although this list of adverse effects may seem somewhat intimidating, keep in mind that some are quite rare. Of course, should these or any other problems arise while you are on medication, it is always a good idea to consult your doctor.

IF YOU DEVELOP	WHAT TO DO
blurred vision ■ eye pain ■ general feeling of unwellness ■ slurred speech ■ hallucinations ■ difficulty in breathing ■ extreme tiredness or weakness ■ clumsiness or unsteadiness ■ loss of appetite ■ pain, numbness, or tingling in hands or feet ■ seizures ■ muscle twitching ■ personality changes ■ nausea or vomiting ■ fever ■ rash ■ swollen lymph glands	**Urgent** Get in touch with your doctor immediately.
dark urine ■ yellowing of eyes or skin ■ ringing in ears ■ memory problems ■ euphoria ■ dizziness ■ upset stomach	**May be serious** Check with your doctor as soon as possible.
dry mouth ■ male breast swelling	If symptoms are disturbing or persist, let your doctor know.

STORAGE INSTRUCTIONS

Store in a cool, dark place (not in a bathroom medicine cabinet).

STOPPING OR INTERRUPTING THERAPY

This medicine should be taken without interruption for the full length of time prescribed by your doctor, even if you begin to feel better. You may have to take isoniazid for one to two years to clear up your tuberculosis infection. It is very important not to miss any doses. If you do miss a dose, take it as soon as possible. If it is almost time for your next dose, skip the missed dose and resume your regular schedule. Do not take two doses at the same time.

SPECIAL CONSIDERATIONS FOR THOSE OVER SIXTY-FIVE

None.

CONDITION: **TUBERCULOSIS**

CATEGORY: **ANTITUBERCULOSIS DRUGS**

GENERIC (CHEMICAL) NAME	BRAND (TRADE) NAME	DOSAGE FORMS AND STRENGTHS
Rifampin	RIFADIN RIMACTANE	Capsules: 150, 300 mg Capsules: 300 mg

DRUG PROFILE

Rifampin is an antibiotic, which both kills and prevents the growth of new bacteria. For the treatment of tuberculosis, it is usually given in combination with another antituberculosis medicine. Rifampin may also be prescribed for a person who is a carrier of meningitis bacteria, even if that person does not have any symptoms of disease, to prevent the spread of meningitis. It is not used for the treatment of meningitis.

BEFORE USING THIS DRUG

Let your doctor know *IF*

You have ever had allergic reactions or other problems with ■ rifampin.

You have ever had any of the following medical problems: ■ alcoholism ■ liver disease.

You are taking any of the following medicines: ■ other medicines for tuberculosis ■ acetaminophen ■ anticoagulants (blood thinners) ■ corticosteroids ■ medicine for diabetes ■ theophylline or related medicine (medicine for asthma) ■ medicine for abnormal heart rhythms ■ medicine for cancer ■ thyroid hormone ■ digitalis (heart medicine) ■ medicine for seizures ■ estrogens or progestins (female hormones) ■ medicine for fungal infections ■ cyclosporine ■ probenecid (medicine for gout) ■ dapsone (medicine for leprosy) ■ beta-blockers (medicine for chest pain or high blood pressure).

SPECIAL RESTRICTIONS WHILE TAKING THIS DRUG

FOOD AND DRUG INTERACTIONS

Other Drugs	Do not take this drug within six hours of the time you take aminosalicylate (another medicine for tuberculosis).
Foods and Beverages	Take this drug on an empty stomach, at least one hour before or two hours after meals.
Alcohol	Avoid alcohol while taking this medicine.

No special restrictions on smoking.

DAILY LIVING

Examinations or Tests	It is important for you to keep all appointments with your doctor, even if you feel well, so that your progress can be checked. Periodic blood tests may be required.
Other Precautions	It is normal for this drug to cause your urine, stool, saliva, sputum, sweat, and tears to turn reddish orange or reddish brown. Since discoloration of the tears may permanently stain soft contact lenses, it is best to avoid wearing soft lenses while you are on this drug. You may continue to wear hard contact lenses.
Helpful Hints	If this medicine upsets your stomach, ask your doctor if you can take it with food.
	If you are unable to swallow capsules, you may open the capsules and mix the contents with applesauce or jelly; you might also ask your pharmacist to make up a liquid preparation for you.

No special restrictions on driving, exertion and exercise, sun exposure, or exposure to excessive heat or cold.

POSSIBLE SIDE EFFECTS

Although this list of adverse effects may seem somewhat intimidating, keep in mind that some are quite rare. Of course, should these or any other problems arise while you are on medication, it is always a good idea to consult your doctor.

IF YOU DEVELOP

difficulty in breathing ■ wheezing ■ flulike symptoms (cough, fever, body aches) ■ dizziness ■ tiredness or weakness ■ headache ■ bloody or cloudy urine ■ decreased urination ■ yellowing of eyes or skin ■ bleeding or bruising ■ sore throat ■ nausea or vomiting ■ loss of appetite

WHAT TO DO

Urgent: Stop taking the drug and get in touch with your doctor immediately.

reddish-orange or reddish-brown discoloration of urine, stool, saliva, sputum, sweat, or tears ■ stomach cramps ■ diarrhea ■ sore mouth or tongue ■ skin redness, rash, or itching

If symptoms are disturbing or persist, let your doctor know.

STORAGE INSTRUCTIONS

Store in a cool, dark place (not in a bathroom medicine cabinet). If your medicine is in a liquid form, it should be kept in the refrigerator, but make sure that it does not freeze. If the color, appearance, or taste of the medicine changes or if the expiration date has passed, discard it immediately. If you are uncertain whether your medicine is all right, consult your pharmacist or doctor.

STOPPING OR INTERRUPTING THERAPY

Rifampin should be taken without interruption for the full length of time prescribed by your doctor (sometimes as long as a year or two), even if you begin to feel better. This will ensure that the tuberculosis clears up completely. If, after two or three weeks, your symptoms either do not improve or worsen, contact your doctor. Be careful not to miss any doses because an irregular dosing schedule may lead to more frequent and serious side effects. If you do miss a dose, take it as soon as possible. If it is almost time for your next dose, skip the missed dose and resume your regular schedule. Do not take two doses at the same time.

SPECIAL CONSIDERATIONS FOR THOSE OVER SIXTY-FIVE

None.

Chapter 10
Disorders of the Skin

SKIN PROBLEMS AND AGING

Skin is much more than just the package we come in. It is, in fact, the body's largest organ, playing key roles in temperature regulation, immunity, and blood circulation.

Like other organs, the skin may be subject to various disorders. Unfortunately, skin problems tend to multiply with age; in one study, two-thirds of people older than seventy had at least one skin problem requiring a doctor's attention.

WHY SKIN CHANGES

Among the normal changes that the skin may undergo over the years are the following:

• Gradually, less sweat and protective oil are secreted by the glands, causing the skin to dry out. The chief result can be itchiness. (One welcome result of reduced sweating, however, is diminished body odor.)

• The inner, structural layer of the skin, the dermis, which contains collagen and elastic fibers, gradually becomes thinner and more fragile. This causes a loss of elasticity and paves the way for wrinkles. (Some doctors prescribe an acne medicine, tretinoin, to decrease skin wrinkling. This agent is described on pages 681–684.)

The loss of elasticity also undermines the support for the small blood vessels that feed the skin. Results can include blue "lakes" of dilated veins (especially around the face, lips, and ears); spider-shaped clusters of vessels on the face, neck, or hands (telangiectasia); and a tendency to bruise.

• The skin becomes more permeable, allowing substances that can irritate or cause allergic reactions to penetrate more readily.

• Changes in the skin's pigmentation can occur with age. "Lentigos," flat brown patches typically found on the face and hands, are a common problem. Such spots are very sensitive to sunlight, which makes them darker.

• Hair growth may also change with aging, resulting in a loss of hair on the scalp. Applying a drug called minoxidil (which, interestingly enough, is a blood-pressure–lowering medicine) to the scalp may stimulate new hair growth, though this drug is not a panacea for baldness. As of this writing, topical minoxidil has not been cleared by the Food and Drug Administration as a hair loss remedy, but you might want to talk with your doctor about the drug's availability and its benefits and risks.

ITCHING

By far the most common symptom that can develop in the skin is itching, or pruritus. It's an unwelcome feature of many of the skin conditions described in the medical guides in this chapter. It can also be a by-product of diseases affecting other parts of the body, including kidney disease, liver disease, and cancer. Itching, however, may simply result from the drying that occurs as skin ages.

Once itching begins, a number of things can make it worse, including exposure of the skin to dry air, contact with irritating or prickly surfaces such as wool, and excessive washing with soap. In addition, anything that dilates the blood vessels, including coffee and alcohol, can increase the blood flow to an itching region and intensify the sensation. Giving in to the impulse to scratch irritates the skin further and leads to more itching; excessive scratching can also open the way to infection.

The first defense against itching—and scratching—is to keep the skin from drying out in the first place. Especially in the winter months, with cold dry air outdoors and hot dry air indoors, make use of moisturizing cream or lotion. At night, turn down the heat and use a humidifier or put pans of water on the radiator.

When you bathe, use a mild soap, such as Dove or Neutrogena. If itchiness develops, don't use soap at all. Bath oils can help moisturize the skin, but at the price of making the tub slippery. Better to do your moisturizing after bathing, by applying such products as Eucerin cream or lotion, Keri lotion, or Neutrogena Emulsion to help lock in moisture.

If dry skin leads to itching, your doctor may prescribe an antihistamine (see the drug charts on pages 684–689) or crotamiton cream or lotion (see the drug chart on page 690). Cool compresses can help soothe a region that has become inflamed from scratching. White petrolatum or hydrogenated vegetable oil with menthol may also help soothe the skin. Avoid creams and sprays containing such anesthetics as benzocaine because they can set the stage for allergic skin reactions.

Let your doctor know if itching continues to be a problem, especially if discoloration or skin eruptions occur. Your doctor may want to reevaluate whether there could be a hidden cause that needs attention.

STASIS DERMATITIS

One skin condition that occurs mainly in older people is stasis dermatitis, or eczema on the legs. Symptoms include red, itchy, raised patches on the legs that may ooze fluid and become crusty. People with stasis dermatitis may have other conditions related to poor blood flow in the legs, such as varicose veins or phlebitis (painful inflammation of a leg vein).

If you have circulation problems in your legs, try to avoid sitting or standing too long in any one position. When you sit or lie down, keep your legs elevated above the level of your hips. Your doctor may advise you to wear support hose, elastic bandages, or pressure stockings to help keep blood from collecting in your legs.

Stasis dermatitis is not a condition you should handle on your own. Your doctor will probably recommend that you use a steroid cream to quell the inflammation (see the drug chart on pages 690–695). Another medicine that may be prescribed is a topical antibiotic, especially if the skin is broken in the affected area (see pages 695–697).

AVOIDING SKIN PROBLEMS

The most important thing you can do to avoid skin damage is to stay out of the sun. When you do spend time outdoors, use a highly protective sunscreen lotion with an SPF (Sun Protection Factor) of at least 15.

Also, avoid prolonged soaking and contact with soaps and detergents. Wear gloves and long sleeves when engaged in hobbies or other activities that could expose you to irritating chemicals. If you need to use an adhesive bandage, coat the skin with one of the new "liquid bandages" first, or ask your pharmacist about bandages with mild adhesive; the stronger adhesives can damage the top layer of skin.

CONDITION: **MISCELLANEOUS SKIN CHANGES**

CATEGORY: **VITAMIN A DERIVATIVES**

GENERIC (CHEMICAL) NAME	BRAND (TRADE) NAME	DOSAGE FORMS AND STRENGTHS
Tretinoin	RETIN-A	Cream: 0.05%, 0.1% Gel: 0.025%, 0.01% Liquid: 0.05%

DRUG PROFILE

Tretinoin, a derivative of vitamin A, is applied to the skin to treat acne. Some doctors also prescribe tretinoin to decrease skin wrinkling, though this use has not yet been approved by the Food and Drug Administration.

BEFORE USING THIS DRUG

Let your doctor know *IF*

You have ever had allergic reactions or other problems with ■ tretinoin ■ vitamin A–like preparations.

You have ever had any of the following medical problems: ■ eczema ■ sunburn.

You are using any of the following medicines: ■ any other skin medicines ■ any preparation containing a peeling agent (such as benzoyl peroxide, resorcinol, salicylic acid, or sulfur) ■ abrasive soaps or cleansers.

SPECIAL RESTRICTIONS WHILE TAKING THIS DRUG

FOOD AND DRUG INTERACTIONS

Other Drugs	To avoid skin irritation, do not apply any of the following types of products on the same areas you are applying tretinoin: other topical medicines including those for acne, abrasive soaps or cleansers, alcohol-

containing preparations, preparations containing peeling agents (such as benzoyl peroxide, resorcinol, salicylic acid, or sulfur), soaps or cosmetics that dry the skin, or medicated cosmetics.

No special restrictions on foods and beverages, alcohol use, or smoking.

DAILY LIVING

Sun Exposure

Skin areas being treated with tretinoin may be more prone to sunburn. Avoid exposure of affected areas to sunlight, including sunlamps. If you must be exposed to the sun, wear protective clothing or apply sunscreen to exposed skin surfaces before going outdoors. Let your doctor know if you should accidentally develop a sunburn.

Excessive Cold

Your skin may become more sensitive to wind and cold temperature while you are using this medicine. It's a good idea to wear protective clothing; let your doctor know if your skin does become windburned or irritated.

Examinations or Tests

It is important for you to keep all appointments with your doctor so your progress can be checked.

Other Precautions

Follow your doctor's instructions and read the patient information brochure carefully. Overuse can cause skin irritation.

Your condition may seem to get worse during the first two or three weeks of treatment. Do not stop using this medicine unless your skin becomes severely irritated or your condition worsens and you've checked with your doctor. Definite improvements may not be seen for three to six weeks.

Be careful not to get this medicine in your eyes or mouth, around your nose, or on any mucous membranes or open wounds.

You may experience a mild stinging sensation or feeling of warmth after application of this medicine.

Helpful Hints

Wash your skin with a mild or hypoallergenic soap and warm water and pat dry. Allow twenty to thirty minutes before applying this medicine to make sure your skin has dried completely. Do not wash your face more than two or three times a day. Avoid using shaving lotions, astringents, and perfume, since these products tend to irritate treated skin. Nonmedicated cosmetics may be used.

If you are using the cream or gel form, put on enough medicine to cover the affected areas and then rub it in gently. Formation of dry flakes while applying the gel indicates that you are using too much. If you are using the solution, apply enough medicine with your fingertips, a gauze pad, or a cotton swab to cover the affected areas. If your skin becomes irritated from this medicine, try using a little less or stop applying it for a day or two until the irritation subsides.

No special restrictions on driving, exertion and exercise, or exposure to excessive heat.

POSSIBLE SIDE EFFECTS

Although this list of adverse effects may seem somewhat intimidating, keep in mind that some are quite rare. Of course, should these or any other problems arise while you are on medication, it is always a good idea to consult your doctor.

IF YOU DEVELOP

severe burning (from sun) or skin redness ■ swelling ■ blisters ■ crusting, darkening, or lightening of treated areas

WHAT TO DO

May be serious Check with your doctor as soon as possible.

| feeling of warmth in treated areas ■ skin peeling ■ mild stinging | If symptoms are disturbing or persist, let your doctor know. |

STORAGE INSTRUCTIONS

Store in a cool, dark place (not in a bathroom medicine cabinet). If your medicine is in a liquid form, make sure that it does not freeze.

STOPPING OR INTERRUPTING THERAPY

If you miss a dose of this medicine, skip the missed dose and resume your regular schedule.

SPECIAL CONSIDERATIONS FOR THOSE OVER SIXTY-FIVE

None.

CONDITION: **ITCHING**

CATEGORY: **ANTIHISTAMINES**

GENERIC (CHEMICAL) NAME	BRAND (TRADE) NAME	DOSAGE FORMS AND STRENGTHS
Diphenhydramine hydrochloride	BENADRYL	Capsules: 25, 50 mg Elixir: 12.5 mg per tsp
Hydroxyzine	ATARAX	Syrup: 10 mg per tsp Tablets: 10, 25, 50, 100 mg
	VISTARIL	Capsules: 25, 50, 100 mg Suspension: 25 mg per tsp

DRUG PROFILE

When you are exposed to a substance to which you are allergic, a chemical called histamine is released into the bloodstream and produces the itchy, watery eyes; runny nose; and rashes that are typical of an allergic reaction. Antihistamines work by blocking the action of histamine. They are used to treat allergies as well as to relieve the symptoms of a cold.

For complete information on these drugs, see pages 633–638.

CONDITION: **ITCHING**

CATEGORY: **ANTIHISTAMINES**

GENERIC (CHEMICAL) NAME	BRAND (TRADE) NAME	DOSAGE FORMS AND STRENGTHS
Trimeprazine tartrate	TEMARIL	Controlled-release capsules: 5 mg Syrup: 2.5 mg per tsp Tablets: 2.5 mg

DRUG PROFILE

Trimeprazine is an antihistamine (see chapter 9, Disorders of the Respiratory System) that is used to relieve the itching associated with hives, rashes, and other skin conditions. When you are exposed to a substance to which you are allergic, a chemical called histamine is released into the bloodstream and produces the symptoms, including itching, that are typical of an allergic reaction. Antihistamines work by blocking the action of histamines.

BEFORE USING THIS DRUG

Let your doctor know *IF*

You have ever had allergic reactions or other problems with ■ trimeprazine ■ other antihistamines ■ phenothiazines (tranquilizers or medicine for nausea).

You have ever had any of the following medical problems: ■ asthma or other lung disease ■ respiratory infections, such as pneumonia ■ heart or blood vessel disease ■ high blood pressure ■ intestinal or urinary blockage ■ other urinary problems ■ enlarged prostate ■ liver disease ■ breast cancer ■ ulcers ■ glaucoma ■ seizures ■ kidney disease ■ overactive thyroid ■ mental illness.

You are taking any of the following medicines: ■ other antihistamines ■ aspirin or aspirinlike medicine ■ medicine for cancer ■ medicine for asthma ■ antibiotics ■ barbiturates ■ muscle relaxants ■ sleep medicines ■ narcotics or other prescription pain-killers ■ tranquilizers ■ medicine for nausea and vomiting ■ medicine for depression ■ diuretics (water pills) ■ medicine for high blood pressure ■ medicine to dilate the blood vessels ■ medicine for seizures ■ antacids ■ appetite suppressants ■ medicine for Parkinson's disease ■ timolol, nadolol, propranolol, metoprolol, atenolol, pindolol, acebutolol, or labetalol (beta-blockers) ■ medicine for hay fever, coughs, or colds ■ vitamin C ■ cimetidine (medicine for ulcers) ■ Antabuse (used in the treatment of alcoholism) ■ digoxin, digitoxin, or digitalis (heart medicines).

SPECIAL RESTRICTIONS WHILE TAKING THIS DRUG

FOOD AND DRUG INTERACTIONS

Other Drugs	Do not take any other drugs, including over-the-counter (OTC) drugs, before checking with your doctor. This drug increases the effects of other drugs that depress the central nervous system, such as other antihistamines; medicine for hay fever, allergies, or colds; sleep medicines; tranquilizers; narcotics or other prescription pain-killers; muscle relaxants; and medicine for seizures. Antihistamines may mask ringing in the ears caused by aspirin. Let your doctor know if you are taking aspirin or aspirinlike drugs.
Alcohol	This drug increases the effect of alcohol, a central nervous system depressant. Avoid alcohol unless your doctor has approved its use.

No special restrictions on foods and beverages or smoking.

DAILY LIVING

Driving	This drug may cause dizziness, drowiness, weakness, loss of alertness, or blurred vision. Be careful

when driving, operating household appliances, or doing any other tasks that require alertness until you know how this drug affects you.

Exertion and Exercise	This drug may cause you to sweat less than normally. Sweating is your body's natural way of cooling down, and not sweating enough can be dangerous. Use caution not to become overheated when you exercise or exert yourself.
Sun Exposure	When this drug is used for a long time, discoloration of the skin may occur, especially in those areas exposed to the sun. It is a good idea to avoid prolonged sun exposure and to apply a sunscreen to exposed skin surfaces before going outdoors.
Excessive Heat	See "Exertion and Exercise"; use caution during hot weather, since overexertion may result in heat stroke. Avoid extremely hot baths or saunas.
Excessive Cold	This drug may disturb your body's ability to regulate its temperature; use care during very cold weather and make sure all exposed parts are well covered. Also, do not swim in extremely cold water.
Examinations or Tests	If you are taking this drug on a long-term basis (several months), it is important for you to keep all appointments with your doctor so that your progress can be checked.
Other Precautions	Tell any doctor or dentist you consult that you are taking this medicine, especially if you will be undergoing any type of surgery. If you are going to be tested for allergies, tell the doctor in charge that you are taking this drug, since it affects the results of allergy tests.

If you are going to have an X-ray examination of the nervous system that requires an injection into the spinal canal, be sure to tell your doctor that you are taking this drug. Because this drug increases the chances of seizures during such a procedure, it will need to be discontinued a short time before and after the examination.

Helpful Hints

If this drug upsets your stomach, taking it with milk, meals, a snack, or water should help.

If your mouth or throat feels dry, chewing sugarless gum or sucking ice chips or sugarless hard candy will help.

Antihistamines sometimes cause insomnia, which can be avoided by taking your last dose several hours before bedtime; check with your doctor about the best dosage schedule for you.

You may feel dizzy, light-headed, or faint when starting out on this type of drug. This should disappear in a few weeks or so. Getting up slowly from a reclining or sitting position should help.

POSSIBLE SIDE EFFECTS

Although this list of adverse effects may seem somewhat intimidating, keep in mind that some are quite rare. Of course, should these or any other problems arise while you are on medication, it is always a good idea to consult your doctor.

IF YOU DEVELOP

seizures ■ unsteadiness or clumsiness ■ severe drowsiness ■ fainting ■ flushing ■ hallucinations ■ difficulty in breathing ■ dilated pupils ■ sleeplessness ■ confusion ■ difficulty in speech ■ difficulty in swallowing ■ nervousness or restlessness ■ irritability ■ excitement or other mood changes ■ muscle weakness or severe muscle stiffness ■ tremors ■ tightness in chest ■ irregular or fast

WHAT TO DO

Urgent Get in touch with your doctor immediately.

heartbeat ■ increased sweating ■ incontinence ■ swelling in throat ■ shuffling walk ■ jerky movements of head and face

fever ■ flulike symptoms (cough, fever, or body aches) ■ sore throat ■ bleeding or bruising ■ tiredness ■ blurred vision or other visual disturbances ■ swelling of hands or feet ■ pain or difficulty in urination ■ rigidity ■ posture changes ■ yellowing of eyes or skin ■ slow, monotonous speech ■ increased skin sensitivity to sunlight ■ nausea or vomiting ■ ringing in the ears ■ nightmares ■ rash ■ upset stomach ■ stomach pain	**May be serious** Check with your doctor as soon as possible.
drowsiness ■ dizziness or light-headedness ■ decreased alertness ■ loss of appetite ■ headache ■ "high" feeling ■ dry mouth, nose, or throat ■ increased appetite ■ weight gain ■ diarrhea ■ constipation ■ diminished sexual desire ■ difficulty in ejaculating ■ stuffy nose ■ thickened phlegm ■ decreased sweating ■ anxiety ■ depression ■ breast pain or swelling ■ mouth sores ■ redness or whiteness inside the mouth ■ cracking of lips and corners of mouth ■ tongue changes ■ loosening of teeth	If symptoms are disturbing or persist, let your doctor know.

STORAGE INSTRUCTIONS

Store in a cool, dark place (not in a bathroom medicine cabinet). If your medicine is in a liquid form, make sure that it does not freeze.

STOPPING OR INTERRUPTING THERAPY

If you miss a dose of this medicine, take it as soon as possible. If it is almost time for your next dose, skip the missed dose and resume your regular schedule. Do not take two doses at the same time.

SPECIAL CONSIDERATIONS FOR THOSE OVER SIXTY-FIVE

Older people taking trimeprazine may be more prone to develop confusion, pain or difficulty in urination, dizziness, drowsiness, fainting, or dry mouth. Nightmares, restlessness, and irritability are also more apt to occur in those over sixty-five. Thus, doctors may start people over sixty-five on a lower dose.

CONDITION: **ITCHING**

CATEGORY: **OTHER DRUGS FOR ITCHING**

GENERIC (CHEMICAL) NAME	BRAND (TRADE) NAME	DOSAGE FORMS AND STRENGTHS
Crotamiton	EURAX	Cream: 10% Lotion: 10%

DRUG PROFILE

Crotamiton is used to treat scabies infestations of the skin. This medicine cures, but does not prevent, scabies. Crotamiton is also sometimes used to relieve severe itching.

For complete information on this drug, see pages 715–717.

CONDITION: **STASIS DERMATITIS, RASH, AND INFLAMMATION**

CATEGORY: **TOPICAL CORTICOSTEROIDS**

GENERIC (CHEMICAL) NAME	BRAND (TRADE) NAME	DOSAGE FORMS AND STRENGTHS
Amcinonide	CYCLOCORT	Cream: 0.1% Ointment: 0.1%
Betamethasone dipropionate	DIPROLENE	Cream: 0.05% Ointment: 0.05%
	DIPROSONE	Cream: 0.05% Lotion: 0.05% Ointment: 0.05% Spray: 0.1%

Betamethasone valerate	VALISONE	Cream: 0.01%, 0.1% Lotion: 0.1% Ointment: 0.1%
Clocortolone pivalate	CLODERM	Cream: 0.1%
Desonide	TRIDESILON	Cream: 0.05% Ointment: 0.05%
Desoximetasone	TOPICORT	Cream: 0.25% Gel: 0.05% Ointment: 0.25%
	TOPICORT LP	Cream: 0.05%
Dexamethasone	AEROSEB-DEX	Spray: 0.01%
Diflorasone diacetate	FLORONE	Cream: 0.05% Ointment: 0.05%
Fluocinolone acetonide	SYNALAR	Cream: 0.025%, 0.01% Ointment: 0.025% Solution: 0.01%
	SYNALAR-HP	Cream: 0.2%
	SYNEMOL	Cream: 0.025%
Fluocinonide	LIDEX	Cream: 0.05% Gel: 0.05% Ointment: 0.05% Solution: 0.05%
	LIDEX-E	Cream: 0.05%
Flurandrenolide	CORDRAN	Lotion: 0.05% Ointment: 0.025%, 0.05%
	CORDRAN SP	Cream: 0.025%, 0.05%

Halcinonide	HALCIDERM	Cream: 0.1%
	HALOG	Cream: 0.025%, 0.1%
		Ointment: 0.1%
		Solution: 0.1%
	HALOG-E	Cream: 0.1%
Hydrocortisone	AEROSEB-HC	Spray: 0.5%
	CORT-DOME	Cream: 0.25%, 0.5%, 1%
		Lotion: 0.125%, 0.25%, 0.5%, 1%
	HYTONE	Cream: 0.5%, 1%, 2.5%
		Lotion: 1%, 2.5%
		Ointment: 1%, 2.5%
Hydrocortisone acetate	CORTEF ACETATE	Ointment: 1%, 2.5%
Hydrocortisone valerate	WESTCORT	Cream: 0.2%
		Ointment: 0.2%
Polymyxin B sulfate, bacitracin zinc, neomycin sulfate, and hydrocortisone	CORTISPORIN Ointment	Ointment: 5,000 units polymyxin B sulfate, 400 units bacitracin zinc, 5 mg neomycin sulfate, and 10 mg hydrocortisone per g
Polymyxin B sulfate, neomycin sulfate, and hydrocortisone acetate	CORTISPORIN Cream	Cream: 10,000 units polymyxin B sulfate, 5 mg neomycin sulfate, and 5 mg hydrocortisone acetate per g
Triamcinolone acetonide	ARISTOCORT	Cream: 0.025%, 0.1%, 0.5%
		Ointment: 0.1%, 0.5%

| ARISTOCORT A | Cream: 0.025%, 0.1%, 0.5% |
| | Ointment: 0.1%, 0.5% |

Many brands of topical hydrocortisone are sold over the counter as well.

DRUG PROFILE

Topical corticosteroids are applied directly to the skin to help alleviate the pain, itching, and swelling of rashes and various other skin conditions. They work by blocking the inflammatory response of the skin to irritations, infections, and allergic reactions.

BEFORE USING THIS DRUG

Let your doctor know *IF*

You have ever had allergic reactions or other problems with ■ any corticosteroids ■ any antibiotics.

You have ever had any of the following medical problems: ■ any other skin problems on the area being treated ■ circulation problems ■ current viral or skin infection, such as chickenpox or herpes ■ tuberculosis ■ perforated ear drum, if the drug is being used to treat an external ear infection.

SPECIAL RESTRICTIONS WHILE TAKING THIS DRUG

FOOD AND DRUG INTERACTIONS

No special restrictions on other drugs, foods and beverages, alcohol use, or smoking.

DAILY LIVING

| Examinations or Tests | If you are using this drug for a prolonged period of time, it is important for you to keep all appointments with your doctor so that your progress can be checked. |

Other Precautions

Use this drug exactly as instructed by your doctor. Do not use it for longer than prescribed or for any other condition than the one for which it has been prescribed.

Do not cover the treated area of skin with bandages or other material unless your doctor tells you to do so. If you have been instructed to make a dressing, follow directions carefully.

Skin reactions are more likely to occur with long-term therapy with topical corticosteroids or if you are using a dressing. Occasionally, skin reactions may occur after therapy has been stopped; let your doctor know if this occurs. Some topical corticosteroids may cause a mild, brief tingling sensation on the area to which they are applied.

No special restrictions on driving, exertion and exercise, sun exposure, or exposure to excessive heat or cold.

POSSIBLE SIDE EFFECTS

Although this list of adverse effects may seem somewhat intimidating, keep in mind that some are quite rare. Of course, should these or any other problems arise while you are on medication, it is always a good idea to consult your doctor.

IF YOU DEVELOP

Signs of further irritation or infection: itching, redness, swelling, blisters, peeling, pain, or any symptoms not present before using the drug

With combination drugs only: hearing problems

WHAT TO DO

May be serious Check with your doctor as soon as possible.

hair growth ■ bruising ■ purplish lines on skin, especially on face, armpits, and groin ■ acne or other facial eruptions ■ whitening of skin ■ inflammation of hair follicles ■ unusual roundness of face	If symptoms are disturbing or persist, let your doctor know.

STORAGE INSTRUCTIONS

Store in a cool, dark place (not in a bathroom medicine cabinet).

STOPPING OR INTERRUPTING THERAPY

If you are using this medicine on a regular schedule and you miss a dose, apply it as soon as possible. If it is almost time for your next dose, skip the missed dose and resume your regular schedule.

SPECIAL CONSIDERATIONS FOR THOSE OVER SIXTY-FIVE

Steroids may cause thinning of the skin, which may be a particular problem for older people whose skin has already grown thinner with age. Doctors may recommend that people over sixty-five apply this medicine less frequently.

CONDITION: **BACTERIAL INFECTIONS**

CATEGORY: **TOPICAL ANTIBIOTICS**

GENERIC (CHEMICAL) NAME	BRAND (TRADE) NAME	DOSAGE FORMS AND STRENGTHS
Gentamicin sulfate	GARAMYCIN	Cream: 0.1% Ointment: 0.1%
Polymyxin B sulfate and bacitracin zinc	POLYSPORIN	Ointment: 10,000 units polymyxin B sulfate and 500 units of bacitracin zinc per g

This type of medicine is available under other brand names; milder strengths are available over the counter.

DRUG PROFILE

Gentamicin works by interfering with bacteria's ability to manufacture protein. Polymyxin B alters the membrane of the bacterial cell so that the bacteria lose essential nutrients. Bacitracin interferes with the bacteria's ability to form new protective cell walls.

BEFORE USING THIS DRUG

Let your doctor know *IF*

You have ever had allergic reactions or other problems with ■ gentamicin ■ polymyxin B sulfate ■ bacitracin zinc ■ aminoglycoside antibiotics ■ preservatives.

You are taking any of the following medicines: ■ other antibiotics.

SPECIAL RESTRICTIONS WHILE TAKING THIS DRUG

FOOD AND DRUG INTERACTIONS

No special restrictions on other drugs, foods and beverages, alcohol use, or smoking.

DAILY LIVING

Precautions	If your skin problem becomes worse or does not improve after a week, check with your doctor.
Helpful Hints	Apply the cream or ointment exactly as instructed by your doctor, using a sterile gauze pad to cover the dressing if indicated. Be careful to avoid contaminating the infected area.

No special restrictions on driving, exertion and exercise, sun exposure, or exposure to excessive heat or cold.

POSSIBLE SIDE EFFECTS

Although this list of adverse effects may seem somewhat intimidating, keep in mind that some are quite rare. Of course should these or any other problems arise while you are on medication, it is always a good idea to consult your doctor.

IF YOU DEVELOP	WHAT TO DO
With preparations containing bacitracin zinc only: rash ■ swelling of lips and face ■ increased sweating ■ tightness in chest ■ extreme dizziness ■ fainting ■ difficulty in breathing	**Urgent** Get in touch with your doctor immediately.
itching, redness, swelling, or other signs of skin irritation that you didn't have before you used the drug	**May be serious** Check with your doctor as soon as possible.

STORAGE INSTRUCTIONS

Store in a cool, dark place (not in a bathroom medicine cabinet).

STOPPING OR INTERRUPTING THERAPY

This medicine should be taken without interruption for the full time prescribed by your doctor, even if your symptoms improve or disappear. If you are using this medicine on a regular schedule and you miss a dose, apply it as soon as possible. If it is almost time for your next dose, skip the missed dose and resume your regular schedule.

SPECIAL CONSIDERATIONS FOR THOSE OVER SIXTY-FIVE

None.

SKIN INFECTIONS AND INFESTATIONS

Of all the uncomfortable and un-sightly ailments the skin is heir to, few are more annoying than the rashes and lesions caused by fungi, yeasts, and mites. Although poor hygiene is commonly blamed for these infections and infestations, the real cause is con-tact with someone or something that harbors an organism capable of grow-ing on or living in human skin. Para-sites and fungi may spread more rap-idly when people are crowded together, but unsanitary conditions are certainly *not* prerequisites for con-tracting any of these organisms.

With a few notable exceptions—such as tinea capitis, a fungal infec-tion of the scalp that mostly affects children—these problems occur with similar frequency in all age groups. The only skin infection that is partic-ularly common in older people is shin-gles, or herpes zoster.

SHINGLES

Unlike other infections mentioned in this guide, shingles is caused by a virus—the varicella-zoster virus, which also causes chickenpox. The varicella virus is one of the herpes viruses, which have the unique ability to lie dormant in the body after an initial infection and become reacti-vated months or even years later.

Scientists believe that varicella vi-ruses stay in certain nerve cells after causing chickenpox and may not cause further problems for long peri-ods of time. Sometimes, however, these dormant viruses become active, inflaming the nerve and causing an outbreak of shingles. No one knows precisely what reactivates the virus, but certain factors such as weakened immunity, trauma to the skin, and spinal surgery often precipitate out-breaks. Two-thirds of shingles cases occur in people over fifty.

Shingles usually begins with pain and itching along the course of the nerve in which the virus has become reactivated. The pain may be constant or intermittent, and it is sometimes accompanied by headache and fever. Several days later, a band of tiny, closely grouped blisters erupt on one side of the body. Seven to ten days after they appear, the blisters dry out and form scablike crusts, which re-main on the skin for two or three weeks. The pain of shingles some-times persists for months or years (this is called post-herpetic neuralgia) after the crusts have fallen off.

Until recently, treatment of shingles was limited to pain relief in the form of analgesics, cool compresses, and calamine lotion. While these measures may still be helpful, the current main-stay of treatment is an antiviral drug called acyclovir. (See the drug chart on pages 720–722.) This drug, which may shorten the shingles outbreak, may be given by mouth or intrave-nously. Treatment usually begins at the first sign of an outbreak and con-tinues until all the lesions have dried. After a shingles outbreak, the varicella virus returns to its dormant state, so a second outbreak may occur.

If you have a shingles outbreak on your face, particularly extending from the side of your nose to your forehead, your doctor may advise hospitalization and intravenous treatment with acyclovir. Shingles in this area can affect the eye, causing serious complications.

FUNGAL INFECTIONS

Fungal infections, which are also called ringworm because of the circular, ridged lesions they produce, are caused by organisms called dermatophytes. People can be infected by a number of different dermatophyte species on different parts of the body.

Tinea Corporis This condition is a fungal infection occurring on any part of the body besides the hands, feet, scalp, beard, or groin. People with such illnesses as leukemia and diabetes run the greatest risk of developing this infection. The rash consists of reddened, itchy, round splotches that may be covered with tiny blisters or bumps. Occasionally, if the rash has been scratched, a bacterial infection may take hold, causing more inflammation and leaking of pus or other fluid. Tinea corporis sometimes clears up on its own, though doctors usually advise use of some soothing ointmeat or lotion. Severe cases are treated with an oral antifungal drug, griseofulvin, which must be taken for four to six weeks. (See the drug chart on pages 705–707.) Doctors will also treat any secondary bacterial infection with antibiotics, such as erythromycin. (See the drug chart on pages 723–726.) The rash may clear more quickly if the skin is kept cool and dry.

Tinea Pedis This condition, also known as athlete's foot, is the most common fungal infection of the skin. Typically, it causes a dry, scaly rash on the feet, starting between the toes and spreading to the soles. Often, tiny blisters that itch, sting, and drain appear, causing inflammation. Some outbreaks of athlete's foot are brief and self-limiting; others—particularly the dry, scaly kind—can last for years despite treatment.

Several over-the-counter and prescription drugs are available for treating athlete's foot. Antifungal ointments, including clotrimazole, haloprogin, and miconazole (see the drug charts on pages 702–704, 708–710, and 713–715), may be helpful, but in severe cases, doctors often prescribe oral griseofulvin. If you have athlete's foot, keep your feet and hands dry and wear well-ventilated shoes and absorbent socks to promote healing.

Tinea Cruris This condition, or jock itch, a fungal infection of the groin, affects men much more often than women. Like athlete's foot, it is frequently caused by a fungus that thrives in warm, moist environments. The rash usually begins in the fold between the buttocks or in the area between the thigh and groin and spreads to cover the upper inner thigh. In men, the skin of the scrotum is almost never affected, which is one of the signs doctors use to distinguish jock itch from other skin infections.

Many doctors recommend treating

jock itch with cool compresses and dusting powder to soothe the itching. Avoiding tightly fitting clothing and wet bathing suits will also help the rash heal. Active, painful infections may require treatment with oral griseofulvin for four to five weeks.

Onychomycosis Fungi and other organisms sometimes take hold in the finger- and toenails, causing an infection called onychomycosis. This infection, which causes the nails to become discolored and crumbly, is often difficult to treat, and recurrences are common. It occurs most often in nails that are already fragile because of injury or because of a generalized illness such as a circulatory disorder. Some doctors treat onychomycosis by removing the diseased nail and prescribing griseofulvin for five to six months if fingernails are involved, or at least eighteen months for infected toenails. Older people whose toenails are affected may be advised to forgo drug treatment in favor of a regimen of foot care that will minimize any discomfort.

Actinomycosis Another unusual infection, actinomycosis, sometimes affects older people. This infection develops when an organism that often inhabits the gums, teeth, and tonsils enters oral tissue through decayed teeth, causing abscesses to form along the jawline. (Hence, the disease is often called "lumpy jaw.") This disorder is treated with such antibiotics as penicillin or tetracycline. (See the drug chart on pages 723–726.)

YEAST INFECTIONS

Candida albicans, a yeast that normally lives in the mouth, gastrointestinal tract, and vagina, sometimes causes a moist, red, itchy rash to develop on the body, particularly in areas where skin surfaces rub together—between the buttocks, beneath the breasts, or in the armpit and groins. *Candida albicans* also causes oral and vaginal infections. Obese people and people with diabetes are especially prone to getting yeast infections.

Yeast infections begin with tiny bumps and blisters that break, drain, and become inflamed. A bacterial infection may also occur.

It is important to keep your skin dry and cool if you have a yeast infection, exposing the affected areas to air and dusting them with powder several times during the day. An oral drug called ketoconazole may be prescribed (see the drug chart on pages 710–712), and clotrimazole (see the drug chart on pages 702–704) applied topically may also be helpful.

LICE AND SCABIES

Three types of lice infest the human. Two set up housekeeping in the hair, while the other lives in the seams of clothing.

Head and body lice are grayish-white bugs that feed on human blood, inject saliva into the skin, and lay seven to ten eggs a day. They are transmitted through hats, combs, and brushes, or, in the case of body lice, clothing and bedding. Bites from these lice produce itchy bumps that the infested person often scratches furiously, paving the way for secondary bacterial infection.

Pubic lice, sometimes called crabs because of their round shape and long, slender front legs, operate in much the same manner as head lice. They are usually transmitted through sexual contact but can be passed on clothing or towels. Bites from these bugs produce blue-gray bumps that are also intensely itchy.

Treatment for both kinds of lice involves application of either lindane cream, lotion, or shampoo, or crotamiton cream or lotion. (See the drug charts on pages 715–719.) Two applications are necessary, one to kill existing lice and the other to eradicate newly hatched eggs (known as nits) a week later. Clothing and bedding must be laundered and, in the case of pubic lice, sex partners must also be treated. Additionally, it may be necessary to take an antibiotic, such as erythromycin (see the drug chart on pages 723–724), if a secondary bacterial infection has developed.

Scabies are tiny mites that lay eggs under the skin, most often in the area of the wrists and hands, though the waist, genitalia, elbows, and feet may also be affected. They are usually transmitted through close personal contact or picked up from clothing or bedding.

Scabies mites produce curved ridges and red, itching bumps. The itching is so severe, especially at night, that most infested people scratch enough to cause secondary irritation.

Lindane and crotamiton are also the agents used to treat scabies. Treatment begins with a bath, followed by application of one of the lotions to all skin below the neck. If one member of your family has scabies, your entire household should be treated.

WOUNDS

Any kind of wound—a cut, puncture, burn, abrasion, scratch, or bite—can become infected with bacteria if it is not properly cleaned or if your immune system is weakened. Wash all skin wounds with soap and water and dab them with a disinfectant. For most wounds, this should be sufficient protection against infection. Any bite (animal or human) and all puncture wounds, however, should be cleaned with special care in a doctor's office. After a bite or puncture wound, it is also necessary to get a tetanus booster if you haven't been immunized against tetanus in the past five years.

OUTLOOK

As annoying and unsightly as skin infections and infestations are, they are also highly treatable, both by medical means and other measures. In some cases, such as for shingles, treatment options are expanding, making it even easier to rid yourself of the infection and pain.

CONDITION: **FUNGAL INFECTIONS**

CATEGORY: **ANTIFUNGAL DRUGS**

GENERIC (CHEMICAL) NAME	BRAND (TRADE) NAME	DOSAGE FORMS AND STRENGTHS
Clotrimazole	LOTRIMIN	Cream: 1% Lotion: 1% Solution: 1%
	MYCELEX	Cream: 1% Lozenges: 10 mg Solution: 1%

DRUG PROFILE

Clotrimazole is used to treat fungal infections. It is given in lozenge (troche) form for the treatment of thrush (white mouth). For skin problems, it can be applied topically as a cream, lotion, or solution. This drug works by altering the permeability of the membrane of the fungal cell so that the fungus loses essential nutrients.

BEFORE USING THIS DRUG

Let your doctor know *IF*

You have ever had allergic reactions or other problems with ■ clotrimazole.

You have ever had the following medical problem: ■ liver disease.

SPECIAL RESTRICTIONS WHILE TAKING THIS DRUG

FOOD AND DRUG INTERACTIONS

No special restrictions on other drugs, foods and beverages, alcohol use, or smoking.

DAILY LIVING

Examinations or Tests	It is important for you to keep all appointments with your doctor so that your progress can be checked. Periodic blood tests or stool samples may be required.
Other Precautions	Tell your doctor if your mouth symptoms do not improve within a week, if your skin problems do not improve within four weeks, or if any problem worsens. Keep the topical forms of this medicine away from your eyes.
Helpful Hints	Allow the lozenges to dissolve slowly and completely in your mouth (this may take fifteen to thirty minutes). Continue to swallow your saliva during this time. Do not chew the lozenges or swallow them whole. When using the cream, lotion, or solution form, apply enough to cover both the affected and surrounding skin areas and rub it in gently. Do not cover it with anything else, unless your doctor tells you to. Make sure to keep the affected areas clean and dry, as this will help them heal as well as prevent reinfection.

No special restrictions on driving, exertion and exercise, sun exposure, or exposure to excessive heat or cold.

POSSIBLE SIDE EFFECTS

Although this list of adverse effects may seem somewhat intimidating, keep in mind that some are quite rare. Of course, should these or any other problems arise while you are on medication, it is always a good idea to consult your doctor.

IF YOU DEVELOP	WHAT TO DO
blisters ■ skin redness ■ itching ■ burning or stinging sensation ■ peeling ■ hives ■ irritation ■ any other skin problem not present before taking this drug	**May be serious** Check with your doctor as soon as possible.
nausea or vomiting ■ stomach cramps ■ diarrhea	If symptoms are disturbing or persist, let your doctor know.

STORAGE INSTRUCTIONS

Store in a cool, dark place (not in a bathroom medicine cabinet). If your medicine is in a liquid form, make sure that it does not freeze.

STOPPING OR INTERRUPTING THERAPY

Use this medicine for the full length of time prescribed by your doctor even if your symptoms begin to improve. This will ensure that the infection clears up completely and that your symptoms do not return. If you miss a dose of this medicine, take it as soon as possible. If it is almost time for your next dose, skip the missed dose and resume your regular schedule. Do not take two doses at the same time.

SPECIAL CONSIDERATIONS FOR THOSE OVER SIXTY-FIVE

None.

CONDITION: **FUNGAL INFECTIONS**

CATEGORY: **ANTIFUNGAL DRUGS**

GENERIC (CHEMICAL) NAME	BRAND (TRADE) NAME	DOSAGE FORMS AND STRENGTHS
Griseofulvin	FULVICIN P/G	Tablets: 125, 165, 250, 330 mg
	FULVICIN-U/F	Tablets: 250, 500 mg
	GRIFULVIN V	Suspension: 125 mg per tsp
		Tablets: 250, 500 mg
	GRISACTIN	Capsules: 125, 250 mg
		Tablets: 500 mg
	GRISACTIN ULTRA	Tablets: 125, 250, 330 mg

DRUG PROFILE

Griseofulvin is a medicine taken by mouth to treat fungal infections of the skin, hair, and nails. This drug works by destroying a part of the fungus cell essential for cell division. Your doctor may prescribe a topical antifungal agent to use along with this medicine.

BEFORE USING THIS DRUG

Let your doctor know *IF*

You have ever had allergic reactions or other problems with ■ griseofulvin ■ penicillin ■ penicillamine (medicine for arthritis).

You have ever had any of the following medical problems: ■ liver disease ■ systemic lupus erythematosus ■ porphyria.

You are taking any of the following medicines: ■ anticoagulants (blood thinners) ■ barbiturates ■ tranquilizers ■ primidone or other medicine for seizures.

SPECIAL RESTRICTIONS WHILE TAKING THIS DRUG

FOOD AND DRUG INTERACTIONS

No special restrictions on other drugs, foods and beverages, alcohol use, or smoking.

DAILY LIVING

Sun Exposure	You may become more sensitive to sunlight while you are taking this medicine. Limit your exposure to bright sunlight or sunlamps until you know how you will react, especially if you normally burn easily. If you have a severe reaction, check with your doctor.
Examinations or Tests	It is important for you to keep all appointments with your doctor so that your progress can be checked. Periodic blood tests may be required.
Other Precautions	It may take several weeks or even months to eradicate the fungus completely, especially if the nails are affected.
Helpful Hints	Make sure to keep the affected areas clean and dry, as this will help them heal, as well as prevent reinfection.
	Taking this medicine with or after meals, especially fatty ones, will help its absorption by the stomach and reduce your chance of upset stomach. Check with your doctor if you are on a low-fat diet.

No special restrictions on driving, exertion and exercise, or exposure to excessive heat or cold.

POSSIBLE SIDE EFFECTS

Although this list of adverse effects may seem somewhat intimidating, keep in mind that some are quite rare. Of course, should these or any other problems arise while you are on medication, it is always a good idea to consult your doctor.

IF YOU DEVELOP	WHAT TO DO
rash, hives, or itching	**Urgent** Get in touch with your doctor immediately.
confusion ■ behavior changes ■ numbness in hands or feet ■ soreness or irritation of mouth or tongue ■ white patches inside mouth ■ fever ■ sore throat	**May be serious** Check with your doctor as soon as possible.
headache ■ fatigue ■ dizziness ■ sleeplessness ■ nausea or vomiting ■ increased thirst ■ diarrhea ■ upset stomach ■ increased skin sensitivity to sunlight ■ gas ■ hearing problems	If symptoms are disturbing or persist, let your doctor know.

STORAGE INSTRUCTIONS

Store in a cool, dark place (not in a bathroom medicine cabinet). If your medicine is in a liquid form, make sure that it does not freeze.

STOPPING OR INTERRUPTING THERAPY

Use this medicine for the full length of time prescribed by your doctor, even if your symptoms begin to improve. This will ensure that the infection clears up completely and that your symptoms do not return. If you miss a dose of this medicine, take it as soon as possible. If it is almost time for your next dose, skip the missed dose and resume your regular schedule. Do not take two doses at the same time.

SPECIAL CONSIDERATIONS FOR THOSE OVER SIXTY-FIVE

None.

CONDITION: **FUNGAL INFECTIONS**

CATEGORY: **ANTIFUNGAL DRUGS**

GENERIC (CHEMICAL) NAME	BRAND (TRADE) NAME	DOSAGE FORMS AND STRENGTHS
Haloprogin	HALOTEX	Cream: 1% Solution: 1%

DRUG PROFILE

Haloprogin is used to treat fungal infections of the skin. It may be used in combination with other medicines if your skin problem is also caused by bacteria or fungi not susceptible to haloprogin. Haloprogin probably works by causing a sloughing off of the skin in which the fungus lives.

BEFORE USING THIS DRUG

Let your doctor know *IF*

You have ever had allergic reactions or other problems with ■ haloprogin.

SPECIAL RESTRICTIONS WHILE TAKING THIS DRUG

FOOD AND DRUG INTERACTIONS

No special restrictions on other drugs, foods and beverages, alcohol use, or smoking.

DAILY LIVING

Examinations or Tests	It is important for you to keep all appointments with your doctor so that your progress can be checked.
Other Precautions	It may take several weeks or even months to eradicate the fungus. If your symptoms do not improve

within four weeks or if they worsen, check with your doctor.

Be careful not to get this medicine in your eyes.

You may feel a mild stinging sensation after applying the solution form of this medicine.

Helpful Hints

Make sure you apply enough of this medicine to cover the affected area, and rub it in gently. Do not cover the area with anything else unless instructed to do so by your doctor.

Make sure to keep the affected areas clean and dry, since this will help them heal as well as prevent reinfection.

No special restrictions on driving, exertion and exercise, sun exposure, or exposure to excessive heat or cold.

POSSIBLE SIDE EFFECTS

Although this list of adverse effects may seem somewhat intimidating, keep in mind that some are quite rare. Of course, should these or any other problems arise while you are on medication, it is always a good idea to consult your doctor.

IF YOU DEVELOP	WHAT TO DO
irritation ■ burning sensation ■ blisters ■ itching ■ worsening of skin condition	**May be serious** Check with your doctor as soon as possible.

STORAGE INSTRUCTIONS

Store in a cool, dark place (not in a bathroom medicine cabinet). If your medicine is in a liquid form, make sure that it does not freeze.

STOPPING OR INTERRUPTING THERAPY

Use this medicine for the full length of time prescribed by your doctor, even if your symptoms begin to improve. This will ensure that the infection clears up completely and that your symptoms do not return. If you miss a dose of this medicine, apply it as soon as possible. If it is almost time for your next dose, skip the missed dose and resume your regular schedule.

SPECIAL CONSIDERATIONS FOR THOSE OVER SIXTY-FIVE

None.

CONDITION: **FUNGAL INFECTIONS**

CATEGORY: **ANTIFUNGAL DRUGS**

GENERIC (CHEMICAL) NAME	BRAND (TRADE) NAME	DOSAGE FORMS AND STRENGTHS
Ketoconazole	NIZORAL	Cream: 2% Suspension: 100 mg per tsp Tablets: 200 mg

DRUG PROFILE

Ketoconazole is used to treat various types of fungal infections. It is usually used in combination with other antifungal medicines. This medicine works by interfering with basic life processes of the fungus cells.

BEFORE USING THIS DRUG

Let your doctor know *IF*

You have ever had allergic reactions or other problems with ■ ketoconazole.

You have ever had any of the following medical problems: ■ achlorhydria (lack of stomach acid) ■ alcoholism ■ liver disease.

You are taking any of the following medicines: ■ acetaminophen ■ oral anticoagulants (blood thinners) ■ medicine for cancer ■ cyclosporine ■ medicine for diabetes ■ rifampin or isoniazid (medicines for tuberculosis) ■ sulfonamides (sulfa drugs) ■ cimetidine or ranitidine (medicine for ulcers) ■ antacids ■ medicine for stomach spasms ■ phenytoin (medicine for seizures) ■ tranquilizers.

SPECIAL RESTRICTIONS WHILE TAKING THIS DRUG

FOOD AND DRUG INTERACTIONS

Alcohol	Drinking alcohol while you are taking this medicine may cause liver problems. Avoid alcohol while you are taking this medicine.

No special restrictions on other drugs, foods and beverages, or smoking.

DAILY LIVING

Driving	This drug may cause drowsiness, light-headedness, dizziness, and loss of alertness and coordination. Be careful when driving, operating household appliances, or doing any other tasks that require alertness until you know how this drug affects you.
Sun Exposure	You may experience increased eye sensitivity to light while taking this drug. Wearing sunglasses if you're exposed to the sun should relieve any discomfort.
Examinations or Tests	It is important for you to keep all appointments with your doctor so that your progress can be checked. Periodic blood, urine, and stool cultures may be required.
Other Precautions	It may take several weeks or even months to eradicate the fungus. If your symptoms do not improve within a few weeks or if they worsen, check with your doctor. If you have cancer or other medical problems that increase your likelihood of developing a fungal infection and your doctor has prescribed this drug for preventive reasons, be especially careful to follow dosage instructions exactly. Be careful not to get this medicine in your eyes.

Helpful Hints

If this medicine upsets your stomach, taking it with a meal or snacks should help.

Make sure to keep the affected areas clean and dry, since this will help them heal as well as prevent reinfection.

No special restrictions on exertion and exercise or exposure to excessive heat or cold.

POSSIBLE SIDE EFFECTS

Although this list of adverse effects may seem somewhat intimidating, keep in mind that some are quite rare. Of course, should these or any other problems arise while you are on medication, it is always a good idea to consult your doctor.

IF YOU DEVELOP	WHAT TO DO
dark or red urine ■ pale stools ■ stomach pain ■ yellowing of eyes or skin ■ extreme tiredness or weakness ■ difficulty in breathing	**Urgent** Get in touch with your doctor immediately.
fever and chills ■ joint pain ■ ringing in ears ■ male breast enlargement and tenderness	**May be serious** Check with your doctor as soon as possible.
loss of appetite ■ nausea or vomiting ■ gas ■ diarrhea ■ itching ■ rash or hives ■ drowsiness ■ dizziness ■ male impotence ■ constipation ■ headache ■ nervousness ■ sleeplessness ■ vivid dreams ■ tingling or burning sensations ■ increased eye sensitivity to light	If symptoms are disturbing or persist, let your doctor know.

STORAGE INSTRUCTIONS

Store in a cool, dark place (not in a bathroom medicine cabinet).

STOPPING OR INTERRUPTING THERAPY

Use this medicine for the full length of time prescribed by your doctor, even if your symptoms begin to improve. This will ensure that the infection clears up completely and that your symptoms do not return. If you miss a dose of this medicine, take it as soon as possible. If it is almost time for your next dose, take the missed dose and wait ten to twelve hours before taking your next dose. Then resume your normal schedule.

SPECIAL CONSIDERATIONS FOR THOSE OVER SIXTY-FIVE

None.

CONDITION: **FUNGAL INFECTIONS**

CATEGORY: **ANTIFUNGAL DRUGS**

GENERIC (CHEMICAL) NAME	BRAND (TRADE) NAME	DOSAGE FORMS AND STRENGTHS
Miconazole	MONISTAT-DERM	Cream: 2% Lotion: 2%

DRUG PROFILE

Miconazole is used to treat fungal infections. This drug works by affecting the membrane and certain enzymes in the fungus cells, which results in destruction of the fungus.

BEFORE USING THIS DRUG

Let your doctor know *IF*

You have ever had allergic reactions or other problems with ■ miconazole.

You are taking any of the following medicines: ■ oral anticoagulants (blood thinners) ■ medicine for seizures.

SPECIAL RESTRICTIONS WHILE TAKING THIS DRUG

FOOD AND DRUG INTERACTIONS

No special restrictions on other drugs, foods and beverages, alcohol use, or smoking.

DAILY LIVING

Examinations or Tests	It is important for you to keep all appointments with your doctor so that your progress can be checked.
Other Precautions	It may take several weeks or even months to eradicate the fungus. If your symptoms do not improve within four weeks or if they worsen, check with your doctor. Keep this medicine away from your eyes.
Helpful Hints	Make sure you apply enough of this drug to cover the affected area, and rub it in gently. Do not cover it with anything else unless instructed to do so by your doctor. It is best to use the lotion, not cream, for areas between folds of skin (e.g., between buttocks, in groin) and rub it in well.

No special restrictions on driving, exertion and exercise, sun exposure, or exposure to excessive heat or cold.

POSSIBLE SIDE EFFECTS

Although this list of adverse effects may seem somewhat intimidating, keep in mind that some are quite rare. Of course, should these or any other problems arise while you are on medication, it is always a good idea to consult your doctor.

IF YOU DEVELOP

irritation ■ burning sensation ■ rash

WHAT TO DO

May be serious Check with your doctor as soon as possible.

STORAGE INSTRUCTIONS

Store in a cool, dark place (not in a bathroom medicine cabinet), and make sure that it does not freeze.

STOPPING OR INTERRUPTING THERAPY

Use this medicine for the full length of time prescribed by your doctor, even if your symptoms begin to improve. This will ensure that the infection clears up completely and that your symptoms do not return. If you miss a dose of this medicine, apply it as soon as possible and resume your regular schedule. If it is almost time for your next dose, skip the missed dose and resume your regular schedule.

SPECIAL CONSIDERATIONS FOR THOSE OVER SIXTY-FIVE

None.

CONDITION: **SCABIES AND LICE**

CATEGORY: **SCABICIDES AND PEDICULICIDES**

GENERIC (CHEMICAL) NAME	BRAND (TRADE) NAME	DOSAGE FORMS AND STRENGTHS
Crotamiton	EURAX	Cream: 10% Lotion: 10%

DRUG PROFILE

Crotamiton is used to treat scabies infestations of the skin. This medicine cures, but does not prevent, scabies. Crotamiton is also sometimes used to relieve severe itching.

BEFORE USING THIS DRUG

Let your doctor know *IF*

You have ever had allergic reactions or other problems with ■ crotamiton ■ other skin medicines.

You have ever had the following medical problem: ■ skin that is severely inflamed or has open sores.

SPECIAL RESTRICTIONS WHILE TAKING THIS DRUG

FOOD AND DRUG INTERACTIONS

No special restrictions on other drugs, foods and beverages, alcohol use, or smoking.

DAILY LIVING

Precautions	Since this drug is poisonous, avoid getting any in your mouth or eyes or in any open scratches, cuts, or sores. Follow your doctor's instructions carefully concerning how much crotamiton to use and how often and for how long to apply it.
Helpful Hints	If you have just taken a bath or shower, make sure your skin is cool and dry before applying this drug.
	Wash all of your recently worn clothing and used bed linens and towels in very hot water or dry-clean them in order to prevent reinfestation of yourself or infestation of other people.

No special restrictions on driving, exertion and exercise, sun exposure, or exposure to excessive heat or cold.

POSSIBLE SIDE EFFECTS

Although this list of adverse effects may seem somewhat intimidating, keep in mind that some are quite rare. Of course, should these or any other problems arise while you are on medication, it is always a good idea to consult your doctor.

IF YOU DEVELOP	WHAT TO DO
burning sensation in the mouth ■ nausea or vomiting ■ stomach pain	**Urgent** Get in touch with your doctor immediately.
rash or irritation that you didn't have before using this medicine	**May be serious** Check with your doctor as soon as possible.

STORAGE INSTRUCTIONS

Store in a cool, dark place (not in a bathroom medicine cabinet), and make sure that it does not freeze.

STOPPING OR INTERRUPTING THERAPY

One treatment (two applications) is usually enough to get rid of lice or scabies. Your doctor will advise you to reapply this medicine only if he or she sees evidence of continued infestation.

SPECIAL CONSIDERATIONS FOR THOSE OVER SIXTY-FIVE

None.

CONDITION: **SCABIES AND LICE**

CATEGORY: **SCABICIDES AND PEDICULOCIDES**

GENERIC (CHEMICAL) NAME	BRAND (TRADE) NAME	DOSAGE FORMS AND STRENGTHS
Lindane	KWELL	Cream: 1% Lotion: 1% Shampoo: 1%

DRUG PROFILE

Lindane cream or lotion is used to treat scabies and lice infestations of the skin. Lindane shampoo is used to treat lice infestation. This medicine cures, but does not prevent, scabies and lice.

BEFORE USING THIS DRUG

Let your doctor know *IF*

You have ever had allergic reactions or other problems with ■ lindane.

You have ever had the following medical problem: ■ seizures.

You are using any of the following medicines: ■ any other skin preparation, including creams, lotions, ointments, or oils.

SPECIAL RESTRICTIONS WHILE TAKING THIS DRUG

FOOD AND DRUG INTERACTIONS

Other Drugs	Other skin preparations such as oils, creams, or lotions may increase the absorption of lindane through your skin, which may be harmful; check with your doctor before using any of these products while using lindane.

No special restrictions on foods and beverages, alcohol use, or smoking.

DAILY LIVING

Precautions	Since lindane is poisonous, avoid getting any in your mouth or eyes or in any open scratches, cuts, or sores. If applying lindane to another person, wear plastic or rubber gloves.
	Follow your doctor's instructions carefully concerning how much lindane to use and how often and for how long to apply it.
	Do not use lindane shampoo in the shower or bath, and do not use it for routine hair cleansing.
Helpful Hints	If you have just taken a bath or shower, make sure your skin is cool and dry before applying lindane cream or lotion.

Wash all of your recently worn clothing and used bed linens and towels in very hot water or dry-clean them in order to prevent reinfestation of yourself or infestation of other people.

No special restrictions on driving, exertion and exercise, sun exposure, or exposure to excessive heat or cold.

POSSIBLE SIDE EFFECTS

Although this list of adverse effects may seem somewhat intimidating, keep in mind that some are quite rare. Of course, should these or any other problems arise while you are on medication, it is always a good idea to consult your doctor.

IF YOU DEVELOP	WHAT TO DO
clumsiness or unsteadiness ■ seizures ■ muscle cramps ■ nervousness or restlessness ■ irritability ■ fast heartbeat ■ vomiting	**Urgent** Get in touch with your doctor immediately.
rash or irritation that you didn't have before using this medicine	**May be serious** Check with your doctor as soon as possible.
itching for several weeks after you stop using this medicine	If symptoms are disturbing or persist, let your doctor know.

STORAGE INSTRUCTIONS

Store in a cool, dark place (not in a bathroom medicine cabinet), and make sure that it does not freeze.

STOPPING OR INTERRUPTING THERAPY

Only one application of this medicine is usually required for cure.

SPECIAL CONSIDERATIONS FOR THOSE OVER SIXTY-FIVE

None.

CONDITION: **VIRAL INFECTIONS**

CATEGORY: **ANTIVIRAL DRUGS**

GENERIC (CHEMICAL) NAME	BRAND (TRADE) NAME	DOSAGE FORMS AND STRENGTHS
Acyclovir	ZOVIRAX	Capsules: 200 mg Ointment: 5%

DRUG PROFILE

Acyclovir is used to treat infections of the external genitalia or skin caused by the herpes simplex virus. This medicine interferes with the ability of the virus to multiply within infected cells. Both the ointment and capsule forms of acyclovir may reduce pain, speed up the healing of sores, and prevent new blisters from forming during the first flare-up of infection. However, only the capsule form is effective for preventing recurrent flare-ups. Some doctors also prescribe oral acyclovir for the treatment of infection with the herpes zoster virus, more commonly known as shingles, though this use has not yet been approved by the Food and Drug Administration.

BEFORE USING THIS DRUG

Let your doctor know *IF*

You have ever had allergic reactions or other problems with ■ acyclovir.

You have ever had the following medical problem:

  ■ *with capsules only:* ■ kidney disease.

You are taking the following medicine:

  ■ *with capsules only:* ■ probenecid (medicine for gout).

SPECIAL RESTRICTIONS WHILE TAKING THIS DRUG

FOOD AND DRUG INTERACTIONS

No special restrictions on other drugs, foods and beverages, alcohol use, or smoking.

DAILY LIVING

Driving	The capsule form of this drug may cause drowsiness, light-headedness, dizziness, and loss of alertness and coordination. Be careful when driving, operating household appliances, or doing any other tasks that require alertness until you know how this drug affects you.
Examinations or Tests	If you are a woman who has genital herpes, your doctor may recommend that you have a Pap smear at least annually to test for cervical cancer.
Other Precautions	If your herpes infection does not begin to improve after you have been taking this medicine for a few days, check with your doctor.
	Your doctor may caution you to refrain from sexual relations during a flare-up of genital herpes.
Helpful Hints	This medicine works best if you use it as soon as you notice such herpes symptoms as pain, burning, or blistering.
	When applying the ointment, wear a rubber glove or finger sheath to avoid spreading the infection from one area to another.

No special restrictions on sun exposure or exposure to excessive heat or cold.

POSSIBLE SIDE EFFECTS

Although this list of adverse effects may seem somewhat intimidating, keep in mind that some are quite rare. Of course, should these or any other problems arise while you are on medication, it is always a good idea to consult your doctor.

IF YOU DEVELOP	WHAT TO DO
rash	**May be serious** Get in touch with your doctor as soon as possible.
headache ■ diarrhea ■ nausea ■ vomiting ■ dizziness ■ joint pain ■ acne ■ loss of appetite ■ sleep disturbances *With ointment only:* mild pain, burning, or stinging ■ itching	If symptoms are disturbing or persist, let your doctor know.

STORAGE INSTRUCTIONS

Store in a cool, dark place (not in a bathroom medicine cabinet). Do not let the ointment freeze.

STOPPING OR INTERRUPTING THERAPY

Use this medicine for the full length of time prescribed by your doctor, even if your symptoms begin to improve. This will ensure that the infection clears up completely and that your symptoms do not return. If you do miss a dose, take it as soon as possible. If it is almost time for your next dose, skip the missed dose and resume your regular schedule. Do not take this medicine more often or for a longer period of time than your doctor has advised.

SPECIAL CONSIDERATIONS FOR THOSE OVER SIXTY-FIVE

None.

CONDITION: **BACTERIAL INFECTIONS**

CATEGORY: **ANTIBIOTICS (ERYTHROMYCINS)**

GENERIC (CHEMICAL) NAME	BRAND (TRADE) NAME	DOSAGE FORMS AND STRENGTHS
Erythromycin	E-MYCIN ERYC ERY-TAB	Tablets: 250, 333 mg Capsules: 125, 250 mg Tablets: 250, 333, 500 mg
Erythromycin estolate	ILOSONE	Capsules: 125, 250 mg Chewable tablets: 125, 250 mg Drops: 100 mg per ml Suspension: 125, 250 mg per tsp Tablets: 500 mg
Erythromycin ethylsuccinate	E.E.S. E-MYCIN E WYAMYCIN E	Chewable tablets: 200 mg Drops: 100 mg per 2.5 ml Suspension: 200, 400 mg per tsp Suspension granules: 200 mg per tsp Tablets: 400 mg Suspension: 200, 400 mg per tsp Suspension: 200, 400 mg per tsp
Erythromycin stearate	ERYTHROCIN Stearate WYAMYCIN S	Tablets: 250, 500 mg Tablets: 250, 500 mg

This type of drug is available under other brand names as well.

DRUG PROFILE

Erythromycins are antibiotics that are used to treat a variety of bacterial infections, including such respiratory tract infections as bronchitis and pneumonia. These drugs suppress the growth of the bacteria and keep them from multiplying by blocking the bacteria's ability to manufacture protein.

For complete information on these drugs, see pages 595–598.

CONDITION: **BACTERIAL INFECTIONS**

CATEGORY: **ANTIBIOTICS (PENICILLINS)**

GENERIC (CHEMICAL) NAME	BRAND (TRADE) NAME	DOSAGE FORMS AND STRENGTHS
Amoxicillin	AMOXIL	Capsules: 250, 500 mg Chewable tablets: 125, 250 mg Suspension: 125, 250 mg per tsp
	LAROTID	Capsules: 250, 500 mg Suspension: 125, 250 mg per tsp
	POLYMOX	Capsules: 250, 500 mg Suspension: 125, 250 mg per tsp
	TRIMOX	Capsules: 250, 500 mg Suspension: 125, 250 mg per tsp
Ampicillin	AMCILL	Capsules: 250, 500 mg Suspension 125, 250 mg per tsp
	OMNIPEN	Capsules: 250, 500 mg Suspension: 125, 250 mg per tsp
	POLYCILLIN	Capsules: 250, 500 mg Suspension: 125, 250, 500 mg per tsp

	SK-AMPICILLIN	Capsules: 250, 500 mg Suspension: 125, 250 mg per tsp
	TOTACILLIN	Capsules: 250, 500 mg Suspension: 125, 250 mg per tsp
Bacampicillin hydrochloride	SPECTROBID	Suspension: 125 mg per tsp Tablets: 400 mg
Carbenicillin indanyl sodium	GEOCILLIN	Tablets: 382 mg
Cloxacillin sodium	TEGOPEN	Capsules: 250, 500 mg Solution: 125 mg per tsp
Cyclacillin	CYCLAPEN-W	Suspension: 125, 250 mg per tsp Tablets: 250, 500 mg
Nafcillin sodium	UNIPEN	Capsules: 250 mg Solution: 250 mg per tsp Tablets: 500 mg
Oxacillin sodium	PROSTAPHLIN	Capsules: 250, 500 mg Solution: 250 mg per tsp
Penicillin G potassium	PENTIDS	Tablets: 200,000, 400,000 units
Penicillin V potassium	LEDERCILLIN VK	Solution: 125, 250 mg per tsp Tablets: 250, 500 mg
	PEN•VEE•K	Solution: 125, 250 mg per tsp Tablets: 250, 500 mg

V-CILLIN K	Solution: 125, 250 mg per tsp Tablets: 125, 250, 500 mg

This type of drug is available under other brand names as well.

DRUG PROFILE

Penicillins are antibiotics that are used to treat a wide variety of bacterial infections, including infections of the ear, nose, and throat and such respiratory tract infections as bronchitis and pneumonia. Penicillins suppress the growth of bacteria by interfering with the bacteria's ability to form new protective cell walls.

For complete information on these drugs, see pages 599–603.

CONDITION: **BACTERIAL INFECTIONS**

CATEGORY: **ANTIBIOTICS (TETRACYCLINES)**

GENERIC (CHEMICAL) NAME	BRAND (TRADE) NAME	DOSAGE FORMS AND STRENGTHS
Tetracycline hydrochloride	ACHROMYCIN V	Capsules: 250, 500 mg Suspension: 125 mg per tsp
	PANMYCIN	Capsules: 250 mg
	ROBITET	Capsules: 250, 500 mg
	SUMYCIN	Capsules: 250, 500 mg Syrup: 125 mg per tsp Tablets: 250, 500 mg

DRUG PROFILE

Tetracyclines are antibiotics that are used to treat a wide variety of bacterial infections, including skin eruptions and bronchitis and pneumonia. These antibiotics suppress the growth of bacteria by interfering with their manufacture of protein.

For complete information on this drug, see pages 591–595.

BENIGN AND MALIGNANT TUMORS OF THE SKIN

Older people often develop skin growths, particularly if they have blond or red hair and light skin and have spent a lot of time outdoors in the sun. While some of these growths are harmless, others may be precursors of serious skin cancers. Therefore, it is important that you see your doctor about any unusual growth or localized change in the texture or color of your skin. If a suspicious-looking growth does turn out to be malignant, early treatment can usually bring about a complete cure.

EPIDERMAL CYSTS

One type of benign growth that often frightens people because it appears as a solid lump is the relatively common epidermal cyst. These cysts, which are caused by the growth of superficial skin cells in deeper layers of the skin, are most often found on the face, neck, chest, or upper back. Usually, the cyst causes no unusual sensation, but if it gets infected from friction or scratching, it may become red and tender. Doctors usually remove an epidermal cyst either by excising, or cutting away, the entire cyst or by opening it and scraping out all the superficial skin cells.

SEBORRHEIC KERATOSES

These benign growths, brought on by long-term exposure to the sun, are the most common tumors among older people. When they first appear, they are sharply defined yellow or brown spots with either smooth or slightly bumpy surfaces. People usually get a crop of seborrheic keratoses rather than just one, and they are usually located on the chest, back, or abdomen. Over time, these early seborrheic keratoses enlarge and thicken.

These small, benign tumors can easily be burned off electrically or frozen off with liquid nitrogen in your doctor's office. Your doctor may choose, in some cases, to take a biopsy of a growth that resembles a seborrheic keratosis to make sure it is not a malignant skin growth.

SENILE SEBACEOUS HYPERPLASIA

This yellowish, rough-surfaced growth is also more common among older people than among other age groups. It is caused by a malformation of the oil-producing glands in the skin, and usually appears on the face, particularly the forehead and nose. These growths can be removed with electrosurgery.

ACTINIC KERATOSES AND SQUAMOUS CELL CARCINOMA

Older men and women who work in the sun often develop actinic keratoses; these are small bumps of reddish, brown, or gray color on the face, lower lip, or the backs of the hands—areas that are seldom covered and thus receive the most ultraviolet radiation. It's extremely important to treat actinic keratoses right away, since about one-fourth of them develop into squamous cell carcinoma. The growths can be removed by scraping, chemical burning, or electrosurgery; if they are particularly large, surgical excision may be necessary. Occasionally, if a large area of skin is involved, doctors treat actinic keratoses with an ointment containing the anticancer drug 5-fluorouracil (see the drug chart on pages 730–732), which is rubbed onto the skin for at least thirty days.

The average age of onset of squamous cell carcinoma—a condition caused by skin exposure—is sixty. People who work with compounds containing arsenic are also prone to this cancer.

Squamous cell carcinomas appear in the same areas of skin as do actinic keratoses. Tumors that do not begin as actinic keratoses start out as firm bumps that slowly enlarge and develop crusty centers that eventually turn into deep, open sores.

If unchecked, any squamous cell carcinoma can invade deeply and spread to cover a large area of skin. To prevent this progression, prompt treatment of precancerous actinic keratoses and early tumors is essential. Small squamous cell lesions that have not invaded deeply can be effectively scraped and burned off. More serious lesions require surgical removal. Occasionally, older people who may not be able to tolerate surgery receive radiation therapy for this form of cancer.

BASAL CELL CARCINOMA

This skin cancer, which is the most common malignancy in white people, is caused by a proliferation of cells from the skin's surface. The same conditions that predispose people to squamous cell carcinoma—exposure to sun and certain chemicals or radiation—also increase the risk of basal cell carcinoma. Fortunately, however, basal cell carcinoma progresses more slowly than squamous cell carcinoma, and 95 percent of cases can be cured.

Several types of basal cell carcinoma have been identified. The most common variety, called noduloulcerative, usually appears on the face; the tumor begins as a small bump, or node, that eventually develops an indented center and ulcerates. In another type, superficial basal cell carcinoma, the lesions are round rough spots with slightly elevated borders. This form of skin cancer is usually a chronic condition developing after long-term exposure to arsenical compounds. Sclerosing basal cell carcinoma, which most often affects the head and neck, is a yellowish-white lesion with no distinct border. It enlarges slowly but, on occasion, invades deeper tissues.

All types of basal cell lesions can be removed by burning or surgical excision. Some tumors are treated with 5-fluorouracil ointment as well (see the drug chart on pages 730–732).

MALIGNANT MELANOMA

This type of cancer has a reputation for being particularly lethal but is actually highly curable—if it is discovered early and treated promptly. There is a 100 percent cure rate for malignant melanomas removed at their earliest stage, before they invade below the outermost layer of the skin. Even when a malignant melanoma invades the first layer of the dermis, the cure rate is 90 percent. Still, of all skin cancer, this is the most serious and most likely to spread to other parts of the body.

Many scientists believe that malignant melanoma, which develops in the pigment-producing cells of the skin, is caused by sun exposure. Some evidence indicates that being in the sun intermittently and getting burned increases the risk for malignant melanoma more than does long-term sun exposure. For unknown reasons, women are more likely to be cured of this disease than are men.

It is estimated that anywhere from 20 percent to 85 percent of malignant melanomas have their origins in already existing moles, which are also called nevi. Typically, a malignant melanoma grows wider on the skin surface for a long period—perhaps as long as ten years—before it invades the deeper skin. It starts as a brown or black spot that is barely raised above the skin's surface. The initial spot may have an irregular border and, as it spreads, its hue may vary from red to blue to black. At the time of invasion, the lesion becomes raised into a lump or node.

Another, less common, type of malignant melanoma, called lentigo maligna melanoma, affects older people primarily. It develops from a benign lesion called a melanotic freckle of Hutchinson—an irregularly shaped brown splotch, usually on the face. Thirty percent to 50 percent of these lesions eventually change to malig-

nant melanoma, a transformation heralded by a roughening of the surface and a darkening of the pigment.

Two other types of malignant melanoma, nodular and acral lentiginous melanoma, are particularly difficult to treat. The nodular type never goes through the typical early growth phase on the skin's surface; instead, it begins as an invasive node. Acral malignant melanoma is difficult to spot because it often occurs on the palms of the hands or soles of the feet, where the skin is thicker and changes are hard to identify. Hence, it is often not detected until it has become invasive.

The mainstay of treatment for all types of malignant melanoma is surgical excision of the tumor. The doctor will examine the excised tumor microscopically to determine how far the disease has progressed; sometimes, if the lesion is particularly thick, the doctor will also take biopsies of nearby lymph nodes to see whether they have been affected. If the disease has spread to other parts of the body, radiation therapy and chemotherapy may be recommended (see the drug charts on pages 730–733).

OUTLOOK

Although many growths on the skin are harmless, all skin tumors should receive immediate medical attention because of the possibility of malignancy. Fortunately, skin cancer is generally curable, but chances are best if detection is early and treatment prompt.

CONDITION: **SKIN CANCER**

CATEGORY: **DRUGS FOR ACTINIC KERATOSES AND SKIN CANCER**

GENERIC (CHEMICAL) NAME	BRAND (TRADE) NAME	DOSAGE FORMS AND STRENGTHS
5-Fluorouracil	EFUDEX	Cream: 5% Solution: 2%, 5%
	FLUOROPLEX	Cream: 1% Solution: 1%

DRUG PROFILE

5-Fluorouracil is used to treat precancerous or cancerous skin conditions. This drug interferes with the manufacture of DNA, which is necessary for the growth and multiplication of cells.

BEFORE USING THIS DRUG

Let your doctor know *IF*

You have ever had allergic reactions or other problems with ■ 5-fluorouracil.

You have ever had the following medical problem: ■ other skin problems.

SPECIAL RESTRICTIONS WHILE TAKING THIS DRUG

FOOD AND DRUG INTERACTIONS

No special restrictions on other drugs, foods and beverages, alcohol use, or smoking.

DAILY LIVING

Sun Exposure   Avoid excessive sun exposure; your skin may become more sensitive to sunlight while you are on this drug and for one to two months after you stop using it. In addition, too much sun may increase the effect of this drug. It is a good idea to apply a sunscreen to exposed skin surfaces before going outdoors.

Examinations or Tests	It is important for you to keep all appointments with your doctor so that your progress can be checked.
Other Precautions	Follow your doctor's instructions carefully concerning how much, how often, and for how long you should use this medicine. The treated skin may become red and sore and peel or scale for several weeks, even after you stop using the medicine. Once the skin heals, the area may remain pink and smooth for another month or two. If the area being treated becomes very uncomfortable, check with your doctor, but do not stop using fluorouracil unless your doctor tells you to.
Helpful Hints	When applying the medicine, use a cotton-tipped applicator or your fingertips to cover the entire affected area with a thin layer. A gauze dressing may be placed over the medicine.
	If you apply this medicine with your fingertips, wash your hands thoroughly afterwards.
	If you are using this medicine on your face, be careful not to get any in your eyes, nose, or mouth.

No special restrictions on driving, exertion and exercise, or exposure to excessive heat or cold.

POSSIBLE SIDE EFFECTS

Although this list of adverse effects may seem somewhat intimidating, keep in mind that some are quite rare. Of course, should these or any other problems arise while you are on medication, it is always a good idea to consult your doctor.

IF YOU DEVELOP	WHAT TO DO
redness and swelling of normal skin	**Urgent** Get in touch with your doctor immediately.
sleeplessness ■ irritability	**May be serious** Check with your doctor as soon as possible.
burning sensation following application ■ rash, scaling, or oozing ■ soreness or tenderness ■ itching ■ increased skin sensitivity to sunlight ■ skin darkening ■ scarring ■ watery eyes ■ sores inside mouth	If symptoms are disturbing or persist, let your doctor know.

STORAGE INSTRUCTIONS

Store in a cool, dark place (not in a bathroom medicine cabinet). If your medicine is in a liquid form, make sure that it does not freeze.

STOPPING OR INTERRUPTING THERAPY

If you miss a dose of this medicine, apply it as soon as possible. If more than a few hours have passed, skip the missed dose and resume your regular schedule. Check with your doctor if you miss more than one dose.

SPECIAL CONSIDERATIONS FOR THOSE OVER SIXTY-FIVE

None.

CONDITION: **SKIN CANCER**

CATEGORY: **CHEMOTHERAPEUTIC AGENTS**

GENERIC (CHEMICAL) NAME	BRAND (TRADE) NAME	DOSAGE FORMS AND STRENGTHS
Cyclophosphamide	CYTOXAN	Tablets: 25, 50 mg

DRUG PROFILE

Cyclophosphamide is used to treat many types of cancer, including leukemia, cancers of the lymph nodes (including Hodgkin's disease), and cancers of the retina, skin, nervous system, ovaries, and breast. This drug slows or stops the spread of cancer, keeping the cancer cells from multiplying.

For complete information on this drug, see pages 886–889.

CONDITION: **SKIN CANCER**

CATEGORY: **CHEMOTHERAPEUTIC AGENTS**

GENERIC (CHEMICAL) NAME	BRAND (TRADE) NAME	DOSAGE FORMS AND STRENGTHS
Methotrexate		Tablets: 2.5 mg

DRUG PROFILE

Methotrexate is used to treat certain types of leukemia, cancer of the lymph nodes, cancer of the breast, and certain cancers of the head, neck, skin, and lung. This drug is also sometimes used to treat severe cases of psoriasis—a skin disorder. Methotrexate slows and halts the growth and spread of cancer cells by interfering with one of the steps in cell growth.

For complete information on this drug, see pages 889–893.

SKIN ALLERGIES AND IRRITATIONS

A number of conditions can develop in the skin as the body responds to allergy-triggering substances and other materials, both man-made and natural. These skin disorders are considered forms of dermatitis, a catchall term meaning "inflammation of the skin." Itchiness, sometimes intense, occurs in all of them. Some also produce reddened, blistery regions that can ooze fluid and become scaly. The treatments for these conditions vary somewhat but are drawn from the same basic groups of medicines.

CONTACT DERMATITIS

If you've ever had poison ivy dermatitis, you've had first-hand experience with the skin disorder known as contact dermatitis—inflammation resulting from skin contact with an offending substance. Depending on the substance involved, contact dermatitis can involve an allergic reaction (as with poison ivy) or a direct irritation. Symptoms can range from redness and hardening of the skin to severe eczema (another term for dermatitis). In older people, the response may be delayed.

Common sources of allergic contact dermatitis include plant products, cosmetics, metals, and dyes. Various household chemicals, as well as those used in hobbies, can bring about irritant contact dermatitis. The allergic form generally requires at least one prior exposure to the substance to cause the immune system to become sensitized. Subsequent encounters then produce the rash, which may appear in minutes or be delayed for many hours. Contact dermatitis can occur anywhere on the body, though it tends to spare the scalp.

Contact dermatitis usually first breaks out at the site of contact and then may spread. Sometimes the source is obvious—for example, when a rash breaks out just where a new piece of jewelry has touched the skin. Other times, though, identifying the source will require some detective work by you and your doctor. Your doctor may recommend having a specialist perform a "patch test," in which a variety of common allergens are applied to a small area of your skin. A rash indicates an allergic reaction.

The severity of contact dermatitis depends in part on how easily the substance can penetrate the skin. Skin that is broken or damaged from frequent contact with soap can be easier to penetrate, as can skin that has grown thinner with age. Contact dermatitis also tends to be worse in winter because of the effects of cold, dry air. With this and all other forms of dermatitis, scratching leads to more itching and can increase the risk of infection.

HAND ECZEMA

This condition is simply contact dermatitis of the hands. It has sometimes been called housewives' dermatitis, but anyone whose hands come in frequent contact with detergents, shampoos, bleaches, cleansers, and other chemicals is a potential candidate.

Hand eczema usually involves direct skin irritation, though a contact allergy is also possible. It can range in severity from redness and roughness to blistering, crusting, and cracking. It usually clears up in a few days if contact is discontinued. However, severe inflammation, especially if accompanied by infection, should be treated by a doctor.

Sensible hand care is the best protection against hand eczema. Whenever possible, wear cotton-lined rubber gloves with additional soft cotton gloves underneath during exposure to an irritating substance. If your hands are frequently immersed in water, be sure to keep a moisturizing lotion nearby, and use it frequently. Superfatted soaps and other cleaning products designed to cut down on the loss of natural skin oils may also help.

ATOPIC DERMATITIS

This intensely itchy form of dermatitis tends to run in families that also have a high incidence of hay fever and allergic asthma. It usually develops in infancy or early childhood, flares up and dies down a number of times over the years, and may disappear for good by the teens or twenties. In some cases, however, it persists throughout life.

A vicious cycle of scratching leading to more itching is common in atopic dermatitis. Strong emotions, extreme temperatures, and contact with scratchy materials can readily reignite the inflammation.

HIVES

Slightly raised, pink wheals with well-defined borders are the hallmark of this condition, also called urticaria. The itchy wheals can appear and disappear within hours, often to be replaced by new wheals elsewhere. Hives generally last for a day or two, though chronic cases can continue for many weeks.

The most common cause of hives is a food allergy. Shellfish, nuts, strawberries, chocolate, and some food additives are common triggers. Some chemicals and drugs, including aspirin and certain opiates and antibiotics, can also produce this skin condition. In some people, physical pressure, a simple scratch, or exposure to cold may lead to hives. Emotional stress can worsen an existing case of hives or can even actually trigger a case.

Hives themselves are usually annoying but harmless. However, in a more severe form of hives called angioedema, swelling develops not just in the top layer of skin but also in the inner layer, or dermis. Sometimes, the swelling becomes severe enough to threaten breathing, requiring immediate medical attention.

DRUG-TRIGGERED SKIN REACTIONS

Medicines, most often antibiotics, can produce hives and other kinds of rashes. The rash may appear within minutes to hours after the drug has been started or may take about a week to develop.

Sometimes, if a person's immune

system is sensitized to a drug, a subsequent exposure can trigger a life-threatening condition known as anaphylactic shock. But if you and your doctor keep close track of any drug allergies you have, the problem can generally be avoided by substituting another medicine.

Sunlight can sometimes set off a rash in people who are on certain medicines. Your doctor may recommend that you stay out of the sun as much as possible while using the drug; an effective sunscreen on the face, hands, and other exposed areas can also help.

TREATMENT

For all the conditions described in this guide, the smartest treatment plan is to steer clear of whatever it is that's causing the problem. But that may not always be possible, either because you don't know what's affecting your skin or because there's no avoiding it.

The two main types of medicine used in treating these conditions are topical steroids (see the drug chart on pages 737–739) and antihistamines (see the drug chart on pages 740–741). Topical steroids help quell redness, itching, and swelling, whatever their cause. Antihistamines counter the effects of histamine (a chemical in your body involved in allergic reactions) and are the drugs of choice in treating hives. Your doctor may also prescribe an antihistamine for contact and atopic dermatitis, especially when an allergy is clearly involved.

Antibiotics are sometimes necessary to prevent or reverse infection in situations in which the skin is broken. Erythromycin is often used for this purpose. (See the drug chart on pages 741–742.) In cases of severe hives, angioedema, or anaphylaxis, an injection of epinephrine may be necessary as part of emergency treatment.

OUTLOOK

Steering clear of poison ivy, while a good idea, is only one approach available to you in dealing with skin allergies and irritations. The medicines used to treat these conditions are quite effective in relieving the inflammation, itchiness, and other typical symptoms. As researchers sharpen their techniques for identifying the offending substances and learn more about the underlying processes, even better treatment methods are likely to evolve.

CONDITION: **ALLERGIC SKIN REACTIONS**

CATEGORY: **TOPICAL CORTICOSTEROIDS**

GENERIC (CHEMICAL) NAME	BRAND (TRADE) NAME	DOSAGE FORMS AND STRENGTHS
Amcinonide	CYCLOCORT	Cream: 0.1% Ointment: 0.1%
Betamethasone dipropionate	DIPROLENE	Cream: 0.05% Ointment: 0.05%
	DIPROSONE	Cream: 0.05% Lotion: 0.05% Ointment: 0.05% Spray: 0.1%
Betamethasone valerate	VALISONE	Cream: 0.01%, 0.1% Lotion: 0.1% Ointment: 0.1%
Clocortolone pivalate	CLODERM	Cream: 0.1%
Desonide	TRIDESILON	Cream: 0.05% Ointment: 0.05%
Desoximetasone	TOPICORT	Cream: 0.25% Gel: 0.05% Ointment: 0.25%
	TOPICORT LP	Cream: 0.05%
Dexamethasone	AEROSEB-DEX	Spray: 0.2 mg per spray
Diflorasone diacetate	FLORONE	Cream: 0.05% Ointment: 0.05%

Fluocinolone acetonide	SYNALAR	Cream: 0.025%, 0.01% Ointment: 0.025% Solution: 0.01%
	SYNALAR-HP	Cream: 0.2%
	SYNEMOL	Cream: 0.025%
Fluocinonide	LIDEX	Cream: 0.05% Gel: 0.05% Ointment: 0.05% Solution: 0.05%
	LIDEX-E	Cream: 0.05%
Flurandrenolide	CORDRAN	Lotion: 0.05% Ointment: 0.025%, 0.05%
	CORDRAN SP	Cream: 0.025%, 0.05%
Halcinonide	HALCIDERM	Cream: 0.1%
	HALOG	Cream: 0.025%, 0.1% Ointment: 0.1% Solution: 0.1%
	HALOG-E	Cream: 0.1%
Hydrocortisone	AEROSEB-HC	Spray: 0.5%
	CORT-DOME	Cream: 0.25%, 0.5%, 1% Lotion: 0.125%, 0.25%, 0.5%, 1%
	HYTONE	Cream: 0.5%, 1%, 2.5% Lotion: 1%, 2.5% Ointment: 1%, 2.5%
Hydrocortisone acetate	CORTEF ACETATE	Ointment: 1%, 2.5%
Hydrocortisone valerate	WESTCORT	Cream: 0.2% Ointment: 0.2%

Polymyxin B sulfate, bacitracin zinc, neomycin sulfate, and hydrocortisone	CORTISPORIN Ointment	Ointment: 5,000 units polymyxin B sulfate, 400 units bacitracin zinc, 5 mg neomycin sulfate, and 10 mg hydrocortisone per g
Polymyxin B sulfate, neomycin sulfate, and hydrocortisone acetate	CORTISPORIN Cream	Cream: 10,000 units polymyxin B sulfate, 5 mg neomycin sulfate, and 5 mg hydrocortisone acetate per g
Triamcinolone acetonide	ARISTOCORT	Cream: 0.025%, 0.1%, 0.5% Ointment: 0.1%, 0.5%
	ARISTOCORT A	Cream: 0.025%, 0.1%, 0.5% Ointment: 0.1%, 0.5%

Many brands of topical hydrocortisone are sold over the counter as well.

DRUG PROFILE

Topical corticosteroids are applied directly to the skin to help alleviate the pain, itching, and swelling of rashes and various other skin conditions. They work by blocking the inflammatory response of the skin to irritations, infections, and allergic reactions.

For complete information on these drugs, see pages 690–695.

CONDITION: **ALLERGIC SKIN REACTIONS**

CATEGORY: **ANTIHISTAMINES**

GENERIC (CHEMICAL) NAME	BRAND (TRADE) NAME	DOSAGE FORMS AND STRENGTHS
Diphenhydramine hydrochloride	BENADRYL	Capsules: 25, 50 mg Elixir: 12.5 mg per tsp
Hydroxyzine	ATARAX VISTARIL	Syrup: 10 mg per tsp Tablets: 10, 25, 50, 100 mg Capsules: 25, 50, 100 mg Suspension: 25 mg per tsp

DRUG PROFILE

When you are exposed to a substance to which you are allergic, a chemical called histamine is released into the bloodstream and produces the itchy, watery eyes; runny nose; and rashes that are typical of an allergic reaction. Antihistamines work by blocking the action of histamine. They are used to treat allergies as well as to relieve the symptoms of a cold.

For complete information on these drugs, see pages 633–638.

CONDITION: **ALLERGIC SKIN REACTIONS**

CATEGORY: **ANTIHISTAMINES**

GENERIC (CHEMICAL) NAME	BRAND (TRADE) NAME	DOSAGE FORMS AND STRENGTHS
Trimeprazine tartrate	TEMARIL	Controlled-release capsules: 5 mg Syrup: 2.5 mg per tsp Tablets: 2.5 mg

DRUG PROFILE

Trimeprazine is an antihistamine (see chapter 9, Disorders of the Respiratory System) that is used to relieve the itching associated with hives, rashes, and other skin conditions. When you are exposed to a substance to which you are allergic, a chemical called histamine is released into the bloodstream and produces the symptoms, including itching, that are typical of an allergic reaction. Antihistamines work by blocking the action of histamines.

For complete information on this drug, see pages 685–689.

CONDITION: **ALLERGIC SKIN REACTIONS**

CATEGORY: **ANTIBIOTICS (ERYTHROMYCINS)**

GENERIC (CHEMICAL) NAME	BRAND (TRADE) NAME	DOSAGE FORMS AND STRENGTHS
Erythromycin	E-MYCIN ERYC ERY-TAB	Tablets: 250, 333 mg Capsules: 125, 250 mg Tablets: 250, 333, 500 mg
Erythromycin estolate	ILOSONE	Capsules: 125, 250 mg Chewable tablets: 125, 250 mg Drops: 100 mg per ml Suspension: 125, 250 mg per tsp Tablets: 500 mg
Erythromycin ethylsuccinate	E.E.S.	Chewable tablets: 200 mg Drops: 100 mg per 2.5 ml Suspension: 200, 400 mg per tsp Suspension granules: 200 mg per tsp Tablets: 400 mg

	E-MYCIN E	Suspension: 200, 400 mg per tsp
	WYAMYCIN E	Suspension: 200, 400 mg per tsp
Erythromycin Stearate	ERYTHROCIN Stearate	Tablets: 250, 500 mg
	WYAMYCIN S	Tablets: 250, 500 mg

This type of drug is available under other brand names as well.

DRUG PROFILE

Erythromycins are antibiotics that are used to treat a variety of bacterial infections, including such respiratory tract infections as bronchitis and pneumonia. These drugs suppress the growth of the bacteria and keep them from multiplying by blocking the bacteria's ability to manufacture protein.

For complete information on these drugs, see pages 595–598.

PSORIASIS, ROSACEA, AND SEBORRHEIC DERMATITIS

The skin conditions known as psoriasis, rosacea, and seborrheic dermatitis are all irritating nuisances of unknown cause. Cures for them have also proven elusive—but these disorders can often be controlled, and you can look and feel as well as ever.

PSORIASIS

Psoriasis, a skin condition that affects one out of fifty people in the United States, can occur for the first time at any age. You may suspect you have it if you notice a raised, sometimes itchy, red patch of skin with silvery scales. These so-called plaques most often appear on the elbows, knees, and scalp but sometimes affect the genital and underarm areas. Because blood supply to the skin diminishes with age, plaques don't become as inflamed in older people as in younger ones. Some people with psoriasis also have fingernails that are pitted or discolored.

Psoriasis is not contagious (passed from person to person), but it may run in families. At least three out of ten people with psoriasis report a family history of the problem. Despite this genetic aspect, some researchers believe that psoriasis doesn't show itself until set off by some aggravating factor. The culprits might include psychological stress, infection, injury to the skin, or vaccination.

It's not hard for a doctor to tell, by looking at the plaques, that the problem is psoriasis. But to confirm the diagnosis, your doctor may stroke this thickened patch of skin with a wooden spatula to dislodge the silvery-white scales that are a sure sign of this annoying disorder.

Many people find that sunlight helps relieve psoriasis. Try a sunlamp if sunlight is scarce, but use it only according to directions. Some doctors prescribe PUVA therapy, a light treatment that uses long-wave ultraviolet light in combination with a drug called methoxsalen.

Steroid creams have been found to be effective in controlling psoriasis (see the drug chart on pages 745–747). Another product, anthralin, may also be used to treat psoriasis of the skin and scalp (see the drug chart on pages 748–750); methotrexate (see the drug chart on pages 752–753) may be prescribed for the most severe cases. However, because psoriasis often recurs, these remedies generally must be used repeatedly.

ROSACEA

Rosacea, formerly known as acne rosacea, has some similarities to the form of acne so embarrassing to adolescents—notably, pimples and oiliness of the skin. But rosacea, which is most common in people over thirty-five, also causes the skin to flush and most often occurs in the middle of the face (mid-forehead, chin, and nose). In fact, a severe form of rosacea that affects men results in enlargement of the nose. Additionally, more than half the people who have rosacea have accompanying eye problems, such as conjunctivitis.

Some researchers had thought that an abnormality of the intestinal tract caused the disease, while others blamed alcohol, spicy foods, stress, or vitamin deficiencies. Recent research shows no evidence that any of these cause rosacea. However, some doctors suggest that people with rosacea avoid spicy foods, caffeine, alcohol, hot drinks, and exposure to extreme heat or cold, since those factors lead to flushing.

A few people will have only one attack of rosacea and then aren't troubled again. But in most cases the condition will get increasingly worse if it's not properly treated. Such antibiotics as tetracycline or minocycline may help improve this harmless but unsightly skin disorder (see the drug chart on page 755). Usually these drugs are taken in high doses for two or three months and then continued in lower doses for another six weeks. This treatment prevents recurrences in about one out of three people. If the condition does recur, low doses of antibiotics are continued. If tetracycline or minocycline doesn't prove effective in your case, your doctor may switch you to a drug called metronidazole. (For more information on this drug, see the chart on page 756).

SEBORRHEIC DERMATITIS

Seborrheic dermatitis is not a single disorder but actually refers to a variety of skin conditions. These range from simple dandruff to dandruff accompanied by inflammation of the scalp to greasy, scaling patches on the chest and eyebrows, behind the ears, and around the nose. Those areas have high concentrations of sebaceous glands, which coat the surface of the skin with an oily substance called sebum. Contrary to popular belief, seborrheic dermatitis does *not* cause baldness, nor is it contagious.

Although the cause of seborrheic dermatitis is unknown, sex hormones appear to play an important role. This skin condition is quite common in older men and postmenopausal women. (Its appearance in older women may reflect a decline in estrogen production by the ovaries.)

Seborrheic dermatitis cannot be cured but can be treated effectively. If you have dandruff, shampoo with a product that contains zinc, selenium, or tar every other day until the dandruff is under control (see the drug charts on pages 750–752 and 753–755); to *keep* it under control, continue to use those shampoos once or twice a week. Hydrocortisone cream can successfully control seborrheic dermatitis on the face or body. (See the drug chart on pages 745–747 for descriptions of appropriate medicines.)

CONDITION: **PSORIASIS**

CATEGORY: **TOPICAL CORTICOSTEROIDS**

GENERIC (CHEMICAL) NAME	BRAND (TRADE) NAME	DOSAGE FORMS AND STRENGTHS
Amcinonide	CYCLOCORT	Cream: 0.1% Ointment: 0.1%
Betamethasone dipropionate	DIPROLENE	Cream: 0.05% Ointment: 0.05%
	DIPROSONE	Cream: 0.05% Lotion: 0.05% Ointment: 0.05% Spray: 0.1%
Betamethasone valerate	VALISONE	Cream: 0.01%, 0.1% Lotion: 0.1% Ointment: 0.1%
Clocortolone pivalate	CLODERM	Cream: 0.1%
Desonide	TRIDESILON	Cream: 0.05% Ointment: 0.05%
Desoximetasone	TOPICORT	Cream: 0.25% Gel: 0.05% Ointment: 0.25%
	TOPICORT LP	Cream: 0.05%
Dexamethasone	AEROSEB-DEX	Spray: 0.01%
Diflorasone diacetate	FLORONE	Cream: 0.05% Ointment: 0.05%

Fluocinolone acetonide	SYNALAR	Cream: 0.025%, 0.01% Ointment: 0.025% Solution: 0.01%
	SYNALAR-HP	Cream: 0.2%
	SYNEMOL	Cream: 0.025%
Fluocinonide	LIDEX	Cream: 0.05% Gel: 0.05% Ointment: 0.05% Solution: 0.05%
	LIDEX-E	Cream: 0.05%
Flurandrenolide	CORDRAN	Lotion: 0.05% Ointment: 0.025%, 0.05%
	CORDRAN SP	Cream: 0.025%, 0.05%
Halcinonide	HALCIDERM	Cream: 0.1%
	HALOG	Cream: 0.025%, 0.1% Ointment: 0.1% Solution: 0.1%
	HALOG-E	Cream: 0.1%
Hydrocortisone	AEROSEB-HC	Spray: 0.5%
	CORT-DOME	Cream: 0.25%, 0.5%, 1% Lotion: 0.125%, 0.25%, 0.5%, 1%
	HYTONE	Cream: 0.5%, 1%, 2.5% Lotion: 1%, 2.5% Ointment: 1%, 2.5%
Hydrocortisone acetate	CORTEF ACETATE	Ointment: 1%, 2.5%
Hydrocortisone valerate	WESTCORT	Cream: 0.2% Ointment: 0.2%

Polymyxin B sulfate, bacitracin zinc, neomycin sulfate, and hydrocortisone	CORTISPORIN Ointment	Ointment: 5,000 units polymyxin B sulfate, 400 units bacitracin zinc, 5 mg neomycin sulfate, and 10 mg hydrocortisone per g
Polymyxin B sulfate, neomycin sulfate, and hydrocortisone acetate	CORTISPORIN Cream	Cream: 10,000 units polymyxin B sulfate, 5 mg neomycin sulfate, and 5 mg hydrocortisone acetate per g
Triamcinolone acetonide	ARISTOCORT	Cream: 0.025%, 0.1%, 0.5% Ointment: 0.1%, 0.5%
	ARISTOCORT A	Cream: 0.025%, 0.1%, 0.5% Ointment: 0.1%, 0.5%

Many brands of topical hydrocortisone are sold over the counter as well.

DRUG PROFILE

Topical corticosteroids are applied directly to the skin to help alleviate the pain, itching, and swelling of rashes and various other skin conditions. They work by blocking the inflammatory response of the skin to irritations, infections, and allergic reactions.

For complete information on these drugs, see pages 690–695.

CONDITION: **PSORIASIS**

CATEGORY: **KERATOLYTIC DRUGS**

GENERIC (CHEMICAL) NAME	BRAND (TRADE) NAME	DOSAGE FORMS AND STRENGTHS
Anthralin	ANTHRA-DERM	Ointment: 0.1%, 0.25%, 0.5%, 1%
	DRITHOCREME	Cream: 0.1%, 0.25%, 0.5%, 1%
	DRITHO-SCALP	Cream: 0.25%, 0.5%

DRUG PROFILE

Anthralin is used to treat psoriasis of the skin and scalp. It works by inhibiting the growth of skin cells in the areas to which it is applied.

BEFORE USING THIS DRUG

Let your doctor know *IF*

You have ever had allergic reactions or other problems with ■ anthralin.

You have ever had the following medical problem: ■ kidney disease.

You are taking any of the following medicines: ■ other medicine for psoriasis (especially coal tar preparations or methoxsalen) ■ oral medicine for diabetes ■ griseofulvin (medicine for fungal infections) ■ nalidixic acid (medicine for urinary tract infections) ■ phenothiazines (tranquilizers) ■ sulfonamides (sulfa medicine) ■ tetracycline (antibiotic) ■ thiazide diuretics (water pills) ■ trioxsalen (medicine for virtiligo).

SPECIAL RESTRICTIONS WHILE TAKING THIS DRUG

FOOD AND DRUG INTERACTIONS

No special restrictions on other drugs, foods and beverages, alcohol use, or smoking.

DAILY LIVING

Precautions	Avoid getting this medicine in your mouth, your eyes, or the inside of your nose or in any open scratches, cuts, or sores.
	Follow your doctor's instructions carefully concerning how much of this medicine to use and how often and for how long to apply it. This medicine can stain your skin and hair, though the stain will fade after you stop using it. It can also stain your clothing and bed linens.
Helpful Hints	Since this medicine can irritate normal skin, surround the affected areas with a ring of petroleum jelly before applying it. Remove any medicine accidentally applied to normal skin.
	Always wash your hands after applying this medicine, or wear plastic gloves. To remove it from your bathtub or shower, wash it off first with hot water and then with a household cleanser.

No special restrictions on driving, exertion and exercise, sun exposure, or exposure to excessive heat or cold.

POSSIBLE SIDE EFFECTS

IF YOU DEVELOP

rash or irritation that you didn't have before using this medicine

WHAT TO DO

May be serious Check with your doctor as soon as possible.

STORAGE INSTRUCTIONS

Store in a cool, dark place (not in a bathroom medicine cabinet), and make sure that it does not freeze.

STOPPING OR INTERRUPTING THERAPY

If you miss a dose of this medicine, apply it as soon as possible. If it is almost time for your next dose, skip the missed dose and resume your regular schedule.

SPECIAL CONSIDERATIONS FOR THOSE OVER SIXTY-FIVE

None.

CONDITION: **ECZEMA, PSORIASIS, SEBORRHEA, AND DANDRUFF**

CATEGORY: **KERATOLYTIC DRUGS (COAL TAR PREPARATIONS)**

GENERIC (CHEMICAL) NAME	BRAND (TRADE) NAME	DOSAGE FORMS AND STRENGTHS
Coal tar	FOTOTAR	Cream: 2%
		Stick: 5%
	ZETAR EMULSION	Lotion: 30%

Numerous coal tar preparations are also available over the counter in a variety of brand names, dosage forms, and strengths.

DRUG PROFILE

Coal tar products are used for relief of the itching, irritation, and skin flaking seen in such conditions as eczema, psoriasis, seborrhea, and dandruff.

BEFORE USING THIS DRUG

Let your doctor know *IF*

You have ever had allergic reactions or other problems with ■ coal tar.

You have ever had any of the following medical problems: ■ sensitivity to sunlight ■ systemic lupus erythematosus ■ skin cancer.

You are taking any of the following medicines: ■ other medicine for psoriasis, especially methoxsalen and anthralin ■ griseofulvin (medicine for fungal infections) ■ nalidixic acid (medicine for urinary tract infections) ■ phenothiazines (tranquilizers) ■ sulfonamides (sulfa drugs) ■ tetracycline (antibiotic) ■ thiazide diuretics (water pills) ■ tretinoin (medicine for acne) ■ trioxsalen (medicine for virtiligo).

SPECIAL RESTRICTIONS WHILE TAKING THIS DRUG

FOOD AND DRUG INTERACTIONS

No special restrictions on other drugs, foods and beverages, alcohol use, or smoking.

DAILY LIVING

Sun Exposure	Avoid sun exposure of any skin area treated with this medicine for twenty-four hours following application unless your doctor tells you otherwise. Use clothing, sunscreens, or sunblocks for protection. Before sun exposure, remove the medicine from your skin. If you have psoriasis, your doctor may recommend sunlight or ultraviolet light treatment in combination with this medicine.
Other Precautions	Avoid getting this medicine in your eyes; in any open scratches, cuts, or sores; or in the anogenital area.
	Follow your doctor's instructions carefully concerning how much of this medicine to use and how often and for how long to apply it. If your problem continues or worsens, check with your doctor.
	This medicine can stain your skin and hair, though the stain will fade after you stop using it. It can also stain your clothing and bed linens.
Helpful Hints	If your skin becomes dry, apply an emollient (a moisturizer) to the treated area one hour after application of this medicine.

No special restrictions on driving, exertion and exercise, or exposure to excessive heat or cold.

POSSIBLE SIDE EFFECTS

IF YOU DEVELOP	WHAT TO DO
rash or irritation that you didn't have before using this medicine	**May be serious** Check with your doctor as soon as possible.
mild stinging upon application of this medicine	If symptoms are disturbing or persist, let your doctor know.

STORAGE INSTRUCTIONS

Store in a cool, dark place (not in a bathroom medicine cabinet). If your medicine is in a liquid form, make sure that it does not freeze.

STOPPING OR INTERRUPTING THERAPY

If you miss a dose of this medicine, apply it as soon as possible. If it is almost time for your next dose, skip the missed dose and resume your regular schedule.

SPECIAL CONSIDERATIONS FOR THOSE OVER SIXTY-FIVE

None.

CONDITION: **PSORIASIS**

CATEGORY: **ANTIPSORIATIC DRUGS**

GENERIC (CHEMICAL) NAME	BRAND (TRADE) NAME	DOSAGE FORMS AND STRENGTHS
Methotrexate		Tablets: 2.5 mg

DRUG PROFILE

Methotrexate is used to treat certain types of leukemia, cancer of the lymph nodes, cancer of the breast, and certain cancers of the head, neck, skin, and lung. This drug is also sometimes used to treat severe cases of psoriasis—a skin disorder. Methotrexate slows and halts the growth and spread of cancer cells by interfering with one of the steps in cell growth.

For complete information on this drug, see pages 889–893.

CONDITION: **DANDRUFF AND SEBORRHEA**

CATEGORY: **ANTISEBORRHEIC DRUGS**

GENERIC (CHEMICAL) NAME	BRAND (TRADE) NAME	DOSAGE FORMS AND STRENGTHS
Selenium sulfide	SELSUN	Lotion: 2.5%
	EXSEL	Lotion: 2.5%

DRUG PROFILE

Selenium sulfide is used to control dandruff and seborrhea of the scalp. It is also sometimes used to treat certain fungal infections of the skin.

BEFORE USING THIS DRUG

Let your doctor know *IF*

You have ever had allergic reactions or other problems with ■ selenium sulfide.

SPECIAL RESTRICTIONS WHILE TAKING THIS DRUG

FOOD AND DRUG INTERACTIONS

No special restrictions on other drugs, foods and beverages, alcohol use, or smoking.

DAILY LIVING

Precautions	Avoid getting this medicine in your eyes or in any open scratches, cuts, or sores.
	Remove all jewelry before using selenium sulfide lotion to avoid possible damage.
Helpful Hints	Rinse your hair thoroughly after applying this medicine to minimize the chance of hair discoloration.

No special restrictions on driving, exertion and exercise, sun exposure, or exposure to excessive heat or cold.

POSSIBLE SIDE EFFECTS

IF YOU DEVELOP	WHAT TO DO
irritation or rash that you didn't have before using this medicine	**May be serious** Check with your doctor as soon as possible.
dryness or oiliness of the hair or scalp ■ hair loss	If symptoms are disturbing or persist, let your doctor know.

STORAGE INSTRUCTIONS

Keep this medicine in a tight container in a cool, dark place (not in a bathroom medicine cabinet), and make sure that it does not freeze.

STOPPING OR INTERRUPTING THERAPY

Although dandruff usually responds well to selenium sulfide products, the problem tends to recur once treatment is stopped. It is best to continue to use this medicine on a regular, relatively infrequent basis (once every one to four weeks) as needed.

SPECIAL CONSIDERATIONS FOR THOSE OVER SIXTY-FIVE

None.

CONDITION: **ROSACEA**

CATEGORY: **ANTIBIOTICS FOR SKIN DISORDERS (TETRACYCLINES)**

GENERIC (CHEMICAL) NAME	BRAND (TRADE) NAME	DOSAGE FORMS AND STRENGTHS
Tetracycline hydrochloride	ACHROMYCIN V	Capsules: 250, 500 mg Suspension: 125 mg per tsp
	PANMYCIN	Capsules: 250 mg
	ROBITET	Capsules: 250, 500 mg
	SUMYCIN	Capsules: 250, 500 mg Syrup: 125 mg per tsp Tablets: 250, 500 mg
Minocycline	MINOCIN	Capsules: 50, 100 mg Suspension: 50 mg per tsp Tablets: 50, 100 mg

DRUG PROFILE

Tetracyclines are antibiotics that are used to treat a wide variety of bacterial infections, including skin eruptions and bronchitis and pneumonia. These antibiotics suppress the growth of bacteria by interfering with their manufacture of protein.

For complete information on these drugs, see pages 591–595.

CONDITION: **ROSACEA**

CATEGORY: **ANTIBIOTICS FOR SKIN DISORDERS**

GENERIC (CHEMICAL) NAME	BRAND (TRADE) NAME	DOSAGE FORMS AND STRENGTHS
Metronidazole	FLAGYL	Tablets: 250, 500 mg

DRUG PROFILE

Metronidazole is an antibiotic that is used to treat trichomoniasis (a vaginal infection) as well as a wide variety of systemic infections including dysentery and infections of the respiratory tract, skin, bones and joints, and stomach.

For complete information on this drug, see pages 809–811.

BEDSORES

Decubitus ulcers, better known as bed-sores, are open wounds that can develop when someone lies or sits in the same position for a long time. Most often, they affect people who are bed-ridden because of a long-term illness or a major disability. But bedsores are more than an unsightly accompaniment to a long stay in bed. These ulcers may become infected, and if they're not treated properly, the infected area may expand.

CAUSES

Bedsores don't occur randomly on different parts of the body. Instead, they tend to develop in certain ulcer sites that vary with the person's position. When someone who is bedridden lies on his or her back, the body's weight presses most heavily at the shoulders, elbows, base of the spine, buttocks, and heels. Lying on one's side produces different pressure points—at the outside of the ankle and the thigh. Being confined to a wheel-chair means still different areas of pressure—on the rim of the pelvic bones and in the lower part of the buttocks.

These areas of pressure are prime targets for bedsores. What happens is that the body weight, pressing down day after day, squeezes the small blood vessels that nourish the skin. The vessels can actually be compressed to the point at which the blood can't continue to flow; the skin, deprived of its blood supply, begins to die, and an ulcer forms. This process can happen to anyone confined to bed or a wheel-chair, but people who have a chronic vascular disease are particularly vulnerable.

DIAGNOSIS

The first sign of a bedsore is a red or purple blotch on the skin over one of the pressure points. It may be painful and feel hot. If the pressure is relieved, the skin will return to normal within a few weeks. Otherwise, the bedsore will get worse. The skin will crack, and blisters will form. Bacteria then usually invade the site, doing further damage as the hole in the skin widens and deepens, opening a channel that can go all the way down to the bone.

PREVENTION AND TREATMENT

Confinement to bed does not necessarily produce bedsores. They may be avoided if the person's position is changed frequently, his or her skin kept clean and dry, and the bedsheets kept absolutely smooth so that wrinkles won't irritate the skin. At the very first sign of a bedsore, you should ask your doctor what to do, since healing is much easier to accomplish before the skin begins to break and blister.

If your doctor is concerned about the possibility of infection—or if bacteria have already invaded the wound—you may be given a prescription for a medicine you can apply right to the affected area. Such topical medicines are described in the drug chart on page 758. In cases where bedsores are neglected and penetrate far below the skin, surgery may be necessary to remove the damaged area and close the opening.

CONDITION: **BEDSORES**

CATEGORY: **TOPICAL ANTIBIOTICS**

GENERIC (CHEMICAL) NAME	BRAND (TRADE) NAME	DOSAGE FORMS AND STRENGTHS
Gentamicin sulfate	GARAMYCIN	Cream: 0.1% Ointment: 0.1%
Polymyxin B sulfate and bacitracin zinc	POLYSPORIN	Ointment: 10,000 units polymyxin B sulfate and 500 units of bacitracin zinc, per gram

This type of medicine is available under other brand names; milder strengths are available over the counter.

DRUG PROFILE

Gentamicin works by interfering with the bacteria's ability to manufacture protein. Polymyxin B alters the membrane of the bacterial cell so that the bacteria lose essential nutrients. Bacitracin interferes with the bacteria's ability to form new protective cell walls.

For complete information on these drugs, see pages 695–697.

Chapter 11
Disorders of the
Genitourinary Tract

URINARY TRACT INFECTION

Infections are among the most common problems of the urinary tract, especially in older people. The organs that may be affected are the kidneys, the bladder, the urethra (the tube that carries urine out of the bladder), and, in men, the prostate gland.

It's possible to have a urinary tract infection and have no symptoms at all. But more commonly, the problem is signalled by one or more of the following problems: a burning sensation when urinating; an urgent need to urinate frequently; blood in the urine; pain in the lower abdomen, groin, or back; and fever. A headache and loss of appetite may also accompany this condition.

CAUSES

The most common cause of urinary tract infections is a bacterium called *Escherichia coli (E. coli* for short), though other bacteria as well as fungi may be involved. *E. coli* normally resides in the colon, but it can migrate to, and multiply in, the urinary tract.

Older people may be especially prone to bacterial invasion of the urinary tract for several reasons. In the first place, the body's immune system, which fights off infection, may not be as efficient as it once was. Therefore, bacteria can multiply more easily.

Physical changes in the urinary tract may also set the stage for infection. In older men, the prostate gland sometimes enlarges and squeezes the urethra; urine therefore pools in the bladder and becomes a breeding ground for bacteria. A loss of bladder muscle strength that leaves women unable to empty their bladders completely can have a similar effect. Although women do not have a prostate gland, the urethra is shorter and closes less tightly, thereby making the bladder more vulnerable to bacteria from the outside. Atrophic vaginitis (see page 798) may add to discomfort.

Other sources of infection may include surgical procedures or urinary catheters, which can irritate the urinary tract and even introduce bacteria into the body. Lurking behind some urinary tract infections is a kidney stone or other blockage to the flow of urine.

DIAGNOSIS

Infections of different areas of the urinary tract have different names: pyelonephritis if the infection is in the kidneys; cystitis if it is in the bladder; urethritis, in the urethra; and prostatitis, in the prostate.

Whatever you call it, a urinary tract infection can make you quite uncomfortable and definitely warrants medical attention. Your doctor will probably want to examine a urine specimen under the microscope to determine precisely what is bothering you and to devise an appropriate treatment plan.

You may be asked simply to produce a specimen by urinating as you ordinarily would. Or the doctor may tell you to cleanse yourself thoroughly, empty your bladder partially, and then release the remaining urine into a specimen bottle. Men may have to use three specimen bottles so that the doctor can do different tests for cystitis, prostatitis, and urethritis.

TREATMENT

Antibiotics are usually quite effective in clearing up urinary tract infections within a week to ten days, though your doctor may prescribe the medicine for two weeks to be certain that the bacteria are all gone. For more information on these drugs, refer to the drug charts on pages 762–778.

Sometimes symptoms return within about two to four weeks of the end of therapy. This happens because the infecting organism was not completely eradicated. Or a new infection may occur caused by a different organism; this usually happens within six months of the original infection. If these relapses or reinfections occur frequently, your doctor may do further tests or prescribe the antibiotic for a longer period of time.

Most doctors choose not to prescribe medicine for older people who have urinary tract infections without any symptoms, since the potential side effects of the medicine outweigh the benefits of treatment in this case. However, if the infection is a symptom of another problem such as a kidney stone or obstruction, that condition will have to be addressed.

OUTLOOK

Urinary tract infections are highly treatable, especially those involving the bladder and urethra. When treatment is started at an early stage, continued for the proper length of time, and resumed or changed appropriately if a relapse occurs, these infections pose no serious threat to health.

CONDITION: **URINARY TRACT INFECTIONS**

CATEGORY: **URINARY ANTI-INFECTIVES**

GENERIC (CHEMICAL) NAME	BRAND (TRADE) NAME	DOSAGE FORMS AND STRENGTHS
Sulfamethoxazole and phenazopyridine hydrochloride	AZO GANTANOL	Tablets: 500 mg sulfamethoxazole and 100 mg phenozopyridine hydrochloride
Sulfisoxazole and phenazopyridine hydrochloride	AZO GANTRISIN	Tablets: 500 mg sulfisoxazole and 50 mg phenazopyridine hydrochloride

DRUG PROFILE

This type of combination drug is used to treat infections of the urinary tract. Sulfamethoxazole and sulfisoxazole are "sulfa" antibiotics, which suppress the growth of bacteria. Phenazopyridine relieves such symptoms of urinary tract infections as pain, burning, and irritation.

BEFORE USING THIS DRUG

Let your doctor know *IF*

You have ever had allergic reactions or other problems with ■ sulfonamides (sulfa drugs) ■ thiazide diuretics (water pills) ■ medicine for diabetes.

You have ever had any of the following medical problems: ■ glucose-6-phosphate dehydrogenase (G-6-PD) deficiency ■ porphyria ■ kidney disease ■ liver disease ■ blood disease ■ asthma or severe allergies.

You are taking any of the following medicines: ■ other sulfa drugs ■ any oral medicine containing para-aminobenzoic acid (PABA) ■ phenytoin (medicine for seizures ■ digoxin, digitoxin, or digitalis (heart medicines) ■ sulfinpyrazone (medicine for gout) ■ aspirin, aspirinlike medicine, or other medicine for pain and inflammation ■ methotrexate (medicine for cancer and severe psoriasis) ■ anti-coagulants (blood thinners) ■ medicine for diabetes ■ tricyclic antidepressants ■ methenamine (other medicine for urinary tract infections) ■ barbiturates.

SPECIAL RESTRICTIONS WHILE TAKING THIS DRUG

FOOD AND DRUG INTERACTIONS

No special restrictions on other drugs, foods and beverages, alcohol use, or smoking.

DAILY LIVING

Sun Exposure	Your skin may become more sensitive to sunlight and more likely to develop a sunburn while you are taking this drug. It is a good idea to avoid too much sun and to apply a sunscreen to exposed skin surfaces before going outdoors.
Examinations or Tests	It is important for you to keep all appointments with your doctor so that your progress can be checked. Blood or urine tests may be required.
Other Precautions	Tell any doctor or dentist you consult that you are taking this medicine, especially if you will be undergoing any type of surgery or diagnostic testing. This medicine causes the urine to turn a reddish-orange color. This effect will disappear when you stop taking it. If you have diabetes, be aware that this drug may affect urine-sugar and ketone tests. Check with your doctor to see whether you should use a different type of test. If your symptoms do not improve within a few days or if they worsen, check with your doctor.

Helpful Hints   For maximum benefit, take this drug on an empty stomach (one hour before or two hours after meals).

Be sure to drink four to six extra glasses of water a day while taking this drug.

No special restrictions on driving, exertion and exercise, or exposure to excessive heat or cold.

POSSIBLE SIDE EFFECTS

Although this list of adverse effects may seem somewhat intimidating, keep in mind that some are quite rare. Of course, should these or any other problems arise while you are on medication, it is always a good idea to consult your doctor.

IF YOU DEVELOP

seizures ■ bluish tinge to skin ■ rash ■ difficulty in breathing

Symptoms of hypoglycemia: ''hot'' feeling, increased sweating, dizziness, unsteadiness, tremors, weakness, blurred vision, hunger, headache, tingling in lips, slurred speech

numbness, tingling, or pain in hands or feet ■ paleness ■ sore throat or fever ■ bleeding or bruising ■ hives, itching, or other skin problems ■ severe headache ■ mouth sores ■ red, itching eyes with runny nose ■ swelling around eyes or neck ■ swelling of the tip of the penis ■ joint pain ■ yellowing of eyes or skin ■ stomach pain ■ blood in urine ■ decreased or increased urination ■ pain or burning sensation in urination ■ low back pain ■ clumsiness ■ depression ■ confusion ■ hallucinations ■ behavior changes ■ tiredness or weakness ■ swelling of tongue or vocal cords ■ ringing or buzzing sound in ears or other hearing problems

WHAT TO DO

Urgent Get in touch with your doctor immediately.

May be serious Check with your doctor as soon as possible.

With Azo Gantrisin only: vomiting, with blood or vomit that looks like coffee grounds ■ bloody or black, tarry stools ■ flushing ■ irregular or fast heartbeat ■ fainting ■ spasms ■ chest pain ■ muscle pain ■ swelling of hands or feet ■ swelling around ears

upset stomach ■ nausea or vomiting ■ increased skin sensitivity to sunlight ■ headache ■ dizziness ■ drowsiness ■ restlessness ■ sleeplessness ■ loss of appetite ■ diarrhea ■ gas ■ skin color changes ■ anxiety

If symptoms are disturbing or persist, let your doctor know.

STORAGE INSTRUCTIONS

Store in a cool, dark place (not in a bathroom medicine cabinet).

STOPPING OR INTERRUPTING THERAPY

This medicine should be taken without interruption for the full length of time prescribed by your doctor, even if you begin to feel better. If you do miss a dose, take it as soon as possible. If it is almost time for your next dose, skip the missed dose and resume your regular schedule. Do not take two doses at the same time.

SPECIAL CONSIDERATIONS FOR THOSE OVER SIXTY-FIVE

Because sulfa drugs are excreted through the kidneys and kidney function commonly decreases with age, doctors may start people over sixty-five on a lower dosage of this drug.

CONDITION: **URINARY TRACT INFECTIONS**

CATEGORY: **URINARY ANTI-INFECTIVES**

GENERIC (CHEMICAL) NAME	BRAND (TRADE) NAME	DOSAGE FORMS AND STRENGTHS
Nalidixic acid	NegGRAM	Suspension: 250 mg per tsp Tablets: 250, 500, 1,000 mg

DRUG PROFILE

Nalidixic acid is used to treat bacterial infections of the urinary tract. This antibiotic drug interferes with the growth of bacteria.

BEFORE USING THIS DRUG

Let your doctor know *IF*

You have ever had allergic reactions or other problems with ■ nalidixic acid ■ oxolinic acid (another urinary antibiotic).

You have ever had any of the following medical problems: ■ seizures ■ cerebral atherosclerosis ■ asthma or other lung disease ■ kidney disease ■ liver disease.

You are taking any of the following medicines: ■ anticoagulants (blood thinners) ■ antacids ■ nitrofurantoin (another urinary antibiotic).

SPECIAL RESTRICTIONS WHILE TAKING THIS DRUG

FOOD AND DRUG INTERACTIONS

Other Drugs	If you are taking an antacid, take it two hours before or after a dose of this medicine.

No special restrictions on foods and beverages, alcohol use, or smoking.

DAILY LIVING

Sun Exposure	This drug may make your skin become more sensitive to sunlight, causing redness and blisters after sun exposure. It is a good idea to avoid prolonged sun exposure and to apply a sunscreen to exposed skin surfaces before going outdoors.
Examinations or Tests	It is important for you to keep all appointments with your doctor so that your progress can be checked. If you are on long-term therapy, periodic blood or urine tests may be required.

Other Precautions	If you have diabetes, be aware that this drug may affect urine-sugar tests. Check with your doctor before increasing your diabetes medicine or altering your diet. If your symptoms do not improve within two days or if they worsen, check with your doctor.
Helpful Hints	For maximum benefit, take this medicine one hour before meals. However, if this medicine upsets your stomach, ask your doctor if you can take it with food or milk.

No special restrictions on driving, exertion and exercise, or exposure to excessive heat or cold.

POSSIBLE SIDE EFFECTS

Although this list of adverse effects may seem somewhat intimidating, keep in mind that some are quite rare. Of course, should these or any other problems arise while you are on medication, it is always a good idea to consult your doctor.

IF YOU DEVELOP

seizures ■ difficulty in breathing ■ personality changes ■ severe drowsiness ■ severe or continuing nausea or vomiting

WHAT TO DO

Urgent Get in touch with your doctor immediately.

blurred or double vision ■ trouble focusing ■ change in color vision ■ increased skin sensitivity to sunlight ■ severe stomach pain ■ sore throat or fever ■ chills ■ bleeding or bruising ■ dark urine ■ yellowing of eyes or skin ■ extreme tiredness or weakness ■ fainting ■ muscle ache ■ joint stiffness ■ excitement ■ confusion ■ depression ■ change in hearing, smell, taste, or touch ■ eye pain or burning ■ jerky eye movements

May be serious Check with your doctor as soon as possible.

diarrhea ■ stomach pain ■ nausea or vomiting
■ rash, hives, or itching ■ dizziness ■ drowsiness
■ headache ■ general feeling of unwellness
■ sleeplessness

If symptoms are disturbing or persist, let your doctor know.

STORAGE INSTRUCTIONS

Store in a cool, dark place (not in a bathroom medicine cabinet). If your medicine is in a liquid form, make sure that it does not freeze.

STOPPING OR INTERRUPTING THERAPY

This medicine should be taken without interruption for the full length of time prescribed by your doctor, even if you begin to feel better. If you do miss a dose, take it as soon as possible. If it is almost time for your next dose and you take three or more doses per day, either space the missed dose and the following dose two to four hours apart or double the following dose.

SPECIAL CONSIDERATIONS FOR THOSE OVER SIXTY-FIVE

None.

CONDITION: **URINARY TRACT INFECTIONS**

CATEGORY: **URINARY ANTI-INFECTIVES**

GENERIC (CHEMICAL) NAME	BRAND (TRADE) NAME	DOSAGE FORMS AND STRENGTHS
Trimethoprim	PROLOPRIM	Tablets: 100, 200 mg
	TRIMPEX	Tablets: 100 mg

DRUG PROFILE

Trimethoprim is used to treat bacterial infections of the urinary tract. This antibiotic suppresses the growth of bacteria.

BEFORE USING THIS DRUG

Let your doctor know *IF*

You have ever had allergic reactions or other problems with ■ trimethoprim.

You have ever had any of the following medical problems: ■ kidney disease ■ liver disease ■ anemia ■ gout ■ malaria.

You are taking any of the following medicines: ■ phenytoin (medicine for seizures and abnormal heart rhythms) ■ anticoagulants (blood thinners) ■ folic acid ■ medicine for diabetes ■ methotrexate (medicine for cancer and severe psoriasis) ■ thiazide diuretics (water pills) ■ medicine for arthritis.

SPECIAL RESTRICTIONS WHILE TAKING THIS DRUG

FOOD AND DRUG INTERACTIONS

No special restrictions on other drugs, foods and beverages, alcohol use, or smoking.

DAILY LIVING

Examinations or Tests	It is important for you to keep all appointments with your doctor so that your progress can be checked.
Other Precautions	If your symptoms do not improve within a few days or if they should worsen, check with your doctor.
Helpful Hints	If this medicine upsets your stomach, taking it with milk, meals, or snacks should help.

No special restrictions on driving, exertion and exercise, sun exposure, or exposure to excessive heat or cold.

POSSIBLE SIDE EFFECTS

Although this list of adverse effects may seem somewhat intimidating, keep in mind that some are quite rare. Of course, should these or any other problems arise while you are on medication, it is always a good idea to consult your doctor.

IF YOU DEVELOP	WHAT TO DO
severe or continuing nausea or vomiting ■ headache ■ dizziness ■ difficulty in breathing	**Urgent** Get in touch with your doctor immediately.
sore throat ■ fever ■ pale skin ■ extreme tiredness ■ bluish nails, lips, or skin ■ bleeding or bruising	**May be serious** Check with your doctor as soon as possible.
rash, itching, or other skin problems ■ nausea or vomiting ■ upset stomach ■ tongue inflammation ■ taste changes ■ diarrhea ■ loss of appetite ■ stomach cramps ■ sore mouth	If symptoms are disturbing or persist, let your doctor know.

STORAGE INSTRUCTIONS

Store in a cool, dark place (not in a bathroom medicine cabinet).

STOPPING OR INTERRUPTING THERAPY

This medicine should be taken without interruption for the full length of time prescribed by your doctor, even if you begin to feel better. If you miss a dose, take it as soon as possible. If it is almost time for your next dose, space the missed dose and following dose ten to twelve hours apart. Then return to your regular schedule.

SPECIAL CONSIDERATIONS FOR THOSE OVER SIXTY-FIVE

None.

CONDITION: **URINARY TRACT INFECTIONS**

CATEGORY: **URINARY ANTI-INFECTIVES**

GENERIC (CHEMICAL) NAME	BRAND (TRADE) NAME	DOSAGE FORMS AND STRENGTHS
Trimethoprim and sulfamethoxazole	BACTRIM	Suspension: 40 mg trimethoprim and 200 mg sulfamethoxazole per tsp Tablets: 80 mg trimethoprim and 400 mg sulfamethoxazole; 160 mg trimethoprim and 800 mg sulfamethoxazole
	SEPTRA	Suspension: 40 mg trimethoprim and 200 mg sulfamethoxazole per tsp Tablets: 80 mg trimethoprim and 400 mg sulfamethoxazole; 160 mg trimethoprim and 800 mg sulfamethoxazole

DRUG PROFILE

This combination drug is used to treat bacterial infections, including those that affect the urinary tract. The antibiotics trimethoprim and sulfamethoxazole work together to suppress the growth of bacteria.

BEFORE USING THIS DRUG

Let your doctor know *IF*

You have ever had allergic reactions or other problems with ■ trimethoprim ■ sulfamethoxazole ■ other sulfonamides (sulfa drugs) ■ thiazide diuretics (water pills) ■ medicine for diabetes.

You have ever had any of the following medical problems: ■ glucose-6-phosphate dehydrogenase (G-6-PD) deficiency ■ folate deficiency ■ anemia ■ porphyria ■ kidney disease ■ liver disease ■ blood disease ■ asthma or other lung disease.

You are taking any of the following medicines: ■ sulfonamides (sulfa drugs) or other urinary antibiotics ■ anticoagulants (blood thinners) ■ any oral medicine containing para-aminobenzoic acid (PABA) ■ medicine for seizures ■ methotrexate (medicine for cancer and severe psoriasis) ■ medicine for diabetes ■ aspirin, aspirinlike medicine, or other medicine for pain and inflammation ■ sulfinpyrazone (medicine for gout) ■ folic acid.

SPECIAL RESTRICTIONS WHILE TAKING THIS DRUG

FOOD AND DRUG INTERACTIONS

Foods and Beverages	Because this medicine can cause folic acid deficiency, be sure to eat a well-balanced diet including plenty of B vitamins.

No special restrictions on other drugs, alcohol use, or smoking.

DAILY LIVING

Sun Exposure	Your skin may become more sensitive to sunlight and more likely to develop a sunburn while you are taking this drug. It is a good idea to avoid too much sun and to apply a sunscreen to exposed skin surfaces before going outdoors.
Examinations or Tests	It is important for you to keep all appointments with your doctor so that your progress can be checked. Periodic urine tests may be required.
Other Precautions	If you have diabetes, be aware that this drug may affect urine-sugar and ketone tests. Check with your doctor to see whether you should use a different type of test. If your symptoms do not improve within a few days or if they worsen, check with your doctor.

Helpful Hints	If this medicine upsets your stomach, taking it with milk, meals, or snacks should help.
	Be sure to drink four to six glasses of water a day while taking this medicine so that your body can easily eliminate the waste products of the medicine.

No special restrictions on driving, exertion and exercise, or exposure to excessive heat or cold.

POSSIBLE SIDE EFFECTS

Although this list of adverse effects may seem somewhat intimidating, keep in mind that some are quite rare. Of course, should these or any other problems arise while you are on medication, it is always a good idea to consult your doctor.

IF YOU DEVELOP	WHAT TO DO
difficulty in breathing ■ sore throat or fever ■ chills ■ extreme tiredness ■ bleeding or bruising ■ joint pain ■ blood in urine if not present earlier ■ dramatically increased or decreased urination ■ swelling in neck ■ severe diarrhea	**Urgent: Stop taking this drug and get in touch with your doctor immediately.**
rash, hives, or other skin problems ■ very pale skin ■ swelling around eyes ■ red, itching eyes ■ tiredness ■ nervousness ■ muscle weakness ■ clumsiness ■ ringing or buzzing sound in ears ■ depression ■ hallucinations ■ yellowing of eyes or skin ■ change in urine or stool color ■ numbness, tingling, or pain in hands or feet ■ bluish nails, lips, or skin ■ low back pain	**May be serious** Check with your doctor as soon as possible.
headache ■ diarrhea ■ dizziness ■ nausea or vomiting ■ stomach pain ■ increased skin sensitivity to sunlight ■ tongue inflammation ■ mouth sores ■ sleeplessness	If symptoms are disturbing or persist, let your doctor know.

STORAGE INSTRUCTIONS

Store in a cool, dark place (not in a bathroom medicine cabinet). If your medicine is in a liquid form, make sure that it does not freeze.

STOPPING OR INTERRUPTING THERAPY

This medicine should be taken without interruption for the full length of time prescribed by your doctor, even if you begin to feel better. If you do miss a dose, space the missed dose between the time you should have taken it and your next scheduled dose or simply double the next scheduled dose and resume your regular schedule.

SPECIAL CONSIDERATIONS FOR THOSE OVER SIXTY-FIVE

Because this medicine is excreted through the kidneys and kidney function commonly decreases with age, doctors may start people over sixty-five on a lower dosage of this medicine.

CONDITION: **URINARY TRACT INFECTIONS**

CATEGORY: **URINARY ANTI-INFECTIVES**

GENERIC (CHEMICAL) NAME	BRAND (TRADE) NAME	DOSAGE FORMS AND STRENGTHS
Methenamine hippurate	HIPREX UREX	Tablets: 1 g Tablets: 1 g
Methenamine mandelate	MANDELAMINE	Granules: 1 g Suspension: 250, 500 mg per tsp Tablets: 0.5, 1 g
Methenamine, methylene blue, phenyl salicylate, benzoic acid, atropine sulfate, and hyoscyamine	URISED	Tablets: 40.8 mg methenamine, 5.4 mg methylene blue, 18.1 mg phenyl salicylate, 4.5 mg benzoic acid, 0.03 mg atropine sulfate, and 0.03 mg hyoscyamine

DRUG PROFILE

Methenamine is used to prevent urinary tract infections from recurring. It is converted into an antibacterial drug in the acidic environment of the urinary tract.

BEFORE USING THIS DRUG

Let your doctor know *IF*

You have ever had allergic reactions or other problems with ■ methenamine ■ tartrazine (FD&C Yellow Dye No. 5) (contained in Hiprex tablets).

You have ever had any of the following medical problems: ■ liver disease.

■ *with Urised only:* ■ heart disease ■ difficulty in urination ■ enlarged prostate ■ glaucoma ■ fecal (stool) impaction or severe constipation.

You are taking any of the following medicines: ■ sulfonamides (sulfa drugs) ■ diuretics (water pills) ■ medicine to make the urine less acidic ■ baking soda ■ any medicine containing potassium citrate, sodium acetate, sodium citrate, or sodium lactate ■ antacids.

■ *with Urised only:* ■ medicine for stomach cramps or pain ■ amantadine (medicine for Parkinson's disease and influenza) ■ antihistamines ■ haloperidol (tranquilizer) ■ phenothiazines (tranquilizers and medicine for nausea) ■ medicine for depression.

SPECIAL RESTRICTIONS WHILE TAKING THIS DRUG

FOOD AND DRUG INTERACTIONS

Other Drugs	Do not take any other drugs, including over-the-counter (OTC) drugs, before checking with your doctor. OTC antacids and allergy or cold medicines may interfere with the action of these drugs.
Foods and Beverages	These drugs are most effective when the urine is very acidic. Foods and beverages that make the urine more acidic include cranberry juice, plums, prunes, and protein-rich foods. Avoid foods and beverages that make the urine alkaline, such as most fruits, especially citrus fruits and juices, milk, cheese, and other dairy products.

No special restrictions on alcohol use or smoking.

DAILY LIVING

Driving

Urised may cause blurred vision or loss of alertness. Be careful when driving, operating household appliances, or doing any other tasks that require alertness until you know how this drug affects you.

Exertion and Exercise

Urised may cause you to sweat less than normally. Sweating is your body's natural way of cooling down, and not sweating enough can be dangerous. Use caution not to become overheated when you exercise or exert yourself.

Excessive Heat

See above; use caution during hot weather, as overexertion may result in heat stroke. Avoid extremely hot baths and saunas.

Examinations or Tests

It is important for you to keep all appointments with your doctor so that your progress can be checked. Periodic blood or urine tests may be required. Your doctor will probably instruct you to test the acidity of your urine with urine acid test paper once a day; follow directions exactly.

Other Precautions

If your symptoms do not improve within a few days or if they should worsen, check with your doctor.

If you are taking Urised, be aware that your urine and stools may be discolored because of the methylene blue component (a dye) in the drug.

Helpful Hints

Taking this medicine after meals and at bedtime may help reduce the chance of upset stomach.

Swallow tablets whole, without crushing or chewing. Dissolve the granules in two to four ounces of water and stir well before drinking.

If your mouth or throat feels dry, chewing sugarless gum or sucking ice chips or sugarless hard candy will help.

No special restrictions on sun exposure or exposure to excessive cold.

POSSIBLE SIDE EFFECTS

Although this list of adverse effects may seem somewhat intimidating, keep in mind that some are quite rare. Of course, should these or any other problems arise while you are on medication, it is always a good idea to consult your doctor.

IF YOU DEVELOP	WHAT TO DO
fever ■ difficulty in breathing	**Urgent** Get in touch with your doctor immediately.
With Urised only: ■ irregular or fast heartbeat ■ dizziness ■ blurred vision ■ hot, dry, flushed skin ■ cessation of urination	
blood in urine ■ lower back pain ■ pain in urination ■ urinary frequency ■ dry mouth ■ swelling of face, feet, or hands ■ muscle cramps ■ ringing or buzzing sound in ears	**May be serious** Check with your doctor as soon as possible.
nausea or vomiting ■ rash, hives, or itching ■ diarrhea ■ stomach cramps ■ loss of appetite ■ mouth sores	If symptoms are disturbing or persist, let your doctor know.

STORAGE INSTRUCTIONS

Store in a cool, dark place (not in a bathroom medicine cabinet). If your medicine is in a liquid form, make sure that it does not freeze.

STOPPING OR INTERRUPTING THERAPY

This medicine should be taken without interruption for the full length of time prescribed by your doctor, even if you begin to feel better. If you do miss a dose, take it as soon as possible. If it is almost time for your next dose and you take two doses a day, space the missed dose and following dose five to six hours apart; if you take three or more doses a day, space the missed dose and the following dose two to four hours apart, or simply double the following dose. Then resume your regular schedule.

SPECIAL CONSIDERATIONS FOR THOSE OVER SIXTY-FIVE

Doctors may start people over sixty-five on a lower-than-usual adult dosage. Older people may be more prone to the side effects of Urised and doctors may wish to check them frequently while they are taking this drug.

CONDITION: **URINARY TRACT INFECTIONS**

CATEGORY: **URINARY ANALGESICS**

GENERIC (CHEMICAL) NAME	BRAND (TRADE) NAME	DOSAGE FORMS AND STRENGTHS
Phenazopyridine hydro-chloride	PYRIDIUM	Tablets: 100, 200 mg
Phenazopyridine hydro-chloride, hyoscyamine hydrobromide, and butabarbital	PYRIDIUM PLUS	Tablets: 150 mg phenazopyridine hydro-chloride, 0.3 mg hyoscyamine hydrobromide, and 15 mg butabarbital

DRUG PROFILE

Phenazopyridine is prescribed to relieve symptoms of urinary tract infections such as pain, burning, irritation, and frequency and urgency of urination.

BEFORE USING THIS DRUG

Let your doctor know *IF*

You have ever had allergic reactions or other problems with ■ phenazopyridine ■ hyoscyamine ■ butabarbital.

You have ever had any of the following medical problems: ■ hepatitis ■ kidney disease ■ glucose-6-phosphate dehydrogenase (G-6-PD) deficiency.

■ *with Pyridium Plus only:* ■ glaucoma ■ porphyria ■ bladder neck obstruction.

You are taking any of the following medicines:

■ *with Pyridium Plus only:* ■ anticoagulants (blood thinners) ■ amantadine (medicine for Parkinson's disease or influenza) ■ antihistamines ■ medicine for hay fever, coughs, or colds ■ narcotics or other prescription pain-killers ■ sleep medicines ■ tranquilizers ■ medicine for seizures ■ medicine for stomach cramps ■ antacids ■ medicine for diarrhea ■ corticosteroids ■ digoxin, digitoxin, or digitalis (heart medicines) ■ griseofulvin (medicine for fungal infections) ■ tetracyclines ■ medicine for depression.

SPECIAL RESTRICTIONS WHILE TAKING THIS DRUG

FOOD AND DRUG INTERACTIONS

Other Drugs	Do not take any other drug, including OTC drugs, before checking with your doctor—especially if you are taking Pyridium Plus. Pyridium Plus increases the effects of drugs that depress the central nervous system, such as antihistamines; medicine for hay fever, allergies, or colds; sleep medicines; tranquilizers; narcotics or other prescription pain-killers; muscle relaxants; and medicine for seizures.
Alcohol	Pyridium Plus increases the effects of alcohol, a central nervous system depressant. Avoid alcohol if you are taking Pyridium Plus unless your doctor has approved its use.

No special restrictions on foods and beverages or smoking.

DAILY LIVING

Driving	Pyridium Plus may cause blurred vision, dizziness, or drowsiness. If you are taking Pyridium Plus, be careful when driving, operating household appliances, or doing any other tasks that require alertness until you know how this drug affects you.
Exertion and Exercise	Pyridium Plus may cause you to sweat less than normally. Sweating is your body's natural way of cooling down, and not sweating enough can be dangerous. Use caution not to become overheated when you exercise or exert yourself.
Excessive Heat	See above; use caution during hot weather, as overexertion may result in heat stroke. Avoid extremely hot baths and saunas.
Other Precautions	These drugs cause the urine to turn a reddish-orange color. This effect will disappear when you stop taking the drug.
	If your symptoms do not improve within a few days or if they worsen, check with your doctor.
	If you have diabetes, be aware that this drug may affect urine-sugar and ketone tests. Check with your doctor to see whether you should use a different type of test.
	Especially for Pyridium Plus: Do not take this drug more often or for a longer period of time than directed by your doctor, since it may become habit forming.
Helpful Hints	If this medicine upsets your stomach, taking it with or immediately after meals should help.

No special restrictions on sun exposure or exposure to excessive cold.

POSSIBLE SIDE EFFECTS

Although this list of adverse effects may seem somewhat intimidating, keep in mind that some are quite rare. Of course, should these or any other problems arise while you are on medication, it is always a good idea to consult your doctor.

IF YOU DEVELOP	WHAT TO DO
pain in urination ■ bluish tinge to skin *With Pyridium Plus only:* difficulty in breathing ■ fast heartbeat ■ hot, dry, flushed skin ■ dry mouth ■ delirium ■ fever■ seizures ■ extreme drowsiness	**Urgent** Get in touch with your doctor immediately.
extreme tiredness ■ skin color changes ■ yellowing of eyes or skin ■ hives *With Pyridium Plus only:* blurred vision ■ nausea or vomiting ■ decreased urination	**May be serious** Check with your doctor as soon as possible.
headache ■ dizziness ■ upset stomach *With Pyridium Plus only:* drowsiness ■ confusion	If symptoms are disturbing or persist, let your doctor know.

STORAGE INSTRUCTIONS

Store in a cool, dark place (not in a bathroom medicine cabinet).

STOPPING OR INTERRUPTING THERAPY

If you miss a dose, take it as soon as possible. If it is almost time for your next dose, skip the missed dose and resume your regular schedule. Do not take two doses at the same time.

SPECIAL CONSIDERATIONS FOR THOSE OVER SIXTY-FIVE

Older people may be more prone to the side effects of Pyridium Plus. Doctors may wish to check people over sixty-five frequently.

URINARY INCONTINENCE

Urinary incontinence—a loss of urinary control—is a problem that commonly accompanies aging, affecting more than two out of every ten older people. It occurs most frequently in older women but strikes men as well. Incontinence can range from the discomfort of slight losses of urine to the distress and disability of severe, frequent wetting.

Most people don't realize that many cases of incontinence can be cured and that the majority of cases can be treated and controlled. This condition is *not* an inevitable result of aging, nor is it a disease. Rather, it is a symptom of an underlying problem, such as a neurologic disorder, or the result of using certain medicines. The three major types of incontinence are discussed below.

STRESS INCONTINENCE

The leakage of urine during activities that put pressure on the bladder, such as coughing or laughing, is called stress incontinence. In women, it may be caused by changes in the anatomy resulting from childbirth or brought on by surgery or by inflammation of the urethra—the canal through which urine flows to the outside. Inflammation may be triggered by infection or by lowered levels of the female hormone estrogen, associated with menopause. Men rarely develop stress incontinence, and when they do, it's usually as a result of surgery. Stress incontinence may be complicated by urge incontinence (see below).

OVERACTIVE BLADDER

Overactive bladder means that the muscular layer lining the bladder is hyperactive, causing the bladder to contract in spasms. This leads to frequent urination, and excessive urination at night. Some causes of this type of incontinence are Parkinson's disease, cancer, infection, cerebrovascular disease, and Alzheimer's disease. If you have an overactive bladder, you may also experience urge incontinence. Urge incontinence refers to the inability to reach the toilet in time. It may accompany an enlarged prostate gland in men. Urge incontinence can also be due to such physical conditions as arthritis or muscle weakness, or such emotional problems as depression and anger (which can be expressed either consciously or unconsciously as incontinence). But it can also occur in otherwise healthy older people. The best approach is to deal with any underlying difficulty, while at the same time making it easy for you to get to the toilet promptly. If you are physically incapacitated, a bedside commode should help.

OVERFLOW INCONTINENCE

In this type of incontinence, small amounts of urine leak frequently from a constantly filled bladder. In men, this is often caused by an enlarged prostate gland, which prevents emptying of the bladder. Some people with diabetes experience overflow incontinence because the bladder cannot contract normally. The use of drugs that relax the bladder may also produce this problem.

DIAGNOSIS

People who have trouble controlling their urination should see a doctor for a complete medical examination. This examination will include a history so the doctor can find out what circumstances, such as coughing or laughing, cause leakage; whether you are able to stop urine flow; and other relevant information, such as medicines you use. Your doctor may ask you to develop an incontinence chart to record the timing of your symptoms. A physical exam will focus on the urinary, reproductive, and neurologic systems. Laboratory tests may also be conducted. Your doctor may then refer you to a urologist, a specialist in diseases of the urinary tract, for further tests.

TREATMENT

Various medicines are available for the treatment of urinary incontinence. Although they must be taken under close medical supervision, they cause remarkable improvement in most people. These remedies are described in the drug charts on pages 784–793.

Certain behavioral conditioning techniques, such as bladder retraining, have proven useful in people with urinary incontinence. These techniques help the person sense bladder filling and delay urination until a toilet is available. If the problem is the result of an enlarged prostate, however, surgical correction may be necessary.

For stress incontinence, some doctors recommend that women perform pelvic floor exercises (Kegel exercises) to strengthen the muscles that help close the bladder outlet. This involves the repeated tightening and then relaxation of these sphincter muscles. Yet another approach to this type of incontinence involves the use of vaginal appliances, such as pessaries and tampons, to raise the urethra. This relieves the problem in some women. If these simple methods fail, surgical correction may be recommended.

Catheterization—inserting a flexible, slender tube into the urethra and collecting the urine in a container—is another treatment alternative. It is generally not done continuously, but intermittently, to reduce the likelihood of urinary infection. In men, the collecting device is sometimes worn externally, over the genitalia, and connected to a drainage bag.

Specially designed absorbent underwear is available, as are layered sheets that will make the person more comfortable. Diapers, however, should be used only as a last resort for a person who's extremely confused. This approach to the problem may be convenient, but it is generally both emotionally and physically damaging.

OUTLOOK

Many people who are incontinent shy away from socializing and try to hide their problem from friends and family. But this condition *can* be managed, even if not totally cured. Once the problem is confronted and medical help sought, modern treatment approaches can ease the discomfort, the inconvenience, and the embarrassment and allow you to live normally.

CONDITION: **URINARY RETENTION**

CATEGORY: **URINARY TRACT STIMULANTS**

GENERIC (CHEMICAL) NAME	BRAND (TRADE) NAME	DOSAGE FORMS AND STRENGTHS
Bethanechol chloride	DUVOID	Tablets: 10, 25, 50 mg
	URECHOLINE	Tablets: 5, 10, 25, 50 mg

DRUG PROFILE

Bethanechol is used to treat urinary retention, that is, difficulty in urinating or in emptying the bladder completely. This drug, which belongs to a class of drugs known as parasympathomimetic agents, stimulates the bladder and relaxes the muscles that control the flow of urine.

BEFORE USING THIS DRUG

Let your doctor know *IF*

You have ever had allergic reactions or other problems with ■ bethanechol.

You have ever had any of the following medical problems: ■ asthma or other lung disease ■ seizures ■ heart or blood vessel disease ■ high or low blood pressure ■ digestive or urinary tract blockage ■ slow heartbeat ■ spastic disease of the digestive tract ■ ulcers ■ overactive thyroid ■ Parkinson's disease or other nerve disorders ■ recent bladder or intestinal surgery.

You are taking any of the following medicines: ■ medicine for myasthenia gravis ■ mecamylamine (medicine for high blood pressure) ■ medicine for abnormal heart rhythms ■ medicine for Parkinson's disease ■ medicine for asthma ■ medicine for irritable bowel syndrome or spastic colon ■ narcotics or other prescription pain-killers.

SPECIAL RESTRICTIONS WHILE TAKING THIS DRUG

FOOD AND DRUG INTERACTIONS

No special restrictions on other drugs, foods and beverages, alcohol use, or smoking.

DAILY LIVING

Driving	This medicine may cause blurred vision or dizziness. Be careful before driving, operating household appliances, or doing any other tasks that require alertness until you know how this drug affects you.
Other Precautions	Tell any doctor or dentist you consult that you are taking this medicine, especially if you will be undergoing any type of surgery.
Helpful Hints	Dizziness or light-headedness may occur, especially when getting up from a reclining or sitting position. Getting up slowly may help this.

To reduce the chance of nausea or vomiting, take this medicine on an empty stomach—one hour before or two hours after meals. |

No special restrictions on exertion and exercise, sun exposure, or exposure to excessive heat or cold.

POSSIBLE SIDE EFFECTS

Although this list of adverse effects may seem somewhat intimidating, keep in mind that some are quite rare. Of course, should these or any other problems arise while you are on medication, it is always a good idea to consult your doctor.

IF YOU DEVELOP	WHAT TO DO
severe dizziness ■ fainting ■ irregular or fast heartbeat ■ bloody diarrhea ■ cold, clammy skin ■ difficulty in breathing ■ tightness in chest	**Urgent** Get in touch with your doctor immediately.
fever ■ difficulty controlling bowel movements ■ blurred vision	**May be serious** Check with your doctor as soon as possible.
diarrhea ■ dizziness ■ headache ■ nausea or vomiting ■ belching ■ stomach pain or cramps ■ flushing or warm skin ■ increased sweating ■ increased salivation ■ tearing ■ urinary urgency ■ increased bowel sounds ■ general feeling of unwellness	If symptoms are disturbing or persist, let your doctor know.

STORAGE INSTRUCTIONS

Store in a cool, dark place (not in a bathroom medicine cabinet).

STOPPING OR INTERRUPTING THERAPY

If you miss a dose of this medicine, take it as soon as possible. If it is more than two hours since the scheduled time of the missed dose, skip it and resume your regular schedule. Do not take two doses at the same time.

SPECIAL CONSIDERATIONS FOR THOSE OVER SIXTY-FIVE

None.

CONDITION: **URINARY INCONTINENCE**

CATEGORY: **ANTISPASMODICS**

GENERIC (CHEMICAL) NAME	BRAND (TRADE) NAME	DOSAGE FORMS AND STRENGTHS
Oxybutynin chloride	DITROPAN	Syrup: 5 mg per tsp Tablets: 5 mg

DRUG PROFILE

Oxybutynin is used to relieve urinary conditions caused by bladder spasms. This drug increases the capacity of the bladder to hold urine, helps control bladder spasms, and delays the desire to urinate.

BEFORE USING THIS DRUG

Let your doctor know *IF*

You have ever had allergic reactions or other problems with ■ oxybutynin.

You have ever had any of the following medical problems: ■ stomach or intestinal problems, including colitis ■ enlarged prostate ■ digestive or urinary tract blockage ■ difficulty in urination ■ recent diarrhea ■ hiatal hernia ■ heart disease ■ abnormal heart rhythms ■ kidney disease ■ liver disease ■ myasthenia gravis ■ overactive thyroid ■ fast heartbeat ■ high blood pressure ■ nerve disorders ■ glaucoma.

You are taking any of the following medicines: ■ any other urinary antibiotics ■ acetaminophen ■ cimetidine (medicine for ulcers) ■ digoxin, digitoxin, or digitalis (heart medicines) ■ medicine for Parkinson's disease ■ thiazide diuretics (water pills) ■ tranquilizers ■ medicine for nausea or vomiting ■ medicine for abnormal heart rhythms ■ medicine for depression ■ antihistamines ■ nadolol, propranolol, timolol, metoprolol, atenolol, or pindolol (beta-blockers).

SPECIAL RESTRICTIONS WHILE TAKING THIS DRUG
FOOD AND DRUG INTERACTIONS

Other Drugs	Do not take any other drugs, including over-the-counter (OTC) drugs, before checking with your doctor. This drug increases the effects of drugs that depress the central nervous system, such as antihistamines; medicine for hay fever, allergies, or colds; sleep medicines; tranquilizers; narcotics or other prescription pain-killers; muscle relaxants; and medicines for seizures.
Alcohol	The combination of this drug with alcohol may increase such side effects as drowsiness or dizziness. Avoid alcohol unless your doctor has approved its use.

No special restrictions on foods and beverages or smoking.

DAILY LIVING

Driving	This drug may cause blurred vision or loss of alertness. Be careful when driving, operating household appliances, or doing any other tasks that require alertness until you know how this drug affects you.
Exertion and Exercise	This drug may cause you to sweat less than normally. Sweating is your body's natural way of cooling down, and not sweating enough can be dangerous. Use caution not to become overheated when you exercise or exert yourself.
Excessive Heat	See above; use caution during hot weather, since overexertion may result in heat stroke. Avoid extremely hot baths and saunas.
Other Precautions	This drug may cause your eyes to become more sensitive to light. Wearing tinted glasses should help ease any discomfort.
Helpful Hints	If your mouth or throat feels dry, chewing sugarless gum or sucking ice chips or sugarless hard candy will help.

No special restrictions on sun exposure or exposure to excessive cold.

POSSIBLE SIDE EFFECTS

Although this list of adverse effects may seem somewhat intimidating, keep in mind that some are quite rare. Of course, should these or any other problems arise while you are on medication, it is always a good idea to consult your doctor.

IF YOU DEVELOP	WHAT TO DO
fever ■ very slow or fast heartbeat ■ agitation ■ excitement ■ restlessness ■ behavior changes ■ flushing ■ loss of balance ■ confusion ■ drowsiness ■ hallucinations ■ difficulty in breathing	**Urgent** Get in touch with your doctor immediately.
eye pain ■ rash or hives ■ difficulty in urination ■ dizziness ■ sleeplessness	**May be serious** Check with your doctor as soon as possible.
constipation ■ decreased sweating ■ drowsiness ■ dry mouth or throat ■ blurred vision ■ changes in pupil size ■ increased eye sensitivity to light ■ nausea or vomiting ■ male impotence ■ bloating	If symptoms are disturbing or persist, let your doctor know.

STORAGE INSTRUCTIONS

Store in a cool, dark place (not in a bathroom medicine cabinet). If your medicine is in a liquid form, make sure that it does not freeze.

STOPPING OR INTERRUPTING THERAPY

If you miss a dose, take it as soon as possible. If it is almost time for your next dose, skip the missed dose and resume your regular schedule. Do not take two doses at the same time.

SPECIAL CONSIDERATIONS FOR THOSE OVER SIXTY-FIVE

Older people may be more prone to the side effects of this drug. Doctors may wish to check people over sixty-five frequently.

CONDITION: **URINARY INCONTINENCE**

CATEGORY: **ANTISPASMODICS**

GENERIC (CHEMICAL) NAME	BRAND (TRADE) NAME	DOSAGE FORMS AND STRENGTHS
Flavoxate hydrochloride	URISPAS	Tablets: 100 mg

DRUG PROFILE

Flavoxate is used to relieve symptoms associated with urinary tract infections such as painful urination, urinary urgency or frequency, urination during the night, bladder pain, and inability to retain urine. This drug acts directly on the muscles of the bladder to stop spasms and increase capacity (the amount of urine the bladder can hold). A urinary antibiotic is usually prescribed along with this drug.

BEFORE USING THIS DRUG

Let your doctor know *IF*

You have ever had allergic reactions or other problems with ■ flavoxate.

You have ever had any of the following medical problems: ■ stomach or intestinal problems ■ urinary tract blockage ■ glaucoma ■ enlarged prostate.

You are taking any of the following medicines: ■ digoxin, digitoxin, or digitalis (heart medicines) ■ tranquilizers ■ medicine for nausea or vomiting ■ medicine for abnormal heart rhythms ■ medicine for depression ■ antihistamines.

SPECIAL RESTRICTIONS WHILE TAKING THIS DRUG

FOOD AND DRUG INTERACTIONS

Other Drugs	Do not take any other drugs, including over-the-counter (OTC) drugs, before checking with your doctor. This drug increases the effects of drugs that depress the central nervous system, such as antihistamines; medicines for hay fever, allergies, or colds; sleep medicines; tranquilizers; narcotics or other pre-

scription pain-killers; muscle relaxants; and medicine for seizures, and may cause you to become drowsy or dizzy.

Alcohol	This drug increases the effect of alcohol, a central nervous system depressant. Avoid alcohol unless your doctor has approved its use.

No special restrictions on foods and beverages or smoking.

DAILY LIVING

Driving	This drug may cause blurred vision, drowsiness, or dizziness. Be careful when driving, operating household appliances, or doing any other tasks that require alertness until you know how this drug affects you.
Exertion and Exercise	This drug may cause you to sweat less than normally. Sweating is your body's natural way of cooling down, and not sweating enough can be dangerous. Use caution not to become overheated when you exercise or exert yourself.
Excessive Heat	See above; use caution during hot weather, since overexertion may result in heat stroke. Avoid extremely hot baths and saunas.
Examinations or Tests	It is important for you to keep all appointments with your doctor so that your progress can be checked.
Other Precautions	This drug may cause your eyes to become more sensitive to light. Wearing tinted glasses should help ease any discomfort.

| Helpful Hints | If your mouth or throat feels dry, chewing sugarless gum or sucking ice chips or sugarless hard candy will help. |
| | If this medicine upsets your stomach, taking it with milk, meals, or snacks should help. |

No special restrictions on sun exposure or exposure to excessive cold.

POSSIBLE SIDE EFFECTS

Although this list of adverse effects may seem somewhat intimidating, keep in mind that some are quite rare. Of course, should these or any other problems arise while you are on medication, it is always a good idea to consult your doctor.

IF YOU DEVELOP	WHAT TO DO
confusion ■ irregular or fast heartbeat	**Urgent** Get in touch with your doctor immediately.
eye pain ■ rash or hives ■ sore throat ■ fever ■ pain in urination ■ inability to concentrate	**May be serious** Check with your doctor as soon as possible.
drowsiness ■ dry mouth or throat ■ blurred vision or other visual disturbances ■ constipation ■ dizziness ■ headache ■ nausea or vomiting ■ nervousness ■ stomach pain ■ difficulty in urination ■ decreased sweating	If symptoms are disturbing or persist, let your doctor know.

STORAGE INSTRUCTIONS

Store in a cool, dark place (not in a bathroom medicine cabinet).

STOPPING OR INTERRUPTING THERAPY

If you miss a dose, take it as soon as possible. If it is almost time for your next dose, skip the missed dose and resume your regular schedule. Do not take two doses at the same time.

SPECIAL CONSIDERATIONS FOR THOSE OVER SIXTY-FIVE

Older people may be more prone to such side effects of this drug as confusion. Doctors may want to check people over sixty-five frequently.

KIDNEY STONES

Although some people save their kidney stones as souvenirs of surgery weathered well, most would prefer to forget the surgery and the stones, as well as the acompanying pain. Kidney stones are actually crystallized deposits of substances—usually calcium phosphate, calcium oxalate, or uric acid—that are normally found in solution in our urine.

In some fortunate people, the crystal deposits may be as small as a grain of sand or piece of gravel and cause little discomfort (other than the urge to urinate more frequently) as they make their way through the urinary tract. Larger stones, some of which may have staghornlike branches, are another story, however. These stones can cause excruciating pain as they pass into the ureter, the duct that transports urine from the kidney to the bladder. Sometimes, the pain is accompanied by inflammation, infection, and fever as well as the appearance of blood in the urine.

CAUSES

Most commonly, stones form because the concentration of calcium or uric acid (or some other offending substance) becomes too high for it to remain dissolved in the urine (just as a heaping spoonful of sugar may refuse to dissolve completely in a cup of tea). As a result, the calcium or uric acid crystallizes out of solution, and the crystals band together to form stones.

Sometimes, the problem can be traced to excess intake of calcium in dairy foods, calcium supplements, or calcium-containing antacids; a diet high in oxalate-containing foods, like rhubarb and spinach; or overuse of vitamin D supplements. Almost never, however, are they caused by ingestion of the normally recommended daily requirement for calcium (800–1,200 mg) and vitamin D (400–600 International Units). Other culprits that may lead to the buildup of calcium stones include prolonged immobilization; overactivity of the parathyroid glands, which sit beside the thyroid; and certain kidney problems. An infection or blockage of the urinary tract is sometimes at the root of stone formation. People who are troubled by gout, a disorder caused by an overabundance of uric acid, may develop uric acid stones. Heredity is also often to blame for kidney stones, as this problem tends to run in families.

DIAGNOSIS

To confirm the diagnosis of kidney stones, doctors usually take X rays of the kidney, ureter, and bladder. A urine sample is also important, to see whether and how the chemical composition, acidity, or bacterial flora of the urine may be contributing to the problem. If you've already passed a kidney stone, your doctor will probably want to analyze its makeup for clues to why you formed the stone.

TREATMENT

Surgery to remove kidney stones is no longer done routinely. It's usually reserved for people whose stones are extremely large, become infected, or are blocking the urinary tract. Surgery will help relieve the acute pain, but stones will continue to form unless the underlying cause is discovered and treated.

A new therapy for people with kidney stones is called extracorporeal shock wave lithotripsy. This is a nonsurgical procedure in which the stones are broken up by shock waves conveyed through a bath of water.

The one treatment prescribed for everyone with kidney stones—regardless of cause—is water. Drinking at least two quarts a day can help prevent new stones from forming and can even help dissolve some types of stones and wash them out of your system.

Other steps may include dietary changes that depend on the chemical makeup of your kidney stones. For example, doctors generally recommend that people who are prone to form calcium stones follow a diet that is low in calcium and vitamin D. Similarly, people with calcium oxalate stones may be told to watch their intake of oxalate-containing foods, such as tea, chocolate, rhubarb, and spinach. People who have calcium phosphate stones are sometimes ad-vised to make their urine more acidic by drinking cranberry juice and taking large doses of vitamin C, while people with uric acid stones may be told to make their urine less acidic by taking sodium bicarbonate or drinking a citrate solution.

Specific medicines may also be prescribed—the diuretic hydrochlorothiazide for some people with calcium stones and allopurinol for those who recurrently form uric acid stones. For more information on these drugs, see the drug charts on pages 796–797.

OUTLOOK

Many people stop taking their medicine and become lax in other parts of their treatment program as soon as their symptoms improve. But treatment must be continued for three to five years. It's considered successful if during that time no new stones are formed, old stones either disappear or stay the same size, pain and infection subside, and kidney function does not deteriorate because of urinary tract blockage. Kidney stones, left untreated, *can* lead to serious problems. But carefully supervised therapy continued for the appropriate length of time can prevent unnecessary surgery and disability.

CONDITION: **KIDNEY STONES**

CATEGORY: **URIC ACID REDUCERS**

GENERIC (CHEMICAL) NAME	BRAND (TRADE) NAME	DOSAGE FORMS AND STRENGTHS
Allopurinol	LOPURIN	Tablets: 100, 300 mg
	ZYLOPRIM	Tablets: 100, 300 mg

DRUG PROFILE

Allopurinol is used in conditions such as gout and kidney stones caused by an excess amount of uric acid in the body. This drug blocks xanthine oxidase, an enzyme necessary for the production of uric acid, and may be used in combination with other drugs.

For complete information on this drug, see pages 454–457.

CONDITION: **KIDNEY STONES**

CATEGORY: **THIAZIDE DIURETICS**

GENERIC (CHEMICAL) NAME	BRAND (TRADE) NAME	DOSAGE FORMS AND STRENGTHS
Hydrochlorothiazide	ESIDRIX	Tablets: 25, 50, 100 mg
	HydroDIURIL	Tablets: 25, 50, 100 mg

DRUG PROFILE

Thiazide and thiazide-type diuretics are often used to help control high blood pressure. They work by increasing the amount of salt and water eliminated by the body (through urination) and by relaxing the walls of the smaller arteries so that they expand. With a smaller volume of blood (because water is eliminated) in a larger amount of space (because the artery walls are expanded), blood pressure decreases. These drugs may also be prescribed for swelling in certain parts of the body (the ankles, for example) because they help the body eliminate excess water. Thiazide diuretics are also used in the treatment of calcium stones because they decrease the amount of calcium eliminated through urination.

For complete information on this drug, see pages 23–27.

ATROPHIC VAGINITIS

Atrophic vaginitis is one of the symptomatic conditions that follow menopause as the ovaries gradually produce less of the female hormone estrogen. The decrease in estrogen production leads to a slowdown in the normal process by which the lining of the vagina sheds old cells and renews itself. In time, the lining of the vagina becomes thin, loses its elasticity and can no longer produce enough natural lubrication. In that fragile state, the vagina may become particularly prone to irritation, injury, and infection.

Whether these changes cause troublesome symptoms varies from woman to woman. Some women may experience itching, burning, and pain, particularly after sexual intercourse. Others may notice a watery or blood-stained discharge or find that they have an unusually frequent and urgent need to urinate. Some actually develop urinary incontinence, the unexpected and unwanted loss of urine.

DIAGNOSIS

To confirm that your discomfort is caused by atrophic vaginitis, your doctor will perform an internal examination and take a Pap smear and cultures, with the goal of ruling out such other problems as an infection or an abnormal growth.

TREATMENT

Fortunately, the irksome symptoms of atrophic vaginitis, as well as other disturbing menopausal symptoms such as hot flashes, can be relieved by taking oral estrogen tablets or by wearing a skin patch that releases estrogen through the skin into the bloodstream. (See the chart on pages 799–800.) Or, your doctor may prescribe estrogen cream to be applied to the vagina. Estrogen cream helps restore the normal thickness, strength, and lubrication of the lining of the vagina.

Estrogen creams are not for everyone. Although only limited amounts of estrogen cream are absorbed by the body, these products may still pose hazards for women who have had blood clots or breast cancer.

Because of the increased fragility of the vagina, it is especially important to treat vaginal fungal infections in women past menopause. (For information on the drugs used to treat these infections, see the charts on pages 804–811.) Let your doctor know if you develop itching, burning, or irritation or a white discharge from the vagina.

OUTLOOK

Daily application of an estrogen cream should clear up the discomfort within a week to ten days. Many experts advise that a woman use the cream daily for three weeks a month, followed by a one-week vacation from estrogen. Others recommend only one or two applications of estrogen cream a week to maintain the improvement. For more information on estrogen cream see the chart on pages 800–803.

CONDITION: **ATROPHIC VAGINITIS**

CATEGORY: **ESTROGENS**

GENERIC (CHEMICAL) NAME	BRAND (TRADE) NAME	DOSAGE FORMS AND STRENGTHS
Conjugated estrogens	PREMARIN	Tablets: 0.3, 0.625, 0.9, 1.25, and 2.5 mg
Chlorotrianisene	TACE	Capsules: 12, 25, 72 mg
Diethylstilbestrol		Tablets: 0.1, 0.25, 0.5, 1, 5 mg
Estradiol	ESTRACE ESTRADERM	Tablets: 1, 2 mg Skin patch: 0.05, 0.1 mg per 24 hours
Estropipate	OGEN	Tablets: 0.75, 1.5, 3, 6 mg
Ethinyl estradiol	ESTINYL	Tablets: 0.02, 0.05, 0.5 mg
Quinestrol	ESTROVIS	Tablets: 100 μg

DRUG PROFILE

Estrogens (female hormones) are used to help treat the bone loss that occurs in women after menopause or after surgical removal of the uterus and/or ovaries, when the body no longer produces natural estrogens. These drugs are also used in other medical conditions such as breast or prostate cancer as well as for atrophic vaginitis (dryness of the vagina) and other symptoms of menopause. It is not known exactly how estrogens prevent bone loss, but they do help the bones absorb the calcium they need to stay healthy. Many studies have shown that estrogen deficiency contributes to bone loss after menopause. Estrogens are usually administered in a cycle: three weeks on therapy and one week off therapy. You may be given a low dose of progesterone along with estrogens, which will help counteract some of estrogen's side effects. Estrogens are used as part of a treatment program for osteoporosis that may include diet, calcium supplements, and exercise. Although estrogens can prevent further bone loss, they cannot rebuild bones or straighten bones that have already become thin.

For complete information on these drugs, see pages 467–472.

CONDITION: **ATROPHIC VAGINITIS**

CATEGORY: **TOPICAL ESTROGENS**

GENERIC (CHEMICAL) NAME	BRAND (TRADE) NAME	DOSAGE FORMS AND STRENGTHS
Conjugated estrogens	PREMARIN	Cream: 0.0625%
Dienestrol	ORTHO DIENESTROL CREAM	Cream: 0.01%
Diethylstilbestrol	DES	Vaginal suppositories: 0.1, 0.5 mg
Estradiol	ESTRACE	Cream: 0.01%
Estropipate	OGEN VAGINAL CREAM	Cream: 0.15%

DRUG PROFILE

Topical estrogens are prescribed for atrophic vaginitis (vaginal dryness) or kraurosis vulvae (dry, sore, or itching vulvae), conditions that sometimes occur after menopause or after surgical removal of the uterus and/or ovaries, when the body no longer produces natural estrogen. These uncomfortable changes can be treated by direct application of estrogens in a cream or vaginal suppository. Although these medicines are applied topically, some drug is absorbed into the bloodstream and may cause side effects similar to those caused by estrogens taken orally.

BEFORE USING THIS DRUG

Let your doctor know *IF*

You have ever had allergic reactions or other problems with ■ estrogens.

> ■ *with Ortho Vaginal Cream only:* ■ tartrazine (FD&C Yellow Dye No. 5) ■ aspirin.

You have ever had any of the following medical problems: ■ asthma ■ circulation disorders or blood clots ■ breast lumps or breast cancer ■ any other kind of cancer ■ diabetes ■ seizures ■ gallbladder disease or gallstones ■ heart disease, including heart attacks ■ high blood pressure or a family history of high blood pressure ■ high blood calcium levels ■ jaundice ■ kidney disease ■ liver disease ■ depression ■ migraine headaches ■ stroke ■ high cholesterol or a family history of high cholesterol.

You are taking any of the following medicines: ■ medicine for seizures ■ barbiturates ■ rifampin (antibiotic) ■ tricyclic antidepressants ■ vitamin C ■ anticoagulants (blood thinners).

SPECIAL RESTRICTIONS WHILE TAKING THIS DRUG

FOOD AND DRUG INTERACTIONS

Smoking	Smoking increases the chance of developing serious side effects such as thromboembolism, heart attack, and stroke with estrogen therapy. If you smoke, try to stop or at least cut down.

No special restrictions on other drugs, foods and beverages, or alcohol use.

DAILY LIVING

Sun Exposure	You may find that you sunburn more easily or that you develop brown, splotchy spots on your skin after exposure to the sun while taking estrogens. Try to minimize sun exposure, and apply a sunscreen to all exposed skin surfaces before going outdoors.

Examinations or Tests	It is important for you to keep all appointments with your doctor so that your progress can be checked. You will probably need periodic gynecologic examinations, including Pap smears. Periodic blood pressure or blood and urine tests may be required while you are on estrogen therapy.
Other Precautions	Tell any doctor or dentist you consult that you are on estrogen therapy, especially if you will be undergoing any type of surgery or any kind of diagnostic testing. If you wear contact lenses, you may find your eyes becoming sensitive to them during estrogen therapy. If this happens, discuss with your eye doctor whether it may be necessary for you to wear eyeglasses while you are on estrogen. Estrogen therapy has been associated with a number of serious side effects. Long-term use of estrogens in women after menopause increases the possibility of developing endometrial cancer. Your doctor may be able to tailor your dosage schedule to minimize such a risk. If your uterus has been surgically removed (hysterectomy), there is no chance of your developing endometrial cancer.
Helpful Hints	If you have been storing the suppository form of this medicine in a warm place, it may be too soft to use. Put it in the refrigerator for half an hour or run cold water over the wrapped suppository before use.

No special restrictions on driving, exertion and exercise, or exposure to excessive heat or cold.

POSSIBLE SIDE EFFECTS

Although this list of adverse effects may seem somewhat intimidating, keep in mind that some are quite rare. Of course, should these or any other problems arise while you are on medication, it is always a good idea to consult your doctor.

IF YOU DEVELOP	**WHAT TO DO**

Possible signs of a blood clot: sharp pain or heavy feeling in chest; sharp pains in groin or legs (especially the calves); weakness or numbness in arms or legs; severe and sudden headache, sometimes with vomiting; visual disturbances; difficulty in speech; sudden dizziness or faintness; unexplained cough

Urgent: Stop taking this drug and get in touch with your doctor immediately.

---

pain, swelling, or tenderness in stomach or side ■ vaginal bleeding ■ vaginal discharge ■ breast lumps ■ discharge from nipples ■ depression ■ uncontrollable jerky movements ■ yellowing of eyes or skin ■ bleeding ■ fever ■ joint pain ■ rash

May be serious Check with your doctor as soon as possible.

---

nausea or vomiting ■ increase or decreased appetite ■ weight gain or loss ■ tenderness and swelling of breasts ■ stomach cramps ■ bloating ■ diarrhea ■ headaches, including migraine headaches ■ dizziness ■ change in sex drive ■ hair growth or loss ■ intolerance to contact lenses or other eye problems ■ increased skin sensitivity to sunlight, including development of brown, splotchy patches ■ reddened skin or other skin problems

If symptoms are disturbing or persist, let your doctor know.

STORAGE INSTRUCTIONS

Store in a cool, dark place (not in a bathroom medicine cabinet). If your medicine is in a liquid form, make sure that it does not freeze. Suppositories should be stored in the refrigerator.

STOPPING OR INTERRUPTING THERAPY

If you miss a dose of this medicine, apply it as soon as possible. If you do not remember until the following day, skip the missed dose and resume your regular schedule. Do not apply two doses at the same time.

SPECIAL CONSIDERATIONS FOR THOSE OVER SIXTY-FIVE

None.

CONDITION: **VAGINAL INFECTIONS**

CATEGORY: **TOPICAL VAGINAL ANTIFUNGAL AGENTS**

GENERIC (CHEMICAL) NAME	BRAND (TRADE) NAME	DOSAGE FORMS AND STRENGTHS
Sulfanilamide	VAGITROL	Vaginal cream: 15%
Sulfanilamide, aminacrine hydrochloride, and allantoin	AVC	Vaginal cream: 15% sulfanilamide, 0.2% aminacrine hydrochloride, and 2% allantoin Vaginal suppositories: 1.05 g sulfanilamide, 0.014 g aminacrine hydrochloride, and 0.14 g allantoin

DRUG PROFILE

These sulfonamides (sulfa drugs) are applied directly in the vagina to treat fungal infections of the vagina (yeast infections).

BEFORE USING THIS DRUG

Let your doctor know *IF*

You have ever had allergic reactions or other problems with ■ sulfonamides (sulfa drugs) ■ furosemide or thiazide diuretics ■ oral medicine for diabetes ■ oral medicine for glaucoma ■ dapsone or sulfoxone (antibiotics).

   ■ *with AVC only:* ■ tartrazine (FD&C Yellow Dye No. 5) (contained in suppository).

SPECIAL RESTRICTIONS WHILE TAKING THIS DRUG

FOOD AND DRUG INTERACTIONS

No special restrictions on other drugs, foods and beverages, alcohol use, or smoking.

DAILY LIVING

Precautions	These drugs usually come with patient instructions, which you should read carefully before use. Unless your doctor instructs you otherwise, this medicine should be applied at bedtime. Ask your doctor about intercourse or douching while on treatment.
Helpful Hints	A sanitary pad may be used to protect your clothing from vaginal discharge. To keep fungal infections from recurring, wear panties and pantyhose with crotches made of cotton rather than of synthetics (such as nylon). If you have been storing the suppository form of this medicine in a warm place, it may be too soft to use. Put it in the refrigerator for half an hour or run cold water over the wrapped suppository before use.

No special restrictions on driving, exertion and exercise, sun exposure, or exposure to excessive heat or cold.

POSSIBLE SIDE EFFECTS

IF YOU DEVELOP

increased discomfort ■ burning sensation ■ rash ■ sore throat ■ fever ■ increased urination

WHAT TO DO

Urgent Get in touch with your doctor immediately.

STORAGE INSTRUCTIONS

Store in a cool, dark place (not in a bathroom medicine cabinet). Suppositories should be stored in the refrigerator.

STOPPING OR INTERRUPTING THERAPY

This medicine should be taken for the full length of time prescribed by your doctor, even if you begin to feel better. This will ensure that the infection clears up completely and that your symptoms don't return. If you miss a dose, simply resume your regular schedule the following day. Do not apply two doses at the same time.

SPECIAL CONSIDERATIONS FOR THOSE OVER SIXTY-FIVE

None.

CONDITION: **VAGINAL INFECTIONS**

CATEGORY: **TOPICAL VAGINAL ANTIFUNGAL AGENTS**

GENERIC (CHEMICAL) NAME	BRAND (TRADE) NAME	DOSAGE FORMS AND STRENGTHS
Clotrimazole	GYNE-LOTRIMIN	Vaginal cream: 1% Vaginal tablets: 100, 500 mg
	MYCELEX-G	Vaginal cream: 1% Vaginal tablets: 100, 500 mg
Miconazole nitrate	MONISTAT 3	Vaginal suppositories: 200 mg
	MONISTAT 7	Vaginal cream: 2% Vaginal suppositories: 100 mg
Nystatin	MYCOSTATIN	Vaginal tablets: 100,000 units

DRUG PROFILE

These antifungal drugs are applied directly in the vagina to treat fungal infections of the vagina (yeast infections).

BEFORE USING THIS DRUG

Let your doctor know *IF*

You have ever had allergic reactions or other problems with ■ clotrimazole ■ miconazole ■ nystatin.

You have ever had any of the following medical problems:

■ *with miconazole only:* ■ diabetes ■ cancer ■ AIDS (acquired immune deficiency syndrome).

SPECIAL RESTRICTIONS WHILE TAKING THIS DRUG

FOOD AND DRUG INTERACTIONS

No special restrictions on other drugs, foods and beverages, alcohol use, or smoking.

DAILY LIVING

Precautions	These drugs usually come with patient instructions, which you should read carefully before use. Unless your doctor instructs you otherwise, this medicine should be applied at bedtime.
	Ask your doctor about intercourse or douching while on treatment.
Helpful Hints	A sanitary pad may be used to protect your clothing from vaginal discharge.
	To keep fungal infections from recurring, wear panties and pantyhose with crotches made of cotton rather than of synthetics (such as nylon).
	If you have been storing the suppository form of this medicine in a warm place, it may be too soft to use. Put it in the refrigerator for half an hour or run cold water over the wrapped suppository before use.

No special restrictions on driving, exertion and exercise, sun exposure, or exposure to excessive heat or cold.

POSSIBLE SIDE EFFECTS

Although this list of adverse effects may seem somewhat intimidating, keep in mind that some are quite rare. Of course, should these or any other problems arise while you are on medication, it is always a good idea to consult your doctor.

IF YOU DEVELOP	WHAT TO DO
vaginal burning, itching, redness, or irritation that was not present before use of the medicine ■ rash or hives	**Urgent** Get in touch with your doctor immediately.
headache ■ pelvic cramps *With clotrimazole only:* increased urination ■ bladder irritation ■ bloating ■ burning and irritation in sexual partner's genitals	**May be serious** Check with your doctor as soon as possible.

STORAGE INSTRUCTIONS

Store in a cool, dark place (not in a bathroom medicine cabinet). Suppositories should be stored in the refrigerator.

STOPPING OR INTERRUPTING THERAPY

This medicine should be used for the full length of time prescribed by your doctor, even if you begin to feel better. This will ensure that the infection clears up completely and that your symptoms don't return. If you miss a dose, simply resume your regular schedule the following day. Do not apply two doses at the same time.

SPECIAL CONSIDERATIONS FOR THOSE OVER SIXTY-FIVE

None.

CONDITION: **VAGINAL INFECTIONS**

CATEGORY: **ANTITRICHOMONAL DRUGS**

GENERIC (CHEMICAL) NAME	BRAND (TRADE) NAME	DOSAGE FORMS AND STRENGTHS
Metronidazole	FLAGYL	Tablets: 250, 500 mg

DRUG PROFILE

Metronidazole is an antibiotic that is used to treat trichomoniasis (a vaginal infection) as well as a wide variety of systemic infections including dysentery and infections of the respiratory tract, skin, bones and joints, and stomach.

BEFORE USING THIS DRUG

Let your doctor know *IF*

You have ever had allergic reactions or other problems with ■ metronidazole.

You have ever had any of the following medical problems: ■ blood disease ■ seizures ■ severe liver disease ■ alcoholism.

You are taking any of the following medicines: ■ anticoagulants (blood thinners) ■ Antabuse (used in the treatment of alcoholism) ■ barbiturates ■ phenytoin (medicine for seizures) ■ cimetidine (medicine for ulcers).

SPECIAL RESTRICTIONS WHILE TAKING THIS DRUG

FOOD AND DRUG INTERACTIONS

Alcohol	Do not drink alcohol while taking this drug and for at least one day before and following the end of therapy. The combination may result in nausea or vomiting, stomach pains, and flushing.

No special restrictions on other drugs, foods and beverages, or smoking.

DAILY LIVING

Examinations or Tests	It is important for you to keep all appointments with your doctor so that your condition can be reevaluated after therapy. Blood tests may be required before and after therapy with this drug.
Other Precautions	If you are being treated for trichomonal infection, your sexual partner should see a doctor, as he may be infected and need treatment as well. Also, it may be necessary to use a condom for a while to prevent both of you from reinfecting each other.
	If your symptoms do not improve within a few days or if they worsen, check with your doctor.
	Let your doctor know if you develop itching, burning, soreness, or general irritation in the genital area; a white vaginal discharge; or a white coating on the inside of your mouth.
Helpful Hints	If this medicine causes upset stomach, taking it with milk, meals, or snacks should help.

No special restrictions on driving, exertion and exercise, sun exposure, or exposure to excessive heat or cold.

POSSIBLE SIDE EFFECTS

Although this list of adverse effects may seem somewhat intimidating, keep in mind that some are quite rare. Of course, should these or any other problems arise while you are on medication, it is always a good idea to consult your doctor.

IF YOU DEVELOP	**WHAT TO DO**
numbness, tingling, pain, or weakness in hands or feet ∎ seizures	**Urgent** Get in touch with your doctor immediately.

clumsiness or unsteadiness ■ rash or hives ■ sore throat ■ fever ■ confusion ■ irritability ■ weakness ■ depression ■ sleeplessness ■ flushing ■ dryness of the vagina or vulva ■ painful intercourse ■ decreased sex drive ■ pain in urination ■ urinary frequency ■ bladder irritation ■ feeling of pressure in the pelvic area	**May be serious** Check with your doctor as soon as possible.
unpleasant taste in mouth ■ nausea or vomiting ■ diarrhea ■ loss of appetite ■ stomach cramps ■ constipation ■ dry mouth ■ mouth sores ■ furry or inflamed tongue ■ dizziness ■ headache ■ stuffy nose ■ dark urine	If symptoms are disturbing or persist, let your doctor know.

STORAGE INSTRUCTIONS

Store in a cool, dark place (not in a bathroom medicine cabinet).

STOPPING OR INTERRUPTING THERAPY

This medicine should be taken for the full length of time prescribed by your doctor, even if you begin to feel better. This will ensure that the infection clears up completely and that your symptoms don't return. If you miss a dose, take it as soon as possible. If it is almost time for your next dose, skip the missed dose and resume your regular schedule.

SPECIAL CONSIDERATIONS FOR THOSE OVER SIXTY-FIVE

None.

Chapter 12
Disorders of the Eye

GLAUCOMA

You may have noticed that you don't see quite as clearly as you used to. The world sometimes has a fuzzy look to it, and your eyes sometimes give you an aching feeling. These may be symptoms of glaucoma, an eye disorder that occurs when too much fluid is trapped inside the eye, causing a buildup of pressure. If glaucoma is not controlled by surgical techniques or drugs described in this section, it can lead to blindness. Glaucoma is, in fact, the leading cause of blindness in the United States.

Present in more than two million people in the United States, glaucoma is most common in men and women over sixty-five, affecting three out of every one hundred people in this age group. Glaucoma tends to run in families, so don't be surprised if a relative of yours had it before you did. This eye condition is also particularly prevalent in people with diabetes.

CAUSES

Your eyes are constantly manufacturing a fluid called aqueous humor, which flows around the lens and through the pupil. In a normal eye, it then drains away through tiny canals in the front of the eye. But in an eye that is affected by glaucoma, that drainage system is blocked. More aqueous humor is continuously produced, but the fluid can't leave the eye. This creates pressure within the eye—pressure that can damage the retina and the optic nerve.

DIAGNOSIS

There are two basic types of glaucoma, each with its own set of symptoms. One type is known as acute angle-closure (or narrow-angle) glaucoma. In this variation, the drainage path is tightly closed, and the pressure from the trapped aqueous humor becomes very high. The results are intense pain, redness of the affected eye, and blurring (halos around lights) or loss of vision. If the pressure from an acute attack is not treated, it can lead to blindness in one to five days.

In the other type, called open-angle (or chronic) glaucoma, the person has virtually no symptoms except for a slow, progressive peripheral vision loss when tested for it. This condition is often referred to as the "sneak thief of sight," since vision is irreversibly lost without the person being aware of even having the disease until it is too late. Over time, permanent damage to the retina and optic nerve occurs. Treatment can keep the condition from becoming worse but cannot restore any loss of vision that has already occurred. Because of this, patients should have their intraocular pressures measured yearly by an ophthalmologist if they have a family history of glaucoma, have diabetes, or are known to have even mildly elevated eye pressure. Otherwise, the eye pressure should be measured every two years. During most routine eye exams by an ophthalmologist, a pressure check is done with an instrument placed on the cornea for a few seconds. This procedure lets the doctor know if the pressure in your eye is too high. The doctor can also look at the drainage pathways in the front of your eye and at the optic nerve and retina to check for any glaucomalike changes.

TREATMENT

Should you experience the symptoms of acute glaucoma described above, go immediately to a doctor or a hospital emergency room, where you will be given eyedrops or other medicine to bring the pressure down. In addition, an eye surgeon might make a tiny opening in your iris to allow the fluid to drain out. This procedure can save your vision. The operation can now be done with the intense light of a laser beam rather than with sharp surgical instruments. The surgeon may recommend a similar operation on the other eye to prevent a second acute attack. (After one attack, the other eye is at an increased risk for a similar attack.)

If you are diagnosed as having glaucoma, and your doctor feels that drug treatment is appropriate, you may be prescribed pills or eyedrops to use at home. Some of the more commonly prescribed medicines used to control glaucoma are listed on pages 816–830.

OUTLOOK

Glaucoma can lead to blindness—whether or not you are aware of its symptoms. However, recognition of its presence can allow treatment to prevent irreversible vision loss. If you see your doctor for regular eye checkups and get medical attention as soon as you experience any symptoms of glaucoma, it's likely that the disease process can be halted before significant or total loss of vision occurs.

CONDITION: **GLAUCOMA**

CATEGORY: **TOPICAL BETA-BLOCKERS**

GENERIC (CHEMICAL) NAME	BRAND (TRADE) NAME	DOSAGE FORMS AND STRENGTHS
Betaxolol hydrochloride	BETOPTIC	Solution: 0.5%
Levobunolol hydrochloride	BETAGAN	Solution: 0.5%
Timolol maleate	TIMOPTIC	Solution: 0.25%, 0.5%

DRUG PROFILE

The topical beta-blockers are prescribed, either alone or in combination with other medicine, to treat glaucoma. They are believed to work by lessening the production of aqueous fluid and thereby reducing increased pressure in the eye.

BEFORE USING THIS DRUG

Let your doctor know *IF*

You have ever had allergic reactions or other problems with ■ any beta-blocker.

You have ever had any of the following medical problems: ■ asthma or other lung disease ■ slow heartbeat ■ diabetes ■ any heart or blood vessel disease ■ overactive thyroid ■ myasthenia gravis.

You are taking any of the following medicines: ■ other medicine for glaucoma ■ other beta-blockers ■ medicine for high blood pressure ■ verapamil (calcium blocker) ■ medicine for asthma or other lung disease ■ medicine for hay fever, allergies, or colds ■ tranquilizers ■ digoxin, digitoxin, or digitalis (heart medicines).

SPECIAL RESTRICTIONS WHILE TAKING THIS DRUG

FOOD AND DRUG INTERACTIONS

Other Drugs	It is especially important to let your doctor know if you are taking the blood-pressure–lowering drug reserpine or the calcium blocker verapamil, since the use of these drugs with a beta-blocker may cause low blood pressure, slow heartbeat, or dizziness.

No special restrictions on foods and beverages, alcohol use, or smoking.

DAILY LIVING

Driving	Do not drive if you are using this drug since it may cause blurred vision. Be careful when operating household appliances or doing any other tasks that require clear vision until you know how this drug affects you.
Exertion and Exercise	Be careful when you exert yourself or exercise since you may become more tired than usual.
Examinations or Tests	It is important for you to keep all appointments with your doctor so that your eye pressure can be checked and your eyes can be examined for any adverse effects from this drug.
Other Precautions	Tell any doctor or dentist you consult that you are taking this medicine, especially if you will be undergoing any type of surgery.
	If you have diabetes, be aware that this medicine may mask the signs of low blood sugar, such as changes in pulse rate or increased blood pressure.

Your eyes may become especially sensitive to light. Wearing tinted glasses should help ease any discomfort.

Helpful Hints	Wash your hands thoroughly before and after each use. After dropping the solution into your eye, apply pressure to the inner corner of your eye with the middle finger for one to two minutes to prevent the medicine from draining into your nose and throat. To prevent contamination, avoid touching the dropper tip to the eye, eyelid, or any other surface, and keep the container tightly closed when not in use.

No special restrictions on sun exposure or exposure to excessive heat or cold.

POSSIBLE SIDE EFFECTS

Although this list of adverse effects may seem somewhat intimidating, keep in mind that some are quite rare. Of course, should these or any other problems arise while you are on medication, it is always a good idea to consult your doctor.

IF YOU DEVELOP	WHAT TO DO
irregular or slow heartbeat ■ dizziness, weakness, light-headedness, or fainting ■ difficulty in breathing ■ confusion ■ headache ■ nausea ■ rash or hives	**Urgent** Get in touch with your doctor immediately.
eye irritation ■ blurred or double vision ■ drooping of the upper eyelids ■ depression ■ lack of coordination ■ lethargy	**May be serious** Check with your doctor as soon as possible.
temporary burning or stinging in eye ■ tearing ■ increased eye sensitivity to light ■ insomnia	If symptoms are disturbing or persist, let your doctor know.

STORAGE INSTRUCTIONS

Store in a cool, dark place (not in a bathroom medicine cabinet) and make sure that it does not freeze.

STOPPING OR INTERRUPTING THERAPY

If you miss a dose and you are taking this medicine more than once a day, apply it as soon as possible and resume your regular schedule. If you miss a dose and you are taking this medicine once a day, apply the missed dose as soon as possible. If you do not remember until the following day, skip the missed dose and resume your regular schedule.

SPECIAL CONSIDERATIONS FOR THOSE OVER SIXTY-FIVE

Older people may be more susceptible to the side effects of this drug. Doctors may want to start people over sixty-five on a lower dosage.

CONDITION: **GLAUCOMA**

CATEGORY: **CARBONIC ANHYDRASE INHIBITORS**

GENERIC (CHEMICAL) NAME	BRAND (TRADE) NAME	DOSAGE FORMS AND STRENGTHS
Acetazolamide	DIAMOX	Controlled-release capsules: 500 mg Tablets: 125, 250 mg
Dichlorphenamide	DARANIDE	Tablets: 50 mg
Methazolamide	NEPTAZANE	Tablets: 50 mg

DRUG PROFILE

These drugs are used as supplemental therapy for glaucoma, along with topical medicines that are applied directly to the eye. They decrease the formation of aqueous humor (the fluid inside the front of the eyeball), thereby reducing the increased pressure inside the eye that is the hallmark of glaucoma. This type of drug has a slight diuretic effect as well; that is, it helps your body rid itself of excess water through increased urination.

BEFORE USING THIS DRUG

Let your doctor know *IF*

You have ever had allergic reactions or other problems with ■ acetazolamide ■ dichlorphenamide ■ methazolamide ■ sulfonamides (sulfa drugs).

You have ever had any of the following medical problems: ■ emphysema or other lung disease ■ potassium or sodium deficiency ■ Addison's disease ■ kidney disease, including kidney stones ■ liver disease ■ diabetes ■ leukemia ■ anemia.

You are taking any of the following medicines: ■ corticosteroids or corticotropin (ACTH) ■ medicine for diabetes ■ digoxin, digitoxin, or digitalis (heart medicines) ■ aspirin or aspirinlike medicine ■ methenamine (medicine to prevent urinary tract infections) ■ phenobarbital ■ lithium ■ diuretics (water pills) ■ amphetamines ■ procainamide or quinidine (medicine for abnormal heart rhythms) ■ tricyclic antidepressants ■ primidone or phenytoin (medicine for seizures) ■ medicine for stomach spasms or cramps.

SPECIAL RESTRICTIONS WHILE TAKING THIS DRUG

FOOD AND DRUG INTERACTIONS

Foods and Beverages	This medicine may decrease potassium levels in your blood. Your doctor may give you special instructions about eating foods or drinking beverages that have a high potassium content (such as bananas and citrus fruit juices), taking a potassium supplement, or using salt substitutes.

No special restrictions on other drugs, alcohol use, or smoking.

DAILY LIVING

Driving	This drug may cause drowsiness. Use caution when driving, operating household appliances, or doing any

other tasks that require alertness until you know how this drug affects you.

Examinations or Tests	It is important for you to keep all appointments with your doctor so that your progress can be checked.
Other Precautions	If you have diabetes, be aware that this medicine may raise blood-sugar levels. If you notice any change when testing sugar levels in your blood or urine, let your doctor know.
Helpful Hints	When first starting on this medicine, you may feel tired or depressed and will probably experience both greater volume and frequency of urination. Until your individual pattern of urination has been established with this medicine, it may be wise to time carefully any activity that will put you out of convenient reach of a bathroom, such as bus or car travel. In addition, taking this medicine at bedtime may interfere with sleep; you should discuss your dosage schedule with your doctor.
	Check with your doctor if you become ill with flulike symptoms, such as cough, fever, or body aches; lose your appetite; vomit; or have diarrhea. This may cause you to lose a great deal of fluid, making it important not to take the diuretic for one or more doses.
	If this medicine upsets your stomach, taking it with meals, milk, or snacks should help.

No special restrictions on exertion and exercise, sun exposure, or exposure to excessive heat or cold.

POSSIBLE SIDE EFFECTS

Although this list of adverse effects may seem somewhat intimidating, keep in mind that some are quite rare. Of course, should these or any other problems arise while you are on medication, it is always a good idea to consult your doctor.

IF YOU DEVELOP	WHAT TO DO
irregular heartbeat ■ tiredness or weakness ■ confusion ■ seizures ■ shortness of breath ■ difficulty in breathing ■ bluish skin ■ bloody or black, tarry stools ■ vomiting, with blood ■ pain in urination ■ blood in urine ■ lower back pain ■ red rash ■ slow blood clotting	**Urgent: Stop using this drug and get in touch with your doctor immediately.**
weak pulse ■ depression ■ nausea or vomiting ■ dry mouth ■ increased thirst ■ drowsiness ■ headache ■ irritability ■ nervousness ■ excitement ■ dizziness ■ clumsiness ■ tremors ■ increased or decreased urination ■ dark urine ■ rash, hives, or itching ■ sore throat or fever ■ bleeding or bruising ■ yellowing of eyes or skin ■ pale stools ■ muscle paralysis	**May be serious** Stop using this drug and check with your doctor as soon as possible.
loss of appetite ■ diarrhea ■ weight loss ■ changes in taste or smell ■ constipation ■ bloating ■ general feeling of unwellness ■ increased skin sensitivity to sunlight ■ numbness or tingling in hands, feet, lips, tongue, or anus ■ development or worsening of nearsightedness	If symptoms are disturbing or persist, let your doctor know.

STORAGE INSTRUCTIONS

Store in a cool, dark place (not in a bathroom medicine cabinet).

STOPPING OR INTERRUPTING THERAPY

If you miss a dose, take it as soon as possible. If it is almost time for your next dose, skip the missed dose and resume your regular schedule. Do not take two doses at the same time.

SPECIAL CONSIDERATIONS FOR THOSE OVER SIXTY-FIVE

None.

CONDITION: **GLAUCOMA**

CATEGORY: **MIOTICS**

GENERIC (CHEMICAL) NAME	BRAND (TRADE) NAME	DOSAGE FORMS AND STRENGTHS
Carbachol	ISOPTO CARBACHOL	Solution: 0.75%, 1.5%, 2.25%, 3%
Demecarium bromide	HUMORSOL	Solution: 0.125%, 0.25%
Echothiopate iodide	PHOSPHOLINE IODIDE	Solution: 0.03%, 0.06%, 0.125%, 0.25%
Isoflurophate	FLOROPRYL	Ointment: 0.025%
Pilocarpine hydrochloride	ADSORBOCARPINE	Solution: 1%, 2%, 4%
	AKARPINE	Solution: 1%, 2%, 3%, 4%
	ALMOCARPINE	Solution: 1%, 2%, 4%
	ISOPTO CARPINE	Solution: 0.25%, 0.5%, 1%, 2%, 3%, 4%, 5%, 6%, 8%, 10%
	OCUSERT	Eye insert medication-release system: 20, 40 μg per hour
	PILOCAR	Solution: 0.5%, 1%, 2%, 3%, 4%, 6%
	PILOPINE HS	Gel: 4%
Pilocarpine nitrate	P.V. CARPINE	Solution: 1%, 2%, 4%

DRUG PROFILE

Miotics are a family of drugs that constrict the pupil and are thought to place tension on the drainage canals at the front of the eye, allowing the fluid to flow out more easily and thereby reducing pressure in the eye.

BEFORE USING THIS DRUG

Let your doctor know *IF*

You have ever had allergic reactions or other problems with ■ carbachol ■ echothiopate iodide ■ pilocarpine ■ preservatives.

You have ever had any of the following medical problems: ■ any injury to or inflammation of the eye ■ asthma ■ heart disease, including recent heart attack ■ ulcers or other problems of the digestive tract ■ urinary tract blockage ■ slow heartbeat ■ low or high blood pressure ■ Parkinson's disease ■ nervous disorders ■ overactive thyroid ■ seizures.

You are using any other eye medications or being treated for myasthenia gravis.

For Phosphaline Iodide only: You are often exposed to organophosphate-type pesticides (i.e., if you are a professional gardener or farmer or if you work at a plant that manufactures such pesticides).

SPECIAL RESTRICTIONS WHILE TAKING THIS DRUG

FOOD AND DRUG INTERACTIONS

Other Drugs	If you are being treated for myasthenia gravis with drugs, your doctor may need to adjust your dosage of these agents while you are on antiglaucoma therapy.

No special restrictions on foods and beverages, alcohol use, or smoking.

DAILY LIVING

Driving	Do not drive if you are using this drug since it may cause blurred vision, especially in dim light. Be careful when operating household appliances or doing any other tasks that require clear vision until you know how this drug affects you.

Other Precautions	Tell any doctor or dentist you consult that you are using this medicine, especially if you will be undergoing any type of surgery. Adverse effects usually disappear within a few days of beginning regular use. If your eye feels painful, try taking aspirin. If side effects fail to subside or if your eye remains irritated, let your doctor know.
Helpful Hints	*If you are using eyedrops:* If you wear soft contact lenses, it is a good idea to remove them before using drops. After dropping the solution into your eye, apply pressure to the inner corner of your eye with your middle finger for one to two minutes to keep the medicine from draining into your nose and throat. Remove any excess solution from around the eyes with a tissue. Wash your hands thoroughly before and after use of this medicine. To prevent contamination, avoid touching the dropper tip to the eye, eyelid, or any other surface and keep the bottle tightly closed when not in use. *If you are using the eye insert system:* Be sure to wash your hands thoroughly before and after inserting the system. You may experience temporary blurred and dim vision after insertion; these effects can be reduced by inserting the system at bedtime. Any discomfort should improve after one to six weeks of therapy.

No special restrictions on exertion and exercise, sun exposure, or exposure to excessive heat or cold.

POSSIBLE SIDE EFFECTS

Although this list of adverse effects may seem somewhat intimidating, keep in mind that some are quite rare. Of course, should these or any other problems arise while you are on medication, it is always a good idea to consult your doctor.

IF YOU DEVELOP

nausea or vomiting ■ diarrhea ■ tremors or weakness ■ stomach pain or cramps ■ increased salivation ■ excessive sweating ■ dizziness ■ tingling sensations ■ slow heartbeat ■ wheezing ■ difficulty in breathing ■ tightness in chest ■ fainting ■ excitement ■ depression ■ clumsiness ■ seizures ■ urinary frequency or incontinence ■ flushing ■ paleness ■ bluish skin ■ flashing lights or floating spots in your field of vision ■ curtain of darkness over part of your vision

WHAT TO DO

Urgent: Stop using this drug and get in touch with your doctor immediately.

---

pain, stinging, or burning in eye ■ blurred or dim vision or other visual disturbances ■ redness or irritation of eyes or edge of eyelids ■ watery eyes ■ twitching of eyelids ■ headache ■ browache ■ increased eye sensitivity to light ■ poor vision in dim light

If symptoms are disturbing or persist, let your doctor know.

STORAGE INSTRUCTIONS

Store in a cool, dark place (not in a bathroom medicine cabinet), and make sure that it does not freeze. Phospholine Iodide should be stored in the refrigerator.

STOPPING OR INTERRUPTNG THERAPY

Take this medicine exactly as prescribed by your doctor. If you miss a dose and you are taking this medicine more than once a day, apply it as soon as possible and resume your regular schedule. If you miss a dose and you take this medicine once a day, apply the missed dose as soon as possible. If you do not remember until the following day, skip the missed dose and resume your regular schedule. If you take this medicine every other day and miss a day, apply the missed dose on the day you remember and skip the following day. If you are using the eye insert system, follow the instructions in the package circular.

SPECIAL CONSIDERATIONS FOR THOSE OVER SIXTY-FIVE

Some older people, especially those with cataracts, will be unable to tolerate miotics; if this is the case, doctors will prescribe another antiglaucoma medicine.

CONDITION: **GLAUCOMA**

CATEGORY: **EPINEPHRINE PREPARATIONS**

GENERIC (CHEMICAL) NAME	BRAND (TRADE) NAME	DOSAGE FORMS AND STRENGTHS
Dipivefrin hydrochloride	PROPINE	Solution: 0.01%
Epinephrine hydrochloride	EPIFRIN	Solution: 0.25%, 0.5%, 1%, 2%
	GLAUCON	Solution: 1%, 2%
Epinephrine bitartrate	AYERST EPITRATE	Solution: 2%
Epinephyl borate	EPINAL	Solution: 0.5%, 1%
	EPPY/N	Solution: 0.5%, 1%, 2%

DRUG PROFILE

These epinephrine preparations are mydriatics—drugs that dilate the pupil—and are used to treat glaucoma. Epinephrine and dipivefrin, which is converted into epinephrine in the eye, are thought to reduce increased pressure in the eye by lessening the production of aqueous fluid and increasing aqueous fluid outflow. Your doctor may prescribe this type of drug to be used either alone or in combination with another medicine.

BEFORE USING THIS DRUG

Let your doctor know *IF*

You have ever had allergic reactions or other problems with ■ epinephrine ■ preservatives.

You have ever had any of the following medical problems: ■ past attack of narrow-angle glaucoma ■ other eye disease ■ cataract surgery ■ heart disease, including abnormal heart rhythm ■ blood vessel disease ■ high blood pressure ■ overactive thyroid.

You are taking any of the following medicines: ■ digoxin, digitoxin, or digitalis (heart medicines) ■ medicine for depression.

SPECIAL RESTRICTIONS WHILE TAKING THIS DRUG

FOOD AND DRUG INTERACTIONS

Other Drugs	There is a greater risk of developing irregular heartbeat when this drug is used with heart medicine (digoxin, digitoxin, or digitalis) or tricyclic antidepressants.
Foods and Beverages	The caffeine in cocoa, chocolate, coffee, tea, and cola drinks may add to the effects of this drug and result in palpitations.

No special restrictions on alcohol use or smoking.

DAILY LIVING

Driving	Do not drive when using this drug since it may cause blurred vision. Be careful when operating household appliances or doing any other tasks that require alertness until you know how this drug affects you.
Examinations or Tests	It is important for you to keep all appointments with your doctor so that your eye pressure can be checked and your eyes can be examined for any adverse effects from this drug.
Other Precautions	Tell any doctor or dentist you consult that you are on this kind of therapy, especially if you will be undergoing any type of surgery.
	If your eye symptoms do not improve or if they worsen, stop using this drug and check with your doctor.

You should not wear soft contact lenses while instilling this drug.

Your eyes may become especially sensitive to light; wearing tinted glasses should help ease any discomfort.

Helpful Hints	Wash your hands thoroughly before and after each use. After dropping the solution into your eye, apply pressure to the inner corner of your eye with the middle finger for one to two minutes to prevent the medicine from draining into your nose and throat. To prevent contamination, avoid touching the dropper tip to the eye, eyelid, or any other surface and keep the container tightly closed when not in use. Although epinephrine usually causes discomfort when it is first instilled, your eye should begin to feel better in a few minutes. Also, if you experience headache or brow-ache, these symptoms may improve with continued treatment.

No special restrictions on exertion and exercise or exposure to excessive heat or cold.

POSSIBLE SIDE EFFECTS

Although this list of adverse effects may seem somewhat intimidating, keep in mind that some are quite rare. Of course, should these or any other problems arise while you are on medication, it is always a good idea to consult your doctor.

IF YOU DEVELOP

irregular, pounding, or fast heartbeat ■ severe pain in the back of the head ■ faintness ■ excessive sweating ■ tremors ■ paleness ■ difficulty in breathing ■ bluish skin ■ chest pain

WHAT TO DO

Urgent: Stop using this drug and get in touch with your doctor immediately.

aching or pain in brow or head ■ aching, pain, stinging, burning, irritation, or watering of the eyes ■ eyelid irritations ■ temporary blurred vision ■ increased eye sensitivity to light ■ black spots floating across your field of vision ■ difficulty seeing at night

If symptoms are disturbing or persist, let your doctor know.

STORAGE INSTRUCTIONS

Store in a cool, dark place (not in a bathroom medicine cabinet), and make sure that it does not freeze.

STOPPING OR INTERRUPTING THERAPY

If you miss a dose of this medicine, apply it as soon as possible. If it is almost time for your next dose, skip the missed dose and resume your regular schedule.

SPECIAL CONSIDERATIONS FOR THOSE OVER SIXTY-FIVE

None.

CONJUNCTIVITIS

Conjunctivitis, popularly called red-eye or pink-eye, is an inflammation of the membrane that covers the eyeball and lines the eyelid. Most of the white of the eye appears red, a color change caused by the dilation of blood vessels in the eye. This condition differs from bloodshot eyes, in which tiny red veins are visible in the whites of the eyes. (The problem, in that case, is usually only lack of sleep or localized eye irritation, from smoke, for example.)

The redness of conjunctivitis may be present in either one eye or in both. Often, the eyes feel itchy and there may be mild discomfort, but usually no pain. Another sign of conjunctivitis is a discharge from the eyes. You may first notice this as a crust on your eyelashes when you wake up in the morning.

CAUSES

Conjunctivitis may be caused by bacterial infections, fungal infections, allergies such as hay fever, or viruses. It can also be brought on by such ailments as arthritis or herpes.

DIAGNOSIS

Your doctor may take a smear from your eye to test for bacteria and examine the cells. Your pattern of symptoms will also provide a clue to the diagnosis. Bacterial conjunctivitis often begins with a discharge of pus from the eye; viral conjunctivitis is likely to be accompanied by a watery discharge and by a painful sensitivity to light, called photophobia; allergic conjunctivitis commonly causes severe itching and accompanying swollen lids.

TREATMENT

To treat conjunctivitis, most doctors prescribe eyedrops or an ointment (see the drug charts pages 833–866). If the source of the problem is a bacterial infection, the drugs will often bring relief in one to three days. But even when the symptoms have disappeared, you should continue to use the antibiotic for as long as the doctor has directed to prevent a relapse. Viral conjunctivitis doesn't respond to antibiotics and takes longer to heal, perhaps one to two weeks (which is the life cycle of the virus). Although antibiotics will not help viral conjunctivitis, the doctor may prescribe them to prevent a secondary infection by bacteria.

Conjunctivitis can be extremely contagious, so when red-eye first appears, you should take some simple precautions to prevent spreading it to a family member. Avoid touching the affected eye; wash your hands frequently; and do not share towels, washcloths, or pillowcases. Launder these linens after each use, if possible. Contact lenses and eye makeup can make conjunctivitis worse—stop using them until the doctor says the infection has cleared. Be sure to sterilize contact lenses carefully before using them again.

OUTLOOK

Symptoms affecting your eyes should be checked by a doctor, but if you're told that conjunctivitis is the cause, you have little to worry about.

If you follow the medical advice your doctor gives you, and the practical advice outlined above, both you and your family should be none the worse for your bout with red-eye.

CONDITION: **INFLAMMATION**

CATEGORY: **OPHTHALMIC CORTICOSTEROIDS**

GENERIC (CHEMICAL) NAME	BRAND (TRADE) NAME	DOSAGE FORMS AND STRENGTHS
Dexamethasone	AK-DEX	Ointment: 0.05% Solution: 0.1%
	DECADRON Phosphate	Ointment: 0.05% Solution: 0.1%
	MAXIDEX	Ointment: 0.05% Suspension: 0.1%
Fluorometholone	FML	Ointment: 0.1% Suspension: 0.1%
	FML Forte	Suspension: 0.25%
Medrysone	HMS	Suspension: 1%
Prednisolone	AK-TATE	Suspension: 1%
	ECONOPRED	Suspension: 0.125%
	ECONOPRED Plus	Suspension: 1%
	INFLAMASE	Solution: 0.125%
	INFLAMASE Forte	Solution: 1%
	PRED Forte	Suspension: 1%
	PRED Mild	Suspension: 0.12%
	PREDATE	Suspension: 1%

DRUG PROFILE

These topical drugs are used to reduce the inflammation and other discomfort associated with such eye conditions as allergies, certain types of conjunctivitis, and uveitis (inflammation of the iris and neighboring parts of the eye).

BEFORE USING THIS DRUG

Let your doctor know *IF*

You have ever had allergic reactions or other problems with ■ corticosteroids ■ sulfites ■ other preservatives.

You have ever had any of the following medical problems: ■ glaucoma ■ cataracts ■ tuberculosis of the eye ■ eye injury ■ any type of eye infection ■ herpes simplex keratitis ■ diabetes (or family history of diabetes) ■ chickenpox or other viral disease ■ fungal infections ■ rheumatoid arthritis.

SPECIAL RESTRICTIONS WHILE TAKING THIS DRUG

FOOD AND DRUG INTERACTIONS

No special restrictions on other drugs, foods and beverages, alcohol use, or smoking.

DAILY LIVING

Driving	Do not drive if you are using this drug since it may cause blurred vision. Be careful when operating household appliances or doing any other tasks that require clear vision until you know how this drug affects you.
Examinations or Tests	Prolonged therapy with ophthalmic corticosteroids may lead to glaucoma or cataracts. It is important for you to keep all appointments with your doctor—particularly if you are on long-term therapy with this drug—so that your eye pressure can be checked and your eyes can be examined for any adverse effects from this drug.
Other Precautions	If your eye symptoms do not improve or if they worsen, check with your doctor. Also, if you develop any signs of infection not present when you first started using this drug, let your doctor know.

The ointment should not be applied while wearing contact lenses.

The use of these drugs slows wound healing, which may be important if you have surgery done in or around the eyes. Let your doctor know that you are taking this drug, if you are undergoing this kind of surgery.

| Helpful Hints | *To use:* After washing your hands thoroughly, pull the lower eyelid down to form a pouch; drop in the solution or squeeze about a one-third-inch strip of ointment into the pouch. Keep your eyes closed for one to two minutes. You may experience a temporary burning or stinging sensation or blurred vision after use of the ointment. |

To prevent contamination, avoid touching either the dropper or tube tip to the eye, eyelid, or any other surface and keep the container tightly closed when not in use. Wipe off the tip of the tube of ointment with a clean tissue before replacing the cap.

No special restrictions on exertion and exercise, sun exposure, or exposure to excessive heat or cold.

POSSIBLE SIDE EFFECTS

Although this list of adverse effects may seem somewhat intimidating, keep in mind that some are quite rare. Of course, should these or any other problems arise while you are on medication, it is always a good idea to consult your doctor.

IF YOU DEVELOP

sudden eye pain ■ loss of vision

WHAT TO DO

Urgent: Stop using this drug and get in touch with your doctor immediately.

blurred vision or other visual disturbances ■ drooping or swelling of eyelids ■ eye pain ■ increased redness of the eyes ■ dilated pupils ■ headache ■ tearing ■ painful rash ■ increased eye sensitivity to light ■ sensation of a foreign body in the eye ■ any sign of eye infection not present before beginning use of this drug	**May be serious** Stop using this drug and check with your doctor as soon as possible.
stinging and burning of the eye	If symptoms are disturbing or persist, let your doctor know.

STORAGE INSTRUCTIONS

Store in a cool, dark place (not in a bathroom medicine cabinet), and make sure that it does not freeze.

STOPPING OR INTERRUPTING THERAPY

If you miss a dose, apply it as soon as possible. If it is almost time for your next dose, skip the missed dose and resume your regular schedule.

SPECIAL CONSIDERATIONS FOR THOSE OVER SIXTY-FIVE

None.

CONDITION: **BACTERIAL INFECTIONS**

CATEGORY: **OPHTHALMIC ANTI-INFECTIVES (AMINOGLYCOSIDES)**

GENERIC (CHEMICAL) NAME	BRAND (TRADE) NAME	DOSAGE FORMS AND STRENGTHS
Gentamicin sulfate	GARAMYCIN	Ointment: 0.3% Solution: 0.3%
	GENOPTIC	Ointment: 0.3% Solution: 0.3%
	GENTACIDIN	Ointment: 0.3% Solution: 0.3%
	GENT-AK	Ointment: 0.3% Solution: 0.3%

Neomycin sulfate, polymyxin B sulfate, gramicidin	AK-SPORE	Solution: neomycin sulfate equivalent to 1.75 mg of neomycin, 10,000 units of polymyxin B sulfate, and 0.025 mg gramicidin per ml
	NEOSPORIN	Solution: neomycin sulfate equivalent to 1.75 mg of neomycin, 10,000 units of polymyxin B sulfate, and 0.025 mg gramicidin per ml
Tobramycin	TOBREX	Ointment: 0.3% Solution: 0.3%

DRUG PROFILE

These antibiotics are applied directly to the eye to treat infections caused by bacteria. They work by interfering with the manufacture of protein inside the bacterial organism.

BEFORE USING THIS DRUG

Let your doctor know *IF*

You have ever had allergic reactions or other problems with ■ gentamicin ■ tobramycin ■ any other aminoglycoside antibiotic, including amikacin, kanamycin, neomycin, netilmicin, or streptomycin ■ preservatives.

You are taking any of the following medicines: ■ other eye preparations.

SPECIAL RESTRICTIONS WHILE TAKING THIS DRUG

FOOD AND DRUG INTERACTIONS

No special restrictions on other drugs, foods and beverages, alcohol use, or smoking.

DAILY LIVING

Driving	Do not drive if you are using this drug since it may cause blurred vision. Be careful when operating household appliances or doing any other tasks that require clear vision until you know how this drug affects you.
Examinations or Tests	It is important for you to keep all appointments with your doctor so that your progress can be checked.
Other Precautions	If your eye symptoms do not improve or if they worsen, check with your doctor. Also, if you develop any signs of eye infection not present when you first started using this drug, let your doctor know.
Helpful Hints	*To use:* After washing your hands thoroughly, pull the lower lid down to form a pouch; drop in the solution or squeeze about a one-third-inch strip of ointment into the pouch. Keep your eyes closed for one to two minutes. You may experience a temporary burning or stinging sensation or blurred vision after use of the ointment.
	To prevent contamination, avoid touching either the dropper or tube tip to the eye, eyelid, or any other surface, and keep the container tightly closed when not in use. Wipe off the tip of the tube of ointment or cream with a clean tissue before replacing the cap.

No special restrictions on exertion and exercise, sun exposure, or exposure to excessive heat or cold.

POSSIBLE SIDE EFFECTS

Although this list of adverse effects may seem somewhat intimidating, keep in mind that some are quite rare. Of course, should these or any other problems arise while you are on medication, it is always a good idea to consult your doctor.

IF YOU DEVELOP

eye irritation ■ itching of eyes ■ swelling of eyelids ■ red eyes ■ watering of the eyes ■ any sign of eye infection not present before beginning use of this drug

WHAT TO DO

May be serious Stop taking this drug and check with you doctor as soon as possible.

---

stinging and burning of the eye

If symptoms are disturbing or persist, let your doctor know.

STORAGE INSTRUCTIONS

Store in a cool, dark place (not in a bathroom medicine cabinet) and make sure that it does not freeze.

STOPPING OR INTERRUPTING THERAPY

If you miss a dose, apply it as soon as possible. If it is almost time for your next dose, however, skip the missed dose and resume your regular schedule.

SPECIAL CONSIDERATIONS FOR THOSE OVER SIXTY-FIVE

None.

CONDITION: **BACTERIAL INFECTIONS**

CATEGORY: **OPHTHALMIC ANTI-INFECTIVES (ERYTHROMYCIN)**

GENERIC (CHEMICAL) NAME	BRAND (TRADE) NAME	DOSAGE FORMS AND STRENGTHS
Erythromycin	AK-MYCIN	Ointment: 0.5%
	ILOTYCIN	Ointment: 0.5%

DRUG PROFILE

This type of antibiotic is applied directly to the eye to treat infections caused by bacteria. It suppresses the growth of bacteria by interfering with the manufacture of protein inside the bacterial organism.

BEFORE USING THIS DRUG

Let your doctor know *IF*

You have ever had allergic reactions or other problems with ■ any form of erythromycin ■ preservatives.

You are taking any of the following medicines: ■ other eye preparations.

SPECIAL RESTRICTIONS WHILE TAKING THIS DRUG

FOOD AND DRUG INTERACTIONS

No special restrictions on other drugs, foods and beverages, alcohol use, or smoking.

DAILY LIVING

Driving	Do not drive if you are using the ointment since it may cause blurred vision. Be careful when operating household appliances or doing any other tasks that require clear vision until you know how this drug affects you.
Examinations or Tests	It is important for you to keep all appointments with your doctor so that your progress can be checked.
Other Precautions	If your eye symptoms do not improve or if they worsen, check with your doctor. Also, if you develop any signs of eye infection not present when you first started using this drug, let your doctor know.

Helpful Hints

To use: Pull the lower eyelid down to form a pouch; squeeze about a one-third-inch strip of ointment into the pouch. Keep your eyes closed for one to two minutes. You may experience a temporary burning or stinging sensation or blurred vision after use of this ointment.

To prevent contamination, avoid touching the tube tip to the eye, eyelid, or any other surface, and keep the container tightly closed when not in use. Wipe off the tip of the tube with a clean tissue before replacing the cap.

No special restrictions on exertion and exercise, sun exposure, or exposure to excessive heat or cold.

POSSIBLE SIDE EFFECTS

Although this list of adverse effects may seem somewhat intimidating, keep in mind that some are quite rare. Of course, should these or any other problems arise while you are on medication, it is always a good idea to consult your doctor.

IF YOU DEVELOP	WHAT TO DO
eye irritation ■ itching of eyes ■ swelling of eyelids ■ red eyes ■ watering of the eyes ■ any sign of eye infection not present before beginning use of this drug	**May be serious** Stop using this drug and check with your doctor as soon as possible.
stinging or burning of eyes	If symptoms are disturbing or persist, let your doctor know.

STORAGE INSTRUCTIONS

Store in a cool, dark place (not in a bathroom medicine cabinet), and make sure that it does not freeze.

STOPPING OR INTERRUPTING THERAPY

If you miss a dose, apply it as soon as possible. If it is almost time for your next dose, skip the missed dose and resume your regular schedule.

SPECIAL CONSIDERATIONS FOR THOSE OVER SIXTY-FIVE

None.

CONDITION: **BACTERIAL INFECTIONS**

CATEGORY: **OPHTHALMIC ANTI-INFECTIVES (SULFONAMIDES)**

GENERIC (CHEMICAL) NAME	BRAND (TRADE) NAME	DOSAGE FORMS AND STRENGTHS
Sulfacetamide sodium	AK-SULF	Ointment: 10% Solution: 10%, 15%
	BLEPH-10	Ointment: 10% Solution: 10%
	ISOPTO-CETAMIDE	Ointment: 10% Solution: 15%
	Sodium SULAMYD	Ointment: 10% Solution: 10%
	SULF-10	Solution: 10%
	SULTEN-10	Solution: 10%
Sulfacetamide sodium and phenylephrine hydrochloride	VASOSULF hydrochloride	Solution: 15% sulfacetamide sodium and 0.125% phenylephrine per ml
Sulfisoxazole	GANTRISIN	Ointment: 4% Solution: 4%

DRUG PROFILE

Ophthalmic sulfonamides (sulfa drugs) are used to treat bacterial infections of the eye such as conjunctivitis and ulcers of the cornea. These antibiotics suppress the growth of bacteria by interfering with the manufacture of folic acid. Phenylephrine, a decongestant drug, relieves redness, watering, and itching by constricting the blood vessels in the eye.

These drugs are sometimes used in combination with other ophthalmic preparations or with oral sulfonamide therapy.

BEFORE USING THIS DRUG

Let your doctor know *IF*

You have ever had allergic reactions or other problems with ■ any sulfonamides (sulfa drugs) ■ furosemide or thiazide diuretics (water pills) ■ oral medicine for diabetes ■ oral medicine for glaucoma ■ sulfites or other preservatives ■ silver preparations.

You are taking any of the following medicines: ■ other eye preparations.

SPECIAL RESTRICTIONS WHILE TAKING THIS DRUG

FOOD AND DRUG INTERACTIONS

No special restrictions on other drugs, foods and beverages, alcohol use, or smoking.

DAILY LIVING

Driving	Do not drive if you are using this drug since it may cause blurred vision. Be careful when operating household appliances or doing any other tasks that require clear vision until you know how this drug affects you.
Examinations or Tests	It is important for you to keep all appointments with your doctor so that your progress can be checked.

Other Precautions

If your eye symptoms do not improve or if they worsen, stop using this drug and check with your doctor. Also, if you develop any signs of eye infection not present when you first started using this drug or if you start to have a pus-filled discharge from the eye, let your doctor know.

Tell any doctor you consult that you are using this drug, if you will be undergoing eye surgery.

Helpful Hints

To use: After washing your hands thoroughly, pull the lower eyelid down to form a pouch; drop in the solution or squeeze about a half-inch to one-inch strip of ointment into the pouch. Keep your eyes closed for one to two minutes.

You may experience a temporary burning or stinging sensation or blurred vision after use of the ointment.

To prevent contamination, avoid touching either the dropper or tube tip to the eye, eyelid, or any other surface, and keep the container tightly closed when not in use. Wipe off the tip of the tube of ointment with a clean tissue before replacing the cap.

No special restrictions on exertion and exercise, sun exposure, or exposure to excessive heat or cold.

POSSIBLE SIDE EFFECTS

Although this list of adverse effects may seem somewhat intimidating, keep in mind that some are quite rare. Of course, should these or any other problems arise while you are on medication, it is always a good idea to consult your doctor.

IF YOU DEVELOP	WHAT TO DO
redness, hives, peeling, scaling, or blisters	**Urgent: Stop using this drug and get in touch with your doctor immediately.**

eye irritation ■ itching of eyes ■ swelling of eyelids ■ red eyes ■ watering of the eyes ■ any sign of eye infection not present before beginning use of this drug	**May be serious** Stop using this drug and check with your doctor as soon as possible.
stinging and burning of the eyes ■ headache ■ browache ■ blurred vision ■ increased eye sensitivity to light	If symptoms are disturbing or persist, let your doctor know.

STORAGE INSTRUCTIONS

Store in a cool, dark place (not in a bathroom medicine cabinet), and make sure that it does not freeze.

STOPPING OR INTERRUPTING THERAPY

If you miss a dose, apply it as soon as possible. If it is almost time for your next dose, skip the missed dose and resume your regular schedule.

SPECIAL CONSIDERATIONS FOR THOSE OVER SIXTY-FIVE

None.

CONDITION: **BACTERIAL INFECTIONS**

CATEGORY: **OPHTHALMIC ANTI-INFECTIVES (TETRACYCLINES)**

GENERIC (CHEMICAL) NAME	BRAND (TRADE) NAME	DOSAGE FORMS AND STRENGTHS
Chlortetracycline hydrochloride	AUREOMYCIN	Ointment: 1%
Tetracycline hydrochloride	ACHROMYCIN	Ointment: 1% Suspension: 1%

DRUG PROFILE

Ophthalmic tetracyclines are used to treat various types of bacterial infections of the eye. These antibiotics suppress the growth of bacteria by interfering with the manufacture of protein inside the bacterial organism. If you are being treated for trachoma, your doctor will probably prescribe an oral antibiotic along with the ophthalmic tetracycline.

BEFORE USING THIS DRUG

Let your doctor know *IF*

You have ever had allergic reactions or other problems with ■ any tetracyclines.

You are taking any of the following medicines: ■ other eye preparations.

SPECIAL RESTRICTIONS WHILE TAKING THIS DRUG

FOOD AND DRUG INTERACTIONS

No special restrictions on other drugs, foods and beverages, alcohol use, or smoking.

DAILY LIVING

Driving	Do not drive if you are using the ointment since it may cause blurred vision. Be careful when operating household appliances or doing any other tasks that require clear vision until you know how this drug affects you.
Examinations or Tests	It is important for you to keep all appointments with your doctor so that your progress can be checked. If your eye symptoms do not improve or if they worsen, stop taking this drug and check with your doctor. Also, if you develop any signs of eye infection not present when you first started using this drug, let your doctor know.

Helpful Hints	*To use:* After washing your hands thoroughly, pull the lower lid down to form a pouch; drop in the solution or squeeze about a one-third-inch strip of ointment into the pouch. Keep your eyes closed for one to two minutes. You may experience a temporary burning or stinging sensation or blurred vision after use of the ointment.
	To prevent contamination, avoid touching either the dropper or tube tip to the eye, eyelid, or any other surface, and keep the container tightly closed when not in use. Wipe off the tip of the tube of ointment with a clean tissue before replacing the cap.

No special restrictions on exertion and exercise, sun exposure, or exposure to excessive heat or cold.

POSSIBLE SIDE EFFECTS

Although this list of adverse effects may seem somewhat intimidating, keep in mind that some are quite rare. Of course, should these or any other problems arise while you are on medication, it is always a good idea to consult your doctor.

IF YOU DEVELOP	WHAT TO DO
eye irritation ■ itching of eyes ■ swelling of the eyelids ■ red eyes ■ watering of the eyes ■ any sign of eye infection not present before beginning use of this drug ■ sensation of a foreign body in the eye	**May be serious** Stop using this drug and check with your doctor as soon as possible.
stinging and burning of the eyes	If symptoms are disturbing or persist, let your doctor know.

STORAGE INSTRUCTIONS

Store in a cool, dark place (not in a bathroom medicine cabinet), and make sure that it does not freeze.

STOPPING OR INTERRUPTING THERAPY

If you miss a dose, apply it as soon as possible. If it is almost time for your next dose, skip the missed dose and resume your regular schedule.

SPECIAL CONSIDERATIONS FOR THOSE OVER SIXTY-FIVE

None.

CONDITION: **BACTERIAL INFECTIONS**

CATEGORY: **OPHTHALMIC ANTI-INFECTIVES (BACITRACIN AND BACITRACIN COMBINATIONS)**

GENERIC (CHEMICAL) NAME	BRAND (TRADE) NAME	DOSAGE FORMS AND STRENGTHS
Bacitracin	BACIGUENT	Ointment: 500 units per g
Bacitracin, neomycin sulfate, and polymyxin B sulfate	MYCITRACIN	Ointment: 500 units bacitracin, 5,000 units polymyxin B sulfate, and neomycin sulfate equivalent to 3.5 mg of neomycin
Bacitracin zinc and polymyxin B sulfate	AK-POLY-BAC	Ointment: 500 units bacitracin zinc and 10,000 units polymyxin B sulfate per g
	POLYSPORIN	Ointment: 500 units bacitracin zinc and 10,000 units polymyxin B sulfate per g

| Bacitracin zinc, polymyxin B sulfate, and neomycin sulfate | NEOSPORIN | Ointment: 400 units bacitracin zinc, 5,000 units polymyxin B sulfate, and neomycin sulfate equivalent to 3.5 mg of neomycin per g |
| | AK-SPORE | Ointment: 400 units bacitracin zinc, 10,000 units polymyxin B sulfate, and neomycin sulfate equivalent to 3.5 mg of neomycin |

DRUG PROFILE

Bacitracin and bacitracin combinations are used for short-term treatment of bacterial infections of the eye. These antibiotics suppress the growth of bacteria by interfering with the manufacture of protein inside the bacterial organism.

BEFORE USING THIS DRUG

Let your doctor know *IF*

You have ever had allergic reactions or other problems with ■ bacitracin ■ neomycin ■ polymyxin.

■ *with products containing neomycin only:* ■ aminoglycoside antibiotics including amikacin, gentamicin, kanamycin, tobramycin, or streptomycin.

You are taking any of the following medicines: ■ other eye preparations.

SPECIAL RESTRICTIONS WHILE TAKING THIS DRUG

FOOD AND DRUG INTERACTIONS

No special restrictions on other drugs, foods and beverages, alcohol use, or smoking.

DAILY LIVING

Driving

Do not drive if you are using this ointment since it may cause blurred vision. Be careful when operating household appliances or doing any other tasks that require clear vision until you know how this drug affects you.

Examinations or Tests

It is important for you to keep all appointments with your doctor so that your progress can be checked.

Other Precautions

If your eye symptoms do not improve or if they worsen, check with your doctor. Also, if you develop any signs of eye infection not present when you first started using this drug, let your doctor know.

Helpful Hints

To use: After washing your hands thoroughly, pull the lower eyelid down to form a pouch; squeeze about a one-third-inch strip of ointment into the pouch. Keep your eyes closed for one to two minutes. You may experience a temporary burning or stinging sensation or blurred vision after use of the ointment.

To prevent contamination, avoid touching the tube tip to the eye, eyelid, or any other surface, and keep the container tightly closed when not in use. Wipe off the tip of the tube with a clean tissue before replacing the cap.

No special restrictions on exertion and exercise, sun exposure, or exposure to excessive heat or cold.

POSSIBLE SIDE EFFECTS

Although this list of adverse effects may seem somewhat intimidating, keep in mind that some are quite rare. Of course, should these or any other problems arise while you are on medication, it is always a good idea to consult your doctor.

IF YOU DEVELOP	WHAT TO DO
difficulty in breathing ■ fainting	**Urgent: Stop using this drug and get in touch with your doctor immediately.**
tightness in chest ■ itching of eyes ■ swelling of lips and face ■ increased sweating ■ inflammation of the eye ■ any sign of eye infection not present before beginning use of this drug ■ rash	**May be serious** Stop using this drug and check with your doctor as soon as possible.

STORAGE INSTRUCTIONS

Store in a cool, dark place (not in a bathroom medicine cabinet), and make sure that it does not freeze.

STOPPING OR INTERRUPTING THERAPY

If you miss a dose, apply it as soon as possible. If it is almost time for your next dose, skip the missed dose and resume your regular schedule.

SPECIAL CONSIDERATIONS FOR THOSE OVER SIXTY-FIVE

None.

CONDITION: **BACTERIAL INFECTIONS**

CATEGORY: **OPHTHALMIC ANTI-INFECTIVES
(CHLORAMPHENICOL)**

GENERIC (CHEMICAL) NAME	BRAND (TRADE) NAME	DOSAGE FORMS AND STRENGTHS
Chloramphenicol	AK-CHLOR CHLOROMYCETIN	Solution: 0.5% Ointment: 1% Powder: to be mixed with distilled water to make 0.16% to 0.5% solution
	CHLOROPTIC	Ointment: 1% Solution: 0.5%
	OPHTHOCHLOR	Solution: 0.5%

DRUG PROFILE

Chloramphenicol is used for short-term treatment of bacterial infections of the eye. These drugs suppress the growth of bacteria by interfering with the manufacture of protein inside the bacterial organism. Your doctor may prescribe an oral antibiotic for you to take as well.

BEFORE USING THIS DRUG

Let your doctor know *IF*

You have ever had allergic reactions or other problems with ■ chloramphenicol ■ sulfites or other preservatives.

SPECIAL RESTRICTIONS WHILE TAKING THIS DRUG

FOOD AND DRUG INTERACTIONS

No special restrictions on other drugs, foods and beverages, alcohol use, or smoking.

DAILY LIVING

Driving	Do not drive if you are using the ointment since it may cause blurred vision. Be careful when operating household appliances or doing any other tasks that require clear vision until you know how this drug affects you.
Examinations or Tests	It is important for you to keep all appointments with your doctor so that your progress can be checked.
Other Precautions	If your eye symptoms do not improve or if they worsen, check with your doctor. Also, if you develop any signs of eye infection not present when you first started using this drug, stop using it and let your doctor know.
Helpful Hints	*To use:* After washing your hands thoroughly, pull the lower lid down to form a pouch; drop in the solution or squeeze about a one-third-inch strip of ointment into the pouch. Keep your eyes closed for one to two minutes. You may experience a temporary burning or stinging sensation or blurred vision after use of the ointment.
	To prevent contamination, avoid touching either the dropper or tube tip to the eye, eyelid, or any other surface, and keep the container tightly closed when not in use. Wipe off the tip of the tube with a clean tissue before replacing the cap.

No special restrictions on exertion and exercise, sun exposure, or exposure to excessive heat or cold.

POSSIBLE SIDE EFFECTS

Although this list of adverse effects may seem somewhat intimidating, keep in mind that some are quite rare. Of course, should these or any other problems arise while you are on medication, it is always a good idea to consult your doctor.

IF YOU DEVELOP	WHAT TO DO
shortness of breath ■ swelling of lips or face ■ fever, chills, or sore throat ■ tiredness ■ paleness ■ delayed blood clotting	**Urgent: Stop using this drug and get in touch with your doctor immediately.**
inflammation, itching, stinging, or burning of the eyes ■ hives, rash, blisters, or changes in skin color ■ any sign of eye infection not present before beginning use of this drug	**May be serious** Stop using this drug and check with your doctor as soon as possible.

STORAGE INSTRUCTIONS

Store in a cool, dark place (not in a bathroom medicine cabinet). If your medicine is in a liquid form, make sure that it does not freeze.

STOPPING OR INTERRUPTING THERAPY

If you miss a dose, apply it as soon as possible. If it is almost time for your next dose, skip the missed dose and resume your regular schedule.

SPECIAL CONSIDERATIONS FOR THOSE OVER SIXTY-FIVE

None.

CONDITION: **VIRAL INFECTIONS**

CATEGORY: **OPHTHALMIC ANTI-INFECTIVES (ANTIVIRAL AGENTS)**

GENERIC (CHEMICAL) NAME	BRAND (TRADE) NAME	DOSAGE FORMS AND STRENGTHS
Idoxuridine	HERPLEX STOXIL	Solution: 0.1% Ointment: 0.5% Solution: 0.1%

| Trifluridine | VIROPTIC | Solution: 1% |
| Vidarabine | VIRA-A | Ointment: 3% |

DRUG PROFILE

These drugs are used for short-term treatment of eye infections caused by the virus herpes simplex. They work by preventing the virus from multiplying.

BEFORE USING THIS DRUG

Let your doctor know *IF*

You have ever had allergic reactions or other problems with ■ idoxuridine ■ trifluridine ■ vidarabine.

SPECIAL RESTRICTIONS WHILE TAKING THIS DRUG

FOOD AND DRUG INTERACTIONS

No special restrictions on other drugs, foods and beverages, alcohol use, or smoking.

DAILY LIVING

Driving	Do not drive if you are using this drug since it may cause blurred vision. Be careful when operating household appliances or doing any other tasks that require clear vision until you know how this drug affects you.
Examinations or Tests	It is important for you to keep all appointments with your doctor so that your progress can be checked.
Other Precautions	If your eye remains irritated, let your doctor know. Do not use this drug for longer than three weeks under any circumstances.

Helpful Hints

To use: After washing your hands thoroughly, pull the lower eyelid down to form a pouch; drop in the solution or squeeze about a half-inch strip of ointment into the pouch (refer to the package instructions for the exact amount). Keep your eyes closed for one to two minutes. You may experience a temporary burning or stinging sensation or blurred vision after use of the ointment.

To prevent contamination, avoid touching either the dropper or tube tip to the eye, eyelid, or any other surface, and keep the container tightly closed when not in use. Wipe off the tip of the tube with a clean tissue before replacing the cap.

No special restrictions on exertion and exercise, sun exposure, or exposure to excessive heat or cold.

POSSIBLE SIDE EFFECTS

Although this list of adverse effects may seem somewhat intimidating, keep in mind that some are quite rare. Of course, should these or any other problems arise while you are on medication, it is always a good idea to consult your doctor.

IF YOU DEVELOP	WHAT TO DO
eye pain or irritation ■ any signs of eye infection not present before beginning use of this drug ■ blurred vision ■ increased eye sensitivity to light	**May be serious** Stop using this drug and check with your doctor as soon as possible.
burning or stinging of the eyes ■ swelling of eyelids ■ dry eyes ■ redness in or around eyes *With vidarabine only:* tearing ■ sensation of a foreign body in the eye	If symptoms are disturbing or persist, let your doctor know.

STORAGE INSTRUCTIONS

Store this medicine in the refrigerator, but make sure that it does not freeze.

STOPPING OR INTERRUPTING THERAPY

If you miss a dose, apply it as soon as possible. If it is almost time for your next dose, skip the missed dose and resume your regular schedule.

SPECIAL CONSIDERATIONS FOR THOSE OVER SIXTY-FIVE

None.

CONDITION: **INFLAMMATION AND INFECTION**

CATEGORY: **OPHTHALMIC CORTICOSTEROID–ANTI-INFECTIVE COMBINATIONS**

GENERIC (CHEMICAL) NAME	BRAND (TRADE) NAME	DOSAGE FORMS AND STRENGTHS
Dexamethasone, neomycin sulfate, and polymyxin B sulfate	AK-TROL	Ointment: 0.1% dexamethasone, 0.5% neomycin sulfate, and 10,000 units polymyxin B sulfate per g Suspension: 0.1% dexamethasone, 0.5% neomycin sulfate, and 10,000 units polymyxin B sulfate per ml
	DEXACIDIN	Ointment: 0.1% dexamethasone, 0.5% neomycin sulfate, and 10,000 units polymyxin B sulfate per g Suspension: 0.1% dexamethasone, 0.5% neomycin sulfate, and 10,000 units polymyxin B sulfate per ml

	MAXITROL	Ointment: 0.1% dexamethasone, 0.5% neomycin sulfate, and 10,000 units polymyxin B sulfate per g Suspension: 0.1% dexamethasone, 0.5% neomycin sulfate, and 10,000 units polymyxin B sulfate per ml
Dexamethasone and neomycin sulfate	NeoDECADRON	Ointment: 0.05% dexamethasone and 0.5% neomycin sulfate per g Solution: 0.1% dexamethasone and 0.5% neomycin sulfate per ml
Hydrocortisone, bacitracin zinc, polymyxin B sulfate, and neomycin sulfate	CORTISPORIN	Ointment: 1% hydrocortisone, 400 units bacitracin zinc, 10,000 units polymyxin B sulfate, and 0.5% neomycin sulfate per g
Hydrocortisone acetate, polymyxin B sulfate, and chloramphenicol	OPHTHOCORT	Ointment: 0.5% mg hydrocortisone acetate, 10,000 units polymyxin B sulfate, and 1% chloramphenicol
Hydrocortisone, polymyxin B sulfate, and neomycin sulfate	CORTISPORIN	Suspension: 1% hydrocortisone, 10,000 units polymyxin B sulfate, and 0.5% neomycin sulfate per ml

	AK-SPORE HC	Suspension: 1% hydrocortisone, 10,000 units polymyxin B sulfate, and 0.5% neomycin sulfate per ml
Prednisolone acetate, polymyxin B sulfate, and neomycin sulfate	POLY-PRED	Suspension: 0.5% prednisolone acetate, 10,000 units polymyxin B sulfate, and 0.5% neomycin sulfate per ml
Prednisolone acetate and sulfacetamide sodium	AK-CIDE	Ointment: 0.5% prednisolone acetate and 10% sulfacetamide sodium per g Suspension: 0.5% prednisolone acetate and 10% sulfacetamide sodium per ml
	BELPHAMIDE	Ointment: 0.2% prednisolone acetate and 10% sulfacetamide sodium per g Suspension: 0.2% prednisolone acetate and 10% sulfacetamide sodium per ml
	CETAPRED	Ointment: 0.25% prednisolone acetate and 10% sulfacetamide sodium per g
	ISOPTO CETAPRED	Suspension: 0.25% prednisolone acetate and 10% sulfacetamide sodium per ml
	VASOCIDIN	Ointment: 0.5% prednisolone acetate and 10% sulfacetamide sodium per g

DRUG PROFILE

These combination drugs are prescribed to treat eye infections, injuries, and other inflammatory conditions. The antibiotic component suppresses the growth of bacteria, while the corticosteroid reduces inflammation and discomfort.

BEFORE USING THIS DRUG

Let your doctor know *IF*

You have ever had allergic reactions or other problems with ■ corticosteroids ■ sulfites or other preservatives ■ neomycin sulfate ■ polymyxin B sulfate.

■ *with sulfacetamide combinations only:* ■ any sulfonamides (sulfa drugs) ■ furosemide or thiazide diuretics (water pills) ■ oral medicine for diabetes ■ oral medicine for glaucoma.

You have ever had any of the following medical problems: ■ any type of eye infection ■ glaucoma ■ cataracts ■ tuberculosis of the eye ■ herpes simplex keratitis ■ recent eye injury (including foreign object in the eye) ■ diabetes (or family history of diabetes) ■ chickenpox or other viral diseases.

You are taking any of the following medicines: ■ any silver preparations for an eye condition.

SPECIAL RESTRICTIONS WHILE TAKING THIS DRUG

FOOD AND DRUG INTERACTIONS

No special restrictions on other drugs, foods and beverages, alcohol use, or smoking.

DAILY LIVING

| Driving | Do not drive if you are using an ointment since it may cause blurred vision. Be careful when operating household appliances or doing any other tasks that require clear vision until you know how this drug affects you. |

Examinations or Tests	It is important for you to keep all appointments with your doctor—particularly if you are on long-term therapy with this drug—so that your eye pressure can be checked and your eyes can be examined for any adverse effects from this drug.
Other Precautions	If your eye symptoms do not improve or it they worsen, check with your doctor. Also, if you develop any signs of eye infection not present when you first started using this drug, let your doctor know.
	If you will be undergoing eye surgery, let your doctor know that you have been using any of these medicines.
Helpful Hints	*To use:* After washing your hands thoroughly, pull the lower eyelid down to form a pouch; drop in the solution or squeeze about a one-third-inch strip of ointment into the pouch. Keep your eyes closed for one to two minutes. You may experience a temporary burning or stinging sensation or blurred vision after use of an ointment.
	To prevent contamination, avoid touching either the dropper or tube tip to the eye, eyelid, or any other surface, and keep the container tightly closed when not in use. Wipe off the tip of the tube with a clean tissue before replacing the cap.

No special restrictions on exertion and exercise, sun exposure, or exposure to excessive heat or cold.

POSSIBLE SIDE EFFECTS

Although this list of adverse effects may seem somewhat intimidating, keep in mind that some are quite rare. Of course, should these or any other problems arise while you are on medication, it is always a good idea to consult your doctor.

IF YOU DEVELOP	WHAT TO DO
severe eye pain ■ blurred vision	**Urgent: Stop using this drug and get in touch with your doctor immediately.**
blurred vision, seeing halos around lights, or other visual disturbances ■ drooping eyelids ■ eye pain or irritation ■ dilated pupils ■ headache or brow-ache ■ herpes ■ itching of the eyelids ■ eye redness or itching ■ any sign of eye infection not present before beginning use of this drug	**May be serious** Stop using this drug and check with your doctor as soon as possible.
burning or stinging of the eyes ■ increased eye sensitivity to light	If symptoms are disturbing or persist, let your doctor know.

STORAGE INSTRUCTIONS

Store in a cool, dark place (not in a bathroom medicine cabinet). If your medicine is in a liquid form, make sure that it does not freeze.

STOPPING OR INTERRUPTING THERAPY

If you miss a dose, apply it as soon as possible. If it is almost time for your next dose, skip the missed dose and resume your regular schedule.

SPECIAL CONSIDERATIONS FOR THOSE OVER SIXTY-FIVE

None.

CONDITION: **IRRITATION**

CATEGORY: **OPHTHALMIC DECONGESTANTS**

GENERIC (CHEMICAL) NAME	BRAND (TRADE) NAME	DOSAGE FORMS AND STRENGTHS
Naphazoline hydrochloride	AK-CON	Solution: 0.1%
	ALBALON	Solution: 0.1%
	MURO'S OPCON	Solution: 0.1%
	NAPHCON	Solution: 0.1%
	VASOCON	Solution: 0.1%
Naphazoline hydrochloride and antazoline phosphate	ALBALON-A	Solution: 0.05% naphazoline hydrochloride and 0.5% antazoline phosphate
	VASOCON-A	Solution: 0.05% naphazoline hydrochloride and 0.5% antazoline phosphate
Naphazoline hydrochloride and pheniramine maleate	AK-CON-A	Solution: 0.025% naphazoline hydrochloride and 0.3% pheniramine maleate
	MURO'S OPCON-A	Solution: 0.025% naphazoline hydrochloride and 0.3% pheniramine maleate
	NAPHCON-A	Solution: 0.025% naphazoline hydrochloride and 0.3% pheniramine maleate
Phenylephrine hydrochloride	NEO-SYNEPHRINE	Solution: 2.5%, 10%

Phenylephrine hydrochloride, pyrilamine maleate, and antipyrine	PREFRIN-A	Solution: 0.12% phenylephrine hydrochloride, 0.1% pyrilamine maleate, and 0.1% antipyrine

DRUG PROFILE

These decongestant drugs are prescribed to relieve the redness, watering, and itching of the eyes associated with minor irritations and allergies. They work by constricting the blood vessels in the eye. The antihistamine components prevent the inflammatory response of the eye to allergens.

BEFORE USING THIS DRUG

Let your doctor know *IF*

You have ever had allergic reactions or other problems with ■ any ophthalmic decongestants.

You have ever had any of the following medical problems: ■ glaucoma ■ recent eye infections or a foreign body in the eye ■ diabetes ■ high blood pressure ■ overactive thyroid ■ any disease of the heart or blood vessels.

You are taking any of the following medicines: ■ monoamine oxidase inhibitors (MAOIs) for depression (in the past two weeks).

■ *with phenylephrine only:* ■ tricyclic antidepressants ■ atenolol, metoprolol, nadolol, pindolol, propranolol, or timolol (beta-blockers) ■ reserpine, guanethidine, or methyldopa (medicine for high blood pressure).

SPECIAL RESTRICTIONS WHILE TAKING THIS DRUG

FOOD AND DRUG INTERACTIONS

Other Drugs	Do not take any other drugs, including over-the-counter (OTC) drugs, before checking with your doctor. The combination of these drugs and certain other medicines—especially monoamine oxidase inhibitors—can result in a severe and dangerous rise in blood pressure.

No special restrictions on foods and beverages, alcohol use, or smoking.

DAILY LIVING

Sun Exposure

Your eyes may become especially sensitive to sunlight; wearing tinted glasses should help ease any discomfort.

Examinations or Tests

If you are hypertensive, it is important to have your blood pressure checked regularly.

Other Precautions

If your eye symptoms do not improve within forty-eight hours or if they worsen, check with your doctor. Avoid frequent, prolonged use of these drugs, as chronic redness of the eyes may develop.

No special restrictions on driving, exertion and exercise, or exposure to excessive heat or cold.

POSSIBLE SIDE EFFECTS

Although this list of adverse effects may seem somewhat intimidating, keep in mind that some are quite rare. Of course, should these or any other problems arise while you are on medication, it is always a good idea to consult your doctor.

IF YOU DEVELOP

irregular, pounding, or fast heartbeat ■ nervousness ■ nausea ■ dizziness ■ weakness ■ drowsiness ■ faintness ■ tremors ■ increased sweating ■ eye pain ■ headache or browache ■ seeing halos around lights

WHAT TO DO

Urgent: Stop using this drug and get in touch with your doctor immediately.

colored spots floating across your field of vision ■ dilated pupils ■ stuffy or runny nose ■ swelling of the eyes ■ worsened eye irritation	**May be serious** Stop using this drug and check with your doctor as soon as possible.
burning or stinging of the eye	If symptoms are disturbing or persist, let your doctor know.

STORAGE INSTRUCTIONS

Store in a cool, dark place (not in a bathroom medicine cabinet), and make sure that it does not freeze.

STOPPING OR INTERRUPTING THERAPY

If you miss a dose, apply it as soon as possible. If it is almost time for your next dose, skip the missed dose and resume your regular schedule. Most of these medicines can be used as needed for eye redness or itching and can be discontinued without adverse effects.

SPECIAL CONSIDERATIONS FOR THOSE OVER SIXTY-FIVE

Older people may be especially susceptible to the effects of these products on the heart and blood vessels. Therefore, it is important that people over sixty-five inform their doctor if they have high blood pressure or a heart condition. In addition, older people may be more prone to the side effect of seeing colored spots floating across the field of vision.

CATARACTS

Clear vision depends on the eye's ability to focus light rays to a point on the retina, a tissue that lines the inside of the back of the eye and relays images to the brain. For light rays to reach the retina at the correct point, they must be bent through two transparent organs—the cornea, which arches like a dome over the iris (the colored part of the eye), and the lens, a pea-shaped organ just behind the iris.

CAUSES

With age, the lens may begin to lose some of its transparency as the result of certain chemical changes in the eye. Cloudy areas, called opacities, may develop. At the same time, the center of the lens—its nucleus—hardens, and the entire lens loses some of its clarity and elasticity. These changes occur in about 80 percent of people over sixty-five, and, for a little less than half of that group, are severe enough to disrupt vision. When a cloudy lens interferes with sight, it is called a cataract.

About two million Americans have cataracts, and, while the condition sometimes affects younger people, 90 percent of cases are age related. Because high blood sugar also has an adverse effect on the lens, diabetics, too, are prone to cataracts. Cataracts are quite unpredictable; for unknown reasons, they progress much more quickly in some people than in others.

DIAGNOSIS

Depending on its exact location in the lens, a cataract may make itself known through a number of different symptoms, some subtle, some greatly annoying. The condition is almost always painless, however, and for many people, the only noticeable change is a gradual deterioration of vision. Some cataract sufferers have said that they seem to be viewing the world through smudged glass.

Cataracts can also cause very distressing double vision. This symptom is the result of a cataract that has some areas that are denser than others. Ironically, another common symptom of cataracts may appear, at first, as an improvement in eyesight—specifically, in near vision, reducing the need for the reading glasses that so many older people rely on. This is due to nuclear sclerosis, which is hardening of the nucleus. This type of cataract, however, may worsen nearsightedness, forcing many people with the condition to change eyeglass or contact lens prescriptions frequently.

Another symptom may be poor vision in bright light, caused by an opacity in the center of the lens's rear surface. This kind of cataract often occurs as a result of long-term use of cortisone, a steroid, to treat disorders such as arthritis and asthma. It may also be due to chronic ocular inflammation, known as uveitis. Finally, an advanced cataract can mute color vision, causing everything to have a yellowish tinge.

TREATMENT

Frequently, when cataracts are first diagnosed, the best course of action is to wait and watch. Your ophthalmologist may be able to reduce the vision problems caused by the cataract with a new prescription for glasses, bifocals, or, rarely, contact lenses. Most of the time, cataract surgery is performed when the person decides it is necessary, although if vision loss is severe enough, the ophthalmologist may recommend an operation. Increased glare may also suggest that earlier surgical intervention be considered.

Certain conditions of the eye make cataract surgery a poor choice for some people. For example, if your retina is already damaged from diabetes, high blood pressure, or a retinal disorder called macular degeneration that is common in older people, your ophthalmologist may not recommend surgery, since the resulting improvement in vision may be minimal.

Three types of cataract surgery are currently performed. The most common type had been intracapsular excision, where the entire lens is removed with a cryoprobe—a pencil probe that freezes itself to the cataract. Most cataract surgeons are now performing extracapsular excision, however, where parts of the cataract are removed separately, starting with the front part of the capsule surrounding the lens. The back portion of the capsule is purposely left behind. Modern microsurgical techniques have made extracapsular surgery safe and effective. The third type of surgery, phacoemulsification, requires the smallest incision of all—only about one-tenth of an inch. The surgeon again removes the front part of the capsule, and then inserts a titanium needle that vibrates at a rapid rate (ultrasound) to pulverize the nucleus. The remaining cortex is then sucked out, and the back portion of the capsule left behind.

Which type of surgery is best for you depends both on the condition of your eye and on your surgeon's preferred technique. Each type is equally effective, since the end result—removal of the cataract—is always the same. However, the types that do not extract the back part of the capsule (extracapsular excision and phacoemulsification) allow a wider choice of intraocular implants—quarter-inch plastic lenses that may be inserted during cataract surgery and are designed to help make up for the loss of your natural lens. Therefore, these techniques are preferred by most cataract surgeons.

For the first twenty-four hours after your operation, you'll have to wear a patch and shield over your eye, and you may, for a few days, experience some pain, tearing, and discharge. After that, complete recovery can take from three or four weeks to three months, depending on the type of operation you had.

During the recovery period, your ophthalmologist may prescribe cortisone drops to clear up inflammation, which may persist for four to six weeks. Any of several brands of cortisone drops, including Pred Forte, Inflamase, Econopred, and Decadron, may be used. (See the drug chart on page 870 for more information.) You may also need antibiotic drops, such as Garamycin, Tobrex, Neosporin, or

Chloroptic, to help prevent infection for a few weeks after surgery. (The drug charts for these products appear on pages 871 and 873.) Also, to control pressure increases within the eye during the first few days after the operation, you might have to use drops such as Timoptic or pills such as Diamox to lower that pressure. (See the drug charts on pages 874–875.)

Surgery takes away your cataract, but it also takes away your lens, which, when functioning properly, holds one-third of the eye's refractory power (which is most important for focusing on near objects). To make up for this loss, you will need glasses, a contact lens, or an intraocular implant. Intraocular implants, which are permanent and rarely have to be changed, are particularly popular in people over forty-five. They are not recommended, however, for young people or people with other serious eye problems.

OUTLOOK

Cataract surgery is one of the most successful types of operations, restoring normal, clear vision to about 95 percent of people who undergo it. Advances in microsurgical techniques have led to this high level of success.

CONDITION: **CATARACTS**

CATEGORY: **OPHTHALMIC CORTICOSTEROIDS**

GENERIC (CHEMICAL) NAME	BRAND (TRADE) NAME	DOSAGE FORMS AND STRENGTHS
Dexamethasone	AK-DEX	Ointment: 0.05%
		Solution: 0.1%
	DECADRON Phosphate	Ointment: 0.05%
		Solution: 0.1%
	MAXIDEX	Ointment: 0.05%
		Suspension: 0.1%
Fluorometholone	FML	Ointment: 0.1%
		Suspension: 0.1%
	FML Forte	Suspension: 0.25%
Medrysone	HMS	Suspension: 1%
Prednisolone	AK-TATE	Suspension: 1%
	ECONOPRED	Suspension: 0.125%
	ECONOPRED Plus	Suspension: 1%
	INFLAMASE	Solution: 0.125%
	INFLAMASE Forte	Solution: 1%
	PRED Forte	Suspension: 1%
	PRED Mild	Suspension: 0.12%
	PREDATE	Suspension: 1%

DRUG PROFILE

These topical drugs are used to reduce the inflammation and other discomfort associated with such eye conditions as allergies, certain types of conjunctivitis, burns, and uveitis (inflammation of the iris and neighboring parts of the eye).

For complete information on these drugs, see pages 833–836.

CONDITION: **CATARACTS**

CATEGORY: **OPHTHALMIC ANTI-INFECTIVES
(AMINOGLYCOSIDES)**

GENERIC (CHEMICAL) NAME	BRAND (TRADE) NAME	DOSAGE FORMS AND STRENGTHS
Gentamicin sulfate	GARAMYCIN	Ointment: 0.3% Solution: 0.3%
	GENOPTIC	Ointment: 0.3% Solution: 0.3%
	GENTACIDIN	Ointment: 0.3% Solution: 0.3%
	GENT-AK	Ointment: 0.3% Solution: 0.3%
Neomycin sulfate, polymyxin B sulfate, gramicidin	AK-SPORE	Solution: neomycin sulfate equivalent to 1.75 mg neomycin, 10,000 units polymyxin B sulfate, and 0.025 mg gramicidin per ml
	NEOSPORIN	Solution: neomycin sulfate equivalent to 1.75 mg neomycin, 10,000 units polymyxin B sulfate, and 0.025 mg gramicidin per ml
Tobramycin	TOBREX	Ointment: 0.3% Solution: 0.3%

DRUG PROFILE

These antibiotics are applied directly to the eye to treat infections caused by bacteria. They work by interfering with the manufacture of protein inside the bacterial organism.

For compete information on these drugs, see pages 836–839.

CONDITION: **CATARACTS**

CATEGORY: **OPHTHALMIC ANTI-INFECTIVES (BACITRACIN AND BACITRACIN COMBINATIONS)**

GENERIC (CHEMICAL) NAME	BRAND (TRADE) NAME	DOSAGE FORMS AND STRENGTHS
Bacitracin	BACIGUENT	Ointment: 500 units per g
Bacitracin, neomycin sulfate, and polymyxin B sulfate	MYCITRACIN	Ointment: 500 units bacitracin, 5,000 units polymyxin B sulfate, and neomycin sulfate equivalent to 3.5 mg of neomycin
Bacitracin zinc and polymyxin B sulfate	AK-POLY-BAC	Ointment: 500 units bacitracin zinc and 10,000 units polymyxin B sulfate per g
	POLYSPORIN	Ointment: 500 units bacitracin zinc and 10,000 units polymyxin B sulfate per g
Bacitracin zinc, polymyxin B sulfate, and neomycin sulfate	NEOSPORIN	Ointment: 400 units bacitracin zinc, 5,000 units polymyxin B sulfate, and neomycin sulfate equivalent to 3.5 mg of neomycin per g
	AK-SPORE	Ointment: 400 units bacitracin zinc, 10,000 units polymyxin B sulfate, and neomycin sulfate equivalent to 3.5 mg of neomycin

DRUG PROFILE

Bacitracin and bacitracin combinations are used for short-term treatment of bacterial infections of the eye. These antibiotics suppress the growth of bacteria by interfering with the manufacture of protein inside the bacterial organism.

For complete information on these drugs, see pages 848–851.

CONDITION: **CATARACTS**

CATEGORY: **OPHTHALMIC ANTI-INFECTIVES (CHLORAMPHENICOL)**

GENERIC (CHEMICAL) NAME	BRAND (TRADE) NAME	DOSAGE FORMS AND STRENGTHS
Chloramphenicol	AK-CHLOR CHLOROMYCETIN	Solution: 0.5% Ointment: 1% Powder: to be mixed with distilled water to make 0.16% to 0.5% solution
	CHLOROPTIC	Ointment: 1% Solution: 0.5%
	OPHTHOCHLOR	Solution: 0.5%

DRUG PROFILE

Chloramphenicol is used for short-term treatment of bacterial infections of the eye. This drug suppresses the growth of bacteria by interfering with the manufacture of protein inside the bacterial organism.

For complete information on this drug, see pages 852–854.

CONDITION: **CATARACTS**

CATEGORY: **TOPICAL BETA-BLOCKERS**

GENERIC (CHEMICAL) NAME	BRAND (TRADE) NAME	DOSAGE FORMS AND STRENGTHS
Betaxolol hydrochloride	BETOPTIC	Solution: 0.5%
Levobunolol hydrochloride	BETAGAN	Solution: 0.5%
Timolol maleate	TIMOPTIC	Solution: 0.25%, 0.5%

DRUG PROFILE

The topical beta-blockers are prescribed, either alone or in combination with other medicine, to treat glaucoma. They are believed to work by lessening the production of aqueous fluid and thereby reducing increased pressure in the eye.

For complete information on these drugs, see pages 816–819.

CONDITION: **CATARACTS**

CATEGORY: **CARBONIC ANHYDRASE INHIBITORS**

GENERIC (CHEMICAL) NAME	BRAND (TRADE) NAME	DOSAGE FORMS AND STRENGTHS
Acetazolamide	DIAMOX	Controlled-release capsules: 500 mg Tablets: 125, 250 mg
Dichlorphenamide	DARANIDE	Tablets: 50 mg

| Methazolamide | NEPTAZANE | Tablets: 50 mg |

DRUG PROFILE

These drugs are used as supplemental therapy for glaucoma, along with topical medicines that are applied directly to the eye. They decrease the formation of aqueous humor (the fluid inside the front of the eyeball), thereby reducing the increased pressure inside the eye that is the hallmark of glaucoma. These drugs have a slight diuretic effect as well; that is, they help your body rid itself of excess water through increased urination.

For complete information on these drugs, see pages 819–822.

Chapter 13
Cancer

CANCER

Cancer is a major threat to health in this country but no longer the inevitable harbinger of death it was once considered. Great progress has been made in the past twenty-five years in both detecting and managing cancer, resulting in improved survival rates associated with some types of the disease.

CAUSES

No one knows exactly how or why a normal cell loses its blueprint for orderly reproduction and starts to multiply abnormally—spreading, invading, and destroying healthy tissue. We do know, however, that certain risk factors, or conditions, may be related to the development of some cancers in some people. For instance, a woman whose mother or sister had breast cancer is considered at risk for developing it herself; childless women are at greater risk for cancers of the reproductive system than are women who were younger than thirty-five when they gave birth. But it's important to remember that not everyone at risk does get cancer, and some people get cancer who were not known to be at any special risk.

We also know that the earlier cancer is found, the more likely it is to be cured or put into a stage of remission, in which it disappears for long periods of time. So it's vital for you to be aware of cancer's warning signals and to consult your doctor promptly if you notice any of them.

DIAGNOSIS AND TREATMENT

Cancer can strike anybody at any age, but certain types of cancer are most often found in people over fifty.

Breast Cancer Changes that might signal breast cancer include a lump or thickening; secretion from the nipples; scaling or puckering of the skin around the nipple; and any alterations in the contour of the breast. The most frequently reported symptom is a breast lump, or tumor. In many cases, this is felt first by the woman herself during a monthly breast self-examination. Most breast lumps are *not* malignant; your doctor may be able to reassure you just by feeling it. Or he or she might biopsy it—that is, remove it surgically, or draw out its contents with a syringe, so that it can be carefully analyzed. Your doctor might also send you for a mammogram, or breast X ray. In fact, experts generally recommend that women past fifty have mammograms once a year in order to discover cancers too small to be found by physical examination.

Breast cancer is most often treated by surgical removal of the breast, the portion of breast that contains the tumor, or the tumor alone. In some cases, the lymph nodes under the arm are also removed. For women with early breast cancer, the trend is definitely toward less radical procedures.

If the breast is not removed, radiation is used to kill any cancer cells remaining in the breast and the area around it. If malignancy has spread to the lymph nodes under the arm, chemotherapy with drugs that kill rapidly dividing cells is usually prescribed. See the drug charts on pages 886–897 for a further discussion of these agents. (Keep in mind that all the drugs referred to in this chapter can be taken at home, by mouth. Other agents are available that are administered by injection in a hospital or a doctor's office.) In older women, hormone therapy aimed at cutting off the supply of estrogen to the cancer is frequently helpful as well. Hormones used to treat advanced cases of breast cancer are frequently helpful as well. These are described in the drug charts on pages 881–885.

Endometrial Cancer Abnormal bleeding or discharge is the primary symptom of this type of cancer, which develops in the tissue lining the uterus. This symptom does not always signal cancer, but it should be reported promptly to your doctor. Early detection of endometrial cancer is possible through regular pelvic exams and Pap tests. (In a Pap test, cells normally shed from the uterus and cervix are examined under the microscope.) The diagnosis is confirmed through biopsy. Treatment is usually removal of the uterus (hysterectomy), sometimes preceded by radiation therapy. In some cases, a synthetic hormone, progestin, which resembles the hormone progesterone, is used to shrink the abnormal endometrium. See the drug chart on pages 883–885 for more information on this drug.

Ovarian Cancer The most common symptom of ovarian cancer is abnormal swelling of the abdomen. Women over forty may also experience persistent stomach discomfort and gas. Diagnosis of ovarian cancer usually includes X rays of the colon, kidneys, and uterus, since an ovarian tumor may change the shape of these organs. To check further, the doctor may perform a procedure known as laparoscopy. This involves inserting a lighted instrument through a small cut in the abdomen so the ovaries can be seen and biopsied. The usual treatment for this type of cancer is removal of one or both ovaries, the fallopian tubes, and the uterus. Radiation and chemotherapy often follow. Drugs used to slow or stop the spread of ovarian cancer are discussed in the drug charts on pages 886–889 and 894–897.

Prostate Cancer Malignancy in this little gland located at the base of the bladder can cause urinary problems in a man—but so can the noncancerous enlargement of the prostate that frequently occurs with age. The doctor might suspect cancer from the way the prostate feels during a rectal examination but will probably perform a biopsy to confirm the diagnosis. Many prostate cancers are not considered dangerous, and no treatment is administered. But they are followed up by annual examinations. If the cancer is the type that might spread rapidly, treatment alternatives include surgery, radiation, and medicines that deprive the tumor of male hormones or introduce female hormones. These drugs are described in the chart on page 885.

Chronic Lymphocytic Leukemia

This cancer creates an excess of immature white cells in the blood that crowd out normal blood cells. Normally the disease comes on slowly, without warning signs. After several years, such symptoms as fatigue, bruising or bleeding, and a decreased ability to fight off infection may develop. This form of leukemia is discovered and diagnosed through blood tests and the analysis of bone marrow. Many times this type of leukemia is asymptomatic and does not require treatment, as it may remain dormant for many years. When leukemia causes symptoms, however, chemotherapy is necessary. For more information on the chemotherapeutic agents used to treat leukemia, see the drug charts on pages 886–906.

Multiple Myeloma

This malignant tumor of the bone marrow, consisting most often of abnormal plasma cells, leads to the destruction of bone. Painful fractures or curving of the spine may be the first apparent symptoms. X rays may show bone loss, and analysis of the bone marrow will confirm the diagnosis. Chemotherapy is used to decrease the number of abnormal cells. Treatment with drugs generally continues for at least twelve months. The drugs used are described in the drug charts on pages 894–897.

Hodgkin's Disease

Although this disease is often considered a young person's disease, it is also common among people over sixty-five. Hodgkin's disease begins in the lymphatic system, which produces certain blood cells and body fluids, filters out bacteria, and temporarily traps cancer cells. The earliest symptom is usually a swollen lymph gland, or node, in the neck, armpit, or groin. Intermittent fevers, night sweats, fatigue, and weight loss may also occur. The first step in diagnosing the condition is a biopsy of the lymph node. If Hodgkin's disease is present, laboratory tests are performed and X rays taken to determine whether the cancer has spread. Treatment generally involves radiation and/or chemotherapy. This therapeutic approach has greatly prolonged the lives of people with advanced Hodgkin's disease. See the drug charts on pages 886–889 for detailed information on the chemotherapeutic agents used to treat this disease.

OUTLOOK

Although many cancers in older people tend to grow slowly, cancer may be fatal at any age, and timely detection is vital to achieve the best outcome. If therapy is initiated early in the course of the illness, the large array of treatment possibilities now at hand offer a good chance of remission or cure.

CONDITION: **BREAST CANCER**

CATEGORY: **HORMONES**

GENERIC (CHEMICAL) NAME	BRAND (TRADE) NAME	DOSAGE FORMS AND STRENGTHS
Tamoxifen citrate	NOLVADEX	Tablets: 10 mg

DRUG PROFILE

Tamoxifen, a hormone, is used to treat advanced cases of breast cancer in post-menopausal women. This drug suppresses growth of the tumor; exactly how it works is not known.

BEFORE USING THIS DRUG

Let your doctor know *IF*

You have ever had allergic reactions or other problems with ■ tamoxifen.

You have ever had any of the following medical problems: ■ cataracts ■ other eye problems.

SPECIAL RESTRICTIONS WHILE TAKING THIS DRUG

FOOD AND DRUG INTERACTIONS

No special restrictions on other drugs, foods and beverages, alcohol use, or smoking.

DAILY LIVING

Examinations or Tests	It is very important for you to keep all appointments with your doctor so that your progress can be monitored and you can be checked for the occurrence of unwanted side effects.

Helpful Hints

This drug may make you vomit or feel nauseated. Eat small, frequent meals to avoid an empty stomach, and keep dry crackers or toast by your bed to nibble on before you get out of bed in the morning. Make sure you get plenty of clear liquids such as carbonated beverages, clear soups, gelatin, and ices or sherbet. Tart foods, such as lemons and sour pickles, may help relieve your nausea. If you vomit shortly after taking a dose of this drug, consult your doctor. Nausea and vomiting often decrease with continued use of this drug. However, if you continue to feel nauseated or to vomit, your doctor may be able to prescribe a drug for your symptoms.

No special restrictions on driving, exertion and exercise, sun exposure, or exposure to excessive heat or cold.

POSSIBLE SIDE EFFECTS

Although this list of adverse effects may seem somewhat intimidating, keep in mind that some are quite rare. Of course, should these or any other problems arise while you are on medication, it is always a good idea to consult your doctor.

IF YOU DEVELOP	WHAT TO DO
blurred vision or other visual disturbances ■ weakness or drowsiness ■ shortness of breath ■ pain or swelling in legs ■ increased bone pain	**May be serious** Check with your doctor as soon as possible.
nausea or vomiting ■ loss of appetite ■ weight gain ■ hot flashes ■ headache ■ dizziness ■ light-headedness ■ depression ■ rash or dry skin ■ itching in genital area ■ vaginal bleeding or discharge	If symptoms are disturbing or persist, let your doctor know.

STORAGE INSTRUCTIONS

Store in a cool, dark place (not in a bathroom medicine cabinet).

STOPPING OR INTERRUPTING THERAPY

Use this medicine exactly as directed by your doctor, because your dosage has been tailored especially to your needs. Frequent side effects of tamoxifen are nausea and vomiting; even if you experience these effects, do not stop taking this medicine without first checking with your doctor. If you miss a dose, skip it and resume your regular schedule, and check with your doctor.

SPECIAL CONSIDERATIONS FOR THOSE OVER SIXTY-FIVE

None.

CONDITION: **BREAST CANCER AND ENDOMETRIAL CANCER**

CATEGORY: **HORMONES**

GENERIC (CHEMICAL) NAME	BRAND (TRADE) NAME	DOSAGE FORMS AND STRENGTHS
Megestrol acetate	MEGACE	Tablets: 20, 40 mg

DRUG PROFILE

Synthetic progestins like megestrol are used to treat advanced cases of cancer of the uterus (endometrial cancer) and of the breast. Synthetic progestins resemble progesterone, one of the two major female sex hormones. It is not known exactly how megestrol works to suppress the growth of tumors.

BEFORE USING THIS DRUG

Let your doctor know *IF*

You have ever had allergic reactions or other problems with ■ megestrol.

You have ever had the following medical problem: ■ thrombophlebitis (inflammation of the veins of the legs).

SPECIAL RESTRICTIONS WHILE TAKING THIS DRUG

FOOD AND DRUG INTERACTIONS

No special restrictions on other drugs, foods and beverages, alcohol use, or smoking.

DAILY LIVING

Examinations or Tests   It is very important for you to keep all appointments with your doctor so that your progress can be monitored and you can be checked for the occurrence of unwanted side effects.

No special restrictions on driving, exertion and exercise, sun exposure, or exposure to excessive heat or cold.

POSSIBLE SIDE EFFECTS

Although this list of adverse affects may seem somewhat intimidating, keep in mind that some are quite rare. Of course, should these or any other problems arise while you are on medication, it is always a good idea to consult your doctor.

IF YOU DEVELOP	WHAT TO DO
severe sudden headaches ■ sudden loss of vision or other visual disturbances ■ chest pain	**Urgent** Get in touch with your doctor immediately.
pain, burning, or tingling in fingers, hands, or elbows ■ pain or swelling of legs, especially calves	**May be serious** Check with your doctor as soon as possible.
weight gain ■ swelling of ankles or feet ■ tiredness or weakness ■ depression ■ hair loss ■ hair growth ■ breast tenderness ■ acne ■ nausea ■ increase or decrease in appetite	If symptoms are disturbing or persist, let your doctor know.

STORAGE INSTRUCTIONS

Store in a cool, dark place (not in a bathroom medicine cabinet).

STOPPING OR INTERRUPTING THERAPY

Use this medicine exactly as directed by your doctor, because your dosage has been tailored especially to your needs. Do not stop taking this medicine without first checking with your doctor. If you miss a dose, skip it and resume your regular schedule, and check with your doctor.

SPECIAL CONSIDERATIONS FOR THOSE OVER SIXTY-FIVE

Older people with reduced liver function may be started on lower dosages of this drug.

CONDITION: **BREAST CANCER AND PROSTATIC CANCER**

CATEGORY: **HORMONES**

GENERIC (CHEMICAL) NAME	BRAND (TRADE) NAME	DOSAGE FORMS AND STRENGTHS
Diethylstilbestrol		Coated tablets: 0.1, 0.25, 0.5, 1, 5 mg Tablets: 1, 5 mg

DRUG PROFILE

Systemic estrogens (female hormones) are used to help treat the bone loss that occurs in women after menopause or after surgical removal of the uterus and/or ovaries, when the body no longer produces natural estrogens. This drug is also used in other medical conditions such as breast cancer or prostate cancer.

For complete information on this drug, see pages 467–472.

CONDITION: **CANCER (VARIOUS TYPES)**

CATEGORY: **CHEMOTHERAPEUTIC AGENTS**

GENERIC (CHEMICAL) NAME	BRAND (TRADE) NAME	DOSAGE FORMS AND STRENGTHS
Cyclophosphamide	CYTOXAN	Tablets: 25, 50 mg

DRUG PROFILE

Cyclophosphamide is used to treat many types of cancer including leukemia, cancers of the lymph nodes (including Hodgkin's disease), and cancers of the retina, skin, nervous system, ovaries, and breast. This drug slows or stops the spread of cancer, keeping the cancer cells from multiplying.

BEFORE USING THIS DRUG

Let your doctor know *IF*

You have ever had allergic reactions or other problems with ■ cyclophosphamide ■ tartrazine (FD&C Yellow Dye No. 5) ■ aspirin.

You have ever had any of the following medical problems: ■ kidney disease ■ liver disease ■ chronic or recurrent infectious disease, such as shingles ■ chickenpox or recent exposure to chickenpox ■ gout ■ diabetes.

You are taking any of the following medicines: ■ any other medicine for cancer ■ medicine for gout ■ corticosteroids ■ sleep medicines ■ medicine for seizures ■ barbiturates ■ diuretics (water pills) ■ insulin ■ estrogens or other sex hormones ■ tranquilizers ■ medicine for bacterial, viral, or fungal infections ■ medicine for malaria ■ medicine for depression ■ cough medicine ■ vitamin A.

You have previously received radiation therapy.

SPECIAL RESTRICTIONS WHILE TAKING THIS DRUG

FOOD AND DRUG INTERACTIONS

Other Drugs	If you have diabetes and are taking insulin, your dosage may have to be adjusted.
	Allopurinol (medicine for gout) may increase the side effects of cyclophosphamide.
	Do not have any vaccinations during therapy or for several weeks after stopping therapy without first checking with your doctor. Because of your lowered resistance, which may persist for one to two months after you stop taking this drug, you may get the infection that the immunization is meant to prevent.
Foods and Beverages	To help your kidneys eliminate waste products of this drug, it is very important to drink seven to twelve glasses of water or other fluid every day.

No special restrictions on alcohol use or smoking.

DAILY LIVING

Examinations or Tests	It is very important for you to keep all appointments with your doctor so that your progress can be monitored and the occurrence of unwanted side effects can be checked. Periodic blood tests may be required.
Other Precautions	This medicine temporarily makes you more susceptible to infections. While taking this medicine, avoid being with people suffering from colds and other infectious diseases. Call your doctor if you develop a fever.

Tell any doctor you consult that you are taking this drug, especially if you will be undergoing any type of skin test.

Helpful Hints

This drug may make you vomit or feel nauseated. Eat small, frequent meals to avoid an empty stomach, and keep dry crackers or toast by your bed to nibble on before you get out of bed in the morning. Make sure you get plenty of clear liquids such as carbonated beverages, clear soups, gelatin, and ices or sherbet. Tart foods, such as lemons and sour pickles, may help relieve your nausea. If you vomit shortly after taking a dose of this drug, consult your doctor. Nausea and vomiting often decrease with continued use of this drug. However, if you continue to feel nauseated, your doctor may be able to prescribe a drug for your symptoms.

No special restrictions on driving, exertion and exercise, sun exposure, or exposure to excessive heat or cold.

POSSIBLE SIDE EFFECTS

Although this list of adverse effects may seem somewhat intimidating, keep in mind that some are quite rare. Of course, should these or any other problems arise while you are on medication, it is always a good idea to consult your doctor.

IF YOU DEVELOP

blood in urine ■ pain in urination or other urinary problems ■ fever, chills, or sore throat ■ fast heartbeat ■ difficulty in breathing ■ cough ■ swelling of feet or legs ■ weight gain ■ side, stomach, or joint pain

After you STOP taking this medicine: blood in urine

WHAT TO DO

Urgent Get in touch with your doctor immediately.

dizziness ■ confusion ■ nervousness ■ headache ■ diarrhea ■ red or white spots in mouth ■ yellowing of eyes or skin ■ swelling of face ■ slow healing of wounds	**May be serious** Check with your doctor as soon as possible.
loss of appetite■ nausea or vomiting ■ tiredness or weakness ■ hair loss ■ darkening of the fingernails ■ changes in skin color ■ rash	If symptoms are disturbing or persist, let your doctor know.

STORAGE INSTRUCTIONS

Store in a cool, dark place (not in a bathroom medicine cabinet).

STOPPING OR INTERRUPTING THERAPY

Use this medicine exactly as directed by your doctor, because your dosage has been tailored especially to your needs. Do not stop taking this medicine without first checking with your doctor. If you miss a dose, skip it and resume your regular schedule, and check with your doctor.

SPECIAL CONSIDERATIONS FOR THOSE OVER SIXTY-FIVE

Since kidney function can decrease with age, it is especially important for older people to drink enough water and other fluids to help their kidneys get rid of waste products of this drug. Older people who are especially prone to anemia and especially susceptible to infectious diseases may need frequent medical checkups while on this drug.

CONDITION: **CANCER (VARIOUS TYPES)**

CATEGORY: **CHEMOTHERAPEUTIC AGENTS**

GENERIC (CHEMICAL) NAME	BRAND (TRADE) NAME	DOSAGE FORMS AND STRENGTHS
Methotrexate		Tablets: 2.5 mg

DRUG PROFILE

Methotrexate is used to treat certain types of leukemia, cancer of the lymph nodes, cancer of the breast, and certain cancers of the head, neck, skin, and lungs. This drug is also sometimes used to treat severe cases of psoriasis—a skin disorder. Methotrexate slows and halts the growth and spread of cancer cells by interfering with one of the steps in cell growth.

BEFORE USING THIS DRUG

Let your doctor know *IF*

You have ever had allergic reactions or other problems with ■ methotrexate.

You have ever had any of the following medical problems: ■ kidney disease ■ liver disease ■ asthma or other lung disease ■ stomach ulcer ■ ulcerative colitis ■ chronic or recurrent infectious diseases, including shingles ■ chickenpox or recent exposure to chickenpox ■ gout ■ anemia or other blood disease.

You are taking any of the following medicines: ■ aspirin or aspirinlike medicine ■ vitamins containing folic acid ■ anticoagulants (blood thinners) ■ medicine for infections ■ medicine for seizures ■ medicine for gout ■ medicine for arthritis ■ medicine for malaria.

You have previously received radiation therapy or medicine for cancer.

SPECIAL RESTRICTIONS WHILE TAKING THIS DRUG

FOOD AND DRUG INTERACTIONS

Other Drugs	While you are taking this medicine, it is important to tell your doctor about all other drugs you may be taking.
	Do not have any vaccinations during therapy or for several weeks after stopping therapy without checking with your doctor. Because of your lowered resistance, which may persist for one to two months after you stop taking the drug, you may get the infection that the immunization is meant to prevent.

Foods and Beverages	To help your kidneys eliminate waste products of this drug, it is very important to drink seven to twelve glasses of water or other liquids every day.
Alcohol	Do not drink alcohol while taking this medicine. This combination may be especially damaging to your liver.

No special restrictions on smoking.

DAILY LIVING

Driving	This medicine may cause drowsiness or dizziness. Be careful when driving, operating household appliances, or doing any other tasks that require alertness until you know how this drug affects you.
Sun Exposure	Your skin may become more sensitive to sunlight and more likely to develop a sunburn, and your eyes may become more sensitive to light. It is a good idea to avoid too much sun, wear tinted sunglasses, and apply a sunscreen to exposed skin surfaces before going outdoors.
Examinations or Tests	Because this medicine is such a powerful drug and affects many different parts of the body, your doctor will perform a number of tests before and during therapy. It is very important for you to keep all appointments with your doctor so that your progress can be monitored and the occurrence of unwanted side effects can be checked.

Other Precautions	This medicine temporarily makes you more susceptible to infections. While taking this medicine, avoid being with people who are suffering from colds and other infectious diseases. Call your doctor if you develop a fever.
Helpful Hints	This drug may make you vomit or feel nauseated. Eat small, frequent meals to avoid an empty stomach, and keep dry crackers or toast by your bed to nibble on before you get out of bed in the morning. Make sure you get plenty of clear liquids such as carbonated beverages, clear soups, gelatin, and ices or sherbet. Tart foods, such as lemons and sour pickles, may help relieve your nausea. If you vomit shortly after taking a dose of this drug, consult your doctor. Nausea and vomiting often decrease with continued use of this drug. However, if you continue to vomit or to feel nauseated, your doctor may be able to prescribe a drug for your symptoms.

No special restrictions on exertion and exercise or exposure to excessive heat or cold.

POSSIBLE SIDE EFFECTS

Although this list of adverse effects may seem somewhat intimidating, keep in mind that some are quite rare. Of course, should these or any other problems arise while you are on medication, it is always a good idea to consult your doctor.

IF YOU DEVELOP

diarrhea ■ stomach pain ■ bloody or black, tarry stools ■ vomiting, with blood or vomit that looks like coffee grounds ■ fever, chills, or sore throat ■ bleeding or bruising ■ red spots on skin ■ sores or bleeding around the mouth ■ irritation or bleeding of gums ■ swelling of the tongue or vocal cords ■ shortness of breath ■ dark or bloody urine ■ seizures

WHAT TO DO

Urgent Get in touch with your doctor immediately.

nausea or vomiting ■ stomach discomfort ■ cough ■ headache ■ drowsiness ■ blurred vision ■ dizziness ■ swelling of feet, ankles, or legs ■ joint pain ■ decreased urination

After you STOP taking this medicine: blurred vision ■ confusion ■ dizziness ■ drowsiness ■ headache ■ tiredness or weakness

May be serious Check with your doctor as soon as possible.

hair loss ■ loss of appetite ■ rash, hives, or itching ■ acne ■ change in skin color ■ increased skin or eye sensitivity to sunlight

If symptoms are disturbing or persist, let your doctor know.

STORAGE INSTRUCTIONS

Store in a cool, dark place (not in a bathroom medicine cabinet).

STOPPING OR INTERRUPTING THERAPY

Use this medicine exactly as directed by your doctor, because your dosage has been tailored especially to your needs. If you miss a dose, skip it and resume your regular schedule, and check with your doctor.

SPECIAL CONSIDERATIONS FOR THOSE OVER SIXTY-FIVE

Since kidney function can decrease with age, it is especially important for older people to drink plenty of water and other fluids to help their kidneys get rid of waste products of this drug. Older people may be especially prone to the side effects of dizziness or drowsiness. Those older people who are especially prone to anemia and especially susceptible to infectious disease may need frequent medical checkups while on this drug.

CONDITION: **CANCER (VARIOUS TYPES)**

CATEGORY: **CHEMOTHERAPEUTIC AGENTS**

GENERIC (CHEMICAL) NAME	BRAND (TRADE) NAME	DOSAGE FORMS AND STRENGTHS
Melphalan	ALKERAN	Tablets: 2 mg

DRUG PROFILE

Melphalan is used to treat breast cancer, multiple myeloma (bone cancer), and cancer of the ovaries that cannot be operated on. This drug slows and halts the growth and spread of cancer cells.

BEFORE USING THIS DRUG

Let your doctor know *IF*

You have ever had allergic reactions or other problems with ■ melphalan ■ chlorambucil (another medicine for cancer).

You have ever had any of the following medical problems: ■ kidney disease, including kidney stones ■ gout ■ chronic or recurrent infectious diseases, including shingles ■ chickenpox or recent exposure to chickenpox.

You are taking any of the following medicines: ■ any other medicine for cancer ■ medicine for gout.

You have previously received radiation therapy or medicine for cancer.

SPECIAL RESTRICTIONS WHILE TAKING THIS DRUG

FOOD AND DRUG INTERACTIONS

Other Drugs	Do not have any vaccinations during therapy or for several weeks after stopping therapy without checking with your doctor. Because of your lowered resistance, which may persist for one to two months after

you stop taking the drug, you may get the infection that the immunization is meant to prevent.

Foods and Beverages	To help your body eliminate waste products of this drug, it is very important to drink seven to twelve glasses of water or other fluids every day.

No special restrictions on alcohol use or smoking.

DAILY LIVING

Examinations or Tests	It is very important for you to keep all appointments with your doctor so that your progress can be monitored and the occurrence of unwanted side effects can be checked. Periodic blood tests may be required.
Other Precautions	This medicine temporarily makes you more susceptible to infections. While taking this medicine, avoid being with people who are suffering from colds and other infectious diseases. Call your doctor if you develop a fever. Let any doctor you consult know you are taking this drug, especially if you will be undergoing any type of skin test.
Helpful Hints	This drug may make you vomit or feel nauseated. Eat small, frequent meals to avoid an empty stomach, and keep dry crackers or toast by your bed to nibble on before you get out of bed in the morning. Make sure you get plenty of clear liquids, such as carbonated beverages, clear soups, gelatin, and ices or sherbet. Tart foods, such as lemons and sour pickles, may help relieve your nausea. If you vomit shortly after taking a dose of this drug, consult your doctor. Nausea and vomiting often decrease with continued

use of this drug. However, if you continue to feel nauseated or to vomit, your doctor may be able to prescribe a drug for your symptoms.

No special restrictions on driving, exertion and exercise, sun exposure, or exposure to excessive heat or cold.

POSSIBLE SIDE EFFECTS

Although this list of adverse effects may seem somewhat intimidating, keep in mind that some are quite rare. Of course, should these or any other problems arise while you are on medication, it is always a good idea to consult your doctor.

IF YOU DEVELOP	WHAT TO DO
rash, hives, or itching ■ bleeding or bruising ■ fever, chills, or sore throat ■ shortness of breath ■ cough ■ side, stomach, or joint pain ■ swelling of feet, ankles, or legs ■ bloody or black, tarry stools ■ chest pain	**Urgent** Get in touch with your doctor immediately.
nausea or vomiting	**May be serious** Check with your doctor as soon as possible.
hair loss ■ diarrhea ■ mouth sores	If symptoms are disturbing or persist, let your doctor know.

STORAGE INSTRUCTIONS

Store in a cool, dark place (not in a bathroom medicine cabinet).

STOPPING OR INTERRUPTING THERAPY

Use this medicine exactly as directed by your doctor, because your dosage has been tailored especially to your needs. Do not stop taking this medicine without first checking with your doctor. If you miss a dose, skip it and resume your regular schedule, and check with your doctor.

SPECIAL CONSIDERATIONS FOR THOSE OVER SIXTY-FIVE

Since kidney function can decrease with age, it is especially important for older people to drink enough water and other fluids to help their kidneys eliminate waste products of this drug. Those older people who are especially prone to anemia and especially susceptible to infectious disease may need frequent medical checkups while on this drug.

CONDITION: **LEUKEMIA**

CATEGORY: **CHEMOTHERAPEUTIC AGENTS**

GENERIC (CHEMICAL) NAME	BRAND (TRADE) NAME	DOSAGE FORMS AND STRENGTHS
Busulfan	MYLERAN	Tablets: 2 mg

DRUG PROFILE

Busulfan is used to treat certain types of leukemia. It works by interfering with the growth of cancer cells—especially in the bone marrow, where many blood cells are manufactured.

BEFORE USING THIS DRUG

Let your doctor know *IF*

You have ever had allergic reactions or other problems with ■ busulfan.

You have ever had any of the following medical problems: ■ kidney disease, including kidney stones ■ chronic or recurrent infectious diseases, such as shingles ■ chickenpox or recent exposure to chickenpox ■ gout ■ asthma or other lung disease ■ anemia.

You are taking the following medicine: ■ medicines for gout.

You have previously received radiation therapy or medicine for cancer.

SPECIAL RESTRICTIONS BEFORE USING THIS DRUG

FOOD AND DRUG INTERACTIONS

Other Drugs	Do not have any vaccinations during therapy or for several weeks after stopping therapy without checking with your doctor. Because of your lowered resistance, which may persist for one to two months after you stop taking the drug, you may get the infection that the immunization is meant to prevent.
Foods and Beverages	To help your body eliminate the waste products of this drug, it is very important to drink seven to twelve glasses of water or other fluids every day.

No special restrictions on alcohol use or smoking.

DAILY LIVING

Examinations or Tests	It is very important for you to keep all appointments with your doctor so that your progress can be monitored and the occurrence of unwanted side effects can be checked. Blood tests may be required before and during therapy.
Other Precautions	This medicine temporarily makes you more susceptible to infections. While taking this medicine, avoid being with people suffering from colds and other infectious diseases. Call your doctor if you develop a fever.
	Let any doctor you consult know you are taking this drug, especially if you will be undergoing any type of skin test.
Helpful Hints	This drug may make you vomit or feel nauseated. Eat small, frequent meals to avoid an empty stomach,

and keep dry crackers or toast by your bed to nibble on before you get out of bed in the morning. Make sure you get plenty of clear liquids such as carbonated beverages, clear soups, gelatin, and ices or sherbet. Tart foods, such as lemons and sour pickles, may help relieve your nausea. If you vomit shortly after taking a dose of this drug, consult your doctor. Nausea and vomiting often decreases with continued use of this drug. However, if you continue to feel nauseated or to vomit, your doctor may be able to prescribe a drug for your symptoms.

No special restrictions on driving, exertion and exercise, sun exposure, or exposure to excessive heat or cold.

POSSIBLE SIDE EFFECTS

Although this list of adverse effects may seem somewhat intimidating, keep in mind that some are quite rare. Of course, should these or any other problems arise while you are on medication, it is always a good idea to consult your doctor.

IF YOU DEVELOP	WHAT TO DO
bleeding or bruising ■ fever, chills, or sore throat ■ shortness of breath ■ cough ■ side, stomach, or joint pain ■ sores or cracks on lips or in mouth ■ swelling of tongue ■ gout ■ yellowing of eyes or skin	**Urgent** Get in touch with your doctor immediately.
swelling of feet, ankles, or legs ■ confusion ■ rash or hives	**May be serious** Check with your doctor as soon as possible.
After you STOP taking this medicine: bleeding or bruising ■ fever ■ cough ■ shortness of breath	
diarrhea ■ nausea or vomiting ■ weight loss ■ loss of appetite ■ drowsiness ■ tiredness or weakness ■ male breast swelling ■ darkening of skin or other skin changes ■ dry mouth, throat, or nose ■ hair loss ■ decreased sweating	If symptoms are disturbing or persist, let your doctor know.

STORAGE INSTRUCTIONS

Store in a cool, dark place (not in a bathroom medicine cabinet).

STOPPING OR INTERRUPTING THERAPY

Use this medicine exactly as directed by your doctor, because your dosage has been tailored especially to your needs. Do not stop taking this medicine without first checking with your doctor. If you miss a dose, skip it and resume your regular schedule, and check with your doctor.

SPECIAL CONSIDERATIONS FOR THOSE OVER SIXTY-FIVE

Since kidney function can decrease with age, it is especially important for older people to drink enough water and other fluids to help their kidneys get rid of the waste products of this drug. Those older people who are especially prone to anemia and especially susceptible to infectious disease may need frequent medical checkups while on this drug.

CONDITION: **LEUKEMIA**

CATEGORY: **CHEMOTHERAPEUTIC AGENTS**

GENERIC (CHEMICAL) NAME	BRAND (TRADE) NAME	DOSAGE FORMS AND STRENGTHS
Mercaptopurine	PURINETHOL	Tablets: 50 mg

DRUG PROFILE

Mercaptopurine is used to treat certain forms of leukemia. It halts the growth and spread of cancer cells by interfering with the ability of these cells to manufacture and use DNA, a building block of all life.

BEFORE USING THIS DRUG

Let your doctor know *IF*

You have ever had allergic reactions or other problems with ■ mercaptopurine.

You have ever had any of the following medical problems: ■ kidney disease ■ liver disease ■ chronic or recurrent infectious disease, such as shingles ■ chickenpox or recent exposure to chickenpox ■ gout ■ anemia.

You are taking the following medicine: ■ medicines for gout, especially allopurinol.

You have previously received radiation therapy or medicine for cancer.

SPECIAL RESTRICTIONS WHILE TAKING THIS DRUG

FOOD AND DRUG INTERACTIONS

Other Drugs	Medicine for gout (especially allopurinol) may worsen some side effects of this drug when the drugs are taken together. Check with your doctor if you are taking medicine for gout.
	Do not have any vaccinations during therapy or for several weeks after stopping therapy without checking with your doctor. Because of your lowered resistance, which may persist for one to two months after you stop taking this drug, you may get the infection that the immunization is meant to prevent.
Foods and Beverages	To help your body eliminate the waste products of this drug, it is very important to drink seven to twelve glasses of water or other fluids every day.
	Although you may lose your appetite or feel sick when taking this drug, it is important to follow a nutritious diet.

No special restrictions on alcohol use or smoking.

DAILY LIVING

Examinations or Tests	Because this drug is very powerful and affects many different parts of the body, your doctor will perform a number of tests before and during therapy. It is very important for you to keep all appointments with your doctor so that your progress can be monitored and the occurrence of unwanted side effects can be checked.
Other Precautions	This medicine temporarily makes you more susceptible to infections. While taking this medicine, avoid being with people who are suffering from colds or other infectious diseases. Call your doctor if you develop a fever.

No special restrictions on driving, exertion and exercise, sun exposure, or exposure to excessive heat or cold.

POSSIBLE SIDE EFFECTS

Although this list of adverse effects may seem somewhat intimidating, keep in mind that some are quite rare. Of course, should these or any other problems arise while you are on medication, it is always a good idea to consult your doctor.

IF YOU DEVELOP	WHAT TO DO
fever, chills, or sore throat ■ bleeding or bruising ■ sides, stomach, or joint pain ■ swelling of feet, ankles, or legs ■ blood in urine ■ decreased urination	**Urgent** Get in touch with your doctor immediately.
diarrhea ■ darkening of skin ■ rash ■ headache ■ sores on lips or in mouth ■ yellowing of eyes or skin	**May be serious** Check with your doctor as soon as possible.
After you STOP taking this medicine: fever, chills, or sore throat ■ bleeding or bruising ■ yellowing of eyes or skin	

loss of appetite ■ nausea or vomiting ■ weakness

If symptoms are disturbing or persist, let your doctor know.

STORAGE INSTRUCTIONS

Store in a cool, dark place (not in a bathroom medicine cabinet).

STOPPING OR INTERRUPTING THERAPY

Use this medicine exactly as directed by your doctor, because your dosage has been tailored especially to your needs. Do not stop taking this medicine without first checking with your doctor. If you miss a dose, skip it and resume your regular schedule, and check with your doctor.

SPECIAL CONSIDERATIONS FOR THOSE OVER SIXTY-FIVE

Since kidney function can decrease with age, it is especially important for older people to drink plenty of water and other fluids to help their kidneys get rid of waste products of this drug. Those older patients who are also especially prone to anemia and especially susceptible to infectious disease may need frequent checkups while on this drug.

CONDITION: **LEUKEMIA**

CATEGORY: **CHEMOTHERAPEUTIC AGENTS**

GENERIC (CHEMICAL) NAME	BRAND (TRADE) NAME	DOSAGE FORMS AND STRENGTHS
Thioguanine		Tablets: 40 mg

DRUG PROFILE

Thioguanine is used to treat certain forms of leukemia. It halts the growth and spread of cancer cells by interfering with the ability of these cells to manufacture and use DNA, a building block of all life.

BEFORE USING THIS DRUG

Let your doctor know *IF*

You have ever had allergic reactions or other problems with ■ thioguanine.

You have ever had any of the following medical problems: ■ kidney disease, including kidney stones ■ liver disease ■ current infection ■ chronic or recurrent infectious disease, such as shingles ■ chickenpox or recent exposure to chickenpox ■ gout.

You are taking the following medicine: ■ medicines for gout, especially allopurinol.

You have previously received radiation therapy or medicine for cancer.

SPECIAL RESTRICTIONS WHILE TAKING THIS DRUG

FOOD AND DRUG INTERACTIONS

Other Drugs	Do not have any vaccinations during therapy or for several weeks after stopping therapy without checking with your doctor. Because of your lowered resistance, which may persist for one to two months after you stop taking the drug, you may get the infection that the immunization is meant to prevent.
Foods and Beverages	To help your body eliminate the waste products of this drug, it is very important to drink seven to twelve glasses of water or other fluids every day.

No special restrictions on other drugs, alcohol use, or smoking.

DAILY LIVING

Examinations or Tests	It is very important for you to keep all appointments with your doctor so that your progress can be monitored and the occurrence of unwanted side effects

can be checked. Blood tests before and during therapy are usually required.

Other Precautions	This medicine temporarily makes you more susceptible to infections. While taking this medicine, avoid being with people suffering from colds or other infectious diseases. Call your doctor if you develop a fever.
Helpful Hints	This drug may make you vomit or feel nauseated. Eat small, frequent meals to avoid an empty stomach, and keep dry crackers or toast by your bed to nibble on before you get out of bed in the morning. Make sure you get plenty of clear liquids such as carbonated beverages, clear soups, gelatin, and ices or sherbet. Tart foods, such as lemons and sour pickles, may help relieve your nausea. If you vomit shortly after taking a dose of this drug, consult your doctor. Nausea and vomiting usually decrease with continued use of this drug. However, if you continue to feel nauseated or to vomit, your doctor may be able to prescribe a drug for your symptoms.

No special restrictions on driving, exertion and exercise, sun exposure, or exposure to excessive heat or cold.

POSSIBLE SIDE EFFECTS

Although this list of adverse effects may seem somewhat intimidating, keep in mind that some are quite rare. Of course, should these or any other problems arise while you are on medication, it is always a good idea to consult your doctor.

IF YOU DEVELOP	WHAT TO DO
fever, chills, or sore throat ■ bleeding or bruising ■ side, stomach, or joint pain ■ swelling of feet, ankles, or legs	**Urgent** Get in touch with your doctor immediately.

diarrhea, sometimes severe ■ nausea or vomiting ■ rash, itching, or skin irritation ■ unsteady walk *After you STOP taking this medicine:* fever, chills, or sore throat ■ bleeding or bruising	**May be serious** Check with your doctor as soon as possible.
loss of ability to sense vibrations	If symptoms are disturbing or persist, let your doctor know.

STORAGE INSTRUCTIONS

Store in a cool, dark place (not in a bathroom medicine cabinet).

STOPPING OR INTERRUPTING THERAPY

Use this medicine exactly as directed by your doctor, because your dosage has been tailored especially to your needs. Do not stop taking this medicine without first checking with your doctor. If you miss a dose, skip it and resume your regular schedule, and check with your doctor.

SPECIAL CONSIDERATIONS FOR THOSE OVER SIXTY-FIVE

Since kidney function can decrease with age, it is especially important for older people to drink enough water and other fluids to help their kidneys get rid of the waste products of this drug. Those older patients who are especially prone to anemia and especially susceptible to infectious disease may need frequent checkups while on this drug.

INDICES

INDEX TO THE COLOR IDENTIFICATION GUIDE

Drugs are listed in this index alphabetically by brand (trade) name and dosage strength. Each entry in this index will direct you to the page (A1 through A38) and row (a through e) where the color picture of the particular drug is located. Only tablets and capsules appear in the Color Identification Guide.

COLOR IDENTIFICATION GUIDE

PINK

SORBITRATE Sublingual 5 mg isosorbide dinitrate	CRYSTODIGIN 0.1 mg digitoxin	DILAUDID 3 mg hydromorphone	LEVOTHROID 200 µg levothyroxine	DIULO 2.5 mg metolazone	DELTASONE 2.5 mg prednisone
PROLIXIN 1 mg fluphenazine	SYNTHROID 200 µg levothyroxine	ESIDRIX 25 mg hydrochlorothiazide	ETRAFON 2-25 perphenazine & amitriptyline	ESTINYL 0.05 mg ethinyl estradiol	ISORDIL Oral 5 mg isosorbide dinitrate
CELESTONE 0.6 mg betamethasone	MICRONASE 2.5 mg glyburide	SER-AP-ES reserpine, hydralazine & hydrochlorothiazide	PARNATE 10 mg tranylcypromine	PROLIXIN 10 mg fluphenazine	DIUPRES-250 reserpine & chlorothiazide
PHENERGAN 50 mg promethazine	METAHYDRIN 2 mg trichlormethiazide	LARODOPA 250 mg levodopa	BUTISOL Sodium 100 mg sodium butabarbital	URECHOLINE 10 mg bethanechol	DIUPRES-500 reserpine & chlorothiazide
SEPTRA trimethoprim & sulfamethoxazole	ELAVIL 100 mg amitriptyline	MELLARIL 200 mg thioridazine	WYAMYCIN S 250 mg erythromycin stearate	RUFEN 400 mg ibuprofen	POLARAMINE 2 mg dexchlorpheniramine maleate

PINK

a

COMBIPRES 0.1 mg
clonidine & chlorthalidone

MEDROL 2 mg
methylprednisolone

LARODOPA 100 mg
levodopa

ERY-TAB 250 mg
erythromycin

AMOXIL 250 mg
Chewable
amoxicillin

b

CHOLEDYL SA
400 mg
oxtriphylline

ERY-TAB 500 mg
erythromycin

E.E.S. 400
erythromycin
ethylsuccinate

WYAMYCIN S 500 mg
erythromycin stearate

ERYTHROCIN
Stearate 500 mg
erythromycin stearate

c

ARISTOCORT 2 mg
triamcinolone

DIAβETA 2.5 mg
glyburide

LOPRESSOR 50 mg
metoprolol tartrate

TEGRETOL 200 mg
carbamazepine

SUMYCIN '250'
tetracycline

d

TRENTAL 400 mg
pentoxifylline

LARODOPA 500 mg
levodopa

SUMYCIN '500'
tetracycline

e

CARAFATE 1 g
sucralfate

BENADRYL 25
Allergy Capsule
diphenhydramine
hydrochloride

BENADRYL 25 mg
diphenhydramine
hydrochloride

DARVON 32 mg
propoxyphene

BENADRYL 50 mg
diphenhydramine
hydrochloride

PINK

a					
SERAX 10 mg oxazepam	PERTOFRANE 25 mg desipramine	LITHONATE 300 mg lithium carbonate	DARVON 65 mg propoxyphene	DILATRATE-SR 40 mg isosorbide dinitrate	SINEQUAN 75 mg doxepin
b					
LARODOPA 250 mg levodopa	MINIPRESS 2 mg prazosin	APRESAZIDE 50/50 hydralazine & hydrochlorothiazide	SINEQUAN 50 mg doxepin	SUMYCIN '250' tetracycline	APRESAZIDE 100/50 hydralazine & hydrochlorothiazide
c					
PROSTAPHLIN 250 mg oxacillin sodium	PROSTAPHLIN 500 mg oxacillin sodium	LARODOPA 500 mg levodopa	SUMYCIN '500' tetracycline	DECADRON 1.5 mg dexamethasone	REGROTON reserpine & chlorthalidone
d					
NAQUA 2 mg trichlormethiazide	INDERAL 60 mg propranolol	TRANXENE 15 mg clorazepate	ILOSONE Chewable 125 mg erythromycin	ILOSONE Chewable 250 mg erythromycin	
e					

RED

a					
ETRAFON-Forte 4-25 perphenazine and amitriptyline	BUTAZOLIDIN 100 mg phenylbutazone	PYRIDIUM 100 mg phenazopyridine	CHOLEDYL 100 mg oxtriphylline	RAUDIXIN 50 mg rauwolfia	DECLOMYCIN 150 mg demeclocycline

b					
RAUDIXIN 100 mg rauwolfia	PYRIDIUM 200 mg phenazopyridine	DECLOMYCIN 300 mg demeclocycline	AZO GANTANOL sulfamethoxazole & phenazopyridine	AZO GANTRISIN sulfisoxazole & phenazopyridine	POLARAMINE 4 mg dexchlorpheniramine maleate

c					
POLARAMINE 6 mg dexchlorpheniramine maleate	PREMARIN 0.625 mg conjugated estrogens	PROCAN SR 1000 mg procainamide	LANOXICAPS 50 μg digoxin	SYMMETREL 100 mg amantadine	PERTOFRANE 50 mg desipramine

d					
RIFADIN 150 mg rifampin	SINEQUAN 10 mg doxepin	DYAZIDE triamterene & hydrochlorothiazide	TRANXENE 7.5 mg clorazepate	DYRENIUM 50 mg triamterene	SERAX 15 mg oxazepam

e					
LARODOPA 100 mg levodopa	SERAX 30 mg oxazepam	RESTORIL 15 mg temazepam	RESTORIL 30 mg temazepam	DYRENIUM 100 mg triamterene	FELDENE 20 mg piroxicam

RED

a				
RIMACTANE 300 mg rifampin	DALMANE 30 mg flurazepam	POLYMOX 250 mg amoxicillin	MEXITIL 150 mg mexiletine	FELDENE 10 mg piroxicam

b				
POLYMOX 500 mg amoxicillin	DURICEF 500 mg cefadroxil	RIFADIN 300 mg rifampin	MEXITIL 200 mg mexiletine	MEPERGAN Fortis meperidine & promethazine

c				
TYLOX oxycodone hydrochloride, oxycodone terephthalate & acetaminophen	FIORINAL with Codeine No. 1 butalbital, aspirin & codeine	POLYCILLIN 500 mg ampicillin	TYLENOL with Codeine No. 4 codeine & acetaminophen	LOPID 300 mg gemfibrozil

Bottom row:

POLYCILLIN 250 mg ampicillin

CLEOCIN HCl 150 mg clindamycin

MEXITIL 250 mg mexiletine

d

e

PURPLE

a					
ESTRACE 1 mg estradiol	BUTISOL Sodium 15 mg sodium butabarbital	LEVOTHROID 125 µg levothyroxine	ZAROXOLYN 2.5 mg metolazone	MELLARIL 15 mg thioridazine	SYNTHROID 75 µg levothyroxine

b					
PBZ-SR 100 mg tripelennamine	PANWARFIN 2 mg warfarin	URISED methenamine, methylene blue, phenyl salicylate, benzoic acid, atropine & hyoscyamine	COUMADIN 2 mg warfarin	PERCODAN-Demi oxycodone & aspirin	HALCION 0.125 mg triazolam

c					
XANAX 1 mg alprazolam	PREMARIN 2.5 mg conjugated estrogens	MANDELAMINE 1 g methenamine mandelate	NITRO-BID 2.5 mg nitroglycerin	CECLOR 250 mg cefaclor	SECTRAL 200 mg acebutolol

d					
MINOCIN 100 mg minocycline	OMNIPEN 250 mg ampicillin	ACHROMYCIN V 250 mg tetracycline	AMOXIL 250 mg amoxicillin	OMNIPEN 500 mg ampicillin	CECLOR 500 mg cefaclor

e					
ACHROMYCIN V 500 mg tetracycline	AMOXIL 500 mg amoxicillin	EUTHROID 120 mg liotrix	PYRIDIUM PLUS phenazopyridine, hyoscyamine & butabarbital	INDERAL 90 mg propranolol	

BLUE

NORPRAMIN 10 mg desipramine	**BLOCADREN 5 mg** timolol	**ZAROXOLYN 5 mg** metolazone	**DIULO 5 mg** metolazone	**ELAVIL 10 mg** amitriptyline
LEVOTHROID 150 µg levothyroxine				
TRANXENE SD 11.25 mg clorazepate	**STELAZINE 1 mg** trifluoperazine	**ESTROVIS 100 µg** quinestrol	**SYNTHROID 150 µg** levothyroxine	**MEGACE 20 mg** megestrol
MICRONASE 5 mg glyburide	**BLOCADREN 10 mg** timolol	**DITROPAN 5 mg** oxybutynin	**KLONOPIN 1 mg** clonazepam	**STELAZINE 2 mg** trifluoperazine
FLAGYL 250 mg metronidazole	**STELAZINE 5 mg** trifluoperazine	**APRESOLINE 50 mg** hydralazine	**APRESOLINE 25 mg** hydralazine	**LIMBITROL** chlordiazepoxide & amitriptyline
STELAZINE 10 mg trifluoperazine	**CORGARD 40 mg** nadolol	**MEGACE 40 mg** megestrol	**METAHYDRIN 4 mg** trichlormethiazide	
		CORGARD 80 mg nadolol	**ESIDRIX 100 mg** hydrochlorothiazide	**COMBIPRES 0.2 mg** clonidine & chlorthalidone
			NORMODYNE 300 mg labetalol	

BLUE

a	HALCION 0.25 mg triazolam	SORBITRATE Oral 40 mg isosorbide dinitrate	SORBITRATE Oral 20 mg isosorbide dinitrate	SINEMET 10-100 levodopa & carbidopa	OGEN 2.5 estropipate	
b	SINEMET 25-250 levodopa & carbidopa	ANAPROX 275 mg naproxen		FLAGYL 500 mg metronidazole		
c	BLOCADREN 20 mg timolol	LOPRESSOR 100 mg metoprolol		ELAVIL 150 mg amitriptyline		
d	CORGARD 120 mg nadolol	CORGARD 160 mg nadolol		ARTANE 5 mg trihexyphenidyl	CENTRAX 10 mg prazepam	
e	TIGAN 100 mg trimethobenzamide	BENTYL 10 mg dicyclomine	INDOCIN 25 mg indomethacin	INDERAL LA 80 mg propranolol	SINEQUAN 25 mg doxepin	APRESAZIDE 25/25 hydralazine & hydrochlorothiazide

BLUE

a	VIBRAMYCIN 50 mg doxycycline	SURMONTIL 100 mg trimipramine	SINEQUAN 100 mg doxepin	SURMONTIL 50 mg trimipramine	VELOSEF '250' cephradine	AMCILL 250 mg ampicillin
b	INDOCIN SR 75 mg indomethacin	VALRELEASE 15 mg diazepam	SURMONTIL 25 mg trimipramine	RONDOMYCIN 150 mg methacycline	INDERAL LA 120 mg propranolol	INDERAL LA 160 mg propranolol
c	TIGAN 250 mg trimethobenzamide	INDOCIN 50 mg indomethacin	ZOVIRAX 200 mg acyclovir	CYCLOSPASMOL 200 mg cyclandelate	RONDOMYCIN 300 mg methacycline	VIBRAMYCIN 100 mg doxycycline
d	AMCILL 500 mg ampicillin	MINIPRESS 5 mg prazosin	SINEQUAN 150 mg doxepin	VELOSEF '500' cephradine	FIORINAL with Codeine No. 3 butalbital, aspirin, caffeine & codeine	NICOBID 500 mg niacin
e	CYCLOSPASMOL 400 mg cyclandelate	INDERAL 20 mg propranolol	DECADRON 0.75 mg dexamethasone	DIABINESE 100 mg chlorpropamide	HYGROTON 50 mg chlorthalidone	TRANXENE 3.75 mg clorazepate

BLUE

TRIAVIL 2-10
perphenazine &
amitriptyline

VALIUM 10 mg
diazepam

ASENDIN 100 mg
amoxapine

DIABINESE 250 mg
chlorpropamide

a

b

c

d

e

GREEN

a					
MELLARIL 10 mg thioridazine	ESTRACE 2 mg estradiol	DILAUDID 1 mg hydromorphone	LEVOTHROID 300 μg levothyroxine	ERGOMAR 2 mg ergotamine tartrate	LIBRITABS 5 mg chlordiazepoxide

b					
HYDROPRES 25 reserpine & hydrochlorothiazide	LEVOTHROID 175 μg levothyroxine	BUTISOL Sodium 30 mg sodium butabarbital	SYNTHROID 300 μg levothyroxine	LIBRITABS 10 mg chlordiazepoxide	LANOXIN 500 μg digoxin

c					
NORPRAMIN 50 mg desipramine	HYDROPRES 50 reserpine & hydrochlorothiazide	CARDIZEM 30 mg diltiazem	DONNATAL No. 2 belladonna alkaloids	ISORDIL Oral Titradose 20 mg isosorbide dinitrate	LIBRITABS 25 mg chlordiazepoxide

d					
PROLIXIN 5 mg fluphenazine	RAUZIDE rauwolfia & bendroflumethiazide	COMPAZINE 5 mg prochlorperazine	SORBITRATE 5 mg Chewable isosorbide dinitrate	SALUTENSIN reserpine & hydroflumethiazide	MELLARIL 100 mg thioridazine

e					
TAGAMET 200 mg cimetidine	COMPAZINE 10 mg prochlorperazine	DONNATAL Extentabs belladonna alkaloids	COMPAZINE 25 mg prochlorperazine	ISORDIL Oral Titradose 40 mg isosorbide dinitrate	ISORDIL Tembids 40 mg isosorbide dinitrate

GREEN

a

OS-CAL 250
calcium carbonate

PARAFON Forte
chlorzoxazone &
acetaminophen

TAGAMET 300 mg
cimetidine

NORGESIC
orphenadrine, aspirin &
caffeine

DONNAZYME
pancreatic enzyme &
digestant combinations

TUMS 750 mg
calcium phosphate

b

BUMEX 0.5 mg
bumetanide

PREMARIN 0.3 mg
conjugated estrogens

SORBITRATE Oral
5 mg
isosorbide dinitrate

OGEN 5
estropipate

PROCAN SR 250 mg
procainamide

c

TAGAMET 800 mg
cimetidine

DIAβETA 5 mg
glyburide

TAGAMET 400 mg
cimetidine

CARDIZEM 90 mg
diltiazem

d

OS-CAL 500
calcium carbonate

BACTRIM
trimethoprim &
sulfamethoxazole

NORGESIC Forte
orphenadrine, aspirin &
caffeine

e

WYGESIC
propoxyphene &
acetaminophen

DISTA 3245

KEFLEX 1 g
cephalexin

LANOXICAPS 200 μg
digoxin

LIBRIUM 5 mg
chlordiazepoxide

GREEN

a				
DONNATAL belladonna alkaloids	CENTRAX 5 mg prazepam	IMODIUM 2 mg loperamide	VISTARIL 50 mg hydroxyzine	VISTARIL 25 mg hydroxyzine
b				
NORPACE CR 100 mg disopyramide	VISTARIL 100 mg hydroxyzine	TUSSIONEX hydrocodone & phenyltoloxamine	ADAPIN 25 mg doxepin	DOPAR 100 mg levodopa
c				
ADAPIN 100 mg doxepin	DOPAR 250 mg levodopa	TRIMOX '250' ampicillin	ADAPIN 50 mg doxepin	MINIZIDE 1 prazosin & polythiazide
d				
KEFLEX 250 mg cephalexin	PHENAPHEN with Codeine No. 4 codeine & acetaminophen	NICOBID 250 mg niacin	FIORINAL butalbital, aspirin & caffeine	MINIZIDE 5 prazosin & polythiazide
e				
DOPAR 500 mg levodopa	UNIPEN 250 mg nafcillin	TRIMOX '500' ampicillin	COTAZYM 25 mg pancrelipase	NITRO-BID 9 mg nitroglycerin

LIBRIUM 25 mg
chlordiazepoxide

LIBRAX
chlordiazepoxide &
clidinium bromide

MINIZIDE 2
prazosin & polythiazide

ANTURANE 200 mg
sulfinpyrazone

TACE 25 mg
chlorotrianisene

GREEN

a	b	c	d	e
NAQUA 4 mg trichlormethiazide				
DECADRON 6 mg dexamethasone				
ATARAX 25 mg hydroxyzine				
TACE 12 mg chlorotrianisene				
KEFLEX 500 mg cephalexin				
Extra-Strength DATRIL 500 mg acetaminophen	INDERAL 40 mg propranolol			

YELLOW

a					
ISORDIL 2.5 mg Sublingual isosorbide dinitrate	CRYSTODIGIN 0.15 mg digitoxin	SANSERT 2 mg methysergide	SORBITRATE Sublingual 10 mg isosorbide dinitrate	DILAUDID 4 mg hydromorphone	DIULO 10 mg metolazone

b					
LANOXIN 125 μg digoxin	MEPHYTON 5 mg vitamin K₁	DARANIDE 50 mg dichlorphenamide	LEVOTHROID 100 μg levothyroxine	ZAROXOLYN 10 mg metolazone	ELAVIL 25 mg amitriptyline

c					
TORECAN 10 mg thiethylperazine	SYNTHROID 100 μg levothyroxine	ETRAFON 2-10 perphenazine & amitriptyline	NORPRAMIN 25 mg desipramine	APRESOLINE 10 mg hydralazine	PANWARFIN 7.5 mg warfarin

d					
ALDOMET 125 mg methyldopa	ISORDIL Chewable 10 mg isosorbide dinitrate	PROLIXIN 2.5 mg fluphenazine	PROLOPRIM 200 mg trimethoprim	ESIDRIX 50 mg hydrochlorothiazide	ISMELIN 10 mg guanethidine

e					
SALUTENSIN-Demi reserpine & hydroflumethiazide	RENESE 2 mg polythiazide	COUMADIN 7.5 mg warfarin	SORBITRATE Chewable 10 mg isosorbide dinitrate	ISOPTIN 80 mg verapamil	PURINETHOL 50 mg mercaptopurine

YELLOW

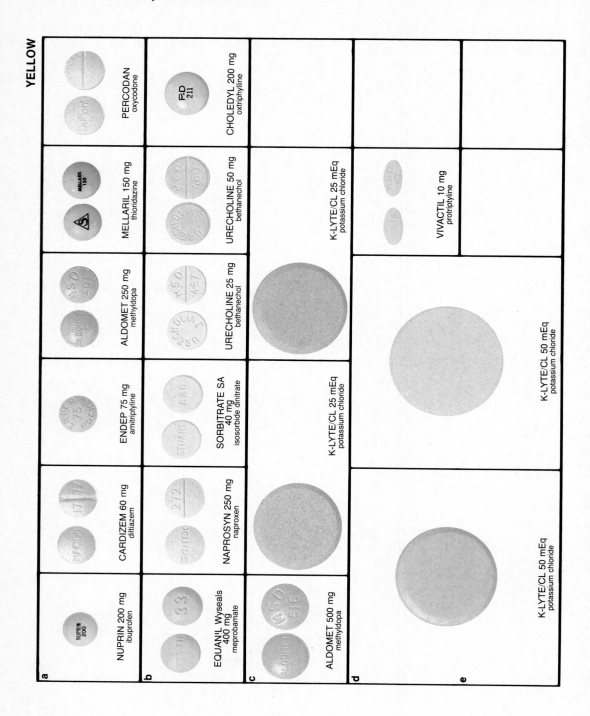

a

NUPRIN 200 mg
ibuprofen

CARDIZEM 60 mg
diltiazem

ENDEP 75 mg
amitriptyline

ALDOMET 250 mg
methyldopa

MELLARIL 150 mg
thioridazine

PERCODAN
oxycodone

b

EQUANIL Wyseals
400 mg
meprobamate

NAPROSYN 250 mg
naproxen

SORBITRATE SA
40 mg
isosorbide dinitrate

URECHOLINE 25 mg
bethanechol

URECHOLINE 50 mg
bethanechol

CHOLEDYL 200 mg
oxtriphylline

c

ALDOMET 500 mg
methyldopa

K-LYTE/CL 25 mEq
potassium chloride

K-LYTE/CL 25 mEq
potassium chloride

K-LYTE/CL 25 mEq
potassium chloride

d

K-LYTE/CL 50 mEq
potassium chloride

K-LYTE/CL 50 mEq
potassium chloride

e

VIVACTIL 10 mg
protriptyline

YELLOW

a	BUMEX 1 mg bumetanide	BRETHINE 2.5 mg terbutaline	MEDROL 24 mg methylprednisolone	SORBITRATE Oral 10 mg isosorbide dinitrate	SINEMET 25-100 levodopa & carbidopa	DARVON-N 100 mg propoxyphene

PREMARIN 1.25 mg
conjugated estrogens

b TONOCARD 400 mg
tocainide

ANTIVERT/50
meclizine

c NegGRAM 1 g
nalidixic acid

PROCAN SR 500 mg
procainamide

PRONESTYL-SR
500 mg
procainamide

NALFON 600 mg
fenoprofen

d ARISTOCORT 1 mg
triamcinolone

ARISTOCORT 8 mg
triamcinolone

NegGRAM 250 mg
nalidixic acid

OGEN 0.625
estropipate

CYCLAPEN-W 250 mg
cyclacillin

e PRONESTYL 250 mg
procainamide

K-TAB 10 mEq
potassium chloride

NegGRAM 500 mg
nalidixic acid

ZANTAC 300 mg
ranitidine

YELLOW

a

BENEMID 0.5 g
probenecid

DYMELOR 500 mg
acetohexamide

NAPROSYN 500 mg
naproxen

HIPREX 1 g
methenamine hippurate

b

GEOCILLIN 382 mg
carbenicillin

BEROCCA Plus
vitamins A, B₁, B₂, B₆, B₁₂; niacin; pantothenic acid; biotin; folic acid; iron; chromium; magnesium; manganese; copper & zinc

CYCLAPEN-W 500 mg
cyclacillin

c

TESSALON 100 mg
benzonatate

LANOXICAPS 100 μg
digoxin

CENTRAX 20 mg
prazepam

NEMBUTAL Sodium
pentobarbital

ADAPIN 10 mg
doxepin

AVENTYL HCl 10 mg
nortriptyline

d

PRONESTYL 250 mg
procainamide

ADAPIN 75 mg
doxepin

CUPRIMINE 250 mg
penicillamine

AVENTYL HCl 25 mg
nortriptyline

LAROTID 500 mg
amoxicillin

GRISACTIN 250 mg
griseofulvin

e

TERRAMYCIN
250 mg
oxytetracycline

TACE 72 mg
chlorotrianisene

DECADRON 0.5 mg
dexamethasone

MIDAMOR 5 mg
amiloride

ENDURONYL
deserpidine &
methyclothiazide

YELLOW

a ATARAX 50 mg hydroxyzine	DILANTIN Infatabs 50 mg phenytoin	SERAX 15 mg oxazepam	FLEXERIL 10 mg cyclobenzaprine	TRIAVIL 4-25 perphenazine & amitriptyline	VALIUM 5 mg diazepam
b INDERAL 80 mg propranolol	CLINORIL 150 mg sulindac	CLINORIL 200 mg sulindac	MAXZIDE triamterene & hydrochlorothiazide	TONOCARD 600 mg tocainide	
c				
d				
e				

ORANGE

a	b	c	d	e
ERGOSTAT Sublingual 2 mg ergotamine tartrate	ENDEP 10 mg amitriptyline	PANWARFIN 2.5 mg warfarin	COUMADIN 2.5 mg warfarin	TRANDATE 300 mg labetalol
DILAUDID 2 mg hydromorphone	LUDIOMIL 50 mg maprotiline	ENDEP 25 mg amitriptyline	NARDIL 15 mg phenelzine	LOPURIN 300 mg allopurinol
CRYSTODIGIN 0.05 mg digitoxin	ETRAFON-A 4-10 perphenazine & amitriptyline	PHENERGAN 12.5 mg promethazine	ENDEP 50 mg amitriptyline	KLOTRIX 10 mEq potassium chloride
PERSANTINE 25 mg dipyridamole	PERSANTINE 50 mg dipyridamole	MARPLAN 10 mg isocarboxazid	TOFRANIL 50 mg imipramine	E-MYCIN 250 mg erythromycin
MINOCIN 50 mg minocycline	KLONOPIN 0.5 mg clonazepam	PERSANTINE 75 mg dipyridamole	ELAVIL 75 mg amitriptyline	SOMA Compound carisoprodol & aspirin
LEVOTHROID 25 μg levothyroxine	MINOCIN 100 mg minocycline	NORPRAMIN 75 mg desipramine	ENDEP 150 mg amitriptyline	AZULFIDINE 500 mg sulfasalazine

ORANGE

MOTRIN 400 mg
ibuprofen

K-LYTE 25 mEq
potassium chloride

K-LYTE 50 mEq
potassium chloride

DARVOCET-N 100
propoxyphene &
acetaminophen

SECONAL Sodium
50 mg
secobarbital

SECONAL Sodium
100 mg
secobarbital

CATAPRES 0.2 mg
clonidine

LUDIOMIL 25 mg
maprotiline

VIVACTIL 5 mg
protriptyline

PROCAN SR 750 mg
procainamide

PRONESTYL 500 mg
procainamide

ROCALTROL 0.5 µg
vitamin D

MINOCIN 50 mg
minocycline

AZULFIDINE EN-tabs
500 mg
sulfasalazine

DARVOCET-N 50
propoxyphene &
acetaminophen

PRONESTYL 375 mg
procainamide

ROCALTROL 0.25 µg
vitamin D

MECLOMEN 50 mg
meclofenamate

ROBAXIN 750 mg
methocarbamol

MOTRIN 800 mg
ibuprofen

MOTRIN 800 mg
ibuprofen

THORAZINE 30 mg
chlorpromazine

THORAZINE 75 mg
chlorpromazine

PAMELOR 10 mg
nortriptyline

a
b
c
d
e

ORANGE

a	NOCTEC 250 mg chloral hydrate	MECLOMEN 100 mg meclofenamate	DALMANE 15 mg flurazepam	ANSPOR 250 mg cephradine	PROCARDIA 10 mg nifedipine	ATROMID-S 500 mg clofibrate
b	PAMELOR 25 mg nortriptyline	BUTAZOLIDIN 100 mg phenylbutazone	PROCARDIA 20 mg nifedipine		PRONESTYL 375 mg procainamide	PAMELOR 75 mg nortriptyline
c	NORPACE 100 mg disopyramide	GRISACTIN 125 mg griseofulvin	DECLOMYCIN 150 mg demeclocycline		THORAZINE 200 mg chlorpromazine	PRONESTYL 500 mg procainamide
d	ERYC 125 mg erythromycin	ERYC 250 mg erythromycin	NOCTEC 500 mg chloral hydrate	ANSPOR 500 mg cephradine	TOLECTIN DS 400 mg tolmetin	DIAMOX 500 mg acetazolamide
e	ILOSONE 250 mg erythromycin	ATARAX 10 mg hydroxyzine	DECADRON 0.25 mg dexamethasone	HYGROTON 25 mg chlorthalidone	ENDURON 2.5 mg methyclothiazide	ENDURON 5 mg methyclothiazide

ORANGE

a				
PAVABID HP 300 mg papaverine				
DESYREL 150 mg trazodone				
TRIAVIL 4-50 perphenazine & amitriptyline				
TRIAVIL 2-25 perphenazine & amitriptyline				
ASENDIN 50 mg amoxapine				

a
b
c
d
e

PEACH

a				
HydroDIURIL 50 mg hydrochlorothiazide	TRANDATE 100 mg labetalol	SYNTHROID 125 µg levothyroxine	SYNTHROID 25 µg levothyroxine	HydroDIURIL 25 mg hydrochlorothiazide	PRO-BANTHINE 15 mg propantheline

b				
VIVOX 100 mg doxycycline	COUMADIN 5 mg warfarin	ANTIVERT/25 Chewable meclizine	DESYREL 50 mg trazodone	PANWARFIN 5 mg warfarin	ESTINYL 0.5 mg ethinyl estradiol

c				
DELTASONE 20 mg prednisone	HydroDIURIL 100 mg hydrochlorothiazide	DUVOID 50 mg bethanechol	LITHOBID 300 mg lithium carbonate	NORPRAMIN 100 mg desipramine	VIBRA-TABS 100 mg doxycycline

d				
EMPRACET with Codeine no. 3 codeine & acetaminophen	ALDORIL methyldopa & hydrochlorothiazide	ZYLOPRIM 300 mg allopurinol	BRONDECON oxtriphylline & guaifenesin	APRESOLINE 100 mg hydralazine	ENDEP 100 mg amitriptyline

e				
XANAX 0.5 mg alprazolam	CATAPRES 0.3 mg clonidine	ERYTHROCIN Stearate 250 mg erythromycin	ROBAXIN 500 mg methocarbamol	GRISACTIN 500 mg griseofulvin	EMPRACET with Codeine no. 4 codeine & acetaminophen

PEACH

MEDROL 8 mg methylprednisolone	MEDROL 32 mg methylprednisolone	OGEN 1.25 estropipate	ALDORIL D30 methyldopa & hydrochlorothiazide		ILOSONE 500 mg erythromycin
MOTRIN 600 mg ibuprofen	REGLAN 10 mg metoclopramide	DOLOBID 250 mg diflunisal		NAPROSYN 375 mg naproxen	
MICRO-K Extencaps potassium chloride	MICRO-K 10 Extencaps potassium chloride	EUTHROID 32 mg liotrix	INDERAL 10 mg propranolol	ASENDIN 150 mg amoxapine	VASOTEC 20 mg enalapril
VASOTEC 10 mg enalapril	TRANXENE 7.5 mg clorazepate	MODURETIC amiloride & hydrochlorothiazide	TRIAVIL 4-10 perphenazine & amitriptyline		

a / b / c / d / e

TAN

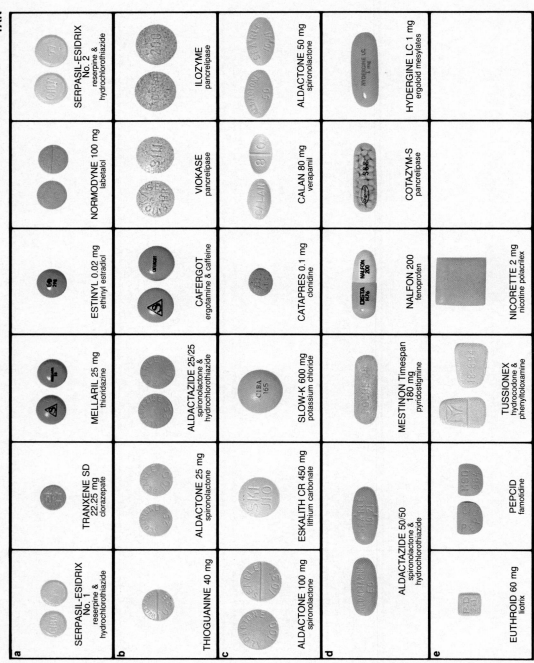

a					
SERPASIL-ESIDRIX No. 1 reserpine & hydrochlorothiazide	TRANXENE SD 22.25 mg clorazepate	MELLARIL 25 mg thioridazine	ESTINYL 0.02 mg ethinyl estradiol	NORMODYNE 100 mg labetalol	SERPASIL-ESIDRIX No. 2 reserpine & hydrochlorothiazide

b					
THIOGUANINE 40 mg	ALDACTONE 25 mg spironolactone	ALDACTAZIDE 25/25 spironolactone & hydrochlorothiazide	CAFERGOT ergotamine & caffeine	VIOKASE pancrelipase	ILOZYME pancrelipase

c					
ALDACTONE 100 mg spironolactone	ESKALITH CR 450 mg lithium carbonate	SLOW-K 600 mg potassium chloride	CATAPRES 0.1 mg clonidine	CALAN 80 mg verapamil	ALDACTONE 50 mg spironolactone

d					
ALDACTAZIDE 50/50 spironolactone & hydrochlorothiazide	MESTINON Timespan 180 mg pyridostigmine	NALFON 200 fenoprofen	COTAZYM-S pancrelipase	HYDERGINE LC 1 mg ergoloid mesylates	

e					
EUTHROID 60 mg liotrix	PEPCID famotidine	TUSSIONEX hydrocodone & phenyltoloxamine	NICORETTE 2 mg nicotine polacrilex		

BROWN

a				
ADVIL 200 mg ibuprofen	THORAZINE 50 mg chlorpromazine	ELAVIL 50 mg amitriptyline	TOFRANIL 25 mg imipramine	THORAZINE 25 mg chlorpromazine	THORAZINE 10 mg chlorpromazine

b				
RIDAURA 3 mg auranofin	ADVIL 200 mg ibuprofen	CHOLEDYL SA 600 mg oxtriphylline	MANDELAMINE 500 mg methenamine mandelate	CALAN 120 mg verapamil	THORAZINE 200 mg chlorpromazine

c				
LAROTID 250 mg amoxicillin	PAVABID 150 mg papaverine	ROBITET '250' tetracycline	NORPACE CR 150 mg disopyramide	TOTACILLIN 250 mg ampicillin	PARLODEL 5 mg bromocriptine

d				
TOFRANIL 10 mg imipramine	SECTRAL 400 mg acebutolol	NALFON 300 mg fenoprofen	ROBITET '500' tetracycline	TOTACILLIN 500 mg ampicillin	NORPACE 150 mg disopyramide

e				

GRAY

PROLOID 32 mg thyroglobulin	PROLOID 65 mg thyroglobulin	LEVOTHROID 75 µg levothyroxine	PROLOID 100 mg thyroglobulin	PROLOID 130 mg thyroglobulin	TEMARIL 2.5 mg trimeprazine

a

PROLOID 32 mg thyroglobulin | PROLOID 65 mg thyroglobulin | LEVOTHROID 75 µg levothyroxine | PROLOID 100 mg thyroglobulin | PROLOID 130 mg thyroglobulin | TEMARIL 2.5 mg trimeprazine

b

PROLOID 200 mg thyroglobulin | ESKALITH 300 mg lithium carbonate | TRANXENE 3.75 mg clorazepate | TEMARIL 5 mg trimeprazine | CUPRIMINE 125 mg penicillamine | TRANXENE 15 mg clorazepate

c

ESKALITH 300 mg lithium carbonate | PANMYCIN 250 mg tetracycline | FIORINAL with Codeine No. 2 butalbital, aspirin, caffeine & codeine | DARVON Compound propoxyphene, aspirin & caffeine | DARVON Compound-65 propoxyphene, aspirin, and caffeine | EUTHROID 180 mg liotrix

d

ENDURONYL Forte deserpidine & methyclothiazide

e

BLACK

	a	b	c	d	e
	LIBRIUM 10 mg chlordiazepoxide	NITRO-BID 6.5 mg nitroglycerin			
	COMPAZINE 10 mg prochlorperazine	PHENAPHEN with Codeine No. 3 codeine & acetaminophen			
	COMPAZINE 15 mg prochlorperazine	PHENAPHEN with Codeine No. 2 codeine & acetaminophen			
	NICOBID 125 mg niacin	VICON Forte multivitamin			
	TEGOPEN 250 mg cloxacillin	TEGOPEN 500 mg cloxacillin			
	COMPAZINE 30 mg prochlorperazine	ULTRACEF 500 mg cefadroxil			

WHITE

ISORDIL 10 mg Sublingual isosorbide dinitrate	COGENTIN 0.5 mg benztropine mesylate	MYLERAN 2 mg busulfan	LOZOL 2.5 mg indapamide	SYNTHROID 50 µg levothyroxine
NITROSTAT 0.4 mg nitroglycerin	ARLIDIN 6 mg nylidrin	VISKEN 5 mg pindolol	MEBARAL 32 mg mephobarbital	LONITEN 10 mg minoxidil
NITROSTAT 0.3 mg nitroglycerin	PRO-BANTHINE 7.5 mg propantheline	DELTASONE 5 mg prednisone	PBZ 25 mg tripelennamine	COGENTIN 2 mg benztropine mesylate
NITROSTAT 0.15 mg nitroglycerin	LOMOTIL diphenoxylate & atropine	DEMEROL 50 mg meperidine	TAVIST 2.68 mg clemastine fumarate	RENESE 1 mg polythiazide
ARMOUR Thyroid 15 mg thyroid, desiccated	ARMOUR Thyroid 30 mg thyroid, desiccated	LEVOTHROID 50 µg levothyroxine	PARLODEL 2.5 mg bromocriptine	HYGROTON 100 mg chlorthalidone
SORBITRATE Sublingual 2.5 mg isosorbide dinitrate	CYTOMEL 5 µg liothyronine	PROVENTIL 2 mg albuterol	VENTOLIN 2 mg albuterol	CYTOMEL 25 µg liothyronine

a   b   c   d   e

WHITE

a	MYSOLINE 50 mg primidone	LONITEN 2.5 mg minoxidil	LANOXIN 250 µg digoxin	ARMOUR Thyroid 60 mg thyroid, desiccated	TENORMIN 50 atenolol	NEPTAZANE 50 mg methazolamide
b	ALKERAN 2 mg melphalan	SYNKAYVITE 5 mg vitamin K₄	HYDERGINE 1 mg ergoloid mesylates	ALUPENT 10 mg metaproterenol	TENORETIC 50 atenolol & chlorthalidone	DEMEROL 100 mg meperidine
c	LASIX 40 mg furosemide	BRICANYL 5 mg terbutaline	BRICANYL 2.5 mg terbutaline	BRETHINE 5 mg terbutaline	PANWARFIN 10 mg warfarin	SERPASIL 0.25 mg reserpine
d	ARLIDIN 12 mg nylidrin	PBZ 50 mg tripelennamine	DONNATAL belladonna alkaloids	KLONOPIN 2 mg clonazepam	PHENERGAN 25 mg promethazine	SERPASIL 0.1 mg reserpine
e	CYTOMEL 50 µg levothyronine	CORTEF 5 mg hydrocortisone	NOLVADEX 10 mg tamoxifen	VISKEN 10 mg pindolol	ISORDIL Oral Titradose 10 mg isosorbide dinitrate	MICRONASE 1.25 mg glyburide

WHITE

a					
ARMOUR Thyroid 90 mg thyroid, desiccated	MEBARAL 100 mg mephobarbital	METAPREL 10 mg metaproterenol	ARTANE 2 mg trihexyphenidyl	DRAMAMINE 50 mg dimenhydrinate	RENESE 4 mg polythiazide

b					
CORTEF 10 mg hydrocortisone	OPTIMINE 1 mg azatadine	PROVENTIL 4 mg albuterol	DIAMOX 125 mg acetazolamide	DELTASONE 10 mg prednisone	VASODILAN 10 mg isoxsuprine

c					
VENTOLIN 4 mg albuterol	COUMADIN 10 mg warfarin	ESIMIL guanethidine & hydrochlorothiazide	TENORMIN 100 atenolol	TOLINASE 100 mg tolazamide	MELLARIL 50 mg thioridazine

d					
AKINETON 2 mg biperiden	HYDERGINE Sublingual 0.5 mg ergoloid mesylates	CYTOXAN 25 mg cyclophosphamide	DIURIL 250 mg chlorothiazide	FULVICIN P/G 125 mg griseofulvin	TRANDATE 200 mg labetalol

e					
ZANTAC 150 ranitidine	ZYLOPRIM 100 mg allopurinol	CORTEF 20 mg hydrocortisone	ARMOUR Thyroid 120 mg thyroid, desiccated	LOPURIN 100 mg allopurinol	PEN·VEE K 250 mg penicillin v potassium

WHITE

a	ORINASE 250 mg tolbutamide	TENORETIC 100 atenolol & chlorthalidone	ANTURANE 100 mg sulfinpyrazone	ALUPENT 20 mg metaproterenol	ISMELIN 25 mg guanethidine	LASIX 80 mg furosemide
b	TYLENOL with Codeine No. 1 codeine & acetaminophen	TEGRETOL Chewable 100 mg carbamazepine	ARTANE 5 mg trihexyphenidyl	LITHOTABS 300 mg lithium carbonate	MILTOWN 200 mg meprobamate	TOLINASE 250 mg tolazamide
c	MESTINON 60 mg pyridostigmine bromide	TYLENOL with Codeine No. 2 codeine & acetaminophen	NORMODYNE 200 mg labetalol	Regular Strength ANACIN-3 325 mg acetaminophen	MYSOLINE 250 mg primidone	ARMOUR Thyroid 180 mg thyroid, desiccated
d	LORELCO 250 mg probucol	Regular Strength TYLENOL 325 mg acetaminophen	GRIFULVIN V 250 mg griseofulvin	NORPRAMIN 150 mg desipramine	VASODILAN 20 mg isoxsuprine	DELTASONE 50 mg prednisone
e	ALDORIL 25 methyldopa & hyrdochlorothiazide	DESYREL 100 mg trazodone	DIURIL 500 mg chlorothiazide	SELDANE 60 mg terfenadine	DIAMOX 250 mg acetazolamide	ARMOUR Thyroid 300 mg thyroid, desiccated

WHITE

a				
URECHOLINE 5 mg bethanechol	FIORINAL butalbital, aspirin & caffeine	FULVICIN U/F 250 mg griseofulvin	ISOPTIN 120 mg verapamil	EQUANIL 400 mg meprobamate	URISPAS 100 mg flavoxate

b				
TYLENOL with Codeine No. 3 codeine & acetaminophen	TYLENOL with Codeine No. 4 codeine & acetaminophen	Maximum Strength ANACIN-3 500 mg acetaminophen	PEN-VEE K 500 mg penicillin v potassium	ARMOUR Thyroid 240 mg thyroid, desiccated	EMPIRIN with Codeine No. 2 codeine & aspirin

c				
EMPIRIN with Codeine No. 3 codeine & aspirin	SOMA 350 mg carisoprodol	EMPIRIN with Codeine No. 4 codeine & aspirin	CYTOXAN 50 mg cyclophosphamide	WIGRAINE ergotamine tartrate with caffeine	TOLECTIN 200 mg tolmetin

d				
METAPREL 20 mg metaproterenol	Extra-Strength DATRIL 500 mg acetaminophen	TOLINASE 500 mg tolazamide	PANADOL 500 mg acetaminophen	FULVICIN U/F 500 mg griseofulvin	FULVICIN P/G 250 mg griseofulvin

e				
CHENIX 250 mg chenodiol	QUINAGLUTE 324 mg quinidine	ROBAXISAL methocarbamol & aspirin	QUINAMM 260 mg quinine	GRIFULVIN V 500 mg griseofulvin	QUINIDEX Extentabs 300 mg quinidine

WHITE

ORINASE 500 mg tolbutamide	**Extra-Strength TYLENOL 500 mg** acetaminophen	**E-MYCIN 333 mg** erythromycin	**PERCOCET** oxycodone hydrochloride & acetaminophen	**MOTRIN 300 mg** ibuprofen	**TUMS 500 mg** calcium phosphate
E.E.S. Chewable 200 mg erythromycin		**HALCION 0.5 mg** triazolam	**LASIX 20 mg** furosemide	**MEDROL 4 mg** methylprednisolone	**COMBIPRES 0.3 mg** clonidine & chlorthalidone
XANAX 0.25 mg alprazolam	**DIUCARDIN 50 mg** hydroflumethiazide	**COGENTIN 1 mg** benztropine mesylate	**ANTIVERT 12.5 mg** meclizine	**LIORESAL 10 mg** baclofen	**MEDROL 16 mg** methylprednisolone
HYDERGINE Sublingual 1 mg ergoloid mesylates	**CAPOTEN 50 mg** captopril	**LUDIOMIL 75 mg** maprotiline	**SORBITRATE Oral 30 mg** isosorbide dinitrate	**ANTIVERT/25** meclizine	**V-CILLIN K 125 mg** penicillin v potassium
TRIMPEX 100 mg trimethoprim	**PREMARIN 0.9 mg** conjugated estrogens	**V-CILLIN K 250 mg** penicillin v potassium	**DEPEN 250 mg** penicillamine	**CAPOTEN 100 mg** captopril	**FULVICIN P/G 165** griseofulvin

a b c d e

WHITE

a

KINESED Chewable
belladonna alkaloids

ERY-TAB 333 mg
erythromycin

V-CILLIN K 500 mg
penicillin v potassium

ALDORIL D50
methyldopa &
hydrochlorothiazide

b

FULVICIN P/G 330
griseofulvin

GRISACTIN Ultra
333 mg
griseofulvin

DURICEF 1 g
cefadroxil

CAPOTEN 12.5 mg
captopril

ARISTOCORT 4 mg
triamcinolone

c

TAVIST-1 1.34 mg
clemastine fumarate

DIAβETA 1.25 mg
glyburide

DYMELOR 250 mg
acetohexamide

LIORESAL 20 mg
baclofen

VICODIN
hydrocodone &
acetaminophen

d

Maximum Strength
ANACIN-3 500 mg
acetaminophen

Extra-Strength
TYLENOL 500 mg
acetaminophen

Regular-Strength
ANACIN-3 500 mg
acetaminophen

MILTOWN 600 mg
meprobamate

PHENAPHEN '650'
with Codeine
codeine & acetaminophen

e

UNIPEN 500 mg
nafcillin

SPECTROBID 400 mg
bacampicillin

ARTHRITIS PAIN
FORMULA
acetaminophen

RUFEN 800 mg
ibuprofen

WHITE

a

CALTRATE 600
calcium

CARDIZEM 120 mg
diltiazem

UREX 1 g
methenamine hippurate

b

ULTRACEF 1 g
cefadroxil

POSTURE 600 mg
calcium phosphate

RUFEN 600 mg
ibuprofen

MINIPRESS 1 mg
prazosin

DILANTIN 100 mg
phenytoin

c

PAMELOR 50 mg
nortriptyline

PANCREASE
pancrelipase

TYLENOL with
Codeine no. 3
codeine & acetaminophen

PANADOL 500 mg
acetaminophen

WYTENSIN 4 mg
guanabenz

ATIVAN 0.5 mg
lorazepam

d

ASENDIN 25 mg
amoxapine

WYTENSIN 8 mg
guanabenz

ATIVAN 1 mg
lorazepam

ATIVAN 2 mg
lorazepam

DECADRON 4 mg
dexamethasone

WYTENSIN 16 mg
guanabenz

e

THALITONE 25 mg
chlorthalidone

DEMI-REGROTON
reserpine & chlorthalidone

VASOTEC 5 mg
enalapril

GLUCOTROL 5 mg
glipizide

EQUANIL 200 mg
meprobamate

CAPOTEN 25 mg
captopril

WHITE

a	b	c	d	e
GRISACTIN Ultra 125 mg griseofulvin				
GRISACTIN Ultra 250 mg griseofulvin				
VALIUM 2 mg diazepam				
GLUCOTROL 10 mg glipizide				

INDEX OF DRUGS

Note: Words in all capital letters are brand-name drugs. Bold-face page numbers in this index refer to the chart that summarizes information about the particular drug.

INDEX OF MEDICAL CONDITIONS

Note: Bold-face page numbers in this index refer to descriptions of medical conditions in the text. Following each medical description are the drug charts that summarize information about the drugs prescribed for a particular condition. Page numbers for the drug charts are given in the table of contents at the beginning of this book.

Scott, Foresman and the American Association of Retired Persons have joined together to bring you

AARP BOOKS

These comprehensive guides, written by experts, will help you manage your money, choose where to live, plan your estate, guard your health, and help those you care about live a better life.

Information You Can Count On!

831. **AARP Pharmacy Service Prescription Drug Handbook.** *$13.95/AARP member price $9.95.*

810. **Alone - Not Lonely:** Independent Living for Women Over Fifty. *$6.95/AARP member price $4.95.*

811. **Travel Easy:** The Practical Guide for People Over 50. *$8.95/AARP member price $6.50.*

812. **Keeping Out of Crime's Way:** The Practical Guide for People Over 50. *$6.95/AARP member price $4.95.*

815. **Cataracts:** The Complete Guide From Diagnosis to Recovery for Patients and Families. *$7.95/AARP member price $5.80.*

805. **The Essential Guide to Wills, Estates, Trusts and Death Taxes.** *$12.95/AARP member price $9.45.*

806. **The Over Easy Foot Care Book.** *$6.95/AARP member price $4.95.*

807. **National Continuing Care Directory:** Retirement Communities with Prepaid Medical Plans. *$13.95/AARP member price $9.95.*

830. **How to Plan Your Successful Retirement.** *$9.95/AARP member price $6.95*

Join AARP today and enjoy valuable benefits.

Join the American Association of Retired Persons, the national organization which helps people like you, age 50 and over, realize their full potential in so many ways! The reward you'll reap with AARP will be many times greater than your low membership dues. And your membership also includes your spouse!

Your AARP benefits

- Modern Maturity magazine
- Legislative work benefiting mature persons
- Nonprofit Pharmacy Service
- Quality Group Health Insurance
- Specially priced Motoring Plan
- Community Volunteer Activities
- Hotel & Car Rental Discounts
- Travel Service
- Tax-Aide Program to help with your taxes

65% of dues is designated for Association publications. Dues outside continental U.S.: $7 one year, $18 three years. Please allow 3 to 6 weeks for receipt of membership kit.

☐ Start my membership in AARP LAAA

☐ one year/$5
☐ three years/$12.50 (saves $2.50)
☐ ten years/$35 (saves $15)

☐ Check or money order enclosed payable to AARP. DO NOT SEND CASH
☐ Please bill me.

Name (please print)

Address   Apt.

City

State   Zip

Date of Birth_____mo/_____day/_____year

☐ Start my membership in NRTA (a division for those in or retired from education) LANA

Other AARP Books of interest...

826. **Think of Your Future** Preretirement Planning Workbook. *$25.00/AARP member price $18.25.*

801. **Planning Your Retirement Housing.** *$8.95/AARP member price $6.50.*

803. **Policy Wise:** The Practical Guide to Insurance Decisions for Older Consumers. *$5.95/AARP member price $4.35.*

804. **It's Your Choice:** The Practical Guide to Planning a Funeral. *$4.95/AARP member price $3.00.*

833. **On the Road in an RV.** *$8.95/AARP member price $6.50.*

825. **A Woman's Guide to Good Health After 50.** *$12.95/AARP member price $9.45.*

822. **Sunbelt Retirement:** The Complete State-by-State Guide. *$11.95/AARP member price $8.50.*

829. **Retirement Edens Outside the Sunbelt.** *$10.95/AARP member price $7.95.*

HOW TO ORDER

To order state book name and number, quantity and price (AARP members: be sure to include your membership no. for discount) and add $1.75 *per entire order* for shipping and handling. *All orders must be prepaid.* For your convenience we accept checks, money orders, VISA and MasterCard (credit card orders must include card no., exp. date and cardholder signature). *Please allow 4 weeks for delivery.*

Send your order today to:

AARP Books, Scott, Foresman and Co., 1865 Miner Street Des Plaines, IL 60016

AARP Books are co-published by AARP and Scott, Foresman and Co., sold by Scott, Foresman and Co., and distributed to bookstores by Little, Brown and Company.
